Laboratory Assessments of Pediatric Leukemia

Weijie Li
Editor

Laboratory Assessments of Pediatric Leukemia

Springer

Editor
Weijie Li
Department of Pathology and
Laboratory Medicine
Children's Mercy Kansas City
University of Missouri-Kansas City
School of Medicine
Kansas City, MO, USA

ISBN 978-3-032-26556-2 ISBN 978-3-032-26557-9 (eBook)
https://doi.org/10.1007/978-3-032-26557-9

This Springer imprint is published by the registered company Springer Nature Switzerland AG
The registered company address is: Gewerbestrasse 11, 6330 Cham, Switzerland

Preface

Leukemia is the most common pediatric cancer, accounting for approximately 25% of all malignancies diagnosed in children. The clinical outcomes of pediatric leukemias have improved significantly in the last several decades. Pediatric acute lymphoblastic leukemia, in particular, has become one of the most successful treatment models in oncology, achieving a cure rate of 90%. The key feature of this model is the personalized treatment approach, which is based on thorough assessments of each case through extensive laboratory testing. These assessments encompass a wide range of laboratory measures related to diagnosis, therapeutic monitoring, risk prediction, and treatment selection. This field is rapidly evolving, with ongoing improvements to existing tests and the introduction of new tests that adopt the latest technological advancements. There is a pressing need for a reference book that covers these assessments for professionals working in this field. This need is the motivation behind writing this book.

This book aims to provide up-to-date, comprehensive coverage of laboratory assessments of pediatric leukemia, encompassing all key topics and recent advances in this field. It consists of 21 chapters. Chapter 1 introduces the diagnosis, classification, and treatment of pediatric leukemia, highlighting the importance of laboratory assessments in clinical practice. Chapters 2, 3, 4, 5, 6, 7, 8, 9, 10, 11, and 12 focus on laboratory tests for pediatric leukemia, ranging from basic complete blood count to cutting-edge long-read sequencing molecular tests. These chapters explain the principles of methodologies, describe and discuss the techniques, key test elements, advantages, limitations, method comparisons, result interpretation, and clinical utility. Chapters 13, 14, and 15 elaborate on the prognostic and predictive biomarkers identified in acute lymphoblastic leukemia and acute myeloid leukemia. Chapters 16, 17, and 18 delve into laboratory tests related to CAR T-cell therapy and hematopoietic stem cell transplantation. Chapter 19 discusses leukemia-related coagulation abnormalities. Finally, Chapters 20 and 21 review two rare types of pediatric leukemia that are minimally or not covered in other chapters.

We hope this book will serve as a comprehensive resource and quick reference guide for pathologists, laboratory directors, laboratory practitioners, and medical researchers who work with pediatric leukemia. We also anticipate that, as a collection of the most up-to-date information on pediatric leukemia, it will be valuable for pediatric oncologists/hematologists, fellows, and residents. Since most of these assessments are not exclusive to pediatric leukemia and are also relevant to adult leukemia and possibly other malignancies, this book will be beneficial for adult oncologists/hematologists as well as other medical professionals or researchers.

Kansas City, MO, USA Weijie Li

Acknowledgments

I am deeply grateful to all the contributors who made this project possible. I truly appreciate their exceptional work and the valuable time they dedicated to this book. On behalf of all the authors, I would like to extend our heartfelt appreciation to our families for their unconditional love, support, and understanding during our many late-night, early-morning, or weekend writing sessions.

We thank the following reviewers (listed in alphabetical order by last name) for their significant contributions to this book through their editing of the manuscripts and valuable suggestions and comments.

Thomas B. Alexander, MD, MPH, University of North Carolina, USA
Yanan Fang, MD, PhD, Montefiore Medical Center, Albert Einstein College of Medicine, USA
Midhat S. Farooqi, MD, PhD, Children's Mercy Kansas City, University of Missouri-Kansas City (UMKC), USA
Kathleen Gallagher, PhD, Massachusetts General Hospital, Harvard University, USA
Alan Gamis, MD, MPH, Children's Mercy Kansas City, UMKC, USA
Laura E. Hogan, MD, Stony Brook Children's, Stony Brook University, USA
Mina Hur, MD, PhD, Konkuk University School of Medicine, Korea
Lisa A. Lansdon, PhD, Children's Mercy Kansas City, UMKC, USA
Gordana Raca, MD, PhD, Children's Hospital Los Angeles, Keck School of Medicine of USC, USA
Laura Ramsey, PhD, Children's Mercy Kansas City, UMKC, USA
Gokce A. Toruner, MD, PhD, The University of Texas MD Anderson Cancer Center, USA
Vincent H.J. van der Velden, PhD, Erasmus MC. Rotterdam, The Netherlands

We are deeply indebted to our technologists, especially those working in cytogenetics, flow cytometry, and hematology laboratories, for their meticulous work, which is central to the subject matter of this book, and for their various forms of support and assistance in the writing of this book.

We also thank our institutions and colleagues for providing invaluable resources and support. I would like to particularly acknowledge the teams in the Department of Pathology and Laboratory Medicine, the Division of Hematology/Oncology and Bone Marrow Transplant, as well as the Medical Writing Center at Children's

Mercy Kansas City, where I have been privileged to work for over 10 years, for their constant support and encouragement for this project. In addition, we thank our leukemia patients, who strive valiantly against this disease every day, inspiring us and giving us the motivation and strength to work hard.

We are also immensely grateful to the publishers, especially Lillie Mae Gaurano (editor of clinical medicine books), Kiruthika Andappan (production editor), and Nithiya Vadivazhagan (project manager) for their enormous assistance in bringing this project to fruition.

Weijie Li

Contents

Editors and Contributors

About the Editor

Weijie Li is a pediatric hematopathologist, board-certified in anatomic pathology, clinical pathology, and hematopathology. He has served as the Director of Hematopathology and Flow Cytometry at Children's Mercy Hospital in Kansas City, United States, for over 10 years. Through many years of practice, he has developed clinical expertise in diagnosing pediatric leukemias, lymphomas, and other hemato-lymphoid diseases, as well as in monitoring therapeutic responses, especially measurable residual disease (MRD) in acute leukemias. His research focuses on diagnostic and prognostic biomarkers of leukemia and lymphoma, MRD detection, and the deregulation of signaling pathways in pediatric leukemia and lymphoma.

Dr. Li is a Professor of Pathology at the University of Missouri-Kansas City School of Medicine and is actively involved in teaching medical students, pathology residents, and hematopathology and hematology-oncology fellows. Moreover, Dr. Li serves as a reviewer for numerous peer-reviewed journals and has published extensively in hematopathology, flow cytometry, and hematology-oncology.

Contributors

Ibrahim Ahmed Division of Hematology, Oncology, and Blood and Marrow Transplant, Children's Mercy Kansas City, University of Missouri-Kansas City School of Medicine, Kansas City, MO, USA

Elizabeth J. Byers Aflac Cancer and Blood Disorders Center, Children's Healthcare of Atlanta, Atlanta, Georgia, USA

Emory University School of Medicine, Atlanta, Georgia, USA

Yang Cao Department of Pathology and Immunology, Washington University School of Medicine, St. Louis, MO, USA

William L. Carroll Division of Pediatric Hematology/Oncology, Department of Pediatrics, NYU Grossman School of Medicine, New York, NY, USA

Perlmutter Cancer Center, NYU Langone Medical Center, New York, NY, USA

Gaurav Chatterjee Hematopathology Department, ACTREC, Tata Memorial Center, HBNI University, Navi Mumbai, Maharashtra, India

Anumeha Chaturvedi Hematopathology Department, Homi Bhabha Cancer Hospital and Research Centre, Visakhapatnam, Andhra Pradesh, India

Weina Chen Department of Pathology, University of Texas Southwestern Medical Center, Dallas, TX, USA

Danielle W. Cohen Division of Pediatric Hematology/Oncology, Department of Pediatrics, NYU Grossman School of Medicine, New York, NY, USA

Linda D. Cooley Department of Pathology and Laboratory Medicine, Children's Mercy Kansas City, University of Missouri-Kansas City School of Medicine, Kansas City, MO, USA

M. Tarek Elghetany Department of Pathology, Baylor College of Medicine, Texas Children's Hospital, Houston, TX, USA

Misha Fan Department of Family Medicine, Thundermist Health Center, Woonsocket, RI, USA

Kevin E. Fisher Department of Pathology, Texas Children's Hospital, Houston, TX, USA

Department of Pathology & Immunology, Baylor College of Medicine, Houston, TX, USA

Luca Guarnera Department of Biomedicine and Prevention, University of Rome Tor Vergata, Rome, Italy

Sahibu Sultan M. Habeebu Department of Pathology and Laboratory Medicine, Children's Mercy, University of Missouri-Kansas City School of Medicine, Kansas City, MO, USA

Kimberly H. Hein Department of Pathology, Baylor College of Medicine, Texas Children's Hospital, Houston, TX, USA

John Herriges Department of Pathology and Laboratory Medicine, Children's Mercy Kansas City, Kansas City, MO, USA

Departments of Pathology and Pediatrics, University of Missouri-Kansas City School of Medicine, Kansas City, MO, USA

Ying-Chen Claire Hou The Steve and Cindy Rasmussen Institute for Genomic Medicine, Nationwide Children's Hospital, Columbus, OH, USA

Department of Pathology and Pediatrics, The Ohio State University, Columbus, OH, USA

Dharmendra Jain Department of Pathology, University of Utah, Salt Lake City, UT, USA

Histocompatibility & Immunogenetics Laboratory, Salt Lake City, UT, USA

Immunology Division, ARUP Laboratories, Salt Lake City, UT, USA

Allison J. Kalinousky Department of Pathology and Laboratory Medicine, Children's Mercy Kansas City, Kansas City, MO, USA

Jessica Krugman Division of Pediatric Hematology/Oncology, Department of Pediatrics, NYU Grossman School of Medicine, New York, NY, USA

Jatinder K. Lamba Department of Pharmacotherapy and Translational Research, College of Pharmacy, University of Florida, Gainesville, FL, USA

UF Health Cancer Center, University of Florida, Gainesville, FL, USA

Eszter Lázár-Molnár Department of Pathology, University of Utah, Salt Lake City, UT, USA

Histocompatibility & Immunogenetics Laboratory, Salt Lake City, UT, USA

Immunology Division, ARUP Laboratories, Salt Lake City, UT, USA

Geling Li Department of Pathology and Laboratory Medicine, Children's of Alabama, Birmingham, AL, USA

Department of Pathology, University of Alabama at Birmingham, Birmingham, AL, USA

Weijie Li Department of Pathology and Laboratory Medicine, Children's Mercy Kansas City, University of Missouri-Kansas City School of Medicine, Kansas City, Missouri, USA

University of Missouri–Kansas City School of Medicine, Kansas City, Missouri, USA

Dmitry A. Lyalin Department of Pathology, Virginia Commonwealth University Health System, Richmond, VA, USA

Sara McElroy, MD Division of Hematology/Oncology/Bone Marrow Transplant, Children's Mercy Kansas City, University of Missouri-Kansas City School of Medicine, Kansas City, MO, USA

Bahareh A. Mojarad Cancer Genetics & Genomics Laboratory, BC Cancer, Vancouver, BC, Canada

Department of Pathology & Laboratory Medicine, Faculty of Medicine, University of British Columbia, Vancouver, BC, Canada

Aravindh Nagarajan Department of Pathology and Laboratory Medicine, Children's Mercy Kansas City, Kansas City, MO, USA

Michelle Nash Division of Pediatric Hematology/Oncology, Stony Brook Children's, Stony Brook, NY, USA

Emily K. O'Donnell Department of Pathology and Laboratory Medicine, Children's Mercy Kansas City, Kansas City, MO, USA

Departments of Pathology and Pediatrics, University of Missouri-Kansas City—School of Medicine, Kansas City, MO, USA

Josephine B. Oehler Computational Biomedicine Lab, College of Science and Engineering, James Cook University, Townsville, QLD, Australia

College of Medicine and Dentistry, James Cook University, Cairns, QLD, Australia

Gabor Oroszi, MD, PhD Department of Pathology and Laboratory Medicine, Children's Mercy Kansas City, University of Missouri-Kansas City School of Medicine, Kansas City, MO, USA

Tiziana Ottone Department of Biomedicine and Prevention, University of Rome Tor Vergata, Rome, Italy

Mrinal M. Patnaik Division of Hematology, Department of Internal Medicine, Mayo Clinic, Rochester, MN, USA

Priscilla Quach Department of Pathology, Nebraska Methodist Hospital, Omaha, NE, USA

Elizabeth A. Raetz Division of Pediatric Hematology/Oncology, Department of Pediatrics, NYU Grossman School of Medicine, New York, NY, USA

Sweta Rajpal Hematopathology Department, ACTREC, Tata Memorial Center, HBNI University, Navi Mumbai, Maharashtra, India

Elena A. Repnikova Department of Pathology and Laboratory Medicine, Children's Mercy Kansas City, University of Missouri-Kansas City School of Medicine, Kansas City, MO, USA

Ulf Schmitz Computational Biomedicine Lab, College of Science and Engineering, James Cook University, Townsville, QLD, Australia

Centre for Tropical Bioinformatics and Molecular Biology, Australian Institute of Tropical Health and Medicine, James Cook University, Cairns, Australia

Centenary Institute, The University of Sydney, Camperdown, Australia

Vivek M. Shastri Department of Pharmacotherapy & Translational Research, College of Pharmacy, University of Florida, Gainesville, FL, USA

Scott C. Smith Department of Pathology, SUNY Upstate Medical University, Syracuse, NY, USA

Madina Sukhanova Department of Pathology, Division of Molecular Pathology, Feinberg School of Medicine, Northwestern University, Chicago, IL, USA

Ryan J. Summers Aflac Cancer and Blood Disorders Center, Children's Healthcare of Atlanta, Atlanta, GA, USA

Emory University School of Medicine, Atlanta, GA, USA

Prashant R. Tembhare Hematopathology Department, ACTREC, Tata Memorial Center, HBNI University, Navi Mumbai, Maharashtra, India

Olga Kagan Weinberg Department of Pathology, University of Texas Southwestern Medical Center, Dallas, TX, USA

Gloria Paz Contreras Yametti Division of Pediatric Hematology/Oncology, Department of Pediatrics, NYU Grossman School of Medicine, New York, NY, USA

Lei Zhang Department of Pathology and Laboratory Medicine, Children's Mercy Kansas City, University of Missouri-Kansas City School of Medicine, Kansas City, MO, USA

Departments of Pathology and Pediatrics, University of Missouri-Kansas City—School of Medicine, Kansas City, MO, USA

Pediatric Leukemia: Diagnosis, Classification, and Treatment

1

Michelle Nash, Elizabeth J. Byers, Ryan J. Summers, and Weijie Li

Introduction

Leukemia is the most common type of cancer in children, with an incidence of nearly 50 per million children under 20 years of age in the United States (US), accounting for approximately 25% of all pediatric malignancies [1, 2]. It includes a heterogeneous group of hematologic malignancies characterized by clonal proliferation of abnormal hematolymphoid cells in the bone marrow

Authors Michelle Nash and Elizabeth J. Byers have equally contributed to this chapter.

M. Nash
Division of Pediatric Hematology/Oncology, Stony Brook Children's, Stony Brook, New York, USA
e-mail: Michelle.Nash@StonyBrookMedicine.edu

E. J. Byers · R. J. Summers
Aflac Cancer and Blood Disorders Center, Children's Healthcare of Atlanta, Atlanta, Georgia, USA

Emory University School of Medicine, Atlanta, Georgia, USA
e-mail: elizabeth.byers@emory.edu; rjsumme@emory.edu

W. Li (✉)
Department of Pathology and Laboratory Medicine, Children's Mercy Kansas City, Kansas City, Missouri, USA

University of Missouri–Kansas City School of Medicine, Kansas City, Missouri, USA
e-mail: wli@cmh.edu

W. Li (ed.), *Laboratory Assessments of Pediatric Leukemia*,
https://doi.org/10.1007/978-3-032-26557-9_1

(BM), often involving peripheral blood (PB), spleen, lymph nodes, and possibly other organs. Leukemia can be classified as acute or chronic based on progression speed. Acute leukemia (AL) progresses rapidly and is predominantly a malignancy of hematolymphoid precursors (blasts). Based on cell origin, AL can be classified as acute lymphoblastic leukemia (ALL), acute myeloid leukemia (AML), or AL of ambiguous lineage (ALAL)/mixed-phenotype AL (MPAL). Chronic leukemia usually progresses slowly and is manifested as the malignancy of mature or maturing hematolymphoid cells, although it originates from mutant hematopoietic stem cells. Leukemias can be further classified into many subtypes by incorporating genetic features, morphology, immunophenotype, and clinical information [3–6].

Most pediatric leukemia cases are AL. According to the data of global cancer statistics in 2022, ALL accounted for 69% of all pediatric leukemia cases worldwide, AML comprised 23%, while MPAL/ALAL and chronic leukemia together represented 8% [7]. B-cell ALL (B-ALL) is the predominant type of ALL in children, accounting for approximately 80% of cases [8]. Chronic myeloid leukemia (CML) and juvenile myelomonocytic leukemia (JMML) are the most common chronic leukemias seen in children. Leukemia displays a slight male predominance in children, with a male-to-female incidence rate ratio of 1.36 in ALL and 1.18 in AML [9].

Over the past several decades, tremendous advances have been made in pediatric leukemia. Our understanding of the biology of different types of leukemia has been significantly enhanced through a huge amount of basic and clinical research. New cytogenetic and molecular testing techniques have been developed quickly. The application of these advanced techniques has significantly improved the efficiency and accuracy of detecting cytogenetic and molecular abnormalities in leukemia, leading to the discovery of many new leukemia subtypes with distinct genetic defects [3–6]. Some of these genetic defects have the potential for molecularly targeted therapy. Technological advances in genetic analysis have also allowed for the identification of many new prognostic and predictive biomarkers in pediatric leukemia [8, 10–12] and more sensitive detection of measurable residual disease (MRD), also known as minimal residual disease. MRD is the strongest independent prognostic biomarker of relapse and prognosis in pediatric ALL. These biomarkers have greatly improved our capacity for individualized risk stratification and the development of risk-adapted therapies.

The advances in technologies and our understanding of leukemia biology have also led to the invention and development of many innovative therapies, including immunotherapies such as monoclonal antibodies, bispecific T-cell engagers, and chimeric antigen receptor (CAR) T-cells, and molecularly targeted therapies such as tyrosine kinase inhibitors and inhibitors targeting other molecules in the altered signaling pathways [13, 14]. Some of these treatments have already demonstrated great success in treating refractory or relapsed cases [13, 14]. The clinical outcomes of all pediatric leukemias have improved significantly. Especially ALL, the most prevalent malignancy in children, which was once considered a fatal disease, is now highly curable, with a 5-year relative survival rate of over

90% in the US [1]. The prognosis of AML lags behind that of ALL, with a 5-year survival rate close to 70% in de novo cases in the US [1]. This chapter provides an overview of the diagnosis, classification, and treatment of pediatric leukemia, with a focus on ALL and AML.

Diagnostic Laboratory Assessments and Diagnosis Based on Morphology and Immunophenotype

Diagnosing AL requires the identification of a significant number of blasts in the BM and/or PB. The diagnostic process typically begins with clinical suspicion and an order for laboratory tests, including a complete blood count (CBC). Since the clinical manifestations of AL, such as fatigue, fever, pale skin, petechiae, and bone pain, are nonspecific, the diagnosis can be delayed. A clinical hematology laboratory should serve as an effective screening checkpoint. Please refer to Chap. 12 for procedures and special considerations in the laboratory screening of pediatric leukemia. Since AL is an aggressive disease that requires prompt treatment, quickly diagnosing AL with an assigned lineage is essential for enabling the clinical team to start treatment. Morphology examination and flow cytometry (FCM) analysis can provide results within 1 or 2 days, allowing for a rapid diagnosis of most AL cases. In contrast, cytogenetic and molecular tests can take one to several weeks, and their results are mainly used for further classification and risk-stratification. A PB specimen can be diagnostic if it shows a high level of blasts, and a BM examination is necessary when the PB contains low-level or no blasts.

JMML is a rare type of leukemia that primarily affects young children and results from the abnormal activation of the RAS pathway. To diagnose JMML, it is essential to correlate clinical information and histopathologic findings with the results of cytogenetic and molecular tests. Please see Chap. 21 for the diagnosis and a more detailed description of JMML. CML and other myeloproliferative neoplasms (MPNs) mostly affect adults and are uncommon in children. The diagnostic approach to these diseases is similar to that of adult cases, relying on a comprehensive workup including genetic testing [15].

Histomorphology Assessment

Morphologically, AL blasts vary greatly, but are typically larger than mature lymphocytes, with loose nuclear chromatin and irregular nuclear contour. ALL lymphoblasts typically show a high nuclear-to-cytoplasmic (N:C) ratio, inconspicuous nucleoli, and scant agranular basophilic cytoplasm (Figs. 1.1a and 1.3a). The morphology of AML blasts varies depending on their differentiation direction and maturation level (Fig. 1.1b–f). The blasts of AML with minimal differentiation or no maturation can look similar to lymphoblasts, or appear larger with more cytoplasm but no cytoplasmic granules or other significant myeloid differentiation except for

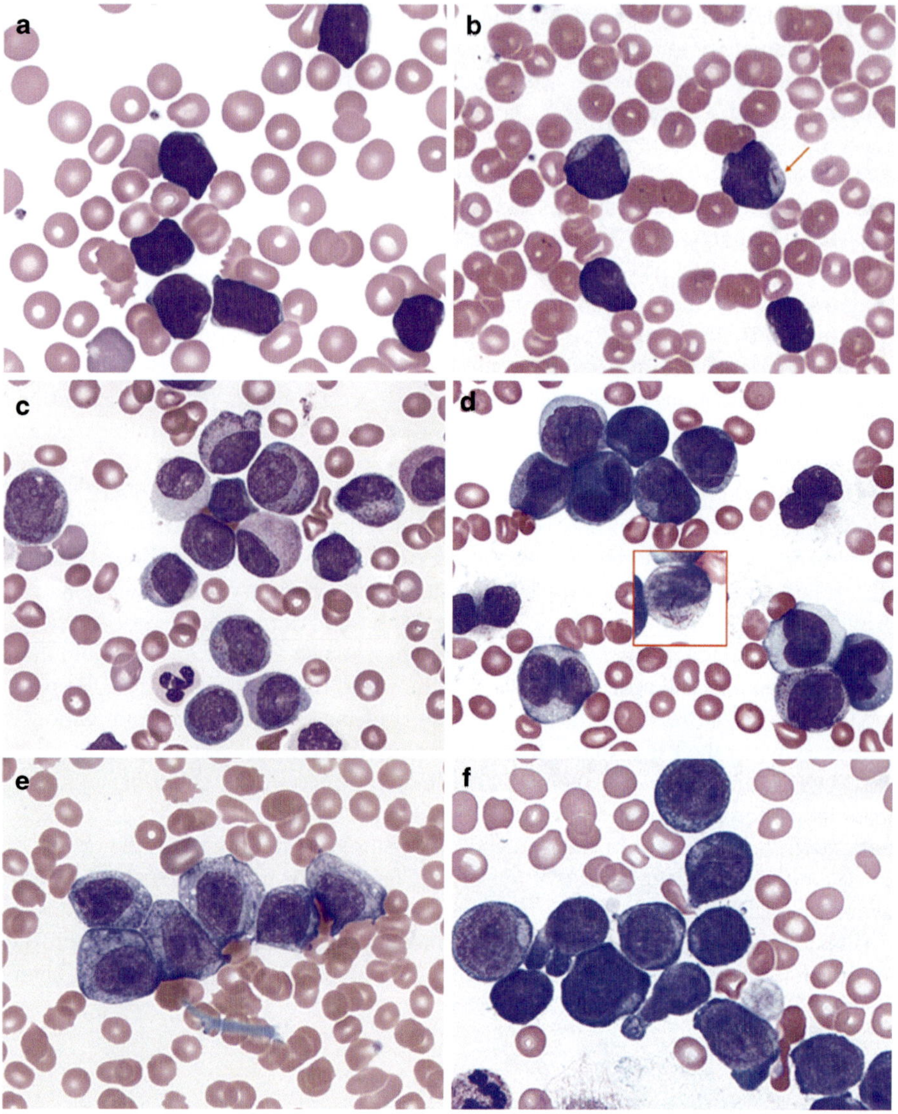

Fig. 1.1 Cytomorphology of the leukemic blasts in different types of acute leukemia: (**a**) acute lymphoblastic leukemia; (**b**) acute myeloid leukemia (AML) with no maturation and an Auer rod pointed by a red arrow; (**c**) hypergranular acute promyelocytic leukemia (APL); (**d**) microgranular APL and a faggot cell with multiple Auer rods in the center red square; (**e**) AML with monocytic differentiation; and (**f**) acute megakaryoblastic leukemia

the presence of Auer rods (Fig. 1.1b). The blasts of AML with maturation often show abundant cytoplasmic azurophilic granules. Acute promyelocytic leukemia (APL) shows abnormal promyelocytes with densely loaded granules (hypergranular variant, Fig. 1.1c) or no/sparse granules (microgranular variant, Fig. 1.1d), and abnormal cells with bundles of Auer rods in the cytoplasm (faggot cells, Fig. 1.1d). The nuclear shape of APL is highly variable and can be bi-lobed or irregularly folded (Fig. 1.1d). Microgranular APL leukemic cells can mimic promonocytes or atypical monocytes, as seen in AML with monocytic differentiation. Monoblasts are usually medium or large in size with round or oval nuclei, delicate lacy nuclear chromatin, prominent nucleoli, and abundant basophilic cytoplasm (Fig. 1.1e). Promonocytes show nuclear indentation and are counted as blast equivalents in AML with monocytic differentiation. Leukemic megakaryoblasts are variable in size, from small to large, and usually contain round or slightly irregular or indented nuclei, fine chromatin, inconspicuous or distinct single or multiple nucleoli, abundant deeply basophilic cytoplasm, and cytoplasmic blebs (Fig. 1.1f). While each type of leukemia has characteristic morphologic features, none of these morphologic features are specific to a particular lineage or a subtype except for Auer rods, the presence of which indicates a myeloid neoplasm.

BM aspirates and/or PB specimens are usually sufficient to make a diagnosis of AL, and BM biopsies are not typically necessary; however, in cases in which a dry

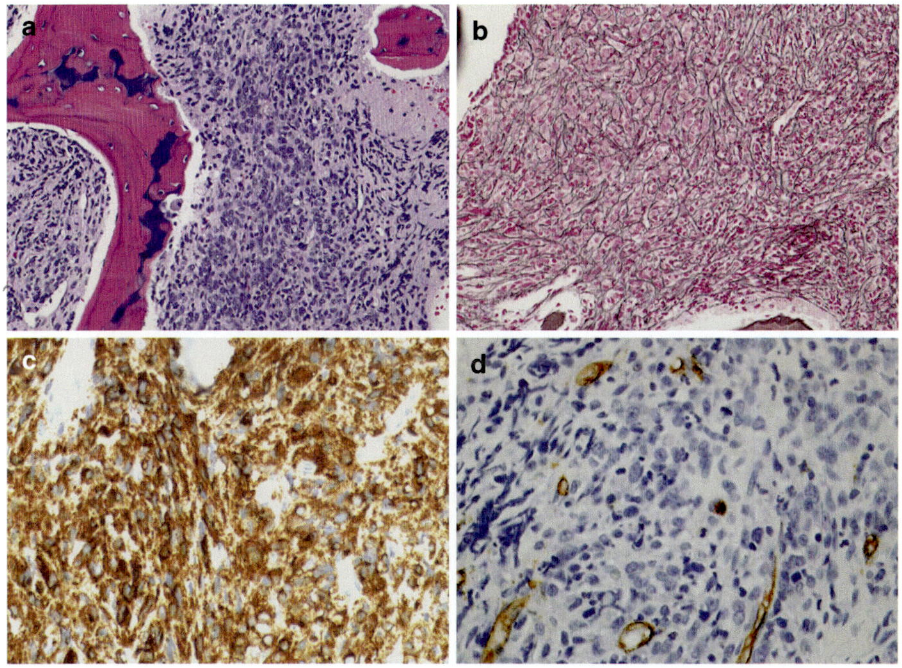

Fig. 1.2 The bone marrow core biopsy of acute megakaryoblastic leukemia shows diffuse infiltration of leukemia cells (**a**, H&E stain, x200), and bone marrow reticulin fibrosis (**b**, reticulin stain, ×200). The blasts are positive for CD61 (**c**, ×400) and negative for CD34 (**d**, ×400)

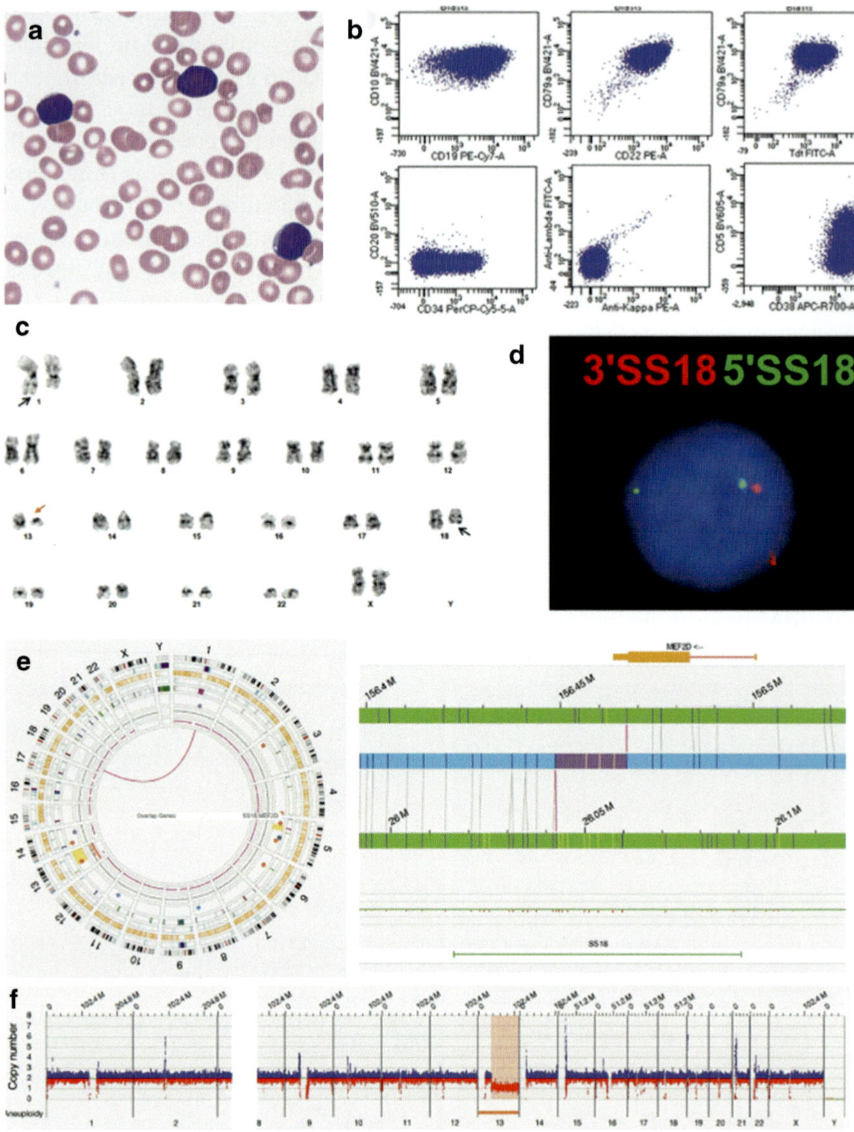

Fig. 1.3 The pathologic findings of an acute leukemia case classified as B-lymphoblastic leukemia with *MEF2D* rearrangement. (**a**) The Wright-Giemsa stained peripheral blood (PB) smear shows three typical lymphoblasts. (**b**) Flow cytometry analysis of PB identifies an abnormal blast population expressing B-cell markers of CD19, CD22, and CD79a; immature markers of CD10, TdT, and CD34 (partial); CD38 and CD5 (partial); and negative for CD20 and surface light chains. (**c**) Karyotyping of PB shows 46,XX,t(1;18)(q22;q11.2) (black arrows) and del(13)(q13) (red arrow). (**d**) Fluorescence in situ hybridization (FISH) analysis on bone marrow (BM) shows SS18 (18q11.2) rearrangement. (**e**) By optical genome mapping (OGM) performed on BM, the circos plot with a de novo assembly shows a translocation between chromosomes 1 and 18 with breakpoints in the *SS18* and *MEF2D* genes. The right panel highlights the breakpoints within *SS18* and at the 3′ end of the *MEF2D* in a zoomed-in view. (**f**) By OGM analysis, the whole genome view shows a deletion on chromosome 13

tap occurs, a BM biopsy becomes important in accurately assessing the percentage of blasts and to perform immunophenotyping by immunohistochemical (IHC) stains. The leukemic megakaryoblasts can secrete growth factors, such as platelet-derived growth factor (PDGF) and transforming growth factor beta (TGF-β), which induce fibroblast proliferation and extracellular matrix production, leading to myelofibrosis [16]. In such cases, BM aspiration may be difficult, and a BM core biopsy is often required for diagnosis (Fig. 1.2). Most BM specimens exhibit hypercellularity and diffuse blast infiltration. Occasionally, a lymph node or other extramedullary tissue is the first specimen examined, typically showing sheets of immature cells, leading to a diagnosis of lymphoblastic lymphoma (LBL) or myeloid sarcoma, depending on the immunophenotype. Rarely, body fluid is the first specimen examined and found to have leukemic cells. For these instances, BM and/or PB should be analyzed afterward to determine whether AL is present.

PB and BM specimens are commonly collected to diagnose JMML and CML. Please see Chap. 21 for the pathologic findings of these specimens in JMML. In the chronic phase of CML, PB typically shows hyperleukocytosis with increased mature granulocytes and their precursors at various stages of maturation. The increased granulocytes show no dysplasia and typically include all three types: neutrophils, eosinophils, and basophils. The BM is usually hypercellular and displays granulocytic hyperplasia and increased megakaryocytes, including frequent small hypolobated forms (dwarf megakaryocytes) [15].

Immunophenotyping and Lineage Assignment

FCM plays a critically important role in diagnosing AL. As a powerful single-cell analysis platform, FCM can efficiently immunophenotype blasts, assign lineage, analyze DNA ploidy, and provide information for subtyping. Please see Chap. 2 for details on how to use FCM to diagnose pediatric leukemia. A comprehensive FCM panel is typically employed to ensure accurate lineage classification and establish a leukemia-associated phenotype that is valuable in MRD monitoring. The panel usually includes markers for T-cell, B-cell, natural killer (NK)-cell, and myeloid lineage, as well as markers of precursors and some nonspecific markers. Based on the identified immunoprofile, the leukemic blasts are assigned to one lineage. ALL usually expresses B-cell or T-cell markers along with immature markers, such as TdT and CD34, and dim CD45 (Fig. 1.3b). Early T-cell precursor ALL (ETP-ALL) is defined by a specific phenotype: CD8−, CD1a−, and CD5− (or dimly + in <75% of blasts), and positive for at least one of the myeloid or stem cell markers. Since AML includes subtypes that exhibit a wide range of differentiation and maturation levels, the immunophenotype of AML shows great variation. Besides the expression of common myeloid markers such as CD13 and CD33, each subtype has a distinct antigen expression profile. In a small subset of cases, the immunophenotype of the blasts cannot be assigned to a single lineage. These cases fall under the category of ALAL [4, 17]. ALAL includes MPAL, acute undifferentiated leukemia (AUL), and ALAL not otherwise specified (NOS). For detailed diagnostic criteria and important considerations in the diagnostic process of these entities, please refer to Chap. 20.

In rare instances, no fresh samples are available for flow cytometry study, and the immunophenotype of the leukemia cells must be determined by IHC and cytochemical stains. Diagnosing AL using these stains can be challenging due to the limited number of evaluable markers and the inability to assess the coexpression of multiple markers, particularly those partially expressed.

Immunophenotyping plays a very limited role in the workup of JMML and CML. FCM analysis of the PB and/or BM specimens is mainly used to quantify blasts and assist in detecting accelerated phase or transformation to AML or ALL. While the phenotypic aberrancies of hematopoietic precursors are commonly detected in these neoplasms [18, 19], the significance of identifying phenotypic alterations is not well characterized.

Diagnosis Based on Morphology and Immunophenotype

Unlike AML, there is no universally accepted blast cutoff number for diagnosing ALL [20]. Although 20% is accepted in Europe and some other regions, 25% is the cutoff used in most treatment protocols in the US. The diagnosis of ALL can be made from a PB or BM specimen when ≥25% abnormal B- or T-lymphoblasts are identified. If low-level (<25%) abnormal lymphoblasts are identified in PB, the diagnosis of ALL then relies on the BM specimen, which often contains ≥25% abnormal lymphoblasts, confirming the diagnosis. There are several scenarios in which low-level (<25%) leukemic blasts are identified in the BM. If there are no or only rare marrow elements and the majority of the nucleated cells are mature leukocytes, the cause is most likely severe hemodilution. In this situation, resampling of the BM is necessary for diagnosis. In BM specimens containing many normal hematopoietic precursors and low-level abnormal lymphoblasts, possible causes include a lymphoblastic lymphoma (LBL) spreading into the BM and the early stage of ALL. In these cases, a whole-body imaging study and follow-up BM examinations are necessary.

A diagnosis of AML can be established from BM and/or PB specimens containing ≥20% abnormal myeloid blasts or blast equivalent cells. In cases with <20% myeloid blasts, the morphology and immunophenotype can only generate a preliminary diagnosis of myeloid neoplasm with differential including AML and myelodysplastic syndrome (MDS). The distinction between AML and MDS will depend on the findings of cytogenetic/molecular tests. The diagnosis of AML can be made with <20% blasts in the presence of most recurrent cytogenetic/molecular abnormalities as listed in Table 1.3. In the absence of these cytogenetic/molecular abnormalities, the diagnosis will be MDS. Patients with APL are at high risk of fatal complications such as disseminated intravascular coagulation (DIC) and intracranial bleeding. Therefore, any patient suspected of having APL, based on morphology and immunophenotype, should be admitted for immediate care. The diagnosis of ALAL/MPAL is made when ≥20% of abnormal blasts with ambiguous immunophenotypic profiles are identified in BM and/or PB specimens.

The morphological assessment and immunophenotyping of PB and/or BM samples cannot definitively diagnose JMML or CML; however, when interpreted in the appropriate clinical context, the findings can indicate the likelihood of these diseases and help prioritize specimens for proper cytogenetic and/or molecular testing.

Cytogenetic and Molecular Testing

Cytogenetic and molecular studies play a critical role in further classification, risk stratification, prognostication, and personalized treatment of AL. The traditional cytogenetic tests, chromosomal analysis (karyotyping), and fluorescence in situ hybridization (FISH) study, which are detailed in Chap. 3, detect structure and copy number alterations (CNAs) within individual cells. These tests have been used clinically in leukemia evaluation for several decades and have demonstrated significant clinical value. However, due to their limitations, these tests alone cannot satisfy the current needs for genetic assessment of pediatric leukemia, particularly with respect to the current leukemia classifications and personalized treatment strategies.

Microarray testing, detailed in Chap. 4, is an innovative technique that has been applied clinically for over 15 years. This test examines DNA extracted from pooled cells and provides a high-resolution assessment of CNAs and copy-neutral loss of heterozygosity (CN-LOH). Recently, optical genome mapping (OGM), detailed in Chap. 6, has been incorporated into the evaluation of pediatric leukemia. Utilizing ultra-high molecular weight DNA, OGM can detect nearly all the abnormalities that are detected by traditional cytogenetic methods, and has a higher resolution and a genome-wide view of structural rearrangements. Both DNA microarray and OGM have provided significant additional values, such as increased resolution and the identification of cryptic genetic abnormalities missed by conventional genetic tests. Next-generation sequencing (NGS), detailed in Chap. 5, including transcriptome sequencing, can detect single nucleotide variants, small insertions and deletions, and MRD, besides other genetic abnormalities identifiable by other methods. NGS has been used in assessing pediatric leukemia for over 10 years and is essential for diagnosing several molecular subtypes. It has also contributed to more accurate genetic subtyping and the identification of potential treatment targets. Long-read sequencing (LRS), detailed in Chap. 7, surpasses conventional short-read sequencing by providing enhanced resolution in detecting complex structural variants, novel mutations, and epigenetic modifications. This technology is currently being implemented to assess pediatric leukemia and is expected to further improve genetic and molecular diagnosis.

Classification of Pediatric Leukemia

WHO (World Health Organization) classification is a widely used system for categorizing leukemia and other tumors, and it provides a unified system to enable people across the world to share their knowledge and research results. This classification system integrates morphology, immunophenotype, genetic findings, and clinical information to generate a diagnosis that deeply reflects tumor biology. It has been kept updated by incorporating the new research findings. The newer edition tends to separate more tumors based on cytogenetic or molecular characteristics. The current edition of the WHO classification of hematolymphoid tumors is the 5th edition (WHO-HEM5), released in 2022 [3–5, 21].

Another classification system of hematolymphoid tumors, the International Consensus Classification (ICC), was also published in the same year as the WHO-HEM5 [6, 22]. The ICC shares similar principles with the WHO-HEM5 in classifying leukemia cases. While there are significant overlaps between the two systems, notable differences exist, especially in the classification of AML. The application of both classification systems in diagnosis increases the burden on hematopathologists, creates confusion among oncologists and patients, complicates the research studies and clinical trials, and ultimately compromises or harms patient care. Hopefully, the two groups can collaborate in the future to merge the two systems into one, regardless of the reasons behind their creation [23, 24].

In practice, most AL cases are classified further in an integrated pathology report when the cytogenetic and molecular testing results are available, usually several weeks after the initial diagnosis. Lack or failure of cytogenetic or molecular testing may preclude WHO/ICC classification.

WHO Classification

Acute Lymphoblastic Leukemia

As ALL and the corresponding LBL share similar biological features, the WHO classification has combined them into a single category: lymphoblastic leukemia/lymphoma (ALL/LBL). The WHO-HEM5 divides B-cell ALL/LBL (B-ALL/LBL) cases into two categories: B-ALL/LBL with recurrent cytogenetic abnormalities, and B-ALL/LBL NOS (Table 1.1). Recurrent cytogenetic abnormalities include two types of aneuploidies (high hyperdiploidy and hypodiploidy), one intrachromosomal amplification (iAMP21), six rearrangements (*ETV6::RUNX1*, *KMT2A* rearrangement, *TCF3::PBX1* fusion, *IGH::IL3* fusion, *TCF3::HLF* fusion, *BCR::ABL1* fusion), and two subtypes based on gene expression profile (*BCR::ABL1*-like features and *ETV6::RUNX1*-like features). Some newly identified genetic abnormalities are subsumed into the category of B-ALL/LBL with other defined cytogenetic alterations, which includes B-ALL/LBL cases with rearrangements involving *DUX4*, *MEF2D*, *ZNF384*, *NUTM1*, or *MYC*, as well as those with *PAX5*alt or *PAX5* p.P80R mutation. Each could represent a new subtype of B-ALL/LBL, though more data are required. As illustrated in Fig. 1.3, a subtype of B-ALL/LBL can be diagnosed in most cases through comprehensive laboratory assessments.

Table 1.1 Classification of B-cell lymphoblastic leukemia/lymphoma (B-ALL/LBL)

5th Ed. WHO Classification	Frequency[a]	Prognosis	International Consensus Classification
B-ALL/LBL, NOS			B-ALL NOS
B-ALL/LBL with recurrent genetic abnormalities:			B-ALL with recurrent genetic abnormalities:
B-ALL/LBL with high hyperdiploidy	25–35%	Favorable	B-ALL, hyperdiploid
B-ALL/LBL with hypodiploidy	<2% near haploid, <1% low-hypodiploid	Adverse	B-ALL, low hypodiploid; B-ALL, near haploid
B-ALL/LBL with iAMP21	~2%	Adverse	B-ALL with iAMP21
B-ALL/LBL with *BCR::ABL1* fusion	2–5%	Adverse, improved with TKIs	B-ALL with t(9;22)(q34.1;q11.2)/*BCR::ABL1* with lymphoid only involvement; B-ALL with t(9;22)(q34.1;q11.2)/BCR::ABL1 with multilineage involvement
B-ALL/LBL with *BCR::ABL1*-like features	10–15%	Adverse, improved with targeted therapy	B-ALL, *BCR::ABL1*-like, ABL-1 class rearranged: B-ALL, *BCR::ABL1*-like; JAK-STAT activated; B-ALL, *BCR::ABL1*-like, NOS
B-ALL/LBL with *KMT2A* rearrangement	70–80% <1YO, 2% in children	Adverse	B-ALL with t(v;11q23.3)/*KMT2A* rearranged
B-ALL/LBL with *ETV6::RUNX1* fusion	25%	Favorable	B-ALL with t(12;21)(p13.2;q22.1)/*ETV6::RUNX1*
B-ALL/LBL with *TCF3::PBX1* fusion	~5%	IntM	B-ALL with t(1;19)(q23.3;p13.3)/*TCF3::PBX1*
B-ALL/LBL with *IGH::IL3* fusion	<1%	IntM	B-ALL with t(5;14)(q31.1;q32.3)/*IL3::IGH*
B-ALL/LBL with *TCF3::HLF* fusion	<1%	Adverse	B-ALL with *HLF* rearrangement

(continued)

Table 1.1 (continued)

5th Ed. WHO Classification	Frequency[a]	Prognosis	International Consensus Classification
B-ALL/LBL with *ETV6::RUNX1*-like features	1–3%	NE	
B-ALL/LBL with other defined genetic alterations:			
B-ALL/LBL with *DUX4* rearrangement	4–7%	Favorable	B-ALL with *DUX4* rearrangement
B-ALL/LBL with *MEF2D* rearrangement	1–4%	Adverse	B-ALL with *MEF2D* rearrangement
B-ALL/LBL with *ZNF384* rearrangement	1–4%	IntM	B-ALL with *ZNF384(362)* rearrangement
B-ALL/LBL with *PAX5*alt	3–9%	IntM	
B-ALL/LBL with *PAX5* p.P80R	1–3%	IntM	B-ALL with mutated *PAX5* P80R
B-ALL/LBL with *NUTM1* rearrangement	1–2%	Favorable	B-ALL with *NUTM1* rearrangement
B-ALL/LBL with *MYC* rearrangement	<1%	Adverse	B-ALL with *MYC* rearrangement
			B-ALL with *UBTF::ATXN7L3/PAN3,CDX2* ("*CDX2/UBTF*")
			B-ALL with mutated *IKZF1* N159Y
			Provisional entities:
			B-ALL, *ETV6::RUNX1*-like
			B-ALL, with *PAX5* alteration
			B-ALL, with mutated *ZEB2* (p.H1038R)/*IGH::CEBPE*
			B-ALL, *ZNF384* rearranged-like
			B-ALL, *KMT2A* rearranged-like

IntM intermediate, *NE* not established, *NOS* not otherwise specified, *TKI* tyrosine kinase inhibitor, *YO* year(s) old

[a]Frequency in pediatric B-ALL/LBL [5]

Table 1.2 Classification of T-cell lymphoblastic leukemia/lymphoma (T-ALL/LBL)

5th Ed. WHO Classification	International Consensus Classification (ICC)
T-ALL/LBL, NOS	T-ALL, NOS
Early T-precursor ALL/LBL	Early T-cell precursor ALL with *BCL11B* rearrangement Early T-cell precursor ALL, NOS
	Provisional entities:
	T-ALL/LBL with *HOXA* dysregulated
	T-ALL/LBL with *SPI1* rearrangement
	T-ALL/LBL with *TLX1* rearrangement
	T-ALL/LBL with *TLX3* rearrangement
	T-ALL/LBL with *NKX2* rearrangement
	T-ALL/LBL with *TAL1-2* rearrangement
	T-ALL/LBL with *LMO1-2* rearrangement
	T-ALL/LBL with other *BHLH* dysregulation

NOS not otherwise specified

B-ALL/LBL with low hypodiploidy or near haploidy is prone to chromosomal doubling, which may lead to misinterpretation of the case as high hyperdiploid B-ALL/LBL and inappropriate prognostication [25]. Accurate diagnosis of these cases requires single nucleotide polymorphism (SNP) microarray or OGM analysis to demonstrate CN-LOH in doubled monosomic chromosomes [26]. Currently, there are no routine cytogenetic or molecular tests capable of detecting the full spectrum of abnormalities seen in B-ALL/LBL with *BCR::ABL1*-like features or *ETV6::RUNX1*-like features, except whole transcriptome sequencing, which can only be conducted at a few large medical centers and rare commercial laboratories [27]. In children, the most common subtypes of B-ALL/LBL are B-ALL/LBL with high hyperdiploidy and B-ALL/LBL with *ETV6::RUNX1* fusion (Table 1.1). Both subtypes are associated with a favorable prognosis. If all recurrent cytogenetic abnormalities are excluded through a comprehensive set of cytogenetic and molecular tests, the case is classified as B-ALL/LBL, NOS. For a detailed description of the diagnostic methodologies and genetic and clinical features of these entities, please refer to Chap. 13.

As shown in Table 1.2, the WHO-HEM5 has not recognized any genetic subtypes of T-ALL/LBL except a subtype defined by phenotype, ETP-ALL/LBL, which accounts for 12–17% of pediatric T-ALL/LBL cases, and shows a gene expression profile resembling that of earlier stages of T-cell precursors [5]. There have been various genetic abnormalities detected in T-ALL/LBL [12, 28]. Some of these abnormalities may represent distinct genetic entities and could be separated into subtypes in the next edition of this classification system. For details regarding these genetic abnormalities and their clinical implications, please see Chap. 14.

Acute Myeloid Leukemia

The classification of AML is more complicated than that of ALL. Clinical information has more influence on assigning the category, for example, a history of MDS directly pointing the case to myelodysplasia-related (MR) AML (AML-MR), or a history of previous cytotoxic therapy pointing the case to the category of secondary myeloid neoplasms. As illustrated in Table 1.3, as in ALL, there are also two basic AML

Table 1.3 Classification of acute myeloid leukemia (AML)

5th Ed. WHO Classification				International Consensus Classification	
AML subtypes	Frequency[a]	Prognosis	Blast%[b]	AML subtypes	Blast%[b]
AML with defining genetic abnormalities:				*AML with recurrent genetic abnormalities:*	
Acute promyelocytic leukemia (APL) with *PML::RARA* fusion	5–10%	Favorable	No	APL with t(15;17)(q24.1;q21.2)/*PML::RARA*; APL with other *RARA* rearrangements	≥10%
AML with *RUNX1::RUNX1T1* fusion	12–15%	Favorable	No	AML with t(8;21)(q22;q22.1) /*RUNX1::RUNX1T1*	≥10%
AML with *CBFB::MYH11* fusion	7–9%	Favorable	No	AML with inv(16)(p13.1q22) or t(16;16)(p13.1;q22)/*CBFB::MYH11*	≥10%
AML with *DEK::NUP214* fusion	0.6–1.7%	Adverse	No	AML with t(6;9)(p22.3;q34.1) /*DEK::NUP214*	≥10%
AML with *BCR::ABL1* fusion	<0.5%	Adverse	≥20%	AML with t(9;22)(q34.1;q11.2) /*BCR::ABL1*	≥20%
AML with *KMT2A* rearrangement	20%	IntM to Adverse	No	AML with t(9;11)(p21.3;q23.3) /*MLLT3::KMT2A*; AML with other *KMT2A* rearrangements	≥10%
AML with *MECOM* rearrangement	2%	Adverse	No	AML with inv(3)(q21.3q26.2) or t(3;3)(q21.3;q26.2)/*GATA2::MECOM*; AML with other MECOM rearrangements	≥10%
AML with *NPM1* mutation	6–8%	Favorable	No	AML with mutated *NPM1*	≥10%
AML with *CEBPA* mutation	5%	Favorable	≥20%	AML with in-frame bZIP *CEBPA* mutations	≥10%
AML, myelodysplasia-related			≥20%	AML with myelodysplasia-related gene mutations; AML with myelodysplasia-related cytogenetic abnormalities	≥20%
				AML with other rare recurring translocations:	
AML with *RBM15::MRTFA* fusion	~0.8%	IntM	No	AML (megakaryoblastic) with t(1;22)(p13.3;q13.1) /*RBM15::MRTF1*	≥10%
AML with *NUP98* rearrangement	2–4.8%	Adverse	No	AML with t(5;11)(q35.2;p15.4/ *NUP98::NSD1*; AML with t(11;12)(p15.4;p13.3) /*NUP98::KMD5A*; AML with *NUP98* and other partners	≥10%

(continued)

Table 1.3 (continued)

5th Ed. WHO Classification				International Consensus Classification	
AML subtypes	Frequency[a]	Prognosis	Blast%[b]	AML subtypes	Blast%[b]
AML with other defined genetic alterations:					
AML with *CBFA2T3::GLIS2* fusion	3%	Adverse	≥20%	AML with inv(16)(p13.3q24.3) /*CBFA2T3::GLIS2*	≥10%
AML with *KAT6A::CREBBP* fusion	0.50%	IntM	≥20%	AML with t(8;16)(p11.2;p13.3) /*KAT6A::CREBBP*	≥10%
AML with *FUS::ERG* fusion	0.40%	Adverse	≥20%	AML with t(16;21)(p11.2;q22.2) /*FUS::ERG*	≥10%
AML with *MNX1::ETV6* fusion	<1%	Adverse	≥20%	AML with t(7;12)(q36.3;p13.2) /*ETV6::MNX1*	≥10%
AML with *NPM1::MLF1* fusion	<0.5%	Adverse	≥20%	AML with t(3;5)(q25.3;q35.1) /*NPM1::MLF1*	≥10%
				AML with t(1;3)(p36.3;q21.3) /*PRDM16::RPN1*	≥10%
				AML with t(10;11)(p12.3;q14.2) /*PICALM::MLLT10*	≥10%
				AML with t(16;21)(q24.3;q22.1) /*RUNX1::CBFA2T3*	≥10%
				AML with mutated *TP53*	≥20%
AML defined by differentiation:				*AML not otherwise specified (NOS):*	
AML with minimal differentiation			≥20%	AML with minimal differentiation	≥20%
AML without maturation			≥20%	AML without maturation	≥20%
AML with maturation			≥20%	AML with maturation	≥20%
Acute basophilic leukemia			≥20%	Acute basophilic leukemia	≥20%
Acute myelomonocytic leukemia			≥20%	Acute myelomonocytic leukemia	≥20%
Acute monocytic leukemia			≥20%	Acute monocytic leukemia	≥20%
Acute erythroid leukemia[c]			30%[d]		
Acute megakaryoblastic leukemia			≥20%	Acute megakaryoblastic leukemia	≥20%

IntM intermediate

[a]Frequency in pediatric AML [5]; [b]Either in peripheral blood or in bone marrow; [c]Acute erythroid leukemia cases are included in AML with mutated TP53 by ICC classification; [d]30% proerythroblasts

subgroups: AML with defining genetic abnormalities and AML defined by differentiation. The defining genetic abnormalities include nine distinct rearrangements: *PML::RARA*, *RUNX1::RUNX1T1*, *CBFB::MYH11*, *DEK::NUP214*, *BCR::ABL1*, *RBM15::MRTFA*, *KMT2A* rearrangement, *NUP98* rearrangement, and *MECOM* rearrangement. A blast count of ≥20% is not required for the diagnosis of all these subtypes except for AML with *BCR::ABL1* fusion. While not mandatory, identifying the fusion partners of *KMT2A*, *NUP98*, and *ECOM* is desirable, as it could provide more accurate prognostic information and help in monitoring MRD. Notably, some rearrangements, especially *NUP98*, can be cryptic and not detected by conventional cytogenetic tests. Also included are two gene mutation subtypes: *NPM1* mutation and *CEBPA* mutation. The 20% blast threshold is needed for diagnosing AML with *CEBPA* mutation, but not for AML with *NPM1* mutation. The *CEBPA* mutation can be biallelic (*biCEBPA*) or involve single mutations located in the basic leucine zipper (bZIP) region (*bZIP-CEBPA*). Among these subtypes, AML with *KMT2A* rearrangements is most common, and its prognosis depends on the partner gene and is usually unfavorable. Core-binding factor AMLs (those with *RUNX1::RUNX1T1* or *CBF::MYH11*) are also common in pediatric AML and are associated with a good prognosis. For more detailed diagnostic methodologies, genetic features, and the clinical implications of these genetic abnormalities, please see Chap. 15.

AML with defining genetic abnormalities also includes AML-MR and AML with other defined genetic alterations. AML-MR is diagnosed under two conditions: AML with a history of MDS or MDS/MPN, and AML with at least one of the MR cytogenetic abnormalities or somatic mutations, which are listed in Table 1.4. The category of AML with other defined genetic alterations provides a

Table 1.4 Defining cytogenetic abnormalities and gene mutations for AML-MR

5th Ed WHO Classification	International Consensus Classification
Cytogenetic abnormalities	*Cytogenetic abnormalities*
Complex karyotype (≥3 abnormalities)	Complex karyotype (≥ 3 abnormalities)
del(5q) or loss of 5q due to t(5q)	del(5q)/t(5q)/add(5q)
monosomy 7, 7q deletion, or loss of 7q	−7/del(7q)
del (12p) or loss of 12p	del(12p)/t(12p)/add(11p)
del (17p) or loss of 17p, i(17q)	i(17q), −17/add(17p) or del(17p)
idic(X)(q13)	idic(X)(q13)
del(11q)	+8
monosomy 13 or del(13q)	del(20q)
Somatic mutations	*Somatic mutations*
ASXL1	*ASXL1*
BCOR	*BCOR*
EZH2	*EZH2*
SF3B1	*SF3B1*
SRSF2	*SRSF2*
STAG2	*STAG2*
U2AF1	*U2AF1*
ZRSR2	*ZRSR2*
	RUNX1

space for newly discovered, often rare, entities, including those with *CBFA2T3::GLIS2*, *KAT6A::CREBBP*, *FUS::ERG*, *MNX1::ETV6*, and *NPM1::MLF1*. More data are needed to determine whether these genetic alterations represent distinct subtypes.

If there are no defining cytogenetic abnormalities or conditions associated with secondary AML, the case is categorized under the group of AML defined by differentiation. Further classification of this group follows the granularity of the French-American-British (FAB) classification system, but employs updated differentiation markers and diagnostic criteria. All subtypes require ≥20% blasts in BM and/or PB except acute erythroid leukemia (AEL), which requires ≥30% proerythroblasts, and patients must not have a history of MPN. Additional distinct criteria are required for each subtype. AML with minimal differentiation requires expression of two or more myeloid antigens and <3% blasts positive for myeloperoxidase (MPO) or Sudan Black B (SBB). AML without maturation requires ≥3% blasts positive for MPO or SBB, no nonspecific esterase (NSE), and <10% granulocytic cells in the BM. AML with maturation requires ≥10% granulocytic cells and <20% monocytic cells in the BM. Acute myelomonocytic leukemia requires ≥20% granulocytic cells and ≥20% monocytic cells in the BM. Acute monocytic leukemia requires ≥80% monocytic cells in the leukemic cells and <20% granulocytic cells in the BM. Diagnosing acute basophilic leukemia requires the presence of metachromasia in leukemic cells on toluidine blue staining, negativity for MPO, SBB, and NSE, and exclusion of mast cell leukemia. The diagnosis of AEL requires erythroid predominance (≥80% erythroblasts in BM) with ≥30% of the erythroblasts being proerythroblasts. Acute megakaryoblastic leukemia (AMKL) is diagnosed based on megakaryocytic differentiation, expressing at least one of the platelet glycoproteins: CD41, CD61, or CD42b.

Secondary Myeloid Neoplasms

As shown in Table 1.5, secondary myeloid neoplasms include three groups: myeloid neoplasms post cytotoxic therapy (pCT), myeloid neoplasms associated with germline predisposition, and myeloid proliferations associated with Down syndrome (DS). The AML cases transformed from MPNs are not included in this category, and they should be called MPN in blast phase. Secondary AML transformed from MDSs or MDS/MPNs is categorized as AML-MR [4, 5, 29]. It is important to consider "pCT" and "associated with germline gene mutation" as disease attribute qualifiers. These qualifiers should be added to the names of AML subtypes, for example, AML with *MECOM* rearrangement pCT, or acute monocytic leukemia with germline *CEBPA* variant. AML-pCT needs to meet the diagnostic criteria of AML as well as a history of chemotherapy or large-field radiation for an unrelated malignancy. As shown in Table 1.5, two clinical types of AML-pCT have been recognized. However, most patients undergo multiple types of therapies, often making the distinctions between these two categories unclear. The clinical manifestations of AML and other myeloid neoplasms with germline predisposition can be categorized into three subgroups, as shown in Table 1.5. Genetic

Table 1.5 The 2022 WHO classification of secondary myeloid neoplasms

Myeloid neoplasm post cytotoxic therapy
AML post cytotoxic therapy, type 1
60–70%, caused by alkylating agents and/or ionizing radiation, present 5–7 years after exposure with a pre-MDS phase; cytogenetic: unbalanced chromosomal abnormalities, often complex karyotypes with loss of 5q, 7q, and 17p, and P53 mutations
AML post cytotoxic therapy, type 2
20–30%, caused by DNA topoisomerase II inhibitors, present 1–3 years after exposure with no pre-MDS phase; cytogenetic: balanced translocations, *KMT2A* rearrangements common
Myeloid neoplasms associated with germline predisposition
Without a preexisting platelet disorder or organ dysfunction
Germline CEBPA P/LP variant (CEBPA-associated familial AML)
Germline DDX41 P/LP variant[a]
Germline TP53 P/LP variant[a] (Li-Fraumeni syndrome)
With preexisting platelet disorder
Germline RUNX1 P/LP variant[a] (familial platelet disorder with associated myeloid malignancy, FPD-MM)
Germline ANKRD26 P/LP variant (Thrombocytopenia 2)
Germline ETV6 P/LP variant[b] (Thrombocytopenia 5)
With potential organ dysfunction
Germline GATA2 P/LP variant (GATA2-deficiency)
Bone marrow failure syndromes
Severe congenital neutropenia (SCN)
Shwachman-Diamond syndrome (SDS)
Fanconi anemia (FA)
Telomere biology disorders (dyskeratosis congenita)
Down syndrome[c]
Germline SAMD9 P/LP variant (MIRAGE syndrome)
Germline SAMD9L P/LP variant (SAMD9L-related ataxia pancytopenia)
Biallelic germline BLM P/LP variant (Bloom syndrome)[a]
RASopathies (Neurofibromatosis type 1, CBL syndrome, Noonan syndrome or Noonan syndrome-like disorders)[a]
Myeloid proliferations associated with Down syndrome
Transient abnormal myelopoiesis (TAM)
Myeloid leukemia associated with Down syndrome (ML-DS)[d]

LP likely pathogenic, *P* pathogenic
[a]Also linked to lymphoid neoplasm; [b]Acute lymphoblastic leukemia (ALL) > myeloid neoplasms; [c]ALL > acute myeloid leukemia in patients over 2 years old; [d]Cases GATA1-negative or over age 4 years should not be included

counseling and family studies are important elements of the diagnostic process for index patients.

Myeloid proliferations associated with DS include two types of abnormal myeloid proliferation in children with DS: transient abnormal myelopoiesis (TAM) and myeloid leukemia associated with DS (ML-DS). Both conditions typically show megakaryoblastic phenotype and somatic mutations in the GATA1 gene at exon 2 or 3. TAM occurs in newborns and usually resolves spontaneously over a period of several weeks to 3 months. In 20–30% of cases, nonremitting AML subsequently develops within 1–3 years [5, 30, 31].

Acute Leukemia of Ambiguous Lineage

ALAL is divided into two groups: ALAL with defining genetic abnormalities and ALAL defined immunophenotypically. The defining genetic abnormalities include *BCR::ABL1* fusion, *KMT2A* rearrangement, *ZNF384* rearrangement, and *BCL11B* rearrangement. These genetic abnormalities are not exclusive to MPAL/ALAL and can be seen in AML and ALL as well. ALAL defined immunophenotypically encompasses B/myeloid MPAL, T/myeloid MPAL, rare types of MPAL, acute undifferentiated leukemia (AUL), and ALAL, NOS. For detailed descriptions and diagnostic considerations regarding these entities, please refer to Chap. 20.

JMML and CML

The WHO-HEM5 includes JMML in the MPN family, which also contains CML and six other entities. For diagnostic criteria and a detailed description of JMML, please see Chap. 21.

The diagnosis of CML is established by identifying granulocytosis in PB and detecting the Philadelphia (Ph) chromosome and/or *BCR::ABL1* using cytogenetic and/or other molecular genetic techniques. BM evaluation is recommended in assessing disease phase and checking for additional cytogenetic abnormalities. The WHO-HEM5 has renamed the accelerated phase of CML as "high-risk chronic phase" and modified the diagnostic criteria for the blast phase. To diagnose the blast phase of CML, the case must meet at least one of three criteria: the presence of ≥20% myeloid blasts in PB or BM, the presence of an extramedullary blast proliferation, and the detection of abnormal lymphoblasts in PB or BM (even if <10%).

International Consensus Classification (ICC) and Its Differences from the 5th Edition of WHO Classification

Acute Lymphoblastic Leukemia

The ICC shows high concordance with the WHO-HEM5 on B-ALL classification, as shown in Table 1.1. The genetic subtypes included in WHO-HEM5 are all recognized in the ICC, although the terminologies are a little bit different. The ICC separates B-ALL with hypodiploidy into two subentities: low hypodiploidy (32–39 chromosomes) and near haploidy (24–31 chromosomes). B-ALL with near haploidy is more common in children. The ICC also separates B-ALL with *BCR::ABL1* into two subentities: cases with lymphoid involvement only and cases with multilineage involvement. The latter subentity requires demonstrating the presence of *BCR::ABL1* fusion in cells of non-B lineage, and it may not be easily distinguished from CML in lymphoid blast phase [32]. Based on the genetic alterations, the ICC further categorizes B-ALL with *BCR::ABL1*-like features into three subentities: *ABL1*-class rearranged, JAK-STAT activated, and NOS. B-ALL/LBL with *ETV6::RUNX1*-like features is a subtype in the WHO-HEM5 but is considered a provisional entity in the ICC. All the new entities listed under the category of B-ALL/LBL with other defined genetic alterations in the WHO-HEM5 are recognized as real genetic subtypes by the ICC, except for B-ALL with *PAX5* alteration, which is also considered a provisional entity. The WHO-HEM5 does not recognize two ICC entities (B-ALL with CDX2/UBTF deregulation and B-ALL with mutated *IKZF1* N159Y) and three ICC provisional entities (B-ALL with *ZEB2 H1038R/IGH::CEBPE*, B-ALL with *ZNF384* rearranged-like, and B-ALL with *KMT2A* rearranged-like).

The ICC has introduced "ETP ALL with *BCL11B* rearrangement" as a new genetic subtype, and identified eight provisional entities of T-ALL/LBL that exhibit alterations involving *HOXA*, *SPI1*, *TLX1*, *TLX3*, *NKX2*, *TAL1-2*, *LMO1-2*, and other *BHLH* transcriptional factors, as shown in Table 1.2. Furthermore, the ICC retains the previous WHO provisional entity of NK cell ALL, which was removed in the WHO-HEM5 [5, 6, 21].

Acute Myeloid Leukemia

The ICC and the WHO-HEM5 diverge significantly in AML classification. One major difference is the blast cutoff numbers required for diagnosing AML of various subtypes. As shown in Table 1.3, the ICC requires ≥10% blasts for diagnosing most genetic subtypes of AML, while the WHO-HEM5 has no minimal blast percentage requirement for most of these genetic subtypes. The ICC concurs with the WHO-HEM5 on a threshold of 20% blasts for diagnosing AML with *BCR::ABL1* fusion and AML-MR. However, the ICC requires ≥10% blasts for AML cases with *CEBPA* mutation, *CBFA2T3::GLIS2* fusion, *KAT6A::CREBBP* fusion, *FUS::ERG* fusion, *MNX1::ETV6* fusion, and *NPM1::MLF1* fusion, whereas the WHO-HEM5 requires ≥20% for these subtypes.

Three of ICC's provisional genetic subtypes are not recognized in the WHO-HEM5. The ICC has created a new subtype, AML with mutated TP53, which requires ≥20% blasts and the presence of mono- or biallelic *TP53* mutation with a variant allele frequency (VAF) of at least 10%. The majority of *TP53*-mutated AML cases have a complex karyotype that fulfills the diagnostic criteria of AML-MR. The ICC has removed "history of MDS or MDS/MPN" as one of the conditions diagnostic of AML-MR, and divided AML-MR into two subentities: AML with MR cytogenetic abnormalities and AML with MR gene mutations. Most cases of AML transformed from MDS or MDS/MPN likely have MR cytogenetic abnormalities and/or gene mutations. Thus, these cases still fall under AML-MR, consistent with the WHO-HEM5. As shown in Table 1.4, categorization of the MR cytogenetic abnormalities and MR gene mutations differ slightly between the two systems. Monosomy 13 or del(13q) and del(11q) are included in the WHO-HEM5 but not in the ICC, while +8 and del(20q) are included in the ICC but not in the WHO-HEM5. RUNX1 is included as one of the MR gene mutations by the ICC but not by the WHO-HEM5. Regarding AML with *CEBPA* mutation, the ICC requires the presence of at least one in-frame bZIP mutation for the diagnosis of "AML with in-frame bZIP *CEBPA* mutations," while the WHO-HEM5 defines "AML with *CEBPA* mutation" more broadly, allowing either any single bZIP mutation or any biallelic mutations [4–6, 29, 33].

The ICC has removed therapy-related AML as a separate category but recommends incorporating prior therapy as a qualifier for the relevant AML subtype. In comparison, the WHO-HEM5 has changed the term to AML-pCT and lists it under the category of secondary myeloid neoplasms. The ICC categorizes AML cases not meeting the diagnostic criteria for a specific genetic subtype as "AML NOS," an equivalent category to the "AML defined by differentiation" in the WHO-HEM5. However, the ICC classifies AEL—a subtype within this category in the WHO-HEM5—as AML with mutated *TP53*, since almost all AEL cases harbor *TP53* mutations.

Acute Leukemia of Ambiguous Lineage

The ICC and WHO-HEM5 are aligned on the classification of ALAL/MPAL. Both systems have recognized *ZNF384* rearrangement and *BCL11B* rearrangement as the new defining genetic abnormalities. However, there are some minor discrepancies between them. The ICC recommends at least 5% abnormal blast population for a diagnosis of bilineal MPAL, while the WHO-HEM5 does not specify a minimum number. In addition, the WHO-HEM5 has introduced intensity criteria for MPAL lineage-defining markers, which are not mentioned in the ICC classification [4–6, 29]. Please see Chap. 20 for more details on the comparison of the two systems on ALAL/MPAL.

Pediatric Disorders and/or Germline Mutation-Associated Disorders

The ICC has created a category of "pediatric disorders and/or germline mutation-associated disorders" to include hematopoietic neoplasms that are either unique to children or associated with a germline mutation. Pediatric-specific neoplasms include JMML, JMML-like neoplasms, Noonan syndrome-like myeloproliferative disorder, and pediatric MDS. There are differences in the diagnostic criteria of JMML between the two systems. Exclusion of *KMT2A* rearrangement is mandatory for diagnosing JMML in the WHO-HEM5, but not in ICC. The WHO-HEM5 accepts noncanonical clonal RAS pathway gene alterations as an alternative genetic criterion and allows for diagnosis based on minor criteria in cases without diagnostic genetic findings. In contrast, the ICC considers the presence of a canonical RAS pathway mutation a mandatory requirement, and categorizes JMML cases meeting the WHO-HEM5 criteria but lacking a RAS-pathway mutation as JMML-like neoplasms. Patients with Noonan syndrome may experience a transient myeloproliferative disorder during their first year of life. Although this disorder can clinically and hematologically resemble JMML, the acquired somatic mutations are absent in these patients.

The ICC uses the term "hematologic neoplasms with germline predisposition" instead of the WHO's "myeloid neoplasms with germline predisposition" to reflect that many involved genes predispose patients not only to myeloid neoplasms but also to lymphoid neoplasms. The ICC has added a new subgroup, acute lymphoblastic leukemia with germline predisposition, which includes ALL patients with germline mutations in the *PAX5* or *IKZF1* gene. This subgroup is not recognized in the WHO-HEM5. In the subgroup of hematologic neoplasms with organ dysfunction, germline *BLM* mutation (Bloom syndrome) is included in the WHO-HEM5 but not in the ICC, while Diamond-Blackfan anemia is included in the ICC but not in the WHO-HEM5. Both systems share the remaining genetic conditions listed in Table 1.5.

Treatment of Pediatric Acute Lymphoblastic Leukemia

As described above, pediatric ALL is a genetically heterogeneous hematologic disease characterized by the proliferation of immature lymphoid cells in the bone marrow, peripheral blood, and other organs. ALL is the most common pediatric leukemia. The use of cytogenetic, immunologic, and molecular laboratory tests is critical in determining risk stratification and treatment regimens in B-ALL. With the use of sophisticated risk stratification and modern-day treatment strategies, overall survival (OS) for children with ALL is greater than 90% [34]. This section will review the current approach to upfront treatment for pediatric ALL, but will not discuss special populations such as those less than 1 year of age, the Down syndrome population, Philadelphia chromosome positive ALL, or those with relapsed or refractory disease.

B-Cell Acute Lymphoblastic Leukemia

Risk Stratification B-ALL

Initial risk stratification for B-ALL is determined at the time of diagnosis by age and initial white blood cell count (WBC). The National Cancer Institute (NCI) Rome risk stratification at diagnosis separates patients into standard risk (SR) (age 1.00–9.99 years, and initial WBC < 50,000/microliter), and high risk (HR) (age ≥ 10 years and/or WBC ≥ 50,000/microliter). Patients younger than 1 year are a special infant subgroup with worse outcomes [35].

After induction therapy, patients are further risk-stratified to determine the ultimate course of treatment. The definitions of risk groups vary among different cooperative groups. However, all groups use a combination of initial risk classification, central nervous system (CNS) disease status, presence of extra-medullary disease, response to therapy, and cytogenetic abnormalities to complete patient risk stratification. Some key high-risk features are outlined in Table 1.6. For more comprehensive coverage of prognostic and predictive biomarkers of B-ALL, please refer to Chap. 13.

Table 1.6 High-risk features of B-ALL

Age ≥ 10 years and/or initial WBC count > 50,000/microliter
Age < 1 year of age
Unfavorable cytogenetics[a]: t(9;22)/*BCR::ABL1* fusion *BCR::ABL1*-like Hypodiploidy (<44 chromosomes) iAMP21 *KMT2A* rearrangements t(17;19)/*TCF3::HLF* fusion
Presence of extramedullary disease, CNS-3 and testicular leukemia, at diagnosis
Poor response to early therapy: MRD ≥ 0.01% at the end of induction

[a]Please see Table 1.1 for the prognostication of more genetic subtypes

Overview of the Treatment of B-ALL

The treatment of pediatric ALL lasts 2–3 years, and there are a variety of successful treatment regimens. While specific approaches can differ among cooperative groups, no single approach has proven to be superior. Broadly speaking, the management of ALL can be grouped into induction, consolidation/late intensification, and maintenance or continuation therapy. The intensity of treatment throughout these phases varies among subsets of children with B-ALL based on their risk stratification.

Induction Therapy: Standard Risk

The initial aim of ALL treatment is the induction of a complete remission.

Induction therapy in SR patients includes a three-drug induction given over a 4-week period. Vincristine is administered weekly for a total of four doses. A 28-day course of oral dexamethasone is given. Asparaginase is the third drug given in induction therapy. Asparaginase depletes leukemic cells of asparagine, leading to apoptosis due to the inability of leukemic cells to synthesize asparagine. Multiple forms of asparaginase are available. There is a pegylated asparaginase (PEG) that allows less frequent dosing and is less immunogenic [36]. Calaspargase pegol is a newer formulation that has a longer half-life than PEG and is used widely in the US now. Asparaginase is associated with silent inactivation and clinically apparent allergic reactions. Silent inactivation can be measured by monitoring asparaginase levels and neutralizing antibodies. In cases where there is either silent inactivation or allergic reactions from these *Escherichia coli*-derived proteins, Erwinia-derived L-asparaginase can be used. Erwinase has a significantly shorter half-life and requires frequent intramuscular administration [37, 38]. Please see Chap. 11 for the pharmacogenomic considerations for asparaginase.

Induction Therapy: High Risk

Induction therapy in HR patients includes a four-drug induction given over a 4-week period. Vincristine is administered weekly for a total of four doses. In patients less than 10 years of age, dexamethasone is given for a total of 14 days. In patients greater than 10 years of age, prednisone is given for 28 days. In comparison to prednisone, dexamethasone has shown superior CNS penetration and is more effective in inducing marrow remission; however, it causes a significant amount of steroid-related complications including life-threatening infections and long-term side effects such as avascular necrosis (AVN). In patients greater than 10 years of age, the risk of AVN is substantially higher, so prednisone is preferred over dexamethasone [39]. HR patients receive asparaginase as the third drug, and the addition of an anthracycline to complete a four-drug induction. Some cooperative groups treat all patients regardless of initial risk stratification with a four-drug induction.

Post-induction Therapy

After the end of induction, when remission has been achieved, the goal of post-induction chemotherapy is to continue to provide leukemic cytoreduction and prevent the emergence of drug-resistant clones. This is accomplished through multiagent chemotherapy given over a course of 6–8 months. The most commonly used post-induction schema is based on a Berlin-Frankfurt-Munster (BFM) backbone and has been adopted by the Children's Oncology Group (COG) [40]. Other cooperative groups may differ in their treatment plans and have variations in the therapy listed below. For example, St. Jude and Dana Farber Cancer Institute rely on a more asparaginase-intensive treatment.

SR patients typically receive a 4-week consolidation that includes vincristine, oral mercaptopurine, and intensive intrathecal (IT) therapy. This phase is followed by interim maintenance (IM1) consisting of escalating doses of low-dose methotrexate given with vincristine. Patients then proceed to an intensive phase of delayed intensification (DI) that includes the drugs used in induction therapy as well as the addition of anthracyclines, cyclophosphamide, cytarabine, and 6-thioguanine. This is followed by a second course of interim maintenance (IM II).

Patients with HR B-ALL require a more intensive post-induction course. Consolidation includes the addition of cyclophosphamide, asparaginase, and cytarabine. IM1 is also intensified with high-dose methotrexate (5000 mg/m^2), rather than escalating lower doses of methotrexate, and is given with vincristine and mercaptopurine [39]. DI and IM II in HR patients are similar to those in SR patients.

Upon completion of these phases of treatment, patients will then begin maintenance therapy.

Immunotherapy in Post-induction Therapy

Blinatumomab, a bispecific T-cell engager that targets CD19, was initially shown to improve outcomes in patients with relapsed disease [41–43]. Given the favorable results in relapsed patients, the recent COG trial AALL1731, for newly diagnosed patients with SR disease, investigated the addition of two nonsequential cycles of blinatumomab to the standard chemotherapy backbone. Disease-free survival (DFS) increased from 88% with chemotherapy alone to 96% with the addition of blinatumomab [44]. This improved survival was similarly shown in adults with newly diagnosed B-ALL through the Eastern Cooperative Oncology Group (ECOG) trial E1910 [45]. Given the benefit shown in both the pediatric and adult populations, blinatumomab has become the standard of care in most patients with SR disease, and many are using it for the treatment of HR disease as well.

Maintenance Therapy

The combination of oral methotrexate and mercaptopurine (6-MP) administered continuously is the cornerstone of maintenance therapy for all cooperative groups. There is some variability in the schedule for administration of vincristine and steroid pulses as well as intrathecal chemotherapy for CNS-directed therapy. Some cooperative groups do not use any vincristine or steroid pulses during maintenance therapy.

Monitoring for compliance is critical in this phase of therapy. A COG study demonstrated that an adherence rate of less than 90% was associated with a significantly increased risk of relapse [46]. Frequent monitoring of blood counts and measurement of mercaptopurine metabolites guides dose modifications.

Additional testing of *TPMT* and *NUDT15* genes should be considered, as host polymorphisms in these genes result in increased sensitivity to 6MP and may warrant dose adjustment to prevent hematologic and hepatotoxicity. For more detailed elaboration of thiopurine pharmacogenomics, please see Chap. 11. The duration of maintenance therapy is approximately 2 years, regardless of biological sex.

Central Nervous System Therapy

In the early decades, central nervous system (CNS) therapy was not incorporated into treatment, and 80% of patients relapsed in the CNS. With the incorporation of CNS-directed therapy into current treatment protocols, the overall risk of CNS relapse is now below 5% [47]. CNS status at diagnosis can be classified into three categories: CNS1, CNS2, and CNS3. The presence and level of leukemic cells in the cerebrospinal fluid (CSF) are determined by cytospin preparation and absolute cell counts.

At diagnosis, approximately 3% of patients have CNS disease. However, the CNS serves as a sanctuary site for leukemia because most systemic chemotherapy has poor CNS penetration. Therefore, all patients will be treated with repetitive administration of intrathecal (IT) chemotherapy during the early intensive phases of treatment, and typically less intensely for the duration of treatment. Patients with CNS disease at diagnosis on most protocols will get once weekly IT chemotherapy during induction until the leukemia cells are no longer identified on cell count and cytospin from the CSF [48]. Cooperative groups differ on the preferred intrathecal agents. Some favor the administration of single-agent methotrexate for IT chemotherapy, while others prefer the use of triple IT, which includes methotrexate, corticosteroid, and cytarabine.

Historically, many patients with ALL with CNS disease underwent craniospinal (CSRT) or cranial irradiation (CRT) therapy, which was highly effective in reducing CNS relapse rates but was fraught with substantial toxicity including secondary malignancy, and neurologic and endocrinologic sequelae. Modern therapy now seeks to eliminate the use of radiation therapy for de novo disease without decreasing cure rates. The ability to maintain cure rates depends upon the intensification of systemic therapy that has the ability to penetrate the blood-brain barrier. The use of high-dose methotrexate in HR patients as well as long-term IT treatment has proved to provide essentially equivalent survival rates compared to the use of CSRT/CRT [49].

Role of Hematopoietic Stem Cell Transplant in B-ALL

Most children with B-ALL do not need a hematopoietic stem cell transplant (HSCT) for cure. However, due to the poor outcome for children with refractory or relapsed disease, HSCT is considered as a potential treatment option.

Role of CAR-T Therapy in B-ALL

Chimeric antigen receptor (CAR) T-cell therapy is a treatment option for pediatric relapsed/refractory B-ALL, as well as HR populations including those with MRD positivity at the end of consolidation, CNS relapse, and relapse in patients with Down syndrome. CAR-T therapy can serve as a bridge to HSCT or as definitive therapy itself. The use of CAR T-cell products has helped achieve a durable response and high rates of complete remission in a subset of patients with historically poor outcomes [50, 51].

T-Cell Acute Lymphoblastic Leukemia

T-ALL accounts for 15% of pediatric ALL and is biologically distinct from its B-ALL counterpart [52]. Outcomes of T-ALL are inferior to those of B-ALL, but with recent advances in therapy, event-free survival (EFS) rates have exceeded 85% [53, 54, 60].

Risk Stratification in T-ALL

Current risk classification in T-ALL is based primarily on MRD responses. Unlike B-ALL, NCI risk and routine cytogenetics are not currently used in treatment risk stratification. Current work is being done to further identify prognostic genetic lesions in T-ALL and their potential use for treatment risk stratification in the future [55, 56]. Please see a more detailed elaboration of these prognostic biomarkers in Chap. 14.

Overview of the Treatment of T-ALL

The kinetics of T-ALL demonstrate a slower disease regression, and overall T-ALL patients have higher rates of induction failure, end of induction MRD positivity, and CNS relapse [57]. Patients with T-ALL require more intensive chemotherapy regimens to achieve similar outcomes to their B-ALL counterparts.

Induction Therapy

All cooperative groups use a four-drug anthracycline-containing induction given over a 4-week period for T-ALL. The need for a four-drug induction on all T-ALL patients was demonstrated in the UKALL2003 trial, which showed that patients with a three-drug induction had an inferior outcome [58]. The medications used in induction for T-ALL are similar to those for B-ALL, including vincristine, dexamethasone, asparaginase, and an anthracycline. A key difference is the primary use of dexamethasone, rather than prednisone. The use of dexamethasone in the COG trial AALL1231 allowed for a reduction in the use of prophylactic cranial radiation therapy without an increase in CNS relapse [54]. The specific type and schedule of anthracyclines in induction differ between cooperative groups; however, there are similar outcomes on the different anthracycline-containing backbones.

Post-induction Therapy

Post-induction therapy for all T-ALL patients remains intensive, particularly given the known slower kinetics of T-ALL clearance and higher rates of CNS relapse.

Over a course of 6–8 months, multiagent chemotherapy using many of the same agents used in post-induction therapy for B-ALL is used. Some key differences in T-ALL treatment include the use of nelarabine and dose-escalating, rather than high-dose methotrexate regimens. COG trial AALL0434 demonstrated unexpectedly that escalating dose methotrexate was superior to the high-dose methotrexate that is used in the HR B-ALL patients [59]. The introduction of nelarabine into T-ALL treatment had a significant impact on the reduction of CNS relapse. Nelarabine is an antimetabolite, a nucleoside analog that inhibits DNA synthesis. Initially, nelarabine was reserved for the relapsed/refractory setting due to concern for neurotoxicity. However, an increased event-free and overall survival with an acceptable toxicity profile was demonstrated on COG AALL0434. Nelarabine is now used upfront throughout multiple phases of therapy, including a maintenance/continuation phase [60].

Maintenance/Continuation Therapy

Maintenance/continuation therapy for T-ALL remains similar to that of B-ALL, except for the addition of nelarabine therapy for most cooperative groups. Nelarabine is typically given for the first three cycles of maintenance and then discontinued.

Role of Hematopoietic Stem Cell Transplant in T-ALL

Most children with T-ALL do not need HSCT for cure. However, due to the very poor outcome for children with MRD positivity at the end of consolidation, or relapse at any time, HSCT with the best available donor should be pursued in these settings.

CNS Treatment

There are varying strategies between cooperative groups for CNS-directed therapy in T-ALL. Historically, prophylactic cranial radiation therapy (CRT) was given to patients with T-ALL due to their high risk of CNS relapse. However, modern treatment protocols have sought to eliminate CRT due to the highly morbid neurocognitive sequelae, endocrinopathies, and secondary malignancies associated with CRT. The addition of intensive chemotherapy backbones with additional doses of asparaginase, the use of dexamethasone, as well as the introduction of nelarabine have decreased the use of CRT [53]. Similar to B-ALL, the use of intrathecal chemotherapy with either methotrexate or methotrexate, cytarabine, and a corticosteroid remains a mainstay of treatment throughout all phases of therapy.

Summary

The treatment of pediatric ALL is one of the great success stories of modern medicine. With significant improvement in overall survival, research now seeks to decrease intensity of chemotherapy in efforts to minimize morbidity and the long-term toxicity seen in survivors of pediatric ALL. The recent addition of immunotherapy may allow us to further decrease the use of cytotoxic chemotherapy as we continue to improve upon and refine the use of immunotherapy in this patient population.

Treatment of Pediatric Acute Myeloid Leukemia

AML is the second most common pediatric leukemia, and accounts for approximately 20% of childhood leukemia cases, with an estimated incidence worldwide of 5–8 per million [61]. AML remains difficult to treat, with an estimated 5-year survival rate of 64.3% in the US, notably with wide-ranging 5-year prognoses for the various subtypes of AML and with a plateau in further improvements over the last several decades [61]. Improvements in outcomes since the 1970s are largely attributed to more intensive chemotherapy regimens, improved supportive care, and improved use of and selection of patients to receive HSCT [62]. Additional improvements for specific subgroups contributing to the improvement in overall survival include the use of all-trans retinoic acid and arsenic trioxide in patients with APL and de-intensification of treatment regimens for children with AML associated with DS [62].

Risk stratification has become increasingly important in the treatment of pediatric AML as a tool to better identify which patients can safely de-intensify therapy to reduce treatment-related morbidity and mortality. The primary factors that determine risk group are cytogenetic features and response to induction therapy as determined by flow cytometry, termed MRD, though stratification schemas vary by cooperative groups and across different trials. For example, the most recent COG trial, AAML1831, uses a revised risk stratification based on a retrospective analysis of outcomes for patients treated on the precursor trial AAML0531 and incorporating molecular data. This new system significantly changes the distribution of risk stratification, with an estimated 33% of patients in AAML0531 classified as high risk based on these prognostic markers compared to a historical 9% in AAML03P1 [63].

This section will review the current treatment approach and recent clinical trials for pediatric AML, with a focus on upfront therapy. We will briefly review the use of HSCT, approaches to specific populations, and treatment of relapsed/refractory disease. This section will not cover the treatment of patients with special subtypes such as APL or Down syndrome-associated AML.

Overview of AML Treatment in the Frontline Setting

The primary goal of treatment of AML is to induce remission (induction), followed by post-remission treatment to reduce relapse risk (consolidation/intensification). Post-remission therapy typically consists of intensified chemotherapy courses or HSCT, depending on both risk stratification and the availability of a suitable donor. Maintenance therapy to maintain remission, a cornerstone of treatment in ALL, has not been shown to improve outcomes in AML, though there is increasing interest in the use of targeted therapies as maintenance treatment in some settings [64–67].

Recent clinical trials for pediatric AML have relied on a conventional chemotherapy backbone of cytarabine and an anthracycline, though the exact backbone used and the number of chemotherapy cycles delivered vary across cooperative groups and risk groups. The United Kingdom Medical Research Council (MRC) AML10 trial established that induction therapy with cytarabine, daunorubicin, and etoposide (ADE) had similar remission rates with lower toxicity in comparison to induction with cytarabine, daunorubicin, and thioguanine [68]. A later trial by the same group, MRC AML15, demonstrated equivalent survival with cytarabine and daunorubicin (AD) compared to ADE [69]. These regimens remain the standard backbone of many of the more recent and ongoing clinical trials.

Recent studies from various cooperative groups are summarized in Table 1.7 below, with much of the recent work focused on intensification of induction courses to improve remission rates or introduction of new chemotherapeutic or immunotherapeutic agents to standard therapy. One example is gemtuzumab ozogamicin (GO), an antibody drug conjugate linking calicheamicin to a CD33-directed monoclonal antibody. The COG trial AAML0531 showed a reduction in post-remission relapses with the addition of GO to standard chemotherapy, with the largest benefit seen in those with low-risk cytogenetics, similar to prior adult studies [70, 71]. For pharmacogenomic considerations of GO treatment, please see Chap. 11.

Special Populations: FLT3 Mutations

Mutations in fms-like tyrosine kinase 3 (FLT3) are less common in pediatric than in adult AML, occurring at a frequency of 10–20% in children compared to 30% of newly diagnosed adults [80–82]. Internal tandem duplication (ITD) activating mutations are the most common and confer a negative prognosis in all age groups, making inhibition of FLT3 an attractive target in both pediatric and adult AML [81, 82]. The COG trial AAML1031 demonstrated improved 3-year EFS, DFS, and relapse risk in patients with FLT3-ITD variants who received the first-generation tyrosine kinase inhibitor sorafenib, though there was no improvement in overall survival [77]. The current COG trial AAML1831 is investigating the use of a newer generation FLT3 inhibitor, gilteritinib, in combination with chemotherapy in patients with FLT3-ITD mutations, though results from this study are not yet available. FLT3 tyrosine kinase domain (TKD) mutations occur less frequently than FLT3-ITD and confer a more favorable prognosis in comparison [83]. The AAML1831 trial is also investigating the addition of gilteritinib for patients with selected FLT3 TKD mutations.

Special Populations: Central Nervous System Disease

Patients with central nervous system involvement in AML have been shown to have lower rates of remission following two induction courses, lower event-free survival, and higher relapse risk compared to those without CNS involvement in COG trials,

Table 1.7 Significant outcomes from recent pediatric AML trials

Trial	Intervention	Significant outcomes	References
St. Jude AML08	Induction I randomization to Clo + Ara-C or HD-ADE	No significant difference in 3-year EFS or OS despite higher rates of MRD positivity at Day 22 in Clo + AraC arm	[72]
AML-BFM 2012	Comparison of clofarabine and etoposide use in first induction course	Improved 3-year OS of 82% and EFS 69% without significant difference between etoposide and clofarabine arm Study closed early due to commercial availability of clofarabine and L-daunorubicin	[73]
MRC AML15	Induction therapy randomized to two courses of DA, ADE, or FLAG-Ida (additional randomization to include GO) Consolidation therapy randomized to MACE/MidAC (MRC standard) vs two courses of HD ARA-C (3 g/m^2 or 1.5 g/m^2)	No significant difference in remission rates between induction regimens Decreased relapse risk with FLAG-Ida but without survival benefit due to increased myelosuppression and death in CR No difference in survival between MACE/MidAC and HD ARA-C consolidation arms with higher myelosuppression and deaths in CR in the MACE/MidAC arm	[74]
COG AAML0531	Randomization to standard 5- course chemotherapy or standard chemotherapy plus GO in induction 1 and intensification 2	Improved EFS but not OS in GO arm Reduction of relapse risk in GO recipients Higher disease-free survival despite increased toxic mortality in remission in GO recipients Superior EFS, similar OS, and reduced relapse risk in patients with KMT2A-r AML	[70, 75]
COG AAML1031	Randomization to standard chemotherapy with or without addition of bortezomib	No improvement in remissions rates, EFS, or OS with bortezomib with higher rates of toxicity Improved EFS for patients with FLT3/ITD+ AML who received sorafenib when adjusted for receipt of HSCT No improvement in survival with mitoxantrone in induction 2 compared to ADE (AAML0531)	[76–78]
COG AAML1831	DA-GO vs CPX-351 and GO in Induction 1	Randomization closed for futility with lower EFS in CPX-351 arm despite similar OS	[79]

ADE cytarabine, daunorubicin, and etoposide, *Clo + Ara-C* clofarabine and cytarabine, *DA* daunorubicin and cytarabine, *DA-GO* daunorubicin, cytarabine, gemtuzumab ozogamicin, *FLAG-Ida* fludarabine, cytarabine, granulocyte colony-stimulating factor, and idarubicin, *GO* gemtuzumab ozogamicin, *HD-ADE* high-dose cytarabine, daunorubicin, and etoposide, *MACE* amsacrine, cytarabine, etoposide, *MidAC* mitoxantrone/cytarabine which used intrathecal cytarabine as CNS-directed therapy [84]. Other groups have shown increased relapse risk with cytarabine alone compared with triple-intrathecal therapy (cytarabine, methotrexate, and hydrocortisone) [85]. The current standard approach at COG centers utilizes triple-intrathecal therapy for all patients. Radiation is no longer used for prophylactic CNS-directed therapy, given significant risks of toxicity associated with craniospinal radiation, with studies failing to show significant benefit [86].

Role of Hematopoietic Stem Cell Transplant

HSCT is a mainstay of consolidation therapy in frontline therapy for patients at increased risk of relapse, though identifying these patients is difficult [87]. There is a general consensus that low-risk patients do not benefit from HSCT; however, the data regarding the benefit for intermediate and high-risk patients remains conflicting [88]. Current recommendations from the American Society for Transplantation and Cellular Therapy include the use of busulfan-based myeloablative conditioning without total body irradiation (TBI) for patients without comorbidities necessitating reduced intensity conditioning [89]. Historical data from multiple cooperative groups have shown improvements in DFS and reduction of relapse risk following HSCT in first remission, though this finding is not consistent across all studies [90–93]. A recent report from the COG evaluating outcomes from HSCT in both AAML0531 and AAML1031 demonstrated 5-year DFS of 49.8% for patients with high-risk cytogenetics who received HSCT, compared to 26% for those patients treated with chemotherapy alone, and similarly improved 5-year DFS of 50.9% compared to 16.9% for HSCT in patients with SR cytogenetics and positive MRD at the end of induction I [94]. The current standard at most North American centers is to utilize HSCT in first remission for patients with HR cytogenetic features or MRD positivity after first induction.

Treatment of Relapsed AML

Despite the improvements that have been made in the treatment of pediatric AML, over 30% of patients will experience relapse [95]. Approaches to relapsed AML and refractory AML (failure to achieve remission following induction courses) aim to achieve a second remission prior to consolidative therapy with HSCT. A full review of available therapies for relapsed disease is beyond the scope of this chapter, but we will highlight some options that may be considered. There is no standard approach to relapsed pediatric AML, and enrollment on a clinical trial should be considered if feasible. Many regimens use high-dose cytarabine in combination with other agents [96]. CPX-351, a liposomal preparation of daunorubicin and cytarabine, demonstrated a tolerable side effect profile and improved response rates compared to historical relapse regimens in a recent COG Phase I/II trial, AAML1421 [97]. Venetoclax is a BCL-2 inhibitor that has been well tolerated, with 70% of patients achieving a complete response in a study at St. Jude Children's Research Hospital [98]. Targeted therapies directed at specific genomic lesions are increasingly being integrated into relapsed therapy, including gilteritinib and sorafenib for FLT3 mutations [99, 100], and revumenib, a menin inhibitor that has demonstrated efficacy in relapsed patients with KMT2A-rearranged or NPM1-altered AML [101]. Gemtuzumab ozogamicin has demonstrated a remission response rate of 37–45% with use in the relapse setting as a single agent or in combination with chemotherapy [102, 103]. Multiple other immunotherapy-based approaches remain under investigation, including monoclonal antibodies, bispecific antibodies, cellular therapies, and immune checkpoint inhibitors [104]. There is evidence that some patients who undergo a second transplant following relapsed disease will achieve long-term remission [105].

Summary

Cooperative group trials have improved survival in pediatric AML over time. Despite these advances, patients with HR or relapsed disease face a poor prognosis. A growing understanding of the cytogenetic and molecular drivers of AML is guiding advances in risk stratification and targeted therapies.

Conclusion

The diagnosis, classification, and treatment of pediatric leukemia have improved significantly over the past decades. These advances have led to tremendously enhanced clinical outcomes. Comprehensive laboratory assessments, especially with the inclusion of genetic testing, play a key role in current diagnosis and personalized treatment. Despite these achievements, there remain many challenges, which include overall high relapse rates and poor prognosis in relapsed cases, significant therapy-related mortality and morbidity, and unequal resource accessibility across the world. Overcoming these challenges will require that we continue to explore novel therapies and optimize individualized treatment to increase therapeutic efficacy, gain deeper remission, and minimize therapy-related side effects. Research should continue delving into the genetic alterations to better understand molecular leukemogenesis and clonal evolution, and uncover new genetic defects for targeted therapies and/or risk-stratification. There should be more international collaboration on clinical trials to shorten the transition time of the new agents from research to clinical stages and provide access to low-resource patients.

References

1. NCCR*Explorer: an interactive website for NCCR cancer statistics [Internet]. National Cancer Institute; 2024. [cited 2025 Aug 13]. Available from: https://nccrexplorer.ccdi.cancer.gov.

2. SEER*Explorer: an interactive website for SEER cancer statistics [Internet]. Surveillance Research Program, National Cancer Institute; 2025. [cited 2025 Aug 13]. Available from: https://seer.cancer.gov/statistics-network/explorer/. Data source(s): SEER Incidence Data, November 2024 Submission (1975–2022), SEER 21 registries.
3. Alaggio R, Amador C, Anagnostopoulos I, et al. The 5th edition of the World Health Organization classification of haematolymphoid tumours: lymphoid neoplasms. Leukemia. 2022;36(7):1720–48. https://doi.org/10.1038/s41375-022-01620-2. Epub 2022 Jun 22.
4. Khoury JD, Solary E, Abla O, et al. The 5th edition of the World Health Organization classification of haematolymphoid tumours: myeloid and histiocytic/dendritic neoplasms. Leukemia. 2022;36(7):1703–19. https://doi.org/10.1038/s41375-022-01613-1. Epub 2022 Jun 22. PMID: 35732831; PMCID: PMC9252913.
5. WHO. WHO Classification of Tumours Editorial Board. Haematolymphoid tumours [Internet]. Lyon: International Agency for Research on Cancer; 2022. (WHO classification of tumours series, 5th ed.; vol. 11). Available from: https://tumourclassification.iarc.who.int/chapters/63.
6. Arber DA, Orazi A, Hasserjian RP, et al. International Consensus Classification of Myeloid Neoplasms and Acute Leukemias: integrating morphologic, clinical, and genomic data. Blood. 2022;140(11):1200–28. https://doi.org/10.1182/blood.2022015850. PMID: 35767897; PMCID: PMC9479031.
7. Daltveit DS, Morgan E, Colombet M, Steliarova-Foucher E, Bendahhou K, Marcos-Gragera R, Rongshou Z, Smith A, Wei H, Soerjomataram I. Global patterns of leukemia by subtype, age, and sex in 185 countries in 2022. Leukemia. 2025;39(2):412–9. https://doi.org/10.1038/s41375-024-02452-y. Epub 2024 Nov 20.
8. Inaba H, Teachey D, Annesley C, et al. Pediatric acute lymphoblastic leukemia, Version 2.2025, NCCN clinical practice guidelines in oncology. J Natl Compr Cancer Netw. 2025;23(2):41–62. https://doi.org/10.6004/jnccn.2025.0006.
9. Williams LA, Richardson M, Marcotte EL, Poynter JN, Spector LG. Sex ratio among childhood cancers by single year of age. Pediatr Blood Cancer. 2019;66(6):e27620. https://doi.org/10.1002/pbc.27620. Epub 2019 Feb 28. PMID: 30815990; PMCID: PMC6472964.
10. Inaba H, Mullighan CG. Pediatric acute lymphoblastic leukemia. Haematologica. 2020;105(11):2524–39. https://doi.org/10.3324/haematol.2020.247031. PMID: 33054110; PMCID: PMC7604619.
11. Umeda M, Ma J, Westover T, et al. A new genomic framework to categorize pediatric acute myeloid leukemia. Nat Genet. 2024;56(2):281–93. https://doi.org/10.1038/s41588-023-01640-3. Epub 2024 Jan 11. PMID: 38212634; PMCID: PMC10864188.
12. Bardelli V, Arniani S, Pierini V, Di Giacomo D, Pierini T, Gorello P, Mecucci C, La Starza R. T-cell acute lymphoblastic leukemia: biomarkers and their clinical usefulness. Genes (Basel). 2021;12(8):1118. https://doi.org/10.3390/genes12081118. PMID: 34440292; PMCID: PMC8394887.
13. Graff Z, Burke MJ, Gossai N. Novel therapies for pediatric acute lymphoblastic leukemia. Curr Opin Pediatr. 2024;36(1):64–70. https://doi.org/10.1097/MOP.0000000000001316. Epub 2023 Nov 22.
14. Karol SE, Gueguen G. Pediatric acute myeloid leukemia—novel approaches. Curr Opin Hematol. 2024;31(2):47–52. https://doi.org/10.1097/MOH.0000000000000795. Epub 2023 Nov 20.
15. El-Sharkawy F, Margolskee E. Pediatric myeloproliferative neoplasms. Clin Lab Med. 2021;41(3):529–40. https://doi.org/10.1016/j.cll.2021.04.010.
16. Kitagawa M, Yoshida S, Ishige I, Minami J, Kuwata T, Tanizawa T, Kamiyama R. Immunolocalization of platelet-derived growth factor, transforming growth factor-beta, and fibronectin in acute megakaryoblastic leukemia manifesting tumor formation. Hum Pathol. 1994;25(7):723–6. https://doi.org/10.1016/0046-8177(94)90307-7.
17. Fuda F, Chen W. Acute Leukemia of Ambiguous Lineage: Diagnosis and Evaluation by Flow Cytometry. Cancers (Basel). 2025;17(5):871. https://doi.org/10.3390/cancers17050871. PMID: 40075717; PMCID: PMC11898493.

18. Bugarin C, Antolini L, Buracchi C, et al. Phenotypic profiling of CD34+ cells by advanced flow cytometry improves diagnosis of juvenile myelomonocytic leukemia. Haematologica. 2024;109(2):521–32. https://doi.org/10.3324/haematol.2023.282805. PMID: 37534527; PMCID: PMC10828789.
19. Frisanco Oliveira A, Tansini A, Toledo TR, Balceiro R, Onofre Vidal D, de Martino Lee ML, Lorand-Metze I, Lopes LF. Immunophenotypic characteristics of juvenile myelomonocytic leukaemia and their relation with the molecular subgroups of the disease. Br J Haematol. 2021;192(1):129–36. https://doi.org/10.1111/bjh.17098. Epub 2020 Sep 23.
20. Belsky JA, Audino AN, Kahwash SB. Separating lymphoblastic lymphoma involving marrow from lymphoblastic leukemia: it is time to update the cutoff number. J Pediatr Hematol Oncol. 2019;41(8):658–9. https://doi.org/10.1097/MPH.0000000000001588.
21. Li W. The 5th Edition of the World Health Organization classification of hematolymphoid tumors. In: Li W, editor. Leukemia [Internet]. Brisbane: Exon Publications; 2022. Chapter 1.
22. Campo E, Jaffe ES, Cook JR, et al. The International Consensus Classification of Mature Lymphoid Neoplasms: a report from the Clinical Advisory Committee. Blood. 2022;140(11):1229–53. https://doi.org/10.1182/blood.2022015851. Erratum in: Blood. 2023;141(4):437. https://doi.org/10.1182/blood.2022019016. PMID: 35653592; PMCID: PMC9479027.
23. Arber DA, Campo E, Jaffe ES. Advances in the classification of myeloid and lymphoid neoplasms. Virchows Arch. 2023;482(1):1–9. https://doi.org/10.1007/s00428-022-03487-1. Epub 2022 Dec 31.
24. Cree IA, The WHO. Classification of haematolymphoid tumours. Leukemia. 2022;36(7):1701–2. https://doi.org/10.1038/s41375-022-01625-x. Epub 2022 Jun 22. PMID: 35732830; PMCID: PMC9252902.
25. Carroll AJ, Shago M, Mikhail FM, et al. Masked hypodiploidy: Hypodiploid acute lymphoblastic leukemia (ALL) mimicking hyperdiploid ALL in children: a report from the Children's Oncology Group. Cancer Genet. 2019;238:62–8. https://doi.org/10.1016/j.cancergen.2019.07.009. Epub 2019 Jul 30. PMID: 31425927; PMCID: PMC6768693.
26. Creasey T, Enshaei A, Nebral K, et al. Single nucleotide polymorphism array-based signature of low hypodiploidy in acute lymphoblastic leukemia. Genes Chromosomes Cancer. 2021;60(9):604–15. https://doi.org/10.1002/gcc.22956. Epub 2021 May 17. Erratum in: Genes Chromosomes Cancer. 2022;61(4):212–4. https://doi.org/10.1002/gcc.23021. PMID: 33938069; PMCID: PMC8600946.
27. Choi JK, Xiao W, Chen X, et al. WHO 5th Edition Classification Project. Fifth Edition of the World Health Organization classification of tumors of the hematopoietic and lymphoid tissues: acute lymphoblastic leukemias, mixed-phenotype acute leukemias, myeloid/lymphoid neoplasms with eosinophilia, dendritic/histiocytic neoplasms, and genetic tumor syndromes. Mod Pathol. 2024;37(5):100466. https://doi.org/10.1016/j.modpat.2024.100466. Epub 2024 Mar 7.
28. Buckley M, Yeung DT, White DL, Eadie LN. T-cell acute lymphoblastic leukaemia: subtype prevalence, clinical outcome, and emerging targeted treatments. Leukemia. 2025;39(6):1294–310. https://doi.org/10.1038/s41375-025-02599-2. Epub 2025 Apr 17. PMID: 40247105; PMCID: PMC12133571.
29. Xiao W, Nardi V, Stein E, Hasserjian RP. A practical approach on the classifications of myeloid neoplasms and acute leukemia: WHO and ICC. J Hematol Oncol. 2024;17(1):56. https://doi.org/10.1186/s13045-024-01571-4. PMID: 39075565; PMCID: PMC11287910.
30. Klusmann JH, Creutzig U, Zimmermann M, et al. Treatment and prognostic impact of transient leukemia in neonates with Down syndrome. Blood. 2008;111(6):2991–8. https://doi.org/10.1182/blood-2007-10-118810. Epub 2008 Jan 8. PMID: 18182574; PMCID: PMC2265448.
31. Gamis AS, Alonzo TA, Gerbing RB, et al. Natural history of transient myeloproliferative disorder clinically diagnosed in Down syndrome neonates: a report from the Children's Oncology Group Study A2971. Blood. 2011;118(26):6752–9; quiz 6996. https://doi.org/10.1182/blood-2011-04-350017. Epub 2011 Aug 17. PMID: 21849481; PMCID: PMC3245202.

32. Duffield AS, Mullighan CG, Borowitz MJ. International Consensus Classification of acute lymphoblastic leukemia/lymphoma. Virchows Arch. 2023;482(1):11–26. https://doi.org/10.1007/s00428-022-03448-8. Epub 2022 Nov 24. PMID: 36422706; PMCID: PMC10646822.
33. Weinberg OK, Porwit A, Orazi A, Hasserjian RP, Foucar K, Duncavage EJ, Arber DA. The International Consensus Classification of acute myeloid leukemia. Virchows Arch. 2023;482(1):27–37. https://doi.org/10.1007/s00428-022-03430-4. Epub 2022 Oct 20.
34. Hunger SP, Mullighan CG. Acute lymphoblastic leukemia in children. N Engl J Med. 2015;373(16):1541–52.
35. Smith M, Arthur D, Camitta B, Carroll AJ, Crist W, Gaynon P, et al. Uniform approach to risk classification and treatment assignment for children with acute lymphoblastic leukemia. J Clin Oncol. 1996;14(1):18–24.
36. Wetzler M, Sanford BL, Kurtzberg J, DeOliveira D, Frankel SR, Powell BL, et al. Effective asparagine depletion with pegylated asparaginase results in improved outcomes in adult acute lymphoblastic leukemia: Cancer and Leukemia Group B Study 9511. Blood. 2007;109(10):4164–7.
37. Salzer WL, Asselin BL, Plourde PV, Corn T, Hunger SP. Development of asparaginase Erwinia chrysanthemi for the treatment of acute lymphoblastic leukemia. Ann N Y Acad Sci. 2014;1329:81–92.
38. Tong WH, Pieters R, Kaspers GJ, te Loo DM, Bierings MB, van den Bos C, et al. A prospective study on drug monitoring of PEGasparaginase and Erwinia asparaginase and asparaginase antibodies in pediatric acute lymphoblastic leukemia. Blood. 2014;123(13):2026–33.
39. Larsen EC, Devidas M, Chen S, Salzer WL, Raetz EA, Loh ML, et al. Dexamethasone and high-dose methotrexate improve outcome for children and young adults with high-risk B-acute lymphoblastic leukemia: a report from Children's Oncology Group Study AALL0232. J Clin Oncol. 2016;34(20):2380–8.
40. Moricke A, Zimmermann M, Reiter A, Henze G, Schrauder A, Gadner H, et al. Long-term results of five consecutive trials in childhood acute lymphoblastic leukemia performed by the ALL-BFM study group from 1981 to 2000. Leukemia. 2010;24(2):265–84.
41. Brown PA, Ji L, Xu X, Devidas M, Hogan LE, Borowitz MJ, et al. Effect of postreinduction therapy consolidation with blinatumomab vs chemotherapy on disease-free survival in children, adolescents, and young adults with first relapse of B-cell acute lymphoblastic leukemia: a randomized clinical trial. JAMA. 2021;325(9):833–42.
42. Hogan LE, Brown PA, Ji L, Xu X, Devidas M, Bhatla T, et al. Children's Oncology Group AALL1331: phase III trial of blinatumomab in children, adolescents, and young adults with low-risk B-cell ALL in first relapse. J Clin Oncol. 2023;41(25):4118–29.
43. Locatelli F, Zugmaier G, von Stackelberg A. Blinatumomab vs chemotherapy among children with relapsed acute lymphoblastic leukemia-reply. JAMA. 2021;326(4):359–60.
44. Gupta S, Rau RE, Loh ML. Blinatumomab in childhood B-cell acute lymphoblastic leukemia. Reply N Engl J Med. 2025;392(22):2286–7.
45. Litzow MR, Sun Z, Mattison RJ, Paietta EM, Roberts KG, Zhang Y, et al. Blinatumomab for MRD-negative acute lymphoblastic leukemia in adults. N Engl J Med. 2024;391(4):320–33.
46. Bhatia S, Landier W, Shangguan M, Hageman L, Schaible AN, Carter AR, et al. Nonadherence to oral mercaptopurine and risk of relapse in Hispanic and non-Hispanic white children with acute lymphoblastic leukemia: a report from the Children's Oncology Group. J Clin Oncol. 2012;30(17):2094–101.
47. McNeer JL, Schmiegelow K. Management of CNS disease in pediatric acute lymphoblastic leukemia. Curr Hematol Malig Rep. 2022;17(1):1–14.
48. Moricke A, Reiter A, Zimmermann M, Gadner H, Stanulla M, Dordelmann M, et al. Risk-adjusted therapy of acute lymphoblastic leukemia can decrease treatment burden and improve survival: treatment results of 2169 unselected pediatric and adolescent patients enrolled in the trial ALL-BFM 95. Blood. 2008;111(9):4477–89.

49. Richards S, Pui CH, Gayon P, Childhood Acute Lymphoblastic Leukemia Collaborative G. Systematic review and meta-analysis of randomized trials of central nervous system directed therapy for childhood acute lymphoblastic leukemia. Pediatr Blood Cancer. 2013;60(2):185–95.
50. Maude SL, Laetsch TW, Buechner J, Rives S, Boyer M, Bittencourt H, et al. Tisagenlecleucel in children and young adults with B-cell lymphoblastic leukemia. N Engl J Med. 2018;378(5):439–48.
51. Talleur AC, Myers R, Annesley C, Shalabi H. Chimeric antigen receptor T-cell therapy: current status and clinical outcomes in pediatric hematologic malignancies. Hematol Oncol Clin North Am. 2022;36(4):701–27.
52. Chiaretti S, Zini G, Bassan R. Diagnosis and subclassification of acute lymphoblastic leukemia. Mediterr J Hematol Infect Dis. 2014;6(1):e2014073.
53. Raetz EA, Teachey DT. T-cell acute lymphoblastic leukemia. Hematology Am Soc Hematol Educ Program. 2016;2016(1):580–8.
54. Teachey DT, Devidas M, Wood BL, Chen Z, Hayashi RJ, Hermiston ML, et al. Children's Oncology Group Trial AALL1231: a phase III clinical trial testing bortezomib in newly diagnosed T-cell acute lymphoblastic leukemia and lymphoma. J Clin Oncol. 2022;40(19):2106–18.
55. Raetz EA, Bhojwani D, Devidas M, Gore L, Rabin KR, Tasian SK, et al. Children's Oncology Group blueprint for research: acute lymphoblastic leukemia. Pediatr Blood Cancer. 2023;70(Suppl 6):e30585.
56. Polonen P, Di Giacomo D, Seffernick AE, Elsayed A, Kimura S, Benini F, et al. The genomic basis of childhood T-lineage acute lymphoblastic leukaemia. Nature. 2024;632(8027):1082–91.
57. Goldberg JM, Silverman LB, Levy DE, Dalton VK, Gelber RD, Lehmann L, et al. Childhood T-cell acute lymphoblastic leukemia: the Dana-Farber Cancer Institute acute lymphoblastic leukemia consortium experience. J Clin Oncol. 2003;21(19):3616–22.
58. Vrooman LM, Stevenson KE, Supko JG, O'Brien J, Dahlberg SE, Asselin BL, et al. Postinduction dexamethasone and individualized dosing of Escherichia Coli L-asparaginase each improve outcome of children and adolescents with newly diagnosed acute lymphoblastic leukemia: results from a randomized study—Dana-Farber Cancer Institute ALL Consortium Protocol 00-01. J Clin Oncol. 2013;31(9):1202–10.
59. Winter SS, Dunsmore KP, Devidas M, Wood BL, Esiashvili N, Chen Z, et al. Improved survival for children and young adults with T-lineage acute lymphoblastic leukemia: results from the Children's Oncology Group AALL0434 methotrexate randomization. J Clin Oncol. 2018;36(29):2926–34.
60. Dunsmore KP, Winter SS, Devidas M, Wood BL, Esiashvili N, Chen Z, et al. Children's Oncology Group AALL0434: a phase III randomized clinical trial testing nelarabine in newly diagnosed T-cell acute lymphoblastic leukemia. J Clin Oncol. 2020;38(28):3282–93.
61. Puumala SE, Ross JA, Aplenc R, Spector LG. Epidemiology of childhood acute myeloid leukemia. Pediatr Blood Cancer. 2013;60(5):728–33.
62. Smith MA, Seibel NL, Altekruse SF, Ries LA, Melbert DL, O'Leary M, et al. Outcomes for children and adolescents with cancer: challenges for the twenty-first century. J Clin Oncol. 2010;28(15):2625–34.
63. Cooper TM, Ries RE, Alonzo TA, Gerbing RB, Loken MR, Brodersen LE, et al. Revised risk stratification criteria for children with newly diagnosed acute myeloid leukemia: a report from the Children's Oncology Group. Blood. 2017;130(Supplement 1):407.
64. Aldoss I, Issa GC, Blachly JS, Thirman MJ, Mannis GN, Arellano ML, et al. Updated results and longer follow-up from the AUGMENT-101 phase 2 study of revumenib in all patients with relapsed or refractory (R/R) KMT2Ar acute leukemia. Blood. 2024;144(Supplement 1):211.

65. Ansar S, Keen MA, Sukaina M, Saeed M, Rehman Z, Rehman R, et al. FLT3 inhibitors as maintenance therapy post allogenic hematopoietic stem cell transplantation in acute myeloid leukemia patients with FLT3 mutations; a systematic review and meta-analysis. Blood. 2024;144(Supplement 1):5197.
66. Perel Y, Auvrignon A, Leblanc T, Vannier JP, Michel G, Nelken B, et al. Impact of addition of maintenance therapy to intensive induction and consolidation chemotherapy for childhood acute myeloblastic leukemia: results of a prospective randomized trial, LAME 89/91. Leucámie Aiqüe Myéloïde Enfant. J Clin Oncol. 2002;20(12):2774–82.
67. Wells RJ, Woods WG, Buckley JD, Odom LF, Benjamin D, Bernstein I, et al. Treatment of newly diagnosed children and adolescents with acute myeloid leukemia: a Children's Cancer Group study. J Clin Oncol. 1994;12(11):2367–77.
68. Hann IM, Stevens RF, Goldstone AH, Rees JK, Wheatley K, Gray RG, et al. Randomized comparison of DAT versus ADE as induction chemotherapy in children and younger adults with acute myeloid leukemia. Results of the Medical Research Council's 10th AML trial (MRC AML10). Adult and Childhood Leukaemia Working Parties of the Medical Research Council. Blood. 1997;89(7):2311–8.
69. Burnett AK, Russell NH, Hills RK, Hunter AE, Kjeldsen L, Yin J, et al. Optimization of chemotherapy for younger patients with acute myeloid leukemia: results of the medical research council AML15 trial. J Clin Oncol. 2013;31(27):3360–8.
70. Gamis AS, Alonzo TA, Meshinchi S, Sung L, Gerbing RB, Raimondi SC, et al. Gemtuzumab ozogamicin in children and adolescents with de novo acute myeloid leukemia improves event-free survival by reducing relapse risk: results from the randomized phase III Children's Oncology Group trial AAML0531. J Clin Oncol. 2014;32(27):3021–32.
71. Hills RK, Castaigne S, Appelbaum FR, Delaunay J, Petersdorf S, Othus M, et al. Addition of gemtuzumab ozogamicin to induction chemotherapy in adult patients with acute myeloid leukaemia: a meta-analysis of individual patient data from randomised controlled trials. Lancet Oncol. 2014;15(9):986–96.
72. Rubnitz JE, Lacayo NJ, Inaba H, Heym K, Ribeiro RC, Taub J, et al. Clofarabine can replace anthracyclines and etoposide in remission induction therapy for childhood acute myeloid leukemia: the AML08 multicenter, randomized phase III trial. J Clin Oncol. 2019;37(23):2072–81.
73. Sendker S, Schneider M, Antoniou E, Neumann D, Niktoreh N, Dirksen U, et al. Improved outcomes and treatment guidance in pediatric therapy-related AML: AML-BFM study group recommendations. Blood Adv. 2025;9(11):2831–41.
74. Burnett AK, Hills RK, Milligan D, Hunter AE, Goldstone AH, Prentice A, et al. Attempts to optimise induction and consolidation chemotherapy in patients with acute myeloid leukaemia: results of the MRC AML15 trial. Blood. 2009;114(22):484.
75. Pollard JA, Guest E, Alonzo TA, Gerbing RB, Loken MR, Brodersen LE, et al. Gemtuzumab ozogamicin improves event-free survival and reduces relapse in pediatric KMT2A-rearranged AML: results from the phase III Children's Oncology Group Trial AAML0531. J Clin Oncol. 2021;39(28):3149–60.
76. Aplenc R, Meshinchi S, Sung L, Alonzo T, Choi J, Fisher B, et al. Bortezomib with standard chemotherapy for children with acute myeloid leukemia does not improve treatment outcomes: a report from the Children's Oncology Group. Haematologica. 2020;105(7):1879–86.
77. Pollard JA, Alonzo TA, Gerbing R, Brown P, Fox E, Choi J, et al. Sorafenib in combination with standard chemotherapy for children with high allelic ratio FLT3/ITD+ acute myeloid leukemia: a report from the Children's Oncology Group Protocol AAML1031. J Clin Oncol. 2022;40(18):2023–35.
78. Elgarten CW, Wood AC, Li Y, Alonzo TA, Brodersen LE, Gerbing RB, et al. Outcomes of intensification of induction chemotherapy for children with high-risk acute myeloid leukemia: a report from the Children's Oncology Group. Pediatr Blood Cancer. 2021;68(12):e29281.

79. Pollard JA, Alonzo TA, Gerbing R, Kutny MA, Hirsch B, Raca G, et al. A phase 3 randomized trial for patients with de novo AML comparing standard therapy including Gemtuzumab Ozogamicin (GO) to CPX-351 with GO—a report from the Children's Oncology Group. Blood. 2024;144(Supplement 1):967.
80. Czogała M, Czogała W, Pawińska-Wąsikowska K, Książek T, Bukowska-Strakova K, Sikorska-Fic B, et al. Characteristics and outcome of FLT3-ITD-positive pediatric acute myeloid leukemia-experience of Polish Pediatric Leukemia and Lymphoma Study Group from 2005 to 2022. Cancers (Basel). 2023;15(18):4557.
81. Kadia TM, Ravandi F, Cortes J, Kantarjian H. Toward individualized therapy in acute myeloid leukemia: a contemporary review. JAMA Oncol. 2015;1(6):820–8.
82. Meshinchi S, Alonzo TA, Stirewalt DL, Zwaan M, Zimmerman M, Reinhardt D, et al. Clinical implications of FLT3 mutations in pediatric AML. Blood. 2006;108(12):3654–61.
83. Mead AJ, Linch DC, Hills RK, Wheatley K, Burnett AK, Gale RE. FLT3 tyrosine kinase domain mutations are biologically distinct from and have a significantly more favorable prognosis than FLT3 internal tandem duplications in patients with acute myeloid leukemia. Blood. 2007;110(4):1262–70.
84. Johnston DL, Alonzo TA, Gerbing RB, Aplenc R, Woods WG, Meshinchi S, et al. Central nervous system disease in pediatric acute myeloid leukemia: A report from the Children's Oncology Group. Pediatr Blood Cancer. 2017;64(12) https://doi.org/10.1002/pbc.26612.
85. Pui CH, Howard SC. Current management and challenges of malignant disease in the CNS in paediatric leukaemia. Lancet Oncol. 2008;9(3):257–68.
86. Creutzig U, Zimmermann M, Bourquin JP, Dworzak MN, Fleischhack G, von Neuhoff C, et al. CNS irradiation in pediatric acute myleoid leukemia: equal results by 12 or 18 Gy in studies AML-BFM98 and 2004. Pediatr Blood Cancer. 2011;57(6):986–92.
87. Horan JT, Alonzo TA, Lyman GH, Gerbing RB, Lange BJ, Ravindranath Y, et al. Impact of disease risk on efficacy of matched related bone marrow transplantation for pediatric acute myeloid leukemia: the Children's Oncology Group. J Clin Oncol. 2008;26(35):5797–801.
88. Niewerth D, Creutzig U, Bierings MB, Kaspers GJ. A review on allogeneic stem cell transplantation for newly diagnosed pediatric acute myeloid leukemia. Blood. 2010;116(13):2205–14.
89. Tarlock K, Sulis ML, Chewning JH, Pollard JA, Cooper T, Gamis A, et al. Hematopoietic cell transplantation in the treatment of pediatric acute myelogenous leukemia and myelodysplastic syndromes: guidelines from the American Society of Transplantation and Cellular Therapy. Transplant Cell Ther. 2022;28(9):530–45.
90. Bleakley M, Lau L, Shaw PJ, Kaufman A. Bone marrow transplantation for paediatric AML in first remission: a systematic review and meta-analysis. Bone Marrow Transplant. 2002;29(10):843–52.
91. Klusmann JH, Reinhardt D, Zimmermann M, Kremens B, Vormoor J, Dworzak M, et al. The role of matched sibling donor allogeneic stem cell transplantation in pediatric high-risk acute myeloid leukemia: results from the AML-BFM 98 study. Haematologica. 2012;97(1):21–9.
92. Stevens RF, Hann IM, Wheatley K, Gray RG. Marked improvements in outcome with chemotherapy alone in paediatric acute myeloid leukemia: results of the United Kingdom Medical Research Council's 10th AML trial. MRC Childhood Leukaemia Working Party. Br J Haematol. 1998;101(1):130–40.
93. Woods WG, Neudorf S, Gold S, Sanders J, Buckley JD, Barnard DR, et al. A comparison of allogeneic bone marrow transplantation, autologous bone marrow transplantation, and aggressive chemotherapy in children with acute myeloid leukemia in remission. Blood. 2001;97(1):56–62.
94. Huang BJ, Meyer LK, Alonzo TA, Wang Y-C, Lamble AJ, Ries RE, et al. Hematopoietic stem cell transplantation outcomes for high-risk AML: a report from the Children's Oncology Group. J Clin Oncol. 2025;43(17):1961–71.
95. Egan G, Tasian SK. Relapsed pediatric acute myeloid leukaemia: state-of-the-art in 2023. Haematologica. 2023;108(9):2275–88.
96. Board PPTE. PDQ childhood acute myeloid leukemia treatment. Updated 04/15/2025. Available from: https://www.cancer.gov/types/leukemia/hp/child-aml-treatment-pdq.

97. Cooper TM, Absalon MJ, Alonzo TA, Gerbing RB, Leger KJ, Hirsch BA, et al. Phase I/II study of CPX-351 followed by fludarabine, cytarabine, and granulocyte-colony stimulating factor for children with relapsed acute myeloid leukemia: a report from the Children's Oncology Group. J Clin Oncol. 2020;38(19):2170–7.
98. Karol SE, Alexander TB, Budhraja A, Pounds SB, Canavera K, Wang L, et al. Venetoclax in combination with cytarabine with or without idarubicin in children with relapsed or refractory acute myeloid leukaemia: a phase 1, dose-escalation study. Lancet Oncol. 2020;21(4):551–60.
99. Perl AE, Martinelli G, Cortes JE, Neubauer A, Berman E, Paolini S, et al. Gilteritinib or chemotherapy for relapsed or refractory FLT3-mutated AML. N Engl J Med. 2019;381(18):1728–40.
100. Inaba H, Rubnitz JE, Coustan-Smith E, Li L, Furmanski BD, Mascara GP, et al. Phase I pharmacokinetic and pharmacodynamic study of the multikinase inhibitor sorafenib in combination with clofarabine and cytarabine in pediatric relapsed/refractory leukemia. J Clin Oncol. 2011;29(24):3293–300.
101. Issa GC, Aldoss I, Thirman MJ, DiPersio J, Arellano M, Blachly JS, et al. Menin inhibition with revumenib for KMT2A-rearranged relapsed or refractory acute leukemia (AUGMENT-101). J Clin Oncol. 2025;43(1):75–84.
102. Aplenc R, Alonzo TA, Gerbing RB, Lange BJ, Hurwitz CA, Wells RJ, et al. Safety and efficacy of gemtuzumab ozogamicin in combination with chemotherapy for pediatric acute myeloid leukemia: a report from the Children's Oncology Group. J Clin Oncol. 2008;26(14):2390–3295.
103. Zwaan CM, Reinhardt D, Zimmerman M, Hasle H, Stary J, Stark B, et al. Salvage treatment for children with refractory first or second relapse of acute myeloid leukaemia with gemtuzumab ozogamicin: results of a phase II study. Br J Haematol. 2010;148(5):768–76.
104. Lamble AJ, Tasian SK. Opportunities for immunotherapy in childhood acute myeloid leukemia. Blood Adv. 2019;3(22):3750–8.
105. Meshinchi S, Leisenring WM, Carpenter PA, Woolfrey AE, Sievers EL, Radich JP, et al. Survival after second hematopoietic stem cell transplantation for recurrent pediatric acute myeloid leukemia. Biol Blood Marrow Transplant. 2003;9(11):706–13.

Flow Cytometry in the Diagnosis of Pediatric Leukemia

2

Weijie Li

Introduction

Leukemia is the most common pediatric malignant disease, with an incidence of approximately 50 new cases per million every year [1–3]. Leukemia results from the clonal proliferation of abnormal lymphoid or hematopoietic cells, involving bone marrow (BM), peripheral blood (PB), spleen, lymph nodes, and possibly other organs. Leukemia can be classified as acute or chronic based on its rate of progression, and further classified as one of many subtypes with incorporation of histomorphology, immunophenotype, and cytogenetic/molecular findings [4–7]. The leukemias in children are mostly acute leukemias, including B-cell acute lymphoblastic leukemia, T-cell acute lymphoblastic leukemia, acute myeloid leukemia (AML), and acute leukemias of mixed or ambiguous lineage. B-cell acute lymphoblastic leukemia is the most common. Certain types of chronic leukemia can occur in children but are overall rare.

Flow cytometry (FCM) is a technology capable of providing rapid multiparameter analysis of single cells or particles. With the tremendous improvement in instrumentation and reagents during the past several decades, FCM has become a very powerful tool applied in many research or clinical fields for a wide variety of purposes [8, 9]. FCM simultaneously measures physical characteristics (size and complexity) and multiple surface/intracellular markers of single cells, allowing for rapid and accurate phenotypic characterization of a cell population. Together with histomorphology and other information, multiparameter FCM can quickly diagnose leukemia and accurately classify leukemia as a subtype as defined by World Health

W. Li (✉)
Department of Pathology and Laboratory Medicine, Children's Mercy Kansas City, Kansas City, Missouri, USA

University of Missouri–Kansas City School of Medicine, Kansas City, Missouri, USA
e-mail: wli@cmh.edu

W. Li (ed.), *Laboratory Assessments of Pediatric Leukemia*,
https://doi.org/10.1007/978-3-032-26557-9_2

Organization (WHO) classification [4–7]. FCM study can also assess the clonality of mature B-cells by evaluating immunoglobulin (Ig) light chain expression, and the clonality of mature αβ T-cells by evaluating T-cell receptor (TCR) Vβ repertoire or TCR β chain constant 1 (TRBC1) expression [10, 11]. In addition, FCM can readily measure DNA content and determine the DNA ploidy of a cell population, which is also helpful in making diagnoses and/or determining prognoses. The fast turnaround time of FCM testing allows for a quick diagnosis or timely selection of the appropriate other ancillary tests.

Compared with immunohistochemistry (IHC), FCM is not only faster, but also capable of easily and efficiently correlating multiple parameters on a single cell. Moreover, FCM can detect the antigen intensity and aberrant antigen expression pattern. The major disadvantage of FCM is the lack of correlation with histomorphology. In addition, FCM requires viable fresh samples, and decreased viability of the specimens often precludes accurate FCM analysis. This chapter provides an overview of the principles and the significant roles of FCM in the diagnosis of leukemias.

Principles and Key Elements of Flow Cytometry

Flow Cytometers

Traditional flow cytometers consist of three main systems: fluidics, optics, and electronics (Fig. 2.1a). The fluidics system is responsible for transporting samples to the flow cell, where the cells form a single file stream and pass the laser beam. A stream of solution (sheath fluid) surrounding the specimen is introduced into the instrument at a higher pressure so that the cells in the specimen form a roughly single-file stream due to the phenomenon called hydrodynamic focusing. The cells or particles in a single-file stream travel through the interrogation point, where they are illuminated by light from one or more lasers. Eventually, the fluid stream is discharged into a waste container (Fig. 2.1a). The optics system consists of light sources (lasers), lenses, filters, and detectors. Lasers illuminate the cells or particles, and dichroic mirrors (DMs) and optical filters (OFs) are used to direct the resulting light signals to the appropriate detectors. DMs allow the light of corresponding wavelengths to pass while reflecting the light of other wavelengths. OFs further narrow the wavelengths reaching a detector. The detectors are usually photomultiplier tubes (PMTs) or photodiode arrays (PDAs) that convert the signals to electrical impulses, which are measured and converted to digital information by the electronics system. The digital information is collected and interpreted by the analysis software [8]. The connected computer system directly interfaces with the flow cytometer and controls its functions. Data analysis can be performed either on the computer connected to the flow cytometer or on other computers that have access to the data.

In contrast to traditional FCM, spectral flow cytometry (SFC) uses a large number of detectors to collect all the fluorescence signals across the entire spectrum from each fluorochrome for each laser. The individual spectral signature of a

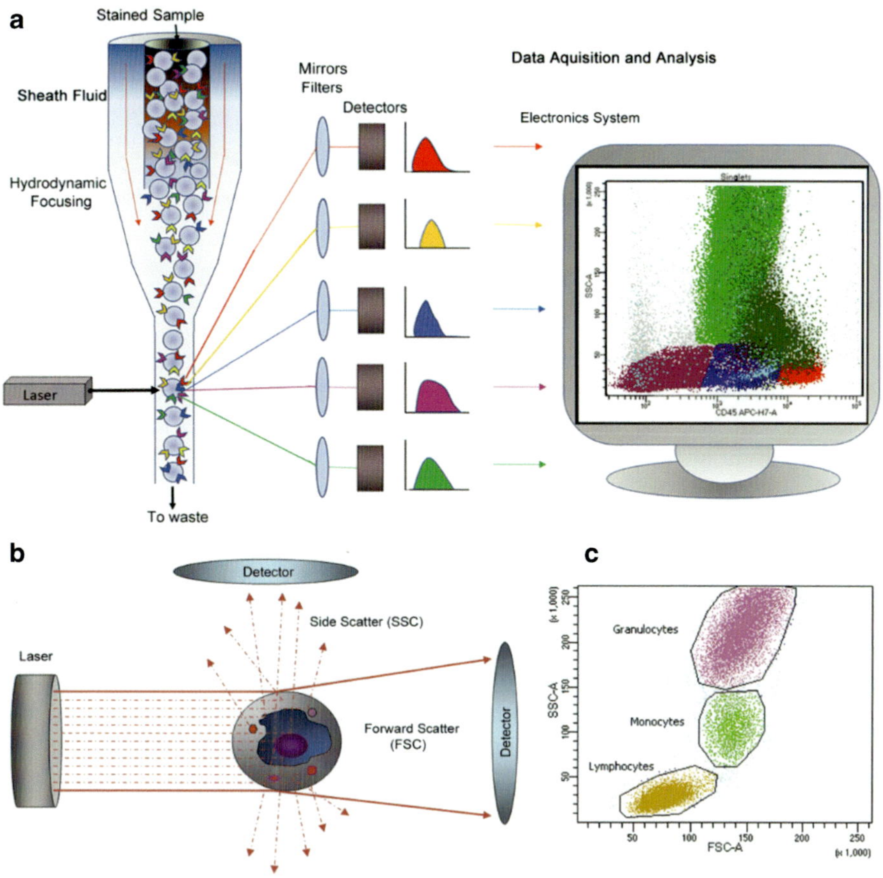

Fig. 2.1 Schematic diagram of how flow cytometry works and the light scatter of cells. (**a**) After a liquid sample with stained cells is injected into a flow cytometer, the cells are forced to form a single-file stream through hydrodynamic focusing. The cells in the single-file stream are illuminated as they travel through a laser beam, and the optical and fluorescence signals of each cell are generated and detected by proper detectors that convert photons to electrical impulses. The electronics system measures the electrical impulses and converts these measurements to digital information that is gathered and interpreted by analysis software in a computer. (**b**) Illustration of forward light scatter (FSC) and side light scatter (SSC) of a cell. (**c**) Differentiation of peripheral blood leukocytes according to forward and side scatter properties

fluorochrome can be identified after the primary fluorescence signals are deconvoluted by a mathematical algorithm. With this fundamental transformation, SFC has the potential to perform simultaneous single-cell analysis of a large number (>40) of parameters [12, 13]. SFC has become a significant player in the cytometry marketplace, and the application of SFC into clinical laboratories and diagnostic processes is expected in the near future. Another high-number-marker (>50) single-cell analysis technique is mass cytometry, which labels antibodies with distinct heavy metal isotopes instead of fluorochromes, detects stained cells by measuring the mass of ions, and separates them based on the specific mass-to-charge ratios of the corresponding ions [14]. Imaging FCM combines the high-throughput capabilities of FCM with morphological analysis of microscopy, representing another significant technological advancement in the field of cytometry [15]. Although these new cytometers overcome the limitations of traditional FCM and provide many advantages, their application comes with many challenges in panel design, optimization, and downstream data analysis and interpretation.

Specimens and Reagents/Antibody Panels

Specimens suitable for FCM analysis include PB, BM, cerebrospinal fluid, serous effusions, fine needle aspirations (FNAs), and fresh unfixed tissue. PB and BM aspirates must be anticoagulated. Sample preparation for FCM analysis varies according to the specimen types and the antigens to be analyzed. The cell suspension generated by mincing tissue should be filtered to remove large particles that may clog the cytometer tubing and/or bind antibodies nonspecifically. In any specimen containing a large amount of PB, the red blood cells should be removed through a lysis process using either a commercially available reagent or a homemade ammonium chloride solution before running the sample in a flow cytometer.

The key reagents for FCM studies are fluorochrome-conjugated antibodies against cell surface, cytoplasmic or nuclear antigens. Table 2.1 lists the antigens commonly evaluated in the workup for hematologic malignancies. How many antibodies and how many tubes to run for a sample depend on the clinical indication and what type of flow cytometer is used. A single-laser flow cytometer can evaluate

Table 2.1 Surface or intracellular antigens commonly assessed by flow cytometry for lineage classification and immunophenotyping of leukemias/lymphomas

Lineage	Antigens
Stem cells	CD34, CD38, CD45
B-cells	CD5, CD10, **CD19**, **CD20**, **CD22**, CD23, CD25, CD34, CD38, CD43, CD45, **CD79a**, CD103, CD200, FMC2, **cIgM**, **Kappa**, **Lambda**, LEF1, TdT
Plasma cells	CD19, CD20, CD38, CD45, CD56, CD117, CD138, **cKappa**, **cLambda**
T-cells/NK cells	CD1a, **CD2**, **CD3**, CD4, **CD5**, CD7, **CD8**, CD10, CD16, CD25, CD26, CD30, CD34, CD45, CD56, **αβ-TCR**, **γδ-TCR**, TdT, **TRBC1**
Myelomonocytic cells	CD4, CD7, CD10, CD11b, CD11c, **CD13**, **CD14**, CD15, CD16, **CD33**, CD34, CD36, CD38, CD45, CD56, **CD64**, **CD65**, CD71, CD117, CD123, **cMPO**, **cLyso**, HLA-DR
Erythroblasts	CD34, CD36, CD38, CD45, CD71, CD117, **CD235a**
Megakaryoblasts	CD33, CD34, CD38, **CD41**, **CD42**, CD45, **CD61**, CD117, HLA-DR

The antigens in bold are lineage-specific markers. *cIgM* cytoplasmic IgM, *cKappa* cytoplasmic kappa, *cLambda* cytoplasmic lambda, *cLyso* cytoplasmic lysozyme, *cMPO* cytoplasmic myeloperoxidase, *HLA-DR* human leukocyte antigen-DR, *LEF1* lymphoid enhancer-binding factor 1, *NK* natural killer, *TCR* T-cell receptor, *TdT* terminal deoxynucleotidyl transferase, *TRBC1* TCR β chain constant 1 three to five antigens simultaneously besides the light scatter properties. A flow cytometer with more lasers can evaluate more antigens at the same time. Eight- to ten-color diagnostic antibody panels for hematologic neoplasms are commonly used currently in the United States. The combination of antibodies in one tube should be properly designed according to the antigens on the cells of interest, fluorochrome characteristics, and clinical purpose. In general, the antibody against a weakly expressed antigen should be conjugated with a bright fluorochrome, and vice versa. Color compensation to minimize the spillover between different fluorochromes is very important in multicolor tubes. For diagnostic purposes, antibodies are typically combined together as panels to answer specific questions about a cell population [16, 17]. The screening panels should evaluate sufficient antigens to distinguish a neoplastic cell population from normal/reactive cells with a high degree of sensitivity.

Light Scatter and Fluorescence Signals

Light scatter and fluorescence are the two types of signals generated and collected for a cell as it travels through the laser beam. Light scatter is used to measure the physical properties of a cell. Forward scatter (FSC) refers to the light scattered at narrow angles to the laser beam, and it is collected by a detector positioned in line with the laser beam on the opposite side of the sample stream (Fig. 2.1b). The FSC is proportional to the surface area or size of the cell. Side scatter (SSC) refers to the light refracted or reflected by cytoplasmic organelles or nuclei of the cell, and it is collected by a detector positioned at approximately 90° to the laser beam. The SSC is proportional to the granularity and internal complexity of a cell (Fig. 2.1b). Together, FSC and SSC signals allow for the separation of cells in a specimen containing heterogeneous cell populations, e.g., three types of leukocytes (granulocytes, monocytes, and lymphocytes) in PB readily separated based on FSC and SSC characteristics (Fig. 2.1c). When a cell crosses the laser beam, the fluorescent dye or fluorochrome attached to the cell is excited by light of a specific wavelength (excitation wavelength); then it absorbs the energy, rises to an even more excited state, and emits light (fluorescence) at a longer wavelength (emission wavelength). In a flow cytometer, the fluorescent signals are detected by the PMTs after being filtered by DMs and OFs. The intensity of the fluorescent signal is proportional to the expression level of the antigen, to which the corresponding fluorescently labeled antibody binds.

Data Acquisition and Analysis

Data acquisition refers to the data collection process. The stained cells are run through a flow cytometer and illuminated by laser light. The resulting signals are then detected by the optics system. The number of cells, also known as events, required for evaluation depends on the purpose of the test and the nature of the specimen. For example, in the evaluation of a PB sample with predominantly leukemic cells, a relatively low number of viable cells (e.g., 20,000/tube) acquired is enough to characterize the phenotype of the leukemia. In contrast, minimal residual disease (MRD) detection usually requires a much larger number of viable cells (e.g., >500,000/tube) acquired to increase the sensitivity for detecting a very small population of residual malignant cells.

FCM data analysis requires specially designed software. Each flow cytometer usually has an associated software for data acquisition and analysis. Independent FCM software, such as FCS Express and FlowJo, with more functions, is also commercially available. The FCM data can be displayed as histograms or dot plots. The histogram is used for displaying a single parameter, while the dot plot is used to display two parameters, and each dot represents one cell or particle. The stronger the signal is, the further along each scale the data are displayed. An antigen is called positive when its associated fluorescent signal is above the negative control (background signal). Since most of the specimens contain heterogeneous cell populations, internal negative control is easily found and used for most antigens. However, due to the possible difference in nonspecific binding and autofluorescence levels, internal control may be misleading. Adding nonspecific Ig of the same isotype may work as a better negative control and is used in some FCM tests.

Gating refers to the process of isolating cell populations within a heterogeneous cell sample according to their physical and phenotypical features and searching for the abnormal cell population. Because normal leukocytes and hematopoietic precursors typically show consistent and reproducible patterns on SSC vs CD45 dot plot, SSC vs CD45 gating is the most commonly used initial step to separate various PB or BM cell populations. An abnormal cell population is identified based on its phenotypical differences from normal. These differences include: (i) abnormal increases or decreases of antigens normally expressed on the cells of interest; (ii) homogeneous expression pattern of antigens that normally show a variable expression pattern; (iii) asynchronous antigen expression; and (iv) aberrant expression of antigens of other cell types. To appreciate these abnormalities, the flow cytometrists must be familiar with the normal antigen expression pattern of all the cell populations in the specimen [18].

Quality Control and Quality Assurance

It is essential to have strict quality assurance (QA) and quality control (QC) practices in an FCM laboratory to maintain consistency in FCM results. Quality control (QC) measures must be performed and documented regularly to ensure optimal instrument performance. Inter-instrument and inter-performer consistency should be evaluated and documented periodically. Any change in the reagents, panels, instruments, or protocols must be carefully validated to ensure that the change does not affect the results. Clinical FCM laboratories should enroll in the available proficiency testing programs for the tests they are performing to ensure that their results are comparable to others. Any discrepancy must be investigated.

Flow Cytometry in the Diagnosis of Acute Leukemias/ Leukemias of Blasts

Acute leukemia is a hematologic malignancy caused by abnormal proliferation of lymphoid or hematopoietic precursors (blasts). The definition of acute leukemia is the presence of a significant number of abnormal blasts in BM, according to the WHO classification [6, 7]. A value of ≥20% myeloblasts of total nucleated cells is required for making the diagnosis of acute myeloid leukemia (AML). Based on the 5th edition of WHO classification [5, 6], the 20% threshold is not needed for an AML diagnosis if the blasts carry *PML::RARA*, *RUNX1-RUNX1T1*, *CBFB-MYH11*, *DEK::NUP214*, *RBM15::MRTFA*, *KMT2A* rearrangement, *MECOM* rearrangement, *NUP98* rearrangement, or *NPM1* mutation. In many treatment protocols in the United States, a value of ≥25% lymphoblasts is needed to make the diagnosis of acute lymphoblastic leukemia (ALL). If the abnormal precursors are localized in tissue, forming a solid mass lesion with effaced tissue architecture, the diagnosis should be lymphoblastic lymphoma (LBL) or myeloid sarcoma, depending on the blast type. LBL shares the same morphology, immunophenotype, and biology with its ALL counterpart, so LBL and corresponding ALL are combined as one group (ALL/LBL) by the current WHO classification [4, 6]. FCM analysis can efficiently identify the abnormal blast population, give blast lineage classification, aid in further WHO classification, and sometimes provide prognostic information [19, 20].

Identification of Blast Population

The identification of a large blast population, such as the ALL cases in Fig. 2.2 and AML cases in Fig. 2.3, is usually straightforward. Blasts usually show low SSC and dim to intermediate CD45 expression, and thus fall in the so-called blast region (low SSC and dim CD45) on CD45 vs SSC dot plot [21]. However, not all the cells in the blast region are leukemic blasts. Basophils and plasmacytoid dendritic cells (PDCs) can also be found here, and normal B-cell precursors (hematogones) and early myeloid precursors are present here as well [18]. The leukemic cells of certain acute leukemias may be seen outside of the blast region, e.g., acute promyelocytic leukemia (APL) typically showing intermediate to high SSC (Fig. 2.3b). Therefore, careful evaluation of the antigen expression profile is always necessary for the identification or separation of the abnormal blast populations, especially in specimens with a low number of blasts. Blasts often differ from mature cells by expressing immature markers and lacking antigens typically present in mature cells. For example, myeloblasts can be distinguished from mature or maturing myeloid cells by the expression of immature markers, such as CD34 and CD117, and the absence of maturation markers, such as CD11b, CD15, and CD16. Neoplastic blasts often have an abnormal phenotype that is different from that of normal hematopoietic precursors. Phenotypic abnormalities include altered expression level or pattern of antigens, aberrant expression of markers of other cell lineages, and asynchronous or dyssynchronous expression of antigens. For example, compared with hematogones

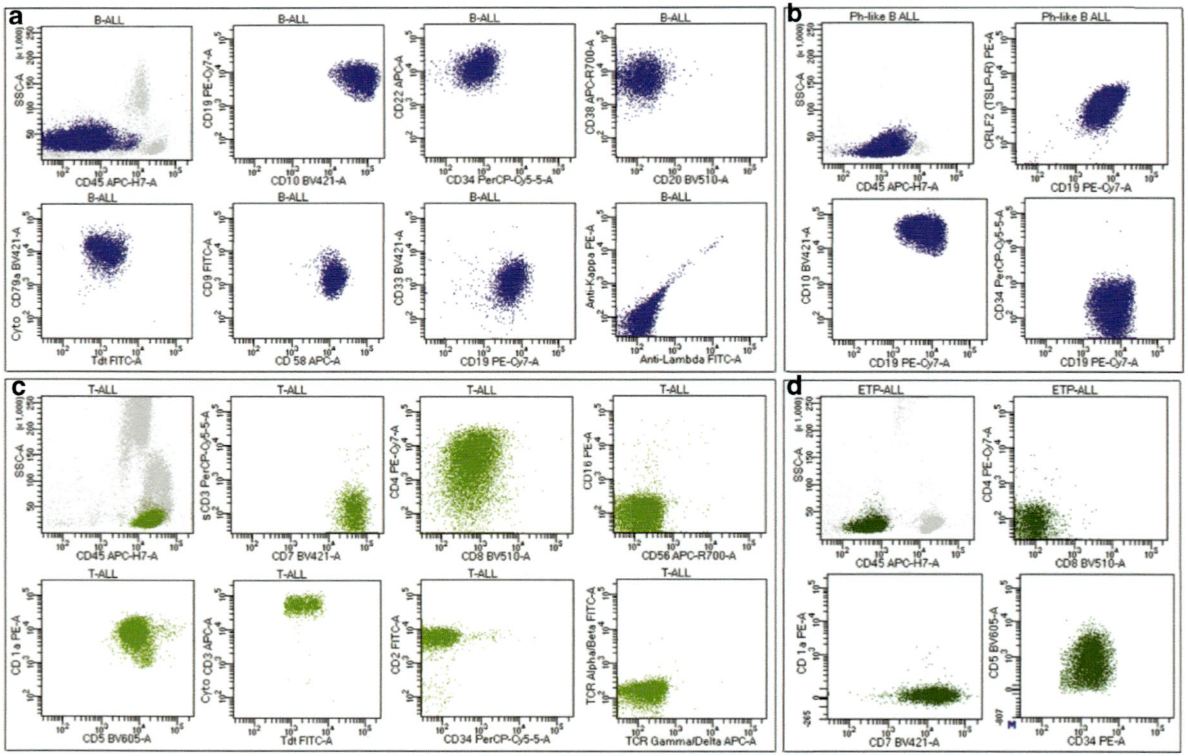

Fig. 2.2 Representative dot plots of acute lymphoblastic leukemia (ALL). (**a**) Precursor B-cell ALL (B-ALL, blue) showing low side scatter, dim to negative CD45, expression of CD19, CD10, CD34, CD22, CD38, cytoplasmic (Cyto) CD79a, TdT, CD9, CD58, CD33, and no expression of CD20, kappa, and lambda. (**b**) Philadelphia-like (Ph-like) B-ALL (blue) showing expression of CRLF2. (**c**) T-cell ALL (T-ALL, green) showing low side scatter, intermediate to bright CD45, expression of CD7, CD4, CD8, CD1a, CD5, Cyto CD3, TdT, CD2, and no expression of surface CD3 (sCD3), CD16, CD56, CD34, TCR alpha beta, and TCR gamma delta. (**d**) Early-T-precursor (ETP) ALL (dark green) being positive for CD7, CD34, CD5 (dim and partial), CD45 (dim to negative), and negative for CD4, CD8, and CD1a

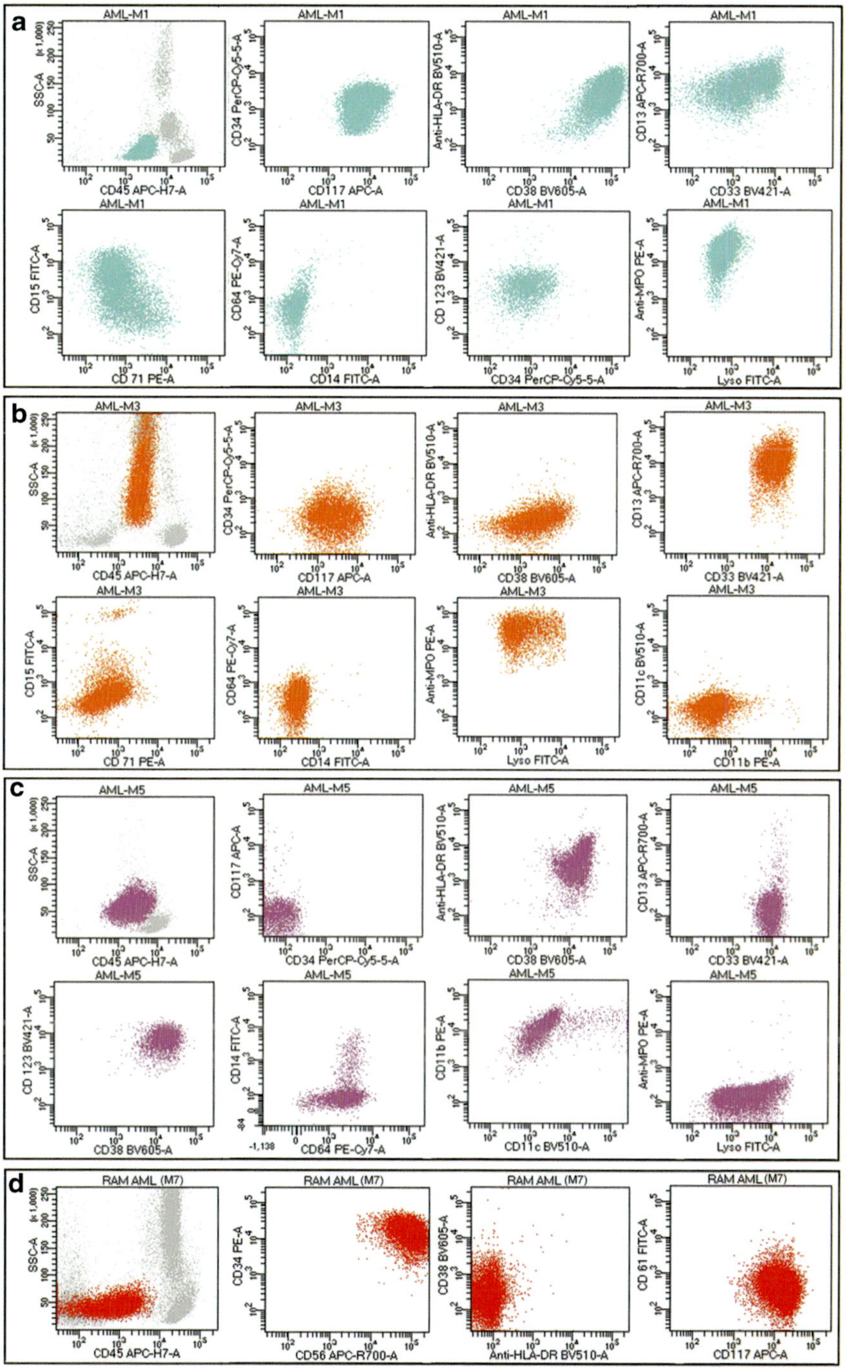
a
AML-M1
SSC-A (x 1,000)
CD45 APC-H7-A
CD34 PerCP-Cy5-5-A
CD117 APC-A
Anti-HLA-DR BV510-A
CD38 BV605-A
CD13 APC-R700-A
CD33 BV421-A
CD15 FITC-A
CD 71 PE-A
CD64 PE-Cy7-A
CD14 FITC-A
CD 123 BV421-A
CD34 PerCP-Cy5-5-A
Anti-MPO PE-A
Lyso FITC-A
b
AML-M3
SSC-A (x 1,000)
CD45 APC-H7-A
CD34 PerCP-Cy5-5-A
CD117 APC-A
Anti-HLA-DR BV510-A
CD38 BV605-A
CD13 APC-R700-A
CD33 BV421-A
CD15 FITC-A
CD 71 PE-A
CD64 PE-Cy7-A
CD14 FITC-A
Anti-MPO PE-A
Lyso FITC-A
CD11c BV510-A
CD11b PE-A
c
AML-M5
SSC-A (x 1,000)
CD45 APC-H7-A
CD117 APC-A
CD34 PerCP-Cy5-5-A
Anti-HLA-DR BV510-A
CD38 BV605-A
CD13 APC-R700-A
CD33 BV421-A
CD 123 BV421-A
CD38 BV605-A
CD14 FITC-A
CD64 PE-Cy7-A
CD11b PE-A
CD11c BV510-A
Anti-MPO PE-A
Lyso FITC-A
d
RAM AML (M7)
SSC-A (x 1,000)
CD45 APC-H7-A
CD34 PE-A
CD56 APC-R700-A
CD38 BV605-A
Anti-HLA-DR BV510-A
CD 61 FITC-A
CD117 APC-A

(normal B-cell precursors in BM), leukemic cells of B-ALL commonly show increased CD10, decreased CD38, aberrant expression of myeloid marker CD13 or CD33, and dyssynchronous co-expression of CD34 and CD20. Knowledge of normal precursor antigen expression patterns is especially important for evaluating post-treatment specimens, which commonly contain normal regenerative precursors and very low-level residual leukemia [22, 23].

Assignment of Blast Lineage

Accurately and quickly classifying an acute leukemia case as AML, B-ALL, or T-ALL is very important for the timely selection of appropriate treatment. Leukemic blasts often show an antigen expression profile resembling a certain cell type and therefore can be assigned to that lineage by FCM analysis. As shown in Fig. 2.2, lymphoblasts of ALL usually show low SSC and a phenotype of precursor B-cells or precursor T-cells. Leukemic blasts from de novo B-ALL are almost always positive for CD19, cytoplasmic CD22, and cytoplasmic CD79a, and negative for surface Ig. Most of the B-ALL cases are positive for surface CD22, CD10, CD38, TdT, and CD24. CD34 is commonly expressed, but its expression is quite variable and often dim or partial. CD45 is usually dim and can be completely negative. CD20 is commonly negative or partially positive. ALL cases can be subclassified based on developmental stage as demonstrated by immunophenotyping, which is currently of little clinical significance and not required to be mentioned in pathology reports. For example, the majority of B-ALL cases express CD10 and are called common ALL (intermediate developmental stage); the B-ALL cases negative for CD10 are classified as pro-B ALL (early stage); the B-ALL cases expressing cytoplasmic μ chain are classified as Pre-B-ALL (late stage). Leukemic blasts from B-ALL can aberrantly express myeloid antigens (usually CD13 and CD33, occasionally CD15) and frequently show abnormal expression patterns of some nonspecific markers such as CD58 and CD9 (Fig. 2.2a). These markers are commonly included in the FCM panel for B-ALL MRD detection. Leukemic blasts of T-ALL are always positive for cytoplasmic CD3, usually positive for TdT, CD7, CD38, and CD45 (dim), and variably positive for other pan T-cell antigens (surface CD3, CD2, CD4, CD5, CD8, T-cell receptor), CD10, and other immature markers (CD1a, CD34, and CD99)

Fig. 2.3 Representative flow cytometry dot plots of acute myeloid leukemia (AML). (**a**) AML-M1 (light blue) showing low side scatter, dim CD45, expression of CD34 (dim), CD117, HLA-DR, CD38, CD13, CD33, CD15, CD71 (partial), CD64 (partial), CD123, and myeloperoxidase (MPO), and no expression of CD14 and lysozyme. (**b**) AML-M3 (acute promyelocytic leukemia) (orange) showing intermediate to high side scatter, intermediate CD45, expression of CD117, CD38, CD13, CD33, CD15 (dim), CD64 (dim and partial), CD71 (partial), MPO, lysozyme (partial), and no expression of CD34, HLA-DR, CD14, CD11b, and CD11c. (**c**) AML-M5 (magenta) showing low to intermediate side scatter, intermediate to bright CD45, expression of HLA-DR, CD38, CD33, CD123, CD64, CD11b, CD11c, lysozyme, CD13 (small subset), CD14 (small subset), and no expression of CD117, CD34, and MPO. (**d**) AML-M7 with RAM phenotype (RAM-AML, red) being positive for CD34, CD56 (bright), CD117, CD61 (dim), CD38 (dim to negative), CD45 (dim to negative), and negative for HLA-DR

(Fig. 2.2c). Some T-ALL cases may aberrantly express CD56, CD79a, CD117, or myeloid markers such as CD13 or CD33. In some cases, especially in the specimens collected after treatment, the immature markers can be very dim or completely absent, and their immature nature has to be determined by the detection of the absence of surface CD3, dual CD4/CD8 positivity, or dual CD4/CD8 negativity [19]. Early-T-cell precursor T-ALL (ETP-ALL, Fig. 2.2d) is defined by a characteristic phenotype: CD8−, CD1a−, CD5−, or dimly+ in <75% blasts, and positive for at least one of the myeloid or stem cell markers (CD11b, CD13, CD33, CD34, CD65, CD117, HLA-DR). ETP-ALL is considered a high-risk T-ALL subtype, especially in adult patients [24]. It is listed as a separate entity in the WHO classification [4, 6, 7].

The morphology and phenotype of AML cases vary greatly according to the differentiation direction and maturation level of the blasts. Leukemic blasts of AML with minimal differentiation (FAB-M0) or AML with no maturation (FAB-M1, Fig. 2.3a) usually show low SSC, express early hematopoietic precursor antigens (CD34, CD38, and HLA-DR), and lack antigens associated with myeloid and monocytic maturation, such as CD11b, CD14, CD15, and CD65. Blasts express at least two myeloid-associated antigens, such as CD13, CD33, and CD117. CD38 and/or HLA-DR expression may be decreased. Rare cases may show asynchronous expression of CD11b or CD15. Myeloperoxidase (MPO) is usually positive in AML-M1, and negative or minimally positive in AML-M0 by FCM. Blasts can aberrantly express CD7, or rarely other lymphoid markers. The leukemic blasts of AML with maturation (FAB-M2) usually express multiple myeloid antigens associated with granulocytic differentiation, such as MPO, CD11b, CD13, CD15, CD33, and CD65. HLA-DR, CD34, CD38, and CD117 are usually positive but can be partially negative. Hypergranular variant of APL (FAB-M3) (Fig. 2.3b) usually shows intermediate to high SSC and is characterized by the absence or minimal expression of HLA-DR and CD34, as well as lack of leukocyte integrins CD11a, CD11b, and CD18. CD13, CD33, CD64, CD117, and MPO are usually positive, while the granulocytic maturation markers CD15 and CD65 are usually negative or weakly positive. In cases with microgranular morphology, CD2 and CD34 are frequently expressed by at least a portion of the leukemic cells. Leukemic blasts from AML with monocytic differentiation variably express the myeloid antigens CD13, CD15, CD33 (often bright), and CD65; they always express some monocytic markers such as CD14, CD64, CD4, CD163, CD11b, CD11c, CD36, and lysozyme. Most cases express HLA-DR, CD38, and CD123. CD34 and CD117 are positive in a subset of cases. MPO is often negative in acute monoblastic leukemia (FAB-M5a, Fig. 2.3c), but may be partially positive in acute monocytic leukemia and acute myelomonocytic leukemia. Glycophorin A is the lineage-specific marker for acute erythroid leukemia (FAB-M6), which is usually also positive for CD71, CD36, and CD117, and negative for CD34 and HLA-DR. CD41, CD61, and CD42b are specific markers for acute megakaryoblastic leukemia (FAB-M7), which is often negative for CD34 and HLA-DR. The abnormal megakaryoblasts are usually positive for CD36 and frequently express CD13, CD33, and CD117, and may aberrantly express CD7, CD4, or CD56. Surface staining of CD41 and CD61 is less specific than their cytoplasmic staining due to possible adherence of platelets to blasts, leading to false positive interpretation [25].

Blastic plasmacytoid dendritic cell neoplasm (BPDCN) expresses CD4, CD56 (bright), CD36, CD38, CD43, CD45, CD71, HLA-DR, as well as plasmacytoid dendritic cell (PDC)-associated markers (CD123, CD303, CD304, TCF4, TCL1) [5, 26]. CD45 expression may range from dim to moderate. SSC of the tumor cells is usually low. CD7 and CD33 are relatively commonly expressed. TdT is positive in approximately one-third of the cases, and occasional cases may express CD117. Based on the WHO diagnostic criteria [5], BPDCN can be diagnosed in the presence of CD123 and one other PDC-associated marker in addition to CD4 and/or CD56, or in the presence of three PDC-associated markers and the absence of CD34 and other cell type-specific markers including CD3, CD14, CD19, lysozyme, and MPO. Given the presence of other hematologic malignancies with a similar phenotype, correlation with histomorphology, clinical information, and IHC studies is always necessary to make a definitive diagnosis of BPDCN.

Lineage classification in some cases can be difficult. There are ~4% of acute leukemia cases with no obvious evidence of differentiation along one cell lineage. These cases can be separated into three groups: mixed-phenotype acute leukemias (MPALs, Fig. 2.4), acute undifferentiated leukemias (AUL), and acute leukemia of ambiguous lineage, not otherwise specified (ALAL NOS). MPAL may have one population of blasts expressing antigens belonging to two lineages (biphenotypic, Fig. 2.4b), or may have two distinct blast populations (bilineal, Fig. 2.4c). There are defined criteria for assigning more than one lineage to a leukemic cell population for WHO classification (Fig. 2.4a) [5, 6]. To qualify for B-cell lineage, the leukemic blasts with strong CD19 expression should have strong expression of at least one of the following: CD10, CD79a, and cytoplasmic CD22, or the leukemic blasts with weak CD19 expression should have at least two of these three other B-cell markers. For CD19 expression to be considered as strong, the intensity of CD19 in at least part of the leukemic blasts should reach 50% of the hematogone level. CD3 (cytoplasmic or surface) is the only lineage-defining marker for T-cells, and its presence at a high intensity (at least partially >50% of mature T-cell level) is enough to classify the blasts as T-cell lineage. Myeloid lineage is determined by the expression of cytoplasmic MPO, which can be detected by FCM, IHC stain, or cytochemical stain. Monocytic lineage is determined by the diffuse expression of at least two of the following: nonspecific esterase, CD11c, CD14, CD64, and lysozyme. The most common combination is a myeloid lineage with a T-cell or B-cell lineage. Other combinations are also possible. No clear cut-off values on the percentage of positive blast cells have been given for these lineage-defining markers. However, current WHO criteria require that the intensity of leukemia cells (at least in part) should exceed 50% of the reference cell level (neutrophil for MPO, mature T-cell for CD3) (Fig. 2.4b). This "50% intensity" criterion is a simplified visual estimate based on a log or biexponential scale instead of mean fluoresce intensity (MFI). MPO may be present at a low level on a small portion of leukemic lymphoblasts. Without other myeloid markers, this kind of MPO expression should not be interpreted as myeloid and lymphoid MPAL [7, 27]. AULs lack lineage-defining antigens and express no

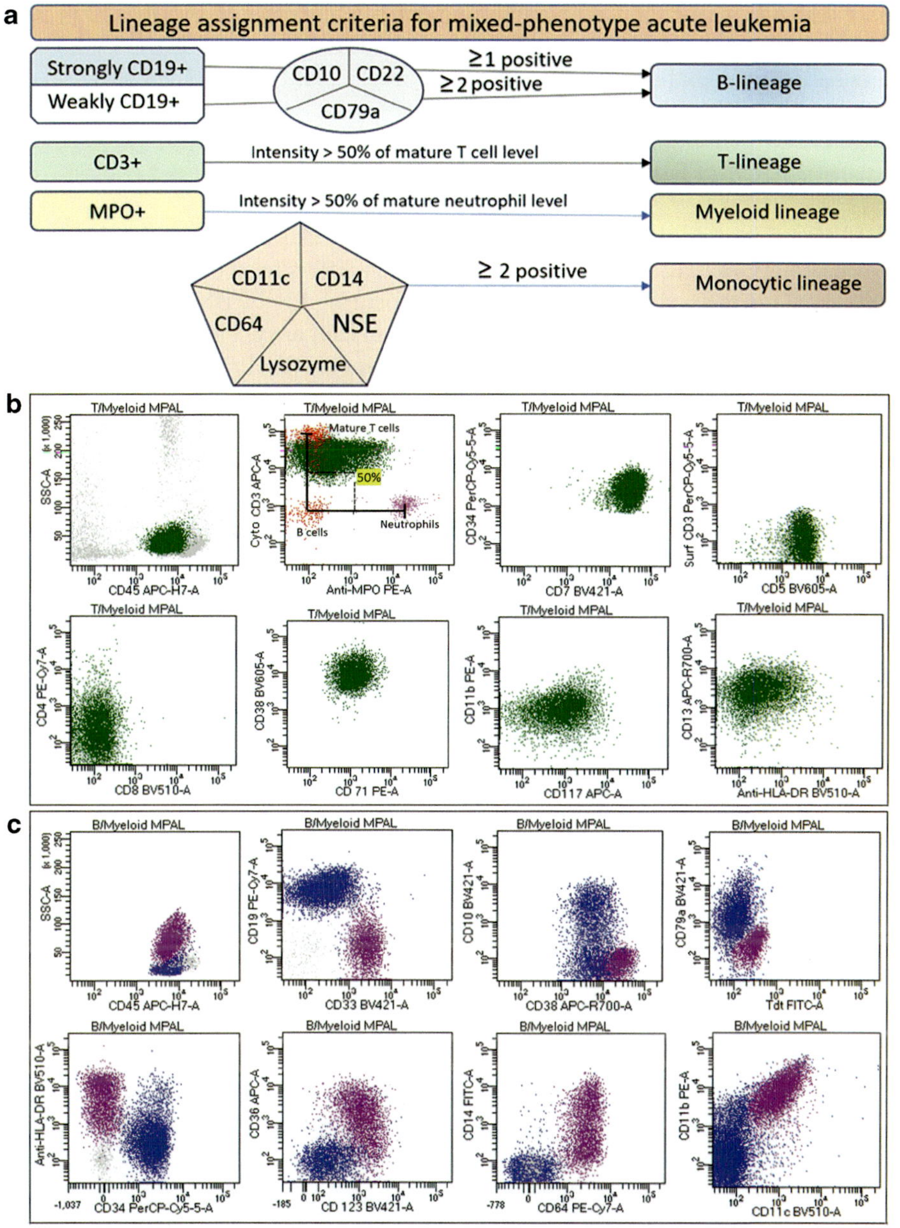

Fig. 2.4 Mixed-phenotype acute leukemia (MPAL). (**a**) WHO lineage assignment criteria for MPAL. MPO, myeloperoxidase; NSE, nonspecific esterase. (**b**) Biphenotypic T-cell/Myeloid MPAL showing one blast population (green) positive for cytoplasmic (Cyto) CD3 (intensity mostly exceeding 50% of mature T-cell level), MPO (intensity partially exceeding 50% of neutrophil level), CD7, CD34, CD5, CD4 (partial), CD38, CD71, CD11b, CD117, CD13, HLA-DR (partial), and negative for surface (Surf) CD3 and CD8. (**c**) Bilineal B-cell/Monocytic MPAL showing two distinct blast populations: one (purple) with low to intermediate side scatter, positive for CD33, CD38, HLA-DR, CD36 (partial), CD123, CD64, CD14 (partial), CD11b, and CD11c, and negative for others; the other (blue) with low side scatter, positive for CD19, CD38, CD10 (partial), CD79a, CD34, CD11b (partial), and negative for others

more than one marker of any given lineage, but often express HLA-DR, CD34, and CD38, and may express TdT. ALAL NOS includes the cases that express some differentiation markers but cannot be classified as ALL, AML, MPAL, or AUL.

Enumeration of Blasts

FCM study can determine the precise percentage of blasts in the samples. However, the percentage of blasts determined by FCM often differs from that identified by the gold standard method—manual differential count of PB or BM aspirate smears. There are several possible explanations for this discrepancy. First, the BM aspirate specimens submitted for FCM analysis are often not the first draw and contain fewer bone marrow spicules with greater dilution with PB. Second, there are likely unlysed erythrocytes in the sample, which increase the denominator for calculating blast percentage. Third, some blasts may be phenotypically difficult to capture and thus not included in the blast population. These are all possible reasons why the blast percentage by FCM may be lower than that by manual differential count. The blast percentage by FCM can also be higher due to a decreased denominator resulting from the loss of nucleated erythroid precursors during the RBC lysis process. In addition, FCM analysis can identify neoplastic cells that might be missed by manual count because of atypical morphology or suboptimal smears. Moreover, the manual count may include some normal immature precursors, such as hematogones, as leukemic blasts. Therefore, it is necessary to perform both FCM and manual count for blast enumeration and investigate the cause of significant discrepancies.

Predicting Cytogenetic Abnormality and Prognosis

Currently, cytogenetic/molecular testing is critical for further WHO classification and risk stratification of acute leukemias. The prognostic value that FCM immunophenotyping provides is most likely attributed to its prediction of certain cytogenetic/molecular subtypes. For example, the Pro-B-ALL immunophenotype is commonly seen in B-ALL with *KMT2A* rearrangement, which is also commonly positive for CD15 and has a very poor prognosis. Pre-B-ALL is often seen in B-ALLs with *TCF3::PBX1 or MEF2D* fusions [28]. CD25 is commonly associated with Philadelphia chromosome-positive B-ALL, a subtype with poor prognosis [29, 30]. The detection of CRLF2 expression (Fig. 2.2b) is associated with *CRLF2* gene alteration that is commonly seen in Philadelphia-like ALL, a subtype associated with inferior prognosis [31]. Surface CD371 expression is specifically associated with B-ALL with *DUX4* rearrangement, a subtype with a very good prognosis [32], which also commonly expresses CD2 [33]. AML with *RUNX1*::*RUNX1T1* fusion commonly expresses B-cell markers, such as CD19 and CD22, and is associated with a favorable prognosis [34]. Aberrant expression of CD2 in APL is associated with *FLT3–ITD* [35]. Nevertheless, FCM immunophenotyping should not be considered as a surrogate tool for the detection of these subtypes due to the lack of

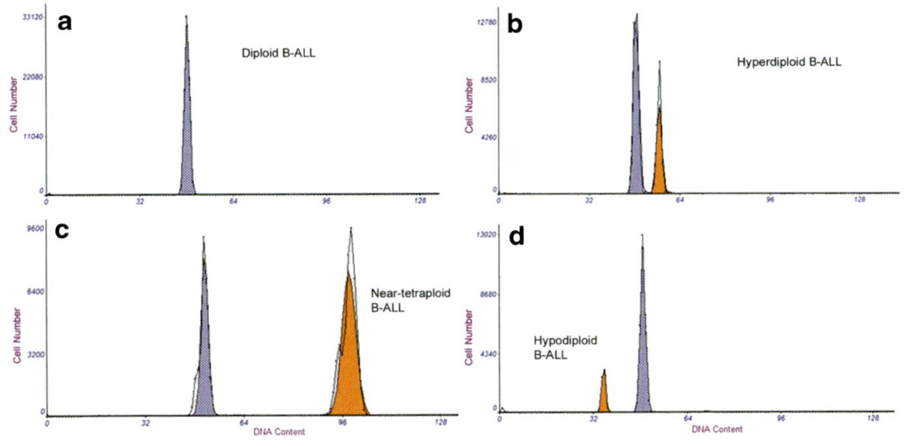

Fig. 2.5 DNA ploidy histogram of precursor B-cell acute lymphoblastic leukemia (B-ALL). (**a**) DNA diploid B-ALL (leukemic cells not separated from normal blood cells). (**b**) DNA hyperdiploid B-ALL (orange color peak, DNA Index = 1.16). (**c**) Near-tetraploid B-ALL (orange color peak, DI = 1.90). (**d**) DNA hypodiploid B-ALL (orange color peak, DI = 0.73)

specificity and sensitivity. As mentioned above, ETP-ALL (Fig. 2.2d) is defined by the typical early-T-precursor immunophenotype and is associated with a poor clinical outcome in adult patients [24]. AML with RAM phenotype (Fig. 2.3d) is defined by the characteristic phenotype (bright CD56 expression, dim to absent CD38, dim to absent CD45, and absent HLA-DR) and is associated with a very poor prognosis [36]. As innovative immunotherapies and targeted therapies are increasingly employed in clinical settings, FCM plays a crucial role in measuring the targeted antigens such as CD19, CD20, CD22, CD33, and CD123, selecting appropriate therapies, and predicting the therapeutic responses.

FCM can measure DNA content and assess DNA ploidy for a cell population. This process involves staining cells with a DNA-binding fluorescent dye and then analyzing fluorescent signals of the cells of interest. A histogram is displayed with different ploidy patterns based on the DNA content of the cells in the sample (Fig. 2.5). DNA ploidy is used for further classification of B-ALL and provides important prognostic information. High hyperdiploidy in B-ALL (DNA index >1.16, Fig. 2.5b) is associated with a very favorable prognosis, while hypodiploidy (DNA index <1, Fig. 2.5d) is associated with a poor prognosis [4, 6, 7].

Flow Cytometry in the Diagnosis of Mature B-Cell Leukemias/ Lymphomas

Mature B-cell neoplasms consist of a heterogeneous group of lymphoid neoplastic diseases derived from B-cells, which can be briefly divided into two groups: Hodgkin lymphoma (HL) and non-Hodgkin lymphoma/leukemia/

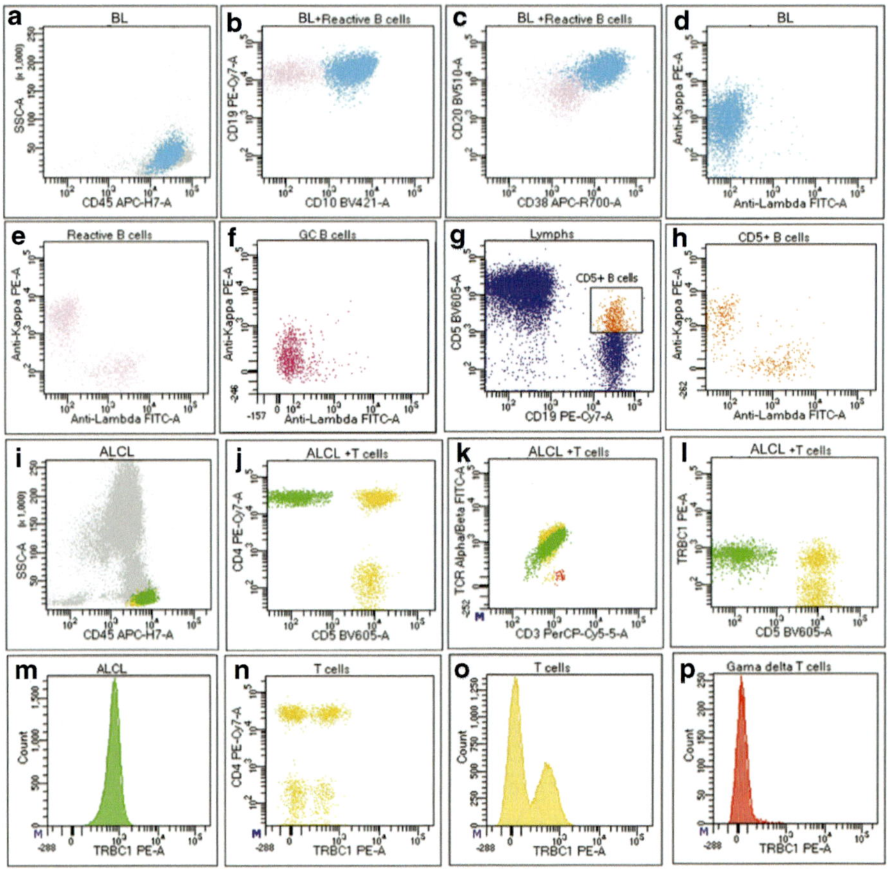

Fig. 2.6 Assessment of clonality of B-cells and T-cells by flow cytometry. Burkitt leukemia (BL, blue) expressing CD45 (**a**), CD19 and CD10 (**b**), CD20 and CD38 (**c**), and showing kappa restriction (**d**). Reactive B-cells (light pink) being polytypic (**e**). Germinal center B-cells (magenta) being partially negative for both kappa and lambda (**f**). Normal CD5+ B-cells (orange, **g**) in the peripheral blood being polytypic (**h**). Anaplastic large cell lymphoma (ALCL, green) being CD45+ (**i**), CD4+ and CD5-(**j**), TCR alpha beta+ and CD3+ (**k**), and expressing TRBC1 only (monotypic, **l**, **m**). Reactive CD4+ and CD4– T-cells (golden) containing mixed TRBC1+ and TRBC1– populations (polytypic, **n**, **o**). Gamma delta T-cells (red) always negative for TRBC1 (**p**)

lymphoproliferative disorders (non-HL). The most common mature B-cell non-HL in children is Burkitt lymphoma (BL), which can present as leukemia (Fig. 2.6a–d) [37]. Diffuse large B-cell lymphoma (DLBCL) may occasionally also have a leukemic phase with significant BM and/or PB involvement. Other mature B-cell non-HLs are very rare in children and often present at an early stage with no leukemic manifestation. The most common leukemia in the Western world, chronic lymphocytic leukemia (CLL), is exceedingly rare in children, as are hairy cell leukemia (HCL) and other adult type mature B-cell non-HLs. FCM analysis can efficiently identify an atypical lymphoid population, differentiate neoplastic cell proliferation from reactive cell proliferation, characterize the phenotype of a neoplastic cell population, and assist in WHO classification. The neoplastic B-cells can be distinguished from normal/reactive B-cells by the identification of two main types of phenotypic abnormalities: immunoglobulin light chain restriction and aberrant antigen expression. These two types of abnormalities are present in most of the non-HL cases and can be efficiently identified by FCM analysis. Due to the large size, low proportion of tumor cells, and T-cell resetting on tumor cells of HL, FCM is not useful in diagnosing HL.

Immunoglobulin Light Chain Restriction/B-Cell Clonality Assessment

Neoplastic B-cells express only one class of light chain (i.e., kappa or lambda) (Fig. 2.6a–d), whereas normal or reactive B-cells always consist of a mixture of kappa-expressing B-cells and lambda-expressing B-cells (Fig. 2.6e). The finding of only one class of light chain (light chain restriction) indicates a monoclonal B-cell proliferation. Light chain restriction may be seen occasionally in nonneoplastic reactive B-cell populations [38]. Therefore, it should not be considered as an equivalent to monoclonality, or by itself diagnostic of neoplasia. Light chain restriction should always be interpreted in combination with clinical information, morphology, and sometimes cytogenetic or molecular testing results. Identification of a large population of light chain-restricted B-cells is usually straightforward and is reflected in an abnormal kappa-to-lambda ratio (Fig. 2.6a–d). However, in the specimens with abundant admixed reactive B-cells, evaluation of the kappa-to-lambda ratio may fail to identify a small clonal population. To increase the sensitivity, separate evaluation of B-cell subsets with distinct phenotypes and/or light scatter characters should be performed. When evaluating small populations of B-cells for light chain restriction, caution should be exercised, because reactive B-cells may include small subsets of phenotypically identical cells. Some germinal center B (GCB) cells may show the absence of both classes of light chain or may have one class of light chain excess, and they should not be interpreted as abnormal CD10+ B-cell population (Fig. 2.6f). It is important to include a prewash step to avoid a false negative result due to soluble antibodies in the samples interfering with the binding of fluorochrome-conjugated antibodies. It should be noted that B-lymphoblasts, plasma cells, and thymic B-cells are negative for surface Ig, and so are their neoplastic counterparts: B-ALL, plasma cell neoplasms (PCNs), and primary mediastinal large B-cell lymphoma.

Aberrant B-Cell Antigen Expression

FCM analysis can identify phenotypic deviations of mature B-cell neoplasms from normal antigen expression patterns of B-cells. The most easily recognized phenotypic aberrancy is the presence of antigens not normally expressed by B-cells. For example, CD5, a T-cell antigen, can be aberrantly expressed in CLL and mantle cell lymphoma (MCL). It should be noted that a small population of mature B-cells normally express CD5. These mature CD5+ B-cells are often found in PB and may also be detected in lymph nodes and other tissue specimens, especially in pediatric patients or patients with autoimmune disease [39]. Therefore, the interpretation of CD5 expression by B-cells needs the correlation with other phenotypic features. The expression of CD5 in normal CD5+ B-cells usually shows a smear pattern, not separated from CD5− B-cells (Fig. 2.6g), and these cells are polytypic (Fig. 2.6h). Another type of phenotypic aberrancy is the abnormal expression of antigens not typically present in the B-cells of a particular subset. For example, normal GCB cells are Bcl-2–, whereas Bcl-2 is positive in most other B-cell subsets. Abnormal Bcl-2 expression is found in most follicular lymphoma (FL) cases, which are derived from GCB cells and express GCB markers CD10 and BCL6. Other phenotypic aberrancies include alteration in the expression level of B-cell-associated antigens. For example, CLL often demonstrates decreased CD20, significantly decreased or absent FMC7, and detectable CD23 [25].

Classification of Mature B-Cell Leukemias/Lymphomas

FCM immunophenotyping plays an important role in the classification of mature B-cell neoplasms. Each type of these diseases has some unique or relatively specific phenotypic features, and FCM findings in combination with histomorphologic features can make the final diagnosis in most cases. Most mature nonplasma cell B-cell neoplasms are positive for B-cell markers CD19, CD20, CD22, CD79a, and surface Ig (sIg), but the expression levels of these markers vary among the neoplasms. The mature B-cell non-HLs in children are predominantly of germinal center B-cell (GCB) origin, including BL, GCB type DLBCL, high-grade B-cell lymphoma with 11q aberration, large B-cell lymphoma with *IRF4* rearrangement, and pediatric type FL [37]. The FCM findings of these lymphomas can be very similar and are unable to be differentiated. Therefore, correlation with histomorphology and sometimes cytogenetic findings is critical to make an accurate classification [37, 40]. Expansion of the panels to include more markers than commonly used B-cell antigens may help differentiate these lymphomas. Compared with DLBCL and other mature B-cell non-HLs, BL likely expresses stronger CD43 and CD83 [41] and is more likely negative for CD44 and CD54 [42]. One study showed that the combination of CD38+ >90%, CD10+ >80%, CD10 median fluorescence intensity ratio >10, bcl-2+ <30%, and Ki-67+ >70% was characteristic of BL, and any deviation from these cut-offs should raise suspicion for other high-grade mature B-cell non-HLs with BL-like morphology [43]. The detection of CD16/56 expression without high CD38 expression favors high-grade B-cell lymphoma with 11q aberration instead of BL [44]. Rare B-ALL cases can show surface light chain restriction, mimicking CD10+ mature B-cell non-HLs. The presence of immature markers (TdT and CD34) and cytomorphology can make the distinction [45]. DLBCL is a heterogeneous group of mature B-cell non-HLs variably positive for B-cell markers with light chain restriction. High FSC is usually present in DLBCL, and it reflects the large size of the tumor cells and can be used as a feature to distinguish DLBCL from small mature B-cell neoplasms.

The common adult mature B-cell non-HLs, such as CLL, usual FL, and marginal zone lymphoma (MZL), are all very rare in children [46, 47]. The diagnosis of any of these diseases in a child deserves the publication of a case report. CLL has a characteristic phenotype: CD20+ (weak), CD22+ (weak), CD23+ (often moderate to strong), FMC-7−, and sIg+ (weak with light chain restriction). This phenotype is enough to make the diagnosis in conjunction with the typical morphology in most of the cases. CD200 is consistently expressed in CLL, but not in mantle cell lymphoma, another CD5+ small lymphocytic neoplasm. The addition of CD200 in the panel has increased the sensitivity to identify CLL, even for the atypical cases [48]. Lymphoid enhancer-binding factor 1 (LEF1) is highly expressed in CLL, but not detected in most other B-cell neoplasms, so it is considered a highly specific marker for CLL [49, 50]. Including LEF1 in the FCM panel will increase the sensitivity and specificity for diagnosing CLL. HCL is rarely reported in children [51]. HCL has a very distinctive phenotype: CD20+ (bright), CD11c+ (bright), CD25+, CD103+, CD22+ (bright), sIg+ (intermediate to bright with light chain restriction), FMC-7+, CD23−, CD5−, and CD10−. This phenotype together with the characteristic morphology is enough to make the diagnosis of HCL. MZL is usually distinguished from HCL by the lack of combined positivity for CD11c, CD25, and CD103, and the lack of bright staining for CD20 and CD22. It is worth remembering that occasionally any subtype of these B-cell neoplasms can have cases with atypical phenotype. Correlation with morphologic features, clinical information, and sometimes cytogenetic/molecular findings is always required for accurate interpretation of FCM results.

Diagnosing Plasma Cell Neoplasms

Plasma cell neoplasms (PCNs) are exceedingly rare in children, with an incidence of 0.06 per million person-years, and are predominantly plasmacytomas [52]. PCNs result from the expansion of a clone of abnormal plasma cells. Plasma cell leukemia (PCL) is a rare form of PCN in which clonal plasma cells account for >20% of total leukocytes in PB. Identification of a clonal plasma cell population with restricted cytoplasmic light chain expression is the basis for the diagnosis of PCN. CD38 and CD138 are the two markers commonly used to identify plasma cells. CD38 is expressed by a spectrum of cell types at a lower intensity than plasma cells. CD138 is more specific for plasma cells but is less sensitive. The neoplastic plasma cells often demonstrate an abnormal CD19−, CD20− phenotype, which is different from most normal CD19+, CD20− plasma cells and CD19+, CD20+ mature B-cell neoplasms. Aberrant CD56 expression is identified in most cases of PCN [53]. Decreased CD38 and/or CD138, abnormal gain of CD28, and loss of CD27 are common in PCN, and some PCN cases express CD117 [54]. Although FCM is very useful in identifying the abnormal plasma cell population and making a distinction between plasma cell neoplasms and other mature B-cell malignancies, the diagnostic utility of FCM is limited by its difficulty in enumerating plasma cells. FCM usually identifies fewer plasma cells than manual count on the smears or IHC stain on biopsy sections. This discrepancy likely results from the sampling difference, loss of plasma cells during sample processing, or a combination of both.

Flow Cytometry in the Diagnosis of Mature T/NK Cell Leukemias/Lymphomas

Mature T-cell or natural killer (NK)-cell neoplasms consist of a heterogeneous group of neoplastic diseases derived from T-cells or NK cells. Mature T-cell or NK-cell leukemias include T-prolymphocytic leukemia (T-PLL), T-large granular lymphocytic leukemia (T-LGL), NK-large granular lymphocytic leukemia (NK-LGL), adult T-cell leukemia/lymphoma (ATLL), aggressive NK-cell leukemia (A-NKL), and Sezary syndrome (SS). These leukemias are all adult diseases and are not present or exceedingly rare in children. The most common mature T/NK cell neoplasm in children is ALK+ anaplastic large cell lymphoma (ALCL), which can extensively involve BM and/or PB, present as leukemia. Systemic Epstein-Barr virus (EBV)+ T-cell lymphoma (TCL) of childhood commonly involves BM and/or PB even though it is named lymphoma. FCM is very useful in the diagnosis and classification of mature T/NK-cell neoplasms. However, it is often more difficult to identify phenotypically abnormal mature T- or NK-cells than abnormal mature B-cells, and FCM immunophenotypic features are usually not specific or diagnostic for any subtype of T/NK-cell neoplasms.

Abnormal mature T-cell or NK-cell populations can often be identified by FCM study through the detection of aberrant antigen expression. With the recent availability of the specific antibody against TRBC1 and TRBC2, the clonality of an alpha beta T-cell population can also be assessed by a one-tube FCM assay [10, 55]. The application of clonality assessment by TRBC1 expression has increased the sensitivity and specificity of FCM analysis in the identification of an abnormal mature T-cell population.

Identification of Restricted Populations of T-Cells or NK Cells/Clonality Assessment

Alteration of CD4/CD8 ratio in T-cells is not a useful indicator of clonality or neoplasia since it can be seen in many reactive or medical conditions. However, a significant deviation of the CD4/CD8 ratio from normal raises concern for the presence of an abnormally restricted T-cell population. For example, an increased CD4/CD8 ratio in PB can lead to further evaluation of the expression of CD26 and CD7 on CD4+ T-cells. Significant loss or absence of CD7 and/or CD26 in the CD4+ T-cell population points to the diagnosis of SS. The traditional FCM method for T-cell clonality assessment is to evaluate the TCR Vβ repertoire. Normal T-cell populations are composed of a mixture of cells expressing variable Vβ family subtypes. T-cell neoplasm is the expansion of a clone of T-cells with restricted Vβ expression. Since there are more than 20 functional Vβ families, this FCM test for TCR Vβ repertoire is complex and labor intensive, and it consumes a large volume of samples and reagents with limited sensitivity. Therefore, it is not widely used for clinical diagnostic purposes. FCM assessment of T-cell clonality has significantly improved with the recent appearance of the antibody specific for TRBC1, one of two mutually exclusive TCR β-chain constant regions. Normal/reactive alpha beta T-cells include a mixture of cells expressing TRBC1 or TRBC2 (TRBC1–) (Fig. 2.6n, o), while the clonal T-cell population is either TRBC1 positive (Fig. 2.6i–m) or negative. This FCM assay has been tested in many mature alpha beta T-cell neoplasms and proved very useful [10, 11]. The panel should include antibodies for TCR αβ and/or TCR γδ besides TRBC1 because TRBC1 is normally negative in γδ T-cells [56], which can serve as an internal negative control (Fig. 2.6p). This assay is not useful for γδ or CD3-negative mature T-cell neoplasms due to the absence of the TCR β chain. With the very recent availability of the TRBC2 antibody and its inclusion in the panel, FCM assessment of TRBC restriction, just like the kappa and lambda Ig light chain restriction analysis, becomes more powerful in the detection of clonal T-cells [55].

NK cells have no TCR, and hence cannot be assessed for clonality using the TCR Vβ/TRBC1 FCM test or PCR for TCR gene rearrangement. FCM analysis of NK-receptor (NKR) expression has been developed to seek evidence of NK-cell clonality [57]. Normal and reactive NK-cell populations express a variety of NKRs, whereas neoplastic NK-cell populations express a more restricted NKR repertoire.

Aberrant T-Cell Antigen Expression

T-cell neoplasms often demonstrate altered expression of T-cell markers, characterized by partial or complete loss of one or more pan-T-cell antigens. Rare extreme cases can lack multiple or all T-cell-associated antigens, showing a "null" phenotype, which can make cell lineage determination very difficult. CD5 and CD7 are the most frequently lost antigens in T-cell neoplasms. It should be noted that a small population of nonneoplastic CD7– T-cells is well recognized in PB, BM, and skin biopsy specimens, and CD7– T-cells may expand in some reactive conditions, such as benign dermatoses. In addition, small subsets of T-cells may lack CD5, for example, CD3+ CD5– γδ T-cells. Some mature T-cell neoplasms can be dual CD4/8– or dual CD4/8+, which is more commonly seen in T-ALL/LBL and can also be seen in some normal/reactive T-cell subsets [18, 58]. Altered staining intensity of T-cell antigens is more frequent than complete loss of them in T-cell and NK-cell neoplasms. However, these changes are more subtle and must be distinguished from the normal or reactive T/NK-cell subsets normally seen with these variations [18, 58]. T/NK-cell neoplasms can also aberrantly express antigens of other cell types, such as CD15, CD13, and CD33. Again, it should be noted that small subsets of normal/

reactive T/NK cells can have markers more specific to other cell types, for example, subsets of NK cells expressing CD19, CD33, or CD117 [18].

Classification of Mature T-Cell or NK Cell Leukemias/Lymphomas

Although phenotypic heterogeneity exists in nearly all of the T-cell neoplasms, the common or typical features can be identified in most of the cases by FCM. ALCL primarily involves lymph nodes and skin but may involve BM, PB, and other sites with variable phenotype and morphology. ALCL is commonly CD4+, CD2+, and CD25+, usually positive for cytotoxic granule-associated proteins and epithelial membrane antigen (EMA), and often lacks multiple other T-cell antigens. IHC stains are usually required for the definite diagnosis of ALCL. CD30 is always positive, diffusely and strongly, with a membrane and Golgi staining pattern. The diagnosis of ALK+ ALCL is established based on the expression of ALK-1 protein or the identification of *ALK* gene rearrangement. SS and Mycosis fungoides (MF) commonly have a CD3+ CD4+ CD26− CD7− T-cell phenotype. CD8+ MF exists and is more commonly seen in the pediatric population with a hypopigmented feature. Systemic EBV+ T-cell lymphoma of childhood is typically CD3+ (dim), CD2+ (bright), CD56−, TIA1+, and CD8+, with partial or complete loss of CD5 and CD7 [6, 59]. The cases transformed from systemic chronic active EBV disease are usually CD4+ [6]. The diagnosis of systemic EBV+ T-cell lymphoma of childhood requires EBV positivity, typical clinical presentation, and the identification of abnormal T-cells. T-LGL usually demonstrates a CD8+ T-cell phenotype with frequent decrease of CD5 and/or CD7 expression. Most T-LGL cases express CD57, CD16, cytotoxic granule-associated proteins granzyme-B, perforin, and TIA-1, while the expression of CD56 is uncommon. A diagnosis of T-LGL is often established by combining this phenotype with morphologic and clinical features. Hepatosplenic T-cell lymphoma (HSTL) is frequently CD4− CD8− (occasionally CD4− CD8+) with expression of CD56 and no expression of CD57 and CD5. Most HSTL cases express TCR $\gamma\delta$, demonstrate a nonactivated cytotoxic phenotype with expression of TIA-1 but no granzyme-B and perforin, and frequently demonstrate the cytogenetic abnormality of isochromosome 7q [60]. Enteropathy-associated T-cell lymphoma (EATL) is usually negative for CD4, CD5, and CD8, positive for CD3, CD7, CD103, and cytotoxic granule-associated proteins TIA-1, granzyme-B, and perforin. EATL is commonly associated with celiac disease. Monomorphic epitheliotropic intestinal T-cell lymphoma (MEITL) shares some similarities in phenotype with EATL, but it is commonly CD8+, CD56+, and shows no clear association with celiac disease [58, 61]. As expected, the phenotype of peripheral T-cell lymphoma (PTCL), NOS is quite heterogeneous and often overlaps with other mature T-cell neoplasms. Other specified T-cell neoplasm entities must be excluded before a diagnosis of PTCL, NOS, can be made.

NK-cell neoplasms, including NK-LGL, A-NKL, extranodal NK/T-cell lymphoma (ENK/TCL), and EBV+ NK-cell lymphoproliferative diseases of childhood, have some overlapping phenotypic features, and it is important to distinguish the more aggressive neoplasms (A-NKL and ENK/TCL) from those with a more indolent course. A-NKL and ENK/TCL share many features, including an NK cell phenotype and the presence of EBV. They are usually positive for CD2, CD56, EBV, and the cytotoxic granule-associated proteins TIA-1, granzyme-B, and perforin. Surface CD3 is negative, but cytoplasmic CD3-epsilon is usually positive. CD4, CD5, and CD57 are often negative [62]. The distinction between them is usually made on clinical grounds. A-NKL presents with BM involvement, circulating neoplastic cells, cytopenias, and constitutional symptoms, while ENK/TCL is a tissue-based mass lesion, commonly seen in the nasal cavity and surrounding area, and demonstrating angiocentric and angiodestructive growth pattern. NK-LGL, previously named as *chronic lymphoproliferative disorder of NK cells*, is characterized by a persistent increase of NK cells in the PB without a clearly identified cause. NK-LGL is rare, not associated with EBV, and usually shows a chronic clinical course with many similarities to T-LGL. By the FCM study, NK-LGL usually demonstrates a mature NK-cell phenotype with dim or absent CD2, CD7, and CD57, and restricted or abnormal NK-cell receptor expression [58].

Flow Cytometry in the Diagnosis of Mature Myeloid Leukemias

Mature myeloid neoplasms are uncommon in children. They are a diverse group of neoplasms composed of neoplastic hematopoietic precursors at different maturation stages. Most of these diseases present as chronic leukemia. The diagnosis of these diseases is based on the combination of clinical information, blood cell counts and morphology, histomorphology of BM, and cytogenetic/molecular testing results. Although the aberrant phenotype of hematopoietic precursors is commonly detected in these neoplasms [63–65], the diagnostic value of FCM immunophenotyping in these neoplasms is limited, and the significance of identifying phenotypic aberrancies in these diseases is not well characterized. For the cases of most myeloproliferative neoplasms, FCM study is mainly used for the quantification of blasts to assist in detecting accelerated phase or transformation to AML. The advantages and limitations of FCM blast quantification are the same as those mentioned above in acute leukemia, and FCM cannot replace manual blast count. Unlike chronic myelomonocytic leukemia (CMML), juvenile myelomonocytic leukemia (JMML) demonstrated no consistent monocyte subset profile [65, 66]. Consequently, flow cytometry monocyte subset partitioning is not useful in diagnosing JMML. CD26 is a marker found on leukemia stem cells (LSCs) in chronic myeloid leukemia (CML), but it is absent on CD34+/CD38− stem cells from healthy individuals and on LSCs from other myeloid neoplasms [67, 68]. A study also indicates that patients with a poorer response to treatment tend to have a higher number of CD26+ LSCs at the time of diagnosis [68]. Therefore, flow cytometry assessment of CD26+ LSCs in CML may provide valuable information for both diagnosis and prognosis.

Conclusion

FCM analysis plays a critically important role in the diagnosis of pediatric leukemias and other hematolymphoid malignancies. It can efficiently identify an abnormal cell population, differentiate the neoplastic cell population from normal/reactive cell populations, characterize the phenotype, give lineage assignment, and provide important information for WHO classification.

Conflict of Interest The author declares no potential conflicts of interest with respect to research, authorship, and/or publication of this manuscript.

Copyright and Permission Statement The author confirms that the materials included in this chapter do not violate copyright laws. Where relevant, appropriate permissions have been obtained from the original copyright holder(s), and all original sources have been appropriately acknowledged or referenced.

References

1. Siegel DA, King J, Tai E, Buchanan N, Ajani UA, Li J. Cancer incidence rates and trends among children and adolescents in the United States, 2001–2009. Pediatrics. 2014;134(4):e945–55. https://doi.org/10.1542/peds.2013-3926.
2. Ward E, DeSantis C, Robbins A, Kohler B, Jemal A. Childhood and adolescent cancer statistics, 2014. CA Cancer J Clin. 2014;64(2):83–103. https://doi.org/10.3322/caac.21219.
3. SEER*Explorer: An interactive website for SEER cancer statistics [Internet]. Surveillance Research Program, National Cancer Institute; 2023 [updated: 2023 Jun 8; cited 2023 Nov 7]. Available from: https://seer.cancer.gov/statistics-network/explorer/. Data source(s): SEER Incidence Data, November 2022 Submission (1975-2020), SEER 22 registries.
4. Alaggio R, Amador C, Anagnostopoulos I, Attygalle AD, Araujo IBO, Berti E, et al. The 5th edition of the World Health Organization classification of haematolymphoid tumours: lymphoid neoplasms. Leukemia. 2022;36(7):1720–48. https://doi.org/10.1038/s41375-022-01620-2. Epub 2022 Jun 22. PMID: 35732829; PMCID: PMC9214472.
5. Khoury JD, Solary E, Abla O, Akkari Y, Alaggio R, Apperley JF, et al. The 5th edition of the World Health Organization classification of haematolymphoid tumours: myeloid and histiocytic/dendritic neoplasms. Leukemia. 2022;36(7):1703–19. https://doi.org/10.1038/s41375-022-01613-1. Epub 2022 Jun 22. PMID: 35732831; PMCID: PMC9252913.
6. WHO Classification of Tumours Editorial Board. Haematolymphoid tumours [Internet]. Lyon: International Agency for Research on Cancer; 2022. (WHO classification of tumours series, 5th ed.; vol. 11). Available from: https://tumourclassification.iarc.who.int/chapters/63.
7. Swerdlow SH, Campo E, Harris NL, et al., editors. World Health Organization classification of tumours of haematopoietic and lymphoid tissues. Revised 4th ed. Lyon: International Agency for Research on Cancer; 2017.
8. Adan A, Alizada G, Kiraz Y, et al. A flow cytometry: basic principles and applications. Crit Rev Biotechnol. 2017;37(2):163–76. https://doi.org/10.3109/07388551.2015.1128876. Epub 2016 Jan 14.
9. McKinnon KM. Flow cytometry: an overview. Curr Protoc Immunol. 2018;120:5.1.1–11. https://doi.org/10.1002/cpim.40. PMID: 29512141; PMCID: PMC5939936.
10. Berg H, Otteson GE, Corley H, et al. Flow cytometric evaluation of TRBC1 expression in tissue specimens and body fluids is a novel and specific method for assessment of T-cell clonality and diagnosis of T-cell neoplasms. Cytometry B Clin Cytom. 2021;100(3):361–9. https://doi.org/10.1002/cyto.b.21881. Epub 2020 Apr 25.

11. Horna P, Shi M, Olteanu H, Johansson U. Emerging role of T-cell receptor constant β chain-1 (TRBC1) expression in the flow cytometric diagnosis of T-cell malignancies. Int J Mol Sci. 2021;22(4):1817. https://doi.org/10.3390/ijms22041817. PMID: 33673033; PMCID: PMC7918842.
12. Nolan JP. The evolution of spectral flow cytometry. Cytometry A. 2022;101(10):812–7. https://doi.org/10.1002/cyto.a.24566. Epub 2022 May 14.
13. Paul Robinson J, Rajwa B. Spectral flow cytometry: fundamentals and future impact. Methods Cell Biol. 2024;186:311–32. https://doi.org/10.1016/bs.mcb.2024.02.022. Epub 2024 Apr 4.
14. Behbehani GK. Immunophenotyping by mass cytometry. Methods Mol Biol. 2019;2032:31–51. https://doi.org/10.1007/978-1-4939-9650-6_2.
15. Dimitriadis S, Dova L, Kotsianidis I, Hatzimichael E, Kapsali E, Markopoulos GS. Imaging flow cytometry: development, present applications, and future challenges. Methods Protoc. 2024;7(2):28. https://doi.org/10.3390/mps7020028. PMID: 38668136; PMCID: PMC11054958.
16. Wood B. 9-color and 10-color flow cytometry in the clinical laboratory. Arch Pathol Lab Med. 2006;130(5):680–90. https://doi.org/10.5858/2006-130-680-CACFCI.
17. Wood BL, Arroz M, Barnett D, et al. 2006 Bethesda International Consensus recommendations on the immunophenotypic analysis of hematolymphoid neoplasia by flow cytometry: optimal reagents and reporting for the flow cytometric diagnosis of hematopoietic neoplasia. Cytometry B Clin Cytom. 2007;72(Suppl 1):S14–22. https://doi.org/10.1002/cyto.b.20363.
18. Li W, Morgan R, Nieder R, et al. Normal or reactive minor cell populations in bone marrow and peripheral blood mimic minimal residual leukemia by flow cytometry. Cytometry B Clin Cytom. 2021;100(5):590–601. https://doi.org/10.1002/cyto.b.21968. Epub 2020 Nov 16.
19. DiGiuseppe JA, Wood BL. Applications of flow cytometric immunophenotyping in the diagnosis and posttreatment monitoring of B and T lymphoblastic leukemia/lymphoma. Cytometry B Clin Cytom. 2019;96(4):256–65. https://doi.org/10.1002/cyto.b.21833. Epub 2019 Jun 24.
20. Weir EG, Borowitz MJ. Flow cytometry in the diagnosis of acute leukemia. Semin Hematol. 2001;38(2):124–38. https://doi.org/10.1016/s0037-1963(01)90046-0.
21. Borowitz MJ, Guenther KL, Shults KE, et al. Immunophenotyping of acute leukemia by flow cytometric analysis. Use of CD45 and right-angle light scatter to gate on leukemic blasts in three-color analysis. Am J Clin Pathol. 1993;100(5):534–40. https://doi.org/10.1093/ajcp/100.5.534. PMID: 8249893.
22. Loken MR, van de Loosdrecht A, Ogata K, et al. Flow cytometry in myelodysplastic syndromes: report from a working conference. Leuk Res. 2008;32(1):5–17. https://doi.org/10.1016/j.leukres.2007.04.020. Epub 2007 Jun 18. PMID: 17576013.
23. McKenna RW, Asplund SL, Kroft SH. Immunophenotypic analysis of hematogones (B-lymphocyte precursors) and neoplastic lymphoblasts by 4-color flow cytometry. Leuk Lymphoma. 2004;45(2):277–85. https://doi.org/10.1080/1042819031000151950. PMID: 15101712.
24. Jain N, Lamb AV, O'Brien S, et al. Early T-cell precursor acute lymphoblastic leukemia/lymphoma (ETP-ALL/LBL) in adolescents and adults: a high-risk subtype. Blood. 2016;127(15):1863–9. https://doi.org/10.1182/blood-2015-08-661702. Epub 2016 Jan 8. PMID: 26747249; PMCID: PMC4915808.
25. Craig FE, Foon KA. Flow cytometric immunophenotyping for hematologic neoplasms. Blood. 2008;111(8):3941–67. https://doi.org/10.1182/blood-2007-11-120535. Epub 2008 Jan 15. PMID: 18198345.
26. Julia F, Dalle S, Duru G, et al. Blastic plasmacytoid dendritic cell neoplasms: clinico-immunohistochemical correlations in a series of 91 patients. Am J Surg Pathol. 2014;38(5):673–80. https://doi.org/10.1097/PAS.0000000000000156. PMID: 24441662.
27. Guy J, Antony-Debré I, Benayoun E, et al. Flow cytometry thresholds of myeloperoxidase detection to discriminate between acute lymphoblastic or myeloblastic leukaemia. Br J Haematol. 2013;161(4):551–5. https://doi.org/10.1111/bjh.12277. Epub 2013 Feb 25. PMID: 23432206.

28. Ohki K, Takahashi H, Fukushima T, Nanmoku T, Kusano S, Mori M, et al. Impact of immunophenotypic characteristics on genetic subgrouping in childhood acute lymphoblastic leukemia: Tokyo Children's Cancer Study Group (TCCSG) study L04–16. Genes Chromosom Cancer. 2020;59(10):551–61. https://doi.org/10.1002/gcc.22858.
29. Gaikwad AS, Donohue RE, Elghetany MT, Sheehan AM, Lu XY, Gramatges MM, et al. Expression of CD25 is a specific and relatively sensitive marker for the Philadelphia chromosome (BCR-ABL1) translocation in pediatric B acute lymphoblastic leukemia. Int J Clin Exp Pathol. 2014;7(9):6225–30. PMID: 25337274; PMCID: PMC4203245.
30. Aricò M, Valsecchi MG, Camitta B, Schrappe M, Chessells J, Baruchel A, et al. Outcome of treatment in children with Philadelphia chromosome-positive acute lymphoblastic leukemia. N Engl J Med. 2000;342(14):998–1006. https://doi.org/10.1056/NEJM200004063421402. PMID: 10749961.
31. Roberts KG, Li Y, Payne-Turner D, et al. Targetable kinase-activating lesions in Ph-like acute lymphoblastic leukemia. N Engl J Med. 2014;371(11):1005–15. https://doi.org/10.1056/NEJMoa1403088. PMID: 25207766; PMCID: PMC4191900.
32. Jeha S, Choi J, Roberts KG, Pei D, Coustan-Smith E, Inaba H, et al. Clinical significance of novel subtypes of acute lymphoblastic leukemia in the context of minimal residual disease-directed therapy. Blood Cancer Discov. 2021;2(4):326–37. https://doi.org/10.1158/2643-3230.BCD-20-0229. PMID: 34250504; PMCID: PMC8265990.
33. Schinnerl D, Mejstrikova E, Schumich A, Zaliova M, Fortschegger K, Nebral K, et al. CD371 cell surface expression: a unique feature of *DUX4*-rearranged acute lymphoblastic leukemia. Haematologica. 2019;104(8):e352–5. https://doi.org/10.3324/haematol.2018.214353. Epub 2019 Jan 31. PMID: 30705095; PMCID: PMC6669149.
34. Chen X, Cherian S. Acute myeloid leukemia immunophenotyping by flow cytometric analysis. Clin Lab Med. 2017;37(4):753–69. https://doi.org/10.1016/j.cll.2017.07.003. Epub 2017 Aug 31. PMID: 29128067.
35. Takenokuchi M, Kawano S, Nakamachi Y, et al. FLT3/ITD associated with an immature immunophenotype in PML-RARα leukemia. Hematol Rep. 2012;4(4):e22. https://doi.org/10.4081/hr.2012.e22. Epub 2012 Oct 16. PMID: 23355940; PMCID: PMC3555210.
36. Eidenschink Brodersen L, Alonzo TA, Menssen AJ, et al. A recurrent immunophenotype at diagnosis independently identifies high-risk pediatric acute myeloid leukemia: a report from Children's Oncology Group. Leukemia. 2016;30(10):2077–80. https://doi.org/10.1038/leu.2016.119. Epub 2016 May 2. PMID: 27133823; PMCID: PMC5136463.
37. Li W. Pathogenesis and pathology of pediatric lymphoma. In: Gallamini A, Juweid M, editors. Lymphoma [Internet]. Brisbane: Exon Publications; 2021. Chapter 1. PMID: 35226433.
38. Kroft SH. Monoclones, monotypes, and neoplasia pitfalls in lymphoma diagnosis. Am J Clin Pathol. 2004;121(4):457–9. https://doi.org/10.1309/RR8A-XUWM-9FYX-178A. PMID: 15080295.
39. Shirai T, Hirose S, Okada T, et al. CD5+ B cells in autoimmune disease and lymphoid malignancy. Clin Immunol Immunopathol. 1991;59(2):173–86. https://doi.org/10.1016/0090-1229(91)90016-4. PMID: 1706969.
40. Zhang L, Brown LE, Bowen LM, McCarthy LC, Cooley LD, Repnikova E, et al. Application of 2016 WHO classification in the diagnosis of paediatric high-grade *MYC*-negative mature B-cell lymphoma with Burkitt-like morphological features. J Clin Pathol. 2020;73(9):563–70. https://doi.org/10.1136/jclinpath-2019-206267. Epub 2020 Jan 21. PMID: 31964683.
41. Cardoso CC, Auat M, Santos-Pirath IM, Rudolf-Oliveira RCM, da Silva JP, Lange BG, et al. The importance of CD39, CD43, CD81, and CD95 expression for differentiating B cell lymphoma by flow cytometry. Cytometry B Clin Cytom. 2018;94(3):451–8. https://doi.org/10.1002/cyto.b.21533. Epub 2017 May 24. PMID: 28509416.
42. Schniederjan SD, Li S, Saxe DF, Lechowicz MJ, Lee KL, Terry PD, et al. A novel flow cytometric antibody panel for distinguishing Burkitt lymphoma from CD10+ diffuse large B-cell lymphoma. Am J Clin Pathol. 2010;133(5):718–26. https://doi.org/10.1309/AJCP0XQDGKFR0HTW. PMID: 20395518.

43. Tsagarakis NJ, Papadhimitriou SI, Pavlidis D, Liapis K, Gortzolidis G, Kostopoulos IV, et al. Contribution of immunophenotype to the investigation and differential diagnosis of Burkitt lymphoma, double-hit high-grade B-cell lymphoma, and single-hit MYC-rearranged diffuse large B-cell lymphoma. Cytometry B Clin Cytom. 2020;98(5):412–20. https://doi.org/10.1002/cyto.b.21887. Epub 2020 Jun 4. PMID: 32497402.
44. Rymkiewicz G, Grygalewicz B, Chechlinska M, Blachnio K, Bystydzienski Z, Romejko-Jarosinska J, et al. A comprehensive flow-cytometry-based immunophenotypic characterization of Burkitt-like lymphoma with 11q aberration. Mod Pathol. 2018;31(5):732–43. https://doi.org/10.1038/modpathol.2017.186. Epub 2018 Jan 12. PMID: 29327714.
45. Kansal R, Deeb G, Barcos M, Wetzler M, Brecher ML, Block AW, et al. Precursor B lymphoblastic leukemia with surface light chain immunoglobulin restriction: a report of 15 patients. Am J Clin Pathol. 2004;121(4):512–25. https://doi.org/10.1309/WTXC-Q5NR-ACVX-TYBY. PMID: 15080303.
46. Quintanilla-Martinez L, Sander B, Chan JK, Xerri L, Ott G, Campo E, et al. Indolent lymphomas in the pediatric population: follicular lymphoma, IRF4/MUM1+ lymphoma, nodal marginal zone lymphoma and chronic lymphocytic leukemia. Virchows Arch. 2016;468(2):141–57. https://doi.org/10.1007/s00428-015-1855-z. Epub 2015 Sep 28. PMID: 26416032.
47. Claviez A, Meyer U, Dominick C, Beck JF, Rister M, Tiemann M. MALT lymphoma in children: a report from the NHL-BFM Study Group. Pediatr Blood Cancer. 2006;47(2):210–4. https://doi.org/10.1002/pbc.20575. PMID: 16123999.
48. Sandes AF, de Lourdes Chauffaille M, Oliveira CR, et al. CD200 has an important role in the differential diagnosis of mature B-cell neoplasms by multiparameter flow cytometry. Cytometry B Clin Cytom. 2014 Mar;86(2):98–105. https://doi.org/10.1002/cyto.b.21128. Epub 2013 Oct 8. PMID: 24243815.
49. Amador-Ortiz C, Goolsby CL, Peterson LC, et al. Flow cytometric analysis of lymphoid enhancer-binding factor 1 in diagnosis of chronic lymphocytic leukemia/small lymphocytic lymphoma. Am J Clin Pathol. 2015;143(2):214–22. https://doi.org/10.1309/AJCPT32JDFIGHFHJ. PMID: 25596247.
50. Menter T, Dirnhofer S, Tzankov A. LEF1: a highly specific marker for the diagnosis of chronic lymphocytic B cell leukaemia/small lymphocytic B cell lymphoma. J Clin Pathol. 2015;68(6):473–8. https://doi.org/10.1136/jclinpath-2015-202862. Epub 2015 Feb 24. PMID: 25713417.
51. Bosma M, Bartels M. Hairy cell leukemia in a child? Blood. 2018;132(11):1216. https://doi.org/10.1182/blood-2018-06-857938. PMID: 30213840.
52. Loap P, Vignon M, Bouscary D, Kirova Y. Pediatric plasma cell neoplasms: a population-based study. Clin Lymphoma Myeloma Leuk. 2022;22(11):841–6. https://doi.org/10.1016/j.clml.2022.07.003. Epub 2022 Jul 11. PMID: 35941071.
53. Lin P, Owens R, Tricot G, Wilson CS. Flow cytometric immunophenotypic analysis of 306 cases of multiple myeloma. Am J Clin Pathol. 2004;121(4):482–8. https://doi.org/10.1309/74R4-TB90-BUWH-27JX. PMID: 15080299.
54. Raja KR, Kovarova L, Hajek R. Review of phenotypic markers used in flow cytometric analysis of MGUS and MM, and applicability of flow cytometry in other plasma cell disorders. Br J Haematol. 2010;149(3):334–51. https://doi.org/10.1111/j.1365-2141.2010.08121.x. Epub 2010 Mar 1. PMID: 20201947.
55. Horna P, Weybright MJ, Ferrari M, et al. Dual T-cell constant β chain (TRBC)1 and TRBC2 staining for the identification of T-cell neoplasms by flow cytometry. Blood Cancer J. 2024;14(1):34. https://doi.org/10.1038/s41408-024-01002-0. PMID: 38424120; PMCID: PMC10904869.
56. Devitt KA, Kern W, Li W, et al. TRBC1 in flow cytometry: assay development, validation, and reporting considerations. Cytometry B Clin Cytom. 2024;106(3):192–202. https://doi.org/10.1002/cyto.b.22175. Epub 2024 May 3. PMID: 38700195.
57. Morice WG, Kurtin PJ, Leibson PJ, Tefferi A, Hanson CA. Demonstration of aberrant T-cell and natural killer-cell antigen expression in all cases of granular lymphocytic leukaemia. Br

J Haematol. 2003;120(6):1026–36. https://doi.org/10.1046/j.1365-2141.2003.04201.x. PMID: 12648073.

58. Craig JW, Dorfman DM. Flow cytometry of T cells and T-cell neoplasms. Clin Lab Med. 2017;37(4):725–51. https://doi.org/10.1016/j.cll.2017.07.002. Epub 2017 Oct 3. PMID: 29128066.
59. Coffey AM, Lewis A, Marcogliese AN, et al. A clinicopathologic study of the spectrum of systemic forms of EBV-associated T-cell lymphoproliferative disorders of childhood: a single tertiary care pediatric institution experience in North America. Pediatr Blood Cancer. 2019;66(8):e27798. https://doi.org/10.1002/pbc.27798. Epub 2019 May 16. PMID: 31099136.
60. Yabe M, Miranda RN, Medeiros LJ. Hepatosplenic T-cell Lymphoma: a review of clinicopathologic features, pathogenesis, and prognostic factors. Hum Pathol. 2018;74:5–16. https://doi.org/10.1016/j.humpath.2018.01.005. Epub 2018 Jan 11. PMID: 29337025.
61. Chen C, Gong Y, Yang Y, Xia Q, Rao Q, Shao Y, et al. Clinicopathological and molecular genomic features of monomorphic epitheliotropic intestinal T-cell lymphoma in the Chinese population: a study of 20 cases. Diagn Pathol. 2021;16(1):114. https://doi.org/10.1186/s13000-021-01173-5. PMID: 34895266; PMCID: PMC8667391.
62. El Hussein S, Patel KP, Fang H, Thakral B, Loghavi S, Kanagal-Shamanna R, et al. Genomic and immunophenotypic landscape of aggressive NK-cell leukemia. Am J Surg Pathol. 2020;44(9):1235–43. https://doi.org/10.1097/PAS.0000000000001518. PMID: 32590457.
63. Kern W, Bacher U, Schnittger S, et al. Multiparameter flow cytometry reveals myelodysplasia-related aberrant antigen expression in myelodysplastic/myeloproliferative neoplasms. Cytometry B Clin Cytom. 2013;84(3):194–7. https://doi.org/10.1002/cyto.b.21068. Epub 2013 Jan 2. PMID: 23283847.
64. Ouyang J, Zheng W, Shen Q, et al. Flow cytometry immunophenotypic analysis of Philadelphia-negative myeloproliferative neoplasms: correlation with histopathologic features. Cytometry B Clin Cytom. 2015;88(4):236–43. https://doi.org/10.1002/cyto.b.21215. Epub 2014 Dec 30. PMID: 25557358.
65. Frisanco Oliveira A, Tansini A, Toledo TR, Balceiro R, Onofre Vidal D, de Martino Lee ML, Lorand-Metze I, Lopes LF. Immunophenotypic characteristics of juvenile myelomonocytic leukaemia and their relation with the molecular subgroups of the disease. Br J Haematol. 2021;192(1):129–36. https://doi.org/10.1111/bjh.17098. Epub 2020 Sep 23. PMID: 32966606.
66. Gadgeel M, Bagla S, Buck S, Shamoun M, Ravindranath Y. CD14/16 monocyte profiling in juvenile myelomonocytic leukemia. Pediatr Blood Cancer. 2020;67(9):e28555. https://doi.org/10.1002/pbc.28555. Epub 2020 Jul 10. PMID: 32648963.
67. Herrmann H, Sadovnik I, Cerny-Reiterer S, et al. Dipeptidylpeptidase IV (CD26) defines leukemic stem cells (LSC) in chronic myeloid leukemia. Blood. 2014;123(25):3951–62. https://doi.org/10.1182/blood-2013-10-536078. Epub 2014 Apr 28. PMID: 24778155.
68. Sicuranza A, Raspadori D, Bocchia M. CD26/DPP-4 in chronic myeloid leukemia. Cancers (Basel). 2022;14(4):891. https://doi.org/10.3390/cancers14040891. PMID: 35205639; PMCID: PMC8870104.

Chromosomal Analysis and Fluorescence In Situ Hybridization (FISH) in the Clinical Study of Pediatric Leukemia

3

Lei Zhang, Misha Fan, and Linda D. Cooley

Introduction

Although the human karyotype has been appreciated since the early twentieth century, the era of clinical cytogenetics is considered to have started in 1956 when the correct chromosome number of 46 in one human cell was established by Tjio and Levan who, by using improved methods (colchicine/hypotonic solutions), found that every human cell has 23 pairs of chromosomes [1]. After that, several additional improvements in techniques were made. One advancement was the introduction of phytohemagglutinin as a mitogen in cell culture by Peter Nowell in 1960 [2], which enabled the use of peripheral blood as a possible specimen for chromosome analysis. Another technical advancement was the development of banding techniques, Q-banding [3, 4] and G-banding [5], in the 1970s, which triggered a cascade of various defined chromosome abnormalities and syndromes. The next revolutionary advancement in cytogenetics was the development of fluorescence in situ hybridization (FISH) technique in the early 1980s, which led to the emergence of the new discipline of molecular cytogenetics. FISH enabled the visualization and mapping of specific DNA sequences on chromosomes with high precision, thus enhancing the ability to detect chromosome abnormalities, particularly in cancer diagnosis and research. In recent years, the integration of conventional chromosome analysis, FISH, and several other innovative technologies (e.g., microarray, optical genome mapping, next generation sequencing) has considerably improved our understanding of cytogenetics as a science.

L. Zhang (✉) · L. D. Cooley
Department of Pathology and Laboratory Medicine, Children's Mercy Kansas City, University of Missouri-Kansas City School of Medicine, Kansas City, MO, USA
e-mail: lzhang@cmh.edu

M. Fan
Department of Family Medicine, Thundermist Health Center, Woonsocket, RI, USA

W. Li (ed.), *Laboratory Assessments of Pediatric Leukemia*,
https://doi.org/10.1007/978-3-032-26557-9_3

Table 3.1 Examples of chromosome abnormalities with diagnostic and prognostic significance [10]

Abnormalities	Associated diagnosis	Prognosis
t(15;17)—*PML::RARA*	APL	Good
inv(16)—*CBFB::MYH11*	AML	Good
t(6;9)—*DEK::NUP214*	AML	Poor
t(9;11)—*KMT2A::MLLT3*	AML	Intermediate
iAMP21	B-ALL	Poor
Hyperdiploidy	B-ALL	Good
Hypodiploidy	B-ALL	Poor
t(1;19)—*TCF3::PBX1*	B-ALL	Intermediate

AML acute myelocytic leukemia, *APL* acute promyelocytic leukemia, *B-ALL* B-cell acute lymphoblastic leukemia, *T-ALL* T-cell acute lymphoblastic leukemia

Cancer cytogenetics started after the discovery of the "Philadelphia" chromosome in 1960 [6], which, for the first time, demonstrated an association between chromosomes and cancer. In 1973, Jane Rowley showed that the "Philadelphia" chromosome actually resulted from the translocation involving chromosomes 9 and 22 [7]. In the same year, the t(8;21) was described in acute myelocytic leukemia (AML) [8]. Over the past five decades, strong evidence has accumulated to demonstrate that cytogenetic studies have been instrumental in detecting nonrandom chromosomal abnormalities associated with cancer diagnosis, treatment, and prognosis, thus moving cancer cytogenetics studies from the bench to clinical practice. Since 2008, the World Health Organization (WHO) has categorized subtypes of acute lymphoblastic leukemia (ALL), AML, as well as other hematological malignancies according to cytogenetic abnormalities [9]. Therefore, cytogenetic analysis of leukemic cells has been an essential part of all newly diagnosed leukemias, and it remains the gold standard for understanding the relationship between clonal evolution and disease progression because it provides a global analysis of the abnormalities in the entire genome of a single cell. Table 3.1 lists examples of chromosome abnormalities with their clinical significance in diagnosis and prognosis [10].

Chromosome analysis (karyotyping) and FISH are the two main methods used in classical cytogenetic studies. Both methods involve microscopic examination of chromosomes in individual cells or tissues fixed on a slide. In this chapter, we will discuss the processes of conventional chromosome and FISH studies related to pediatric leukemia, from specimen types and processing to chromosome abnormalities, abnormal FISH patterns, and reporting. Given that a standardized nomenclature [11] is critical for an accurate and consistent description of chromosome and FISH abnormalities and constitutes a necessary portion of the cytogenetic laboratory report, we will also review commonly used nomenclature for abnormalities frequently seen in pediatric leukemias.

Conventional Chromosome Study

Cytogenetics is the study of chromosome morphology, structure, function, behavior, and inheritance. Obtaining metaphase chromosomes requires cells that are actively dividing or can be stimulated to divide in cultures. The specimen source and quality, as well as specimen collection/handling, can have great influence on whether the cells will grow and divide, and on the quality of the resulting metaphase cells and their chromosomes. In this section, we will review the cytogenetic workflow, followed by chromosome recognition, chromosome abnormalities identification, and reporting.

Specimen Collection and Handling

Bone Marrow Aspirates Bone marrow is the preferred sample type for investigation of most hematologic disorders. Collection containers must be sterile and contain preservative-free sodium heparin. Room temperature is often recommended for specimen storage and transportation. Specimens to be cultured must never be frozen or exposed to excessive heat. Refrigeration is helpful for some specimens that may have a risk for contamination. The first few milliliters of the bone marrow tap is the best portion for cytogenetic study because it contains the highest percentage of cells. Subsequent taps are likely to be diluted by blood and contain fewer actively dividing cells. Re-siting the needle, through the same puncture, gives better results than trying to get more material from the same site. Bone marrow specimens can be transported with or without medium. However, use of medium may reduce the likelihood of the sample clotting or drying out [12–14].

Bone Marrow Core Biopsy Usually, a bone marrow core biopsy is obtained when the white cell count of the marrow aspirate is inadequate for cytogenetic studies. The collection requirements for bone marrow biopsy are essentially the same as for bone marrow aspirate. The bone marrow biopsy should be transported to the laboratory as soon as possible, at room temperature, and in growth medium.

Neoplastic Blood Unstimulated blood can be used for cytogenetic study if it contains at least 5% of circulating blasts and marrow is not available or has failed [12–14]. Mitogen-stimulated blood can be used to establish the patient's constitutional karyotype and to help clarify the origin, whether germline or somatic, of identified abnormalities. The collection requirements for blood samples are essentially the same as for bone marrow.

Lymph Node, Thymus, or Solid Tissue Biopsies Biopsies of tissues may contain leukemia or tumor cells that can be used for cytogenetic studies to aid in the diagnoses of lymphoblastic lymphoma or myeloid sarcoma. Small specimens should be collected and transported in sterile culture vessels containing growth or tissue culture medium (not formalin). Sterile saline is not optimal but can be used if no other choices are available [13, 15]. Larger specimens may be sent to the laboratory for dissection. Specimens should be delivered to the laboratory as soon as possible, well protected from temperature extremes.

Pleural Fluid and Ascitic Fluid Fluid samples should be collected and transported aseptically. Culture medium is not required [16].

Leukapheresis Specimen Leukapheresis samples from a leukemia patient may contain a very high white blood cell (WBC) count and can be used for cytogenetic study.

Cultures, Harvesting, Slide Preparation, and Banding

In general, chromosome preparation requires the four principal steps for bone marrow and peripheral blood: (1) cell culture to promote malignant cell growth and division; (2) harvest of the dividing cells at metaphase; (3) slide preparation; and (4) chromosome banding [12, 13, 17].

At least two different cultures should be set up for bone marrow and neoplastic blood if sample volume allows to provide more opportunities to capture the malignant cell population. Cell divisions from different lineages tend to occur at different times, thus an important factor in obtaining a successful result is using various culture times. Culture types may include (1) direct harvest, (2) overnight culture, (3) 24-hour culture, and (4) 48- or 72-h culture, depending on the working diagnoses and lineage origin (e.g., myeloid versus lymphoid). Longer culture periods are generally not advised because the abnormal tumor cells may be lost over time. Among pediatric leukemias, ALL is known to be challenging for most clinical cytogeneticists due to low mitotic index and poor chromosome morphology [18]; thus, setting up several cultures is a first step for good results.

Cell harvest starts with adding a mitotic inhibitor to obtain adequate numbers of cells in metaphase. Colcemid, an analog of colchicine, is used in most cytogenetics laboratories as a mitotic inhibitor. After incubation with colcemid, a hypotonic solution is added to swell the cells. A fixative (3:1 methanol to acetic acid) is added to stop the action of the hypotonic solution and fix the cells in the swollen state.

Slide preparation involves dropping the fixed cells from cultures onto glass slides for subsequent staining and banding. Optimized temperature, humidity, and airflow are three major factors to ensure adequate spreading of the chromosomes.

Chromosome banding is a process of pretreating the slides with trypsin and then staining with Giemsa (G-banding). The trypsin digests certain proteins on the chromosomes and produces a characteristic pattern of light and dark bands after staining that allows for identification of every chromosome. G-banding is the most widely used routine banding method. The dark bands are A-T-rich, late-replicating, heterochromatic regions of the chromosomes, whereas the light bands are C-G-rich, early replicating, euchromatic regions. Other banding methods include Q-banding (Quinacrine banding), which produces bright and dull fluorescence corresponding to the dark and light bands in G-banding; R-banding (Reverse banding), which produces the opposite or reverse of G-banding and Q-banding patterns; and other banding methods staining selective chromosome regions, such as C-banding (Constitutive heterochromatin banding), T-banding (Telomere banding), and NOR staining (Silver Staining for Nucleolar Organizer Regions).

Chromosome Organization, Structure, and Analysis

Once chromosome preparations have been banded, chromosomes are ready to be analyzed for both numerical and structural aberrations.

Chromosome is an organized chromatin structure that appears rod-shaped in cells during mitosis. *Chromatin* consists of genomic DNA complexed with histone and nonhistone proteins. Several levels of DNA organization allow the gradual condensation of chromatin from its homogenous appearance in interphase to microscopically visible chromosomes during cell division [19]. The DNA double helix is the first level of condensation. Next, the DNA helix winds around a *histone core* (constituted of two copies each of the four core histones H2A, H2B, H3, and H4) to form a *nucleosome*, the basic structural unit of chromatin. Between two nucleosomes is a spacer. Repeated winding around histone cores gives rise to the nucleosome fiber, also called "beads on a string". The nucleosome fiber is further coiled into a *solenoid* fiber, which is 30-nm in diameter and visible under the electronic microscope. Solenoid fiber appears to be the fundamental unit of chromatin and can be packed into loops or domains attached to the nonhistone protein matrix within the nucleus. These loops/domains are thought to be the functional units of the genome. The looped domains coil further to give rise to the chromosomes that are visible under the light microscope during cell division. Chromosomes reach their most condensed state during the metaphase stage (Fig. 3.1).

The human genome in a somatic cell consists of 46 chromosomes arranged in 23 pairs. The autosomes are numbered from 1 to 22 in descending order of length; the sex chromosomes are referred to as X and Y. Members of a pair of chromosomes are *homologues*, one inherited from the father and the other from the mother carrying matching genetic information. A chromosome complement can be referred to as *karyotype* in terms of the number, morphology, and content of the chromosomes that make up its genome [20]. Genomic DNAs replicate during S-phase; therefore, every chromosome seen in mitosis consists of two *sister chromatids* linked at the centromere. Each sister chromatid is comprised of a compacted double helix of DNA. An important landmark of every chromosome is the *centromere*, a primary constriction dividing the chromosome into two arms, a short arm designated as *p* and a long arm designated as *q*. A functional chromosome must have one, and only one, centromere. Based on the position of the centromere, chromosomes are classified into three types: metacentric chromosomes with a centrally located centromere;

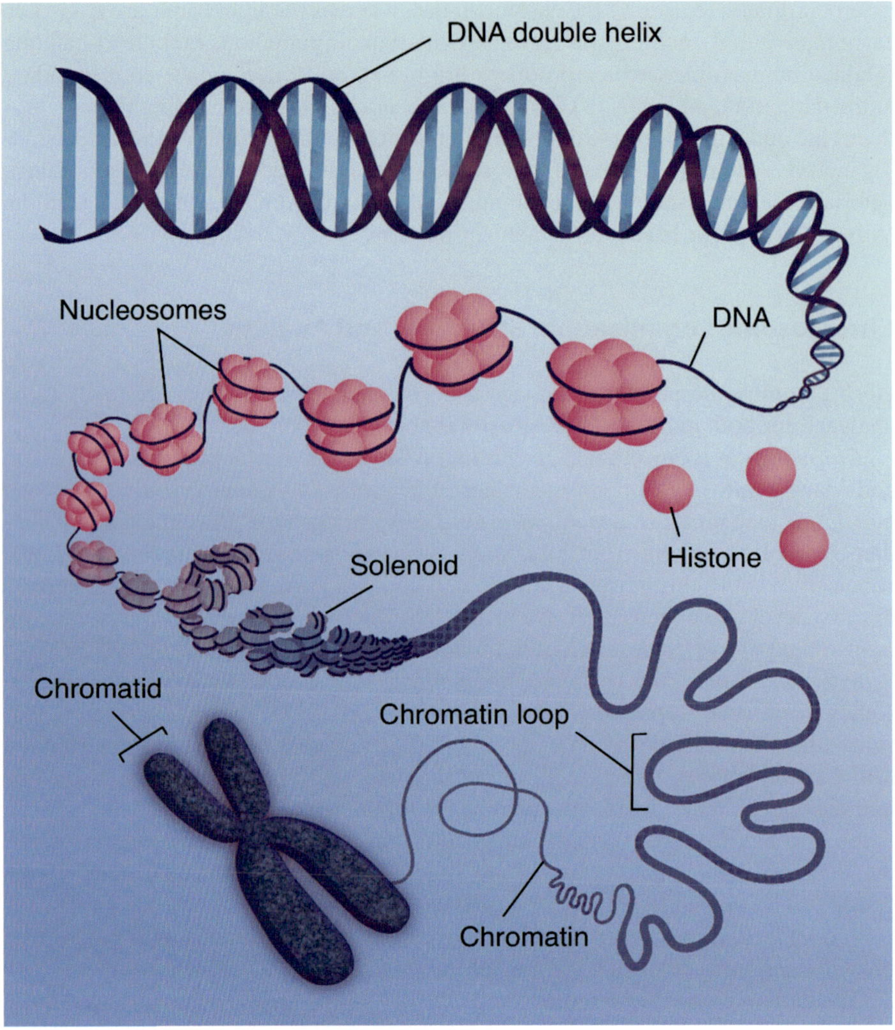

Fig. 3.1 The levels of DNA organization

submetacentric chromosomes with an off-center centromere; and acrocentric chromosomes with the centromere near one end. Another important chromosome landmark is the telomere, which contains tandem repeats of the hexamer TTAGGG over 3–20 kb at the ends of the chromosome [21]. Telomeres can protect chromosome ends from end-to-end fusion of chromosomes as well as degradation after chromosome breakage.

Two types of chromatin, euchromatin and heterochromatin, are spatially segregated in different genomic compartments in the nucleus. Euchromatin is loosely organized, gene-rich, more accessible to transcription, and stains lightly with G-banding techniques. Heterochromatin is typically highly condensed, gene-poor, transcriptionally silent, and stains dark with G-banding [22, 23]. After G-banding, each of the 24 human chromosomes has a unique banding pattern that is distinct from all other chromosomes and nonvariant from individual to individual (unless there is a chromosome abnormality). Between the centromere and telomere of each chromosome are regions that are numbered outward from the centromere. The regions are divided into bands, which can be further divided into sub-bands as banding resolution increases. Therefore, to precisely describe a location within a specific chromosome, four defining factors must be present: chromosome number, chromosome arm, region number, and band number. For example, 10q21 refers to chromosome 10, long arm, region 2, and band 1. If high-resolution banding is achieved, further sub-bands can be described using a decimal point after the band designation, like 10q21.2. The total number of bands countable in a haploid set of autosomes plus the sex chromosomes is used to describe the band level. The International System for Human Cytogenomic Nomenclature (ISCN 2024) describes five levels of resolution [11]; from 300-band low-level to 550-band intermediate-level that provides sufficient resolution for detection of chromosomal aberrations to 850-band high-level resolution obtained from prometaphase cells that allows visualization of microabnormalities.

Karyotype Nomenclature and Chromosome Abnormalities

The International System of Cytogenomic Nomenclature (ISCN) provides a standard nomenclature that unambiguously characterizes a given person's chromosome complement. The description of any human karyotype begins with the total number of chromosomes followed by the sex chromosome complement with a comma separating these two components. Thus, normal male and female karyotypes are written as 46,XY and 46,XX. Any aberrations are listed after the sex chromosomes separated by a comma. A standard set of abbreviations and nomenclature are used to describe the nature of the abnormality.

All general chromosome aberrations can be found in pediatric leukemias as acquired genetic abnormalities, including numerical and structural chromosome changes.

Numerical abnormalities can be ploidy errors or losses/gains of specific chromosomes. Haploid refers to one set of nonhomologous chromosomes. An exact multiple of the haploid chromosome number (n) is called euploid. Normal human somatic cells are diploid (2n, 2 × 23). Polyploid refers to any multiple of 23 (n) greater than diploid (e.g., triploid [3n: 69,XXY], tetraploid [4n: 92,XXYY], pentaploid [5n: 115,XXXYY], etc.). Any other chromosome number that is not a multiple of 23 is aneuploid. "Hypo" range refers to a loss of no greater than 11 chromosomes and "hyper" range refers to a gain of no greater than 11 chromosomes from the corresponding ploidy. For example, the karyotype 43,X,-X,-2,-11[20] is hypodiploid and the karyotype 71,XXY,+12,+21[20] is hypertriploid.

Structural chromosome abnormalities can be classified as balanced and unbalanced rearrangements. In balanced rearrangements, the genome has the normal complement of chromosome material. In a balanced translocation, one chromosome exchanges a segment of its arm with another chromosome. In an inversion, a segment of a chromosome is inverted end to end. In an insertion, a segment is removed from one chromosome and inserted into a different chromosome (nonreciprocal type of translocation). Note that apparent balanced rearrangements may be unbalanced at the molecular level. A good example is the t(9;22)(q34;q11.2) associated with ALL, which can be completely balanced or have subtle deletions at one or both breakpoints. In the karyotype description, the first parentheses explain the participating chromosomes and the second parentheses depict the breakpoints of the involved chromosomes. Translocations may not be limited to two chromosomes; thus, multiple chromosomes can be involved in one complex event resulting in three-way or multi-way translocations.

Unbalanced rearrangements are associated with a gain or loss of genomic material, including but not limited to the following.

Deletion (del): Deletions involve loss of a chromosome segment that can be interstitial (within a chromosome arm) or terminal (at the end of a chromosome).

Duplication (dup): Duplications are associated with gain of genomic material and can be tandem or inverted. Triplication and quadruplication also exist.

Derivative chromosome (der): Derivative chromosomes are generated by either unbalanced rearrangements that may involve more than two chromosomes or multiple aberrations within a single chromosome. For example, karyotype 46,XY,der(22)t(9;22)(q34;q11.2) indicates that one copy of chromosome 22 is a derivative chromosome resulting from an unbalanced translocation between 9q and 22q, with gain of a segment from 9q34 to 9qter and loss of a segment from 22q11.2 to 22qter, with the presence of two normal copies of chromosome 9 and only one normal copy of chromosome 22.

Additional material (add): When unknown, additional material is attached to one end of a chromosome or replaces a terminal segment of a chromosome; the "add" symbol is used to describe the abnormalities.

Ring chromosome (r): When chromosomes lose telomeres, the broken ends of chromosomes can reunite to form a ring structure. The original chromosome of the ring may not always be recognizable by banding pattern.

Marker chromosome (mar): Unidentified chromosomes are called marker chromosomes. Both markers and rings are frequently in mosaic state.

Isochromosomes (i): An isochromosome has one arm missing and the other arm duplicated, resulting in a mirror image banding pattern.

Dicentric chromosome (dic): A dicentric chromosome has two centromeres and usually results from a translocation with loss of the acentric counterparts.

Double minute (dmin): Every metaphase chromosome must have a centromere to attach to the spindle fiber apparatus during cell division. However, one exception to this rule is the formation of small "double minute" chromosomes (dmins). These dmins are commonly the site of gene amplification (e.g., *MYC* or *KMT2A* amplification in neoplasms) [24].

Homogeneously staining region (hsr): An hsr appears as unbanded, inserted material within a chromosome arm and generally indicates gene amplification [24].

Jumping translocation: One breakpoint reoccurs clonally in translocation with different chromosome partners in different cells.

In cancers, some abnormalities may represent the primary clonal changes and may be found as the sole karyotypic abnormality as is often found with leukemia types [25]. Some aberrations may be secondary findings related to the primary clone. The most basic clone in a series of related clonal progression is called the *stemline* (sl) and is written first in the karyotype. Subclones are called *sidelines* (sdl or sdl1, sdl2, etc.), which are written following the stemline with increasing complexity, irrespective of their frequency. The different cell lines are separated by a forward slash (/). For example, the karyotype 46,XY,t(9;22)(q34;q11.2)[4]/47,sl,+19[3]/48,sdl1,+19,+der(22)[8]/46,XY[5] indicates that the t(9;22) is a stemline (sl) abnormality with gain of chromosome 19 in the sideline 1 (sdl1) and further gain of another derivative chromosome 22 in the sideline 2. When rearrangements are too complex or clonal evolution too convoluted to describe the scenario meaningfully, a *composite karyotype* (cp) may be used to describe each clonal event, even though the abnormalities have not presented in every cell. In these situations, a range for chromosome count would be used when there is a variation between cells. For example, karyotype 49–51,XX,+4,+6+10,+12,+21[cp15] indicates that not all gained chromosomes are present in all abnormal cells.

Incomplete (inc) is another term in cancer karyotype description. Some leukemias may produce metaphase cells with very low resolution and poor morphology, which prevents complete analysis of the chromosomes. The incomplete designation can be placed at the end of the karyotype string for these situations. For example, the karyotype 46,XY,add(1)(q25),inc[20] indicates that the karyotype is likely to contain unidentified numerical and structural changes.

Although cancer cytogenetic study focuses on acquired clonal abnormalities, constitutional aberrations may also be identified if present. In these situations, the karyotypes use a "c" to distinguish a constitutional event from acquired abnormalities. For example, the karyotype 50,XX,+4,+10,+14,+21c indicates that the extra copy of chromosome 21 is not a part of the clone but constitutional in origin.

Fluorescence In Situ Hybridization Study

Fluorescence in situ hybridization (FISH) is a molecular diagnostic technique that utilizes a cloned piece of DNA labeled with fluorescent dye to examine the presence or absence of a particular DNA sequence, or to evaluate the number or organization of a chromosome or chromosomal region in place in the cells, or in situ. It evolved from ISH by replacing nonfluorescence-labeled probes with fluorescence-labeled probes, which made it possible to achieve a high sensitivity in a simple and quick assay [26]. The FISH technique was introduced to the clinical cytogenetics laboratory in the late 1980s with higher resolution and flexibility [27, 28]. The convergence of traditional cytogenetics and FISH as a molecular technology has led to the term “molecular cytogenetics” as a synonym for FISH [29, 30]. FISH applications have grown since then and become an integral part of the clinical cytogenetics laboratory. It has been accepted as standard-of-care for pediatric leukemia to follow the standards and guidelines set by the American College of Medical Genetics and Genomics (ACMG) and the Clinical Laboratory Standards Institutes (CLSI) [31, 32].

Basic FISH Process

Excellent references are available that describe various FISH protocols [33, 34]. Briefly, the sample DNA (metaphase chromosomes or interphase nuclei) is first fixed on slides, a labeled probe is added, and then both probe and sample DNA are denatured. When the denatured probe and target DNA reanneal into double-stranded DNA, the probe hybridizes with the sample DNA at the target site. The probe signal can be visualized with a fluorescence microscope, so the sample can be evaluated for the presence or absence of the signal (Fig. 3.2).

Probe Types

The DNA sequence of probes can come from virtually any locus of the genome and can vary in size from typically 10 kb or more to whole chromosome “paint” probes [35]. Most FISH probes fall into one of three categories: unique sequence, repetitive sequence, and whole chromosome.

Unique sequence probes are gene-specific or locus-specific probes designed to detect the presence, absence, extra copies, or the location of a particular gene. These probes are widely used for detection of gains/amplifications or losses of specific regions or loci in leukemia. The unique sequence probe can be in a single color but is often in a probe set that contains an internal control probe of a second color. These probes have also been designed in specific ways to increase the detection specificity/sensitivity for translocations or rearrangements involving specific loci. One such design uses *dual-color dual-fusion probes*. These probes are mixtures of two single probes—each designed for one locus involved in a translocation and labeled with a different fluorescent dye. A translocation will be observed as two fusion signals from both the translocation junction and the reciprocal of the translocation junction, such as t(15;17) (*PML::RARA*) in acute promyelocytic leukemia (Fig. 3.3a, b). The limitation of this design is that variant translocations may be difficult to detect. Another design uses *dual-color break-apart probes* to identify translocations where one chromosome can recombine with multiple potential partners. Two probes are designed to bind to the sequences flanking the translocation breakpoint, with a different probe color on each side. When a translocation occurs, the two probes separate from fusion to two single colors (Fig. 3.3c–e). This design allows evaluation of

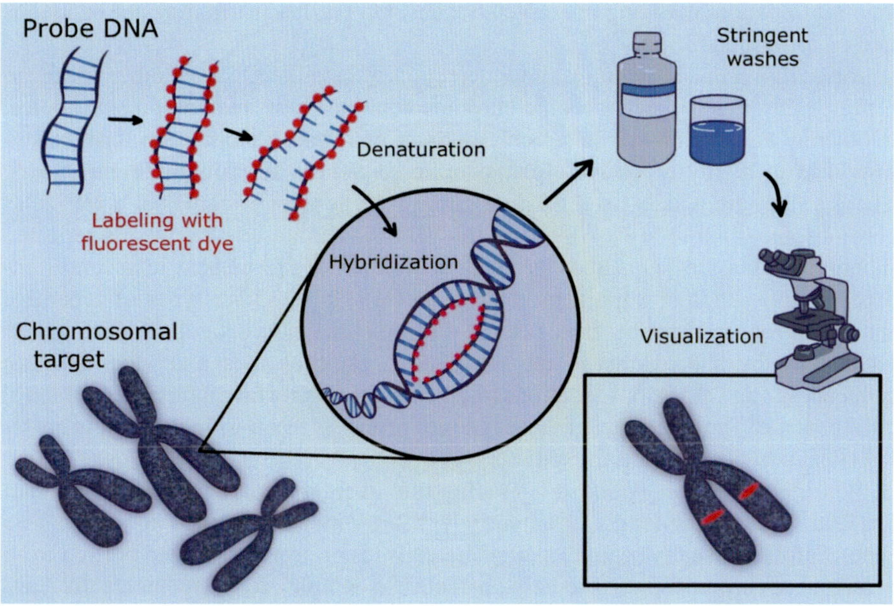

Fig. 3.2 FISH process. From left to right: the probe DNA is labeled with a fluorophore (red, green, blue, etc.); the probe and target (in this case a segment of DNA sequence on a chromosome, but interphase cells are also appropriate) are denatured and then annealed; the cells are counter-stained to show the chromatin location of the probe under a fluorescence microscope

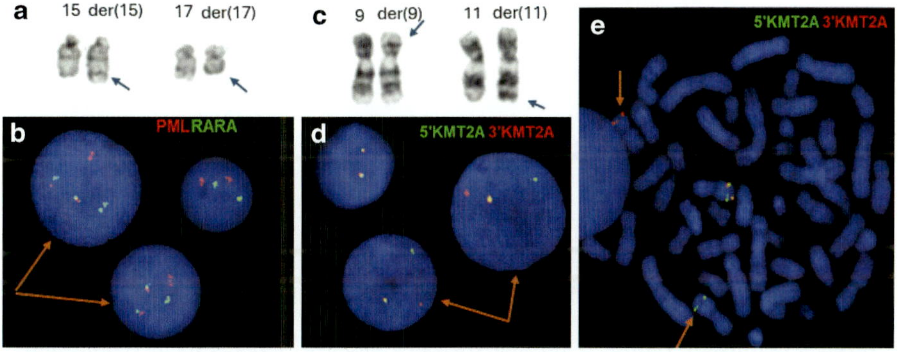

Fig. 3.3 (**a**) t(15;17)(q24;q21) on chromosome analysis; (**b**) *PML* (red) and *RARA* (green) dual-color dual-fusion probes show 2f1r1g signal pattern in abnormal nuclei (arrows); (**c**) t(9;11)(p21;q23) on chromosome analysis; (**d**) *KMT2A* break-apart probes show separation of 5′KMT2A (green) and 3′KMT2A (red) in abnormal nuclei; (**e**) One metaphase shows 3′KMT2A (red) move to 9p with 5’KMT2A (green) remain on 11q

any translocation involving the targeted locus, but partner genes may not be identified or confirmed [36].

Repetitive sequence probes allow detection of satellite DNA or other localized repeated DNA elements at specific chromosomal locations, including centromeres, telomeres, and regions of heterochromatin. Centromeric probes are designed to hybridize to highly repetitive alpha satellite sequences surrounding centromeres. These probes are widely used for determining the number of copies of a particular chromosome (gain or loss). Alpha satellite DNA is composed of tandemly repeated monomers; thus the sequences targeted by the probes are present in several hundreds or thousands of copies, producing strong signals. Other types of repetitive sequences for which probes have been developed include the beta satellite sequences located in the short arms of the acrocentric chromosomes and other satellite sequences found at various locations, including the heterochromatic region of the Y chromosome. The limitation of these types of probes is that they may result in cross-hybridization of other chromosomes.

Whole chromosome paint probe is a mixture of single-copy DNA sequences that are located along the length of an entire chromosome (or chromosome arm). This type of probe is usually used on metaphase cells to confirm a suspected portion from a derivative chromosome, or to help characterize complex rearrangements that cannot be resolved by banding pattern alone. This type of probe cannot detect small deletions or duplications.

Another strategy in FISH analysis is to use multicolor FISH by combining different unique sequence probes and a centromere probe or chromosome paint probe. Simultaneous use of a set of probes with different colors can yield more information than carrying out separate assays. For example, adding a chromosome 8 centromere probe to the t(9;22) dual-color dual-fusion probes can indicate whether the cells with t(9;22) also carry trisomy 8, or whether t(9;22) and trisomy 8 are in the same or different cell lines.

Specimens

FISH can be performed on a variety of specimen types. Metaphase preparations from cultured cells that are routinely used for cytogenetic analysis are optimal preparations for FISH studies (e.g., cultures from previously described bone marrow aspirates, neoplastic blood, bone marrow core biopsy, biopsies from lymph node, thymus, solid tumor tissue). The benefits of using the same preparations for chromosome and FISH analysis include the ability to obtain a concentrated monolayer of cells to permit examination of many cells quickly. If clinically indicated, FISH can be performed on a specimen that is harvested directly (without culturing), allowing same-day hybridization.

Given that FISH can also be performed on interphase cells, the specimen types for FISH in leukemia testing can be broadened to include bone marrow smears, cytospins, formalin-fixed paraffin-embedded (FFPE) tissues, and touch imprints. Cytospin preparations are typically made from cytologic specimens that have been centrifuged to concentrate the cell pellet. FFPE specimens permit evaluation of tissue that was not sent for chromosome analysis and for which fresh tissue is no longer available. A hematoxylin-and-eosin (H&E)-stained slide must accompany the specimen, and a board-certified anatomic pathologist must review the H&E and mark the areas to be scored. Because nuclear truncation is common for FFPE slides of ~3 μm to 5 μm thickness and nuclear overlap is also common in FFPE tissue, interpretation of FISH results from enumeration probes (real loss versus nuclear truncating) and dual-fusion probes (real fusion or signals overlapping) should be carried out with caution. Touch imprints usually avoid the nuclear overlap and truncation in FFPE tissue, providing an alternative for FISH on myeloid sarcoma or other solid tumors. A limitation to touch imprints is the failure of the neoplastic cells to adhere to the slide, which may be due to fibrosis, resulting in the absence of tumor cells in the submitted specimen.

Result Analysis

Probes have been developed for the most common recurrent abnormalities in leukemia, including gene losses, gains, amplifications, and fusions. Fusions can be indicated by the presence of dual-fusion signals or break-apart signals, depending on the probe type used. Unlike G-banding, FISH does not provide a "whole genome view." Instead, FISH can generate information specific to only probed loci and can evaluate hundreds of cells in a short time. Thus, the sensitivity of FISH analysis, in which at least 200 interphase cells are typically evaluated, is higher than that of G-banding analysis (20 metaphase cells). Therefore, FISH analysis can not only detect/confirm clonal abnormalities but also monitor therapy response/minimal residual disease (MRD). FISH is also able to detect abnormalities involving only small portions of a chromosome that may not be visible on chromosome analysis, for example, less than 1 Mb in size, and in some cases, less than 50 kb.

Metaphase FISH analysis can provide information regarding not only the number of signals, but also the chromosomal position of the fluorescence signals. Of note, small duplications are better appreciated in interphase cells and may not be resolved by metaphase FISH due to the highly condensed nature of metaphase chromosome, which results in merging of the closely located duplicated signals into a single signal.

FISH Nomenclature

As for chromosome karyotype, the ISCN also provides a standard nomenclature for description of FISH signal patterns. Metaphase FISH nomenclature starts with "ish," followed by a space, the chromosome abnormality, then FISH abnormalities with probe name and "−" or "+" in parentheses. For example, ish del(5)(q31)(EGR1−) indicates loss of one copy of the *EGR1* locus due to a 5q deletion. Interphase nomenclature starts with "nuc ish," followed by a space, probe name(s) in parentheses, multiplication sign (×), signal number seen, and nuclei number analyzed in square brackets. For example, nuc ish (ABL1,BCR) × 2[200] indicates that interphase FISH shows two signals for each of *ABL1* and *BCR* genes in 200 nuclei scored. Table 3.2 lists the commonly used abbreviations and examples in FISH nomenclature.

Table 3.2 Common symbols and abbreviations used in FISH nomenclature

Abbreviation	Interpretation	Example
ish	In situ hybridization, refers to metaphase FISH	ish 14q32(IGH)×2
nuc ish	Nuclear or nonmitotic cells in situ hybridization	nuc ish(ABL1,BCR)×2[200]
minus sign (−)	Loss of a probe signal	ish del(5)(q31)(EGR1−)[50/200] Deletion of *EGR1* is present in 50 out of 200 nuclei analyzed
plus sign (+)	Presence of a probe signal	ish der(4)(3′KMT2A+) 3′*KMT2A* probe signal is present on the derivative chromosome 4
multiplication sign (×)	Precedes the number of signals observed	nuc ish (ABL1,BCR)×2[200]
con	Connection (fusion) of signals	nuc ish(MYH11,CBFB)×3(MYH11 con CBFB)×2[150/200] *MYH11/CBFB* dual-color dual-fusion probes show two *MYH11::CBFB* fusion signals in 150 out of 200 nuclei analyzed
sep	Separation of signals	nuc ish (KMT2A×2)(5′KMT2A sep 3′KMT2A)×1[150/200] *KMT2A* break-apart probes show one copy of *KMT2A* gene rearranged by presence of separation of 5′*KMT2A* probe from 3′*KMT2A* probe
amp	Amplification	nuc ish (MYCN)amp Amplification of the *MYCN* locus beyond that which can be accurately counted
dim	Diminished signal	ish 13q14(S13S319)dim A less intense signal (diminished) is observed at 13q14 appearing smaller than the signal on the homologous 13q14 locus
enh	Enhanced signal	ish 13q14(S13S319)enh An enhanced signal is observed at 13q14 appearing larger than the one on the homologous 13q14 locus

Summary

Conventional cytogenetics using regular banded chromosomal analysis remains a basic straightforward technique to review the entire human genome on a single-cell basis, and the best way to view clonal evolution. Limitations of chromosome analysis include low resolution (below 5–8 Mb), requirement for cell growth and metaphase cells, trained personnel, and potential issues such as culture artifact. Some of these limitations have been greatly reduced by incorporating automation into the cytogenetics laboratory, especially the recently developed artificial intelligence (AI)-assisted chromosome analysis and capturing. AI has streamlined cytogenetics by removing numerous technologist-required steps in the karyotyping process, resulting in faster turnaround times and improved accuracy [37, 38]. FISH technology provides rapid results with much higher resolution and specificity than G-banded chromosome analysis, but it does not allow for efficient analysis of the entire genome and is limited by probe availability. The combined use of chromosome and FISH analyses complements each other, leading to precise detection of genetic alterations in leukemia. Cancer cytogenetics has been further reinforced by the application of additional molecular technologies in clinical diagnosis, such as microarray, optical genome mapping, whole genome sequencing, and long-read sequencing. For detailed descriptions of these new genetic tests, please see Chaps. 4, 5, 6, and 7. Each technology has its advantages and limitations; thus, cytogenetic technologies will continue to be indispensable tools for the diagnosis and treatment guidance in leukemia.

References

1. Tjio HJ. The chromosome numbers of man. Hereditas. 1956;42:1–6.
2. Nowell P. Phytohaemagglutinin: an initiatior of mitosis in cultures of normal human leukocytes. Cancer Res. 1960;20:219–22.
3. Caspersson T, Zech L, Johansson C. Differential binding of alkylating fluorochromes in human chromosomes. Exp Cell Res. 1970;60(3):315–9.
4. Caspersson T. The 24 fluorescence pattern of the human metaphase chromosomes—distinguishing charactersand variability. Hereditas. 1971;61:89–102.
5. Drets ME, Shaw MW. Specific banding patterns of human chromosomes. Proc Natl Acad Sci USA. 1971;68(9):2073–7.
6. Hungerford PND. Chromosome studies on normal and leukemic human leukocytes. J Natl Cancer Inst. 1960;25(1):85–109.
7. Rowley JD. Letter: a new consistent chromosomal abnormality in chronic myelogenous leukaemia identified by quinacrine fluorescence and Giemsa staining. Nature. 1973;243(5405):290–3.
8. Rowley J. Identification of a translocation with quinacrine fluorescence in a patient with acute leukemia. Ann Genet. 1973;16:109–12.
9. Khoury JD, Solary E, Abla O, Akkari Y, Alaggio R, Apperley JF, et al. The 5th edition of the World Health Organization classification of haematolymphoid tumours: myeloid and histiocytic/dendritic neoplasms. Leukemia. 2022;36(7):1703–19.
10. Board. WCoTE. Haematolymphoid tumours [Internet]. Lyon: International Agency for Research on Cancer; 2025. (WHO classification of tumours series, 5th ed.; vol. 11). Available from: https://tumourclassification.iarc.who.int/chapters/63.

11. Hastings RJ, Moore S, Chia N, editors. ISCN 2024: An International System for Human Cytogenomic Nomenclature (2024). S. Karger AG; 2024.
12. Heerema NA. Cytogenetic analysis of hematologic malignant diseases. In: Arsham MS, Barch MJ, Lawce HJ, editors. The AGT cytogenetics laboratory manual. 4th ed. Wiley; 2017.
13. Keagle MBGSL. Basic cytogenetics laboratory procedures. In: Keagle MB, Gersen SL, editors. The principles of clinical cytogenetics. New York/Heidelberg/Dordrecht/London: Springer; 2013.
14. Swansbury GJ. Cytogenetic technique for human leukemia. In: Pollard JW, Walker JM, editors. Methods in molecular biology volume 5: animal cell culture. The Humana Press Inc; 1990.
15. Nelson M. Cytogenetic methods and findings in human solid tumors. In: Arsham MS, Barch MJ, Lawce HJ, editors. The AGT cytogenetics laboratory manual. 4th ed. Wiley; 2017.
16. Gole LA, Anandakumar C, Bongso A, Chua TM, Wong YC, Ratnam SS. Analysis of cystic hygroma, ascitic, and pleural fluids by conventional lymphocyte culture and fluorescent in situ hybridization. Prenat Diagn. 1997;17(12):1151–7.
17. Hui EKC, Wan TSK, Ng MHL. Chromosome preparation for myeloid malignancies. In: Wan TSK, editor. Cancer cytogenetics methods and protocols. Springer Science+Business Media LLC; 2017.
18. Garipidou VS-WL. The use of fl uorodeoxyuridine synchronization for cytogenetic investigation of acute lymphoblastic leukemia. Cancer Genet Cytogenet. 1991;52:107–11.
19. Sharma T, editor. Trends in chromosome research. New Delhi: Narosa Publishing House; 1990.
20. Hamosh AaSSW. Introduction to the human genome. In: Cohn, RDC, Scherer SW, Hamosh A, editors. Thompson & Thompson genetics and genomics in medicine. 9th ed. Elsevier; 2024.
21. Moyzis RK, Buckingham JM, Cram LS, Dani M, Deaven LL, Jones MD, et al. A highly conserved repetitive DNA sequence, (TTAGGG)n, present at the telomeres of human chromosomes. Proc Natl Acad Sci USA. 1988;85(18):6622–6.
22. Tamaru H. Confining euchromatin/heterochromatin territory: jumonji crosses the line. Genes Dev. 2010;24(14):1465–78.
23. Morrison O, Thakur J. Molecular complexes at euchromatin, heterochromatin and centromeric chromatin. Int J Mol Sci. 2021;22(13).
24. Rayeroux KC, Campbell LJ. Gene amplification in myeloid leukemias elucidated by fluorescence in situ hybridization. Cancer Genet Cytogenet. 2009;193(1):44–53.
25. Heim S, Mitelman F, editors. Cancer cytogenetics. Wiley-Blackwell; 2009.
26. Pinkel D, Straume T, Gray JW. Cytogenetic analysis using quantitative, high-sensitivity, fluorescence hybridization. Proc Natl Acad Sci USA. 1986;83(9):2934–8.
27. Levsky JM, Singer RH. Fluorescence in situ hybridization: past, present and future. J Cell Sci. 2003;116(Pt 14):2833–8.
28. Pinkel D. Cytogenetic analysis by in situ hybridization with fluorescently labeled nucleic acid probes. Cold Spring Harb Symp Quant Biol. 1986;51:151–7.
29. Liehr T. Molecular cytogenetics in the era of chromosomics and cytogenomic approaches. Front Genet. 2021;12:720507.
30. Cheng L, Zhang S, Wang L, MacLennan GT, Davidson DD. Fluorescence in situ hybridization in surgical pathology: principles and applications. J Pathol Clin Res. 2017;3(2):73–99.
31. Mascarello JT, Hirsch B, Kearney HM, Ketterling RP, Olson SB, Quigley DI, et al. Section E9 of the American College of Medical Genetics technical standards and guidelines: fluorescence in situ hybridization. Genet Med. 2011;13(7):667–75.
32. James T. Mascarello LDC, Patricia K, Dowling M, Carcia MV, Jewell SS, Philip R, Rao PN, Sheppard E, South ST, Tsuchiya K, Wiktor A, Wolff DJ. Fluorescence in situ hybridization methods for clinical laboratories; approved guideline—second edition. 2013.
33. Volpi EV, Bridger JM. FISH glossary: an overview of the fluorescence in situ hybridization technique. Biotechniques. 2008;45(4):385–6, 8, 90 passim.
34. Weise A, Mrasek K, Ewers E, Mkrtchyan H, Kosyakova N, Liehr T. Diagnostic applications of fluorescence in situ hybridization. Expert Opin Med Diagn. 2009;3(4):453–60.
35. Wan TS. Cancer cytogenetics: an introduction. Methods Mol Biol. 2017;1541:1–10.

36. Buckingham L. editor. Molecular diagnostics: fundamentals, methods, and clinical applications. F. A. Davis Company; 2019.
37. Rosenblum LS, Holmes J, Taghiyev AF. The emergence of artificial intelligence-guided karyotyping: a review and reflection. Genes (Basel) 2025;16(6).
38. Miller C, Thurston J, Cohen N. Incorporating automation in a cytogenetics laboratory: three practitioners' perspectives on benefits and limitations. Mol Cytogenet. 2025;18(1):12.

DNA Microarray in the Clinical Study of Pediatric Leukemia

4

Allison J. Kalinousky, Aravindh Nagarajan, and Elena A. Repnikova

Introduction

The term "microarray" was introduced in 1995. Initial works demonstrated the capability of this technology to simultaneously monitor the expression of many genes. The sample array was prepared by high-speed robotic printing of DNA sequences on a glass slide [1]. These arrays were utilized for research purposes only. It was not until the early 2000s when DNA-based microarrays began to be used as clinical diagnostic tests [2]. Unlike the expression microarrays, these types of arrays could detect changes in DNA copy number, loss of heterozygosity (LOH), and ploidy changes [3]. By 2011, this method had established itself as the primary approach for the clinical evaluation of copy number alterations in patients exhibiting developmental delays, congenital malformations, autism, and dysmorphic features [4, 5]. Shortly after, technical guidelines and standards for diagnosis of neoplastic disorders were developed by the American College of Medical Genetics and Genomics (ACMG) [6]. Based on comprehensive evidence, the findings from microarray analysis significantly contributed to the diagnosis and cytogenetic risk assessment in oncological specimens [7–10]. Consequently, the integration of microarray testing into the standard clinical diagnosis of hematologic malignancies

Authors Allison J. Kalinousky and Aravindh Nagarajan have equally contributed to this chapter.

A. J. Kalinousky · A. Nagarajan
Department of Pathology and Laboratory Medicine, Children's Mercy Kansas City, Kansas City, MO, USA

E. A. Repnikova (✉)
Department of Pathology and Laboratory Medicine, Children's Mercy Kansas City, University of Missouri–Kansas City School of Medicine, Kansas City, MO, USA
e-mail: erepnikova@cmh.edu

W. Li (ed.), *Laboratory Assessments of Pediatric Leukemia*, https://doi.org/10.1007/978-3-032-26557-9_4

at the time of initial diagnosis and during relapses, alongside traditional karyotyping, can provide a wealth of additional valuable information [11].

Key Principles of the Microarray Technology

The main features of microarray technology include denaturation of DNA from the sample of interest, followed by fragmentation of DNA and labeling of the fragments with fluorescent dye. The fragmented DNA is then added onto the chip, where it is hybridized to complementary DNA sequences called probes. The microarray chip is then scanned to measure the fluorescence signal at each spot (Fig. 4.1). The measurement of the fluorescence from the hybridized DNA sequence enables the determination of copy number of a particular DNA segment [12].

There are two types of copy number microarrays, also known as chromosomal microarrays, that are used in clinical diagnostics: Comparative Genomic Hybridization (CGH) and Single Nucleotide Polymorphism (SNP).

CGH Microarray

Array comparative genomic hybridization (aCGH) offers improved detection of chromosomal aneuploidies, deletions, and duplications compared to traditional karyotyping, resulting in a higher diagnostic yield. This method measures the quantity of genomic DNA segment in a patient's sample and compares it with the genomic DNA segment in a control sample [13]. In the first step of the aCGH procedure, DNA is extracted from both the patient and control samples, then enzymatically digested into smaller fragments, and labeled with distinct fluorescent dyes. The differentially labeled DNA samples are mixed in equal proportions and hybridized to the microarray chip containing probes. The sizes of these probes can range

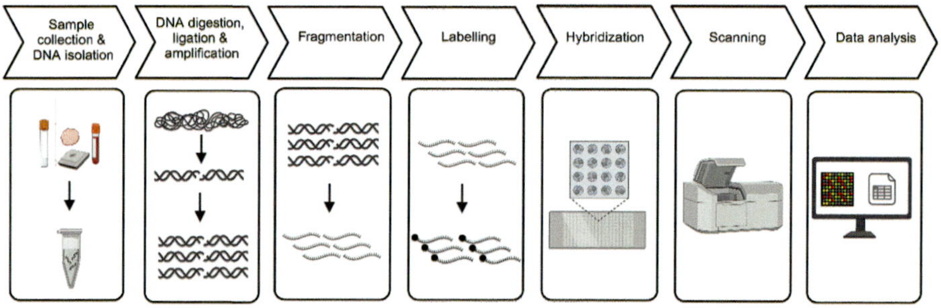

Fig. 4.1 Basic steps of the general microarray workflow. The initial step is to collect the specimen. The next steps includes DNA extraction, followed by DNA digestion, amplification, and further fragmentation with labeling. DNA fragments are then hybridized overnight to an array chip. After incubation, chips are washed and lastly scanned using a scanner, then analyzed using software for copy number calls and regions with loss of heterozygosity

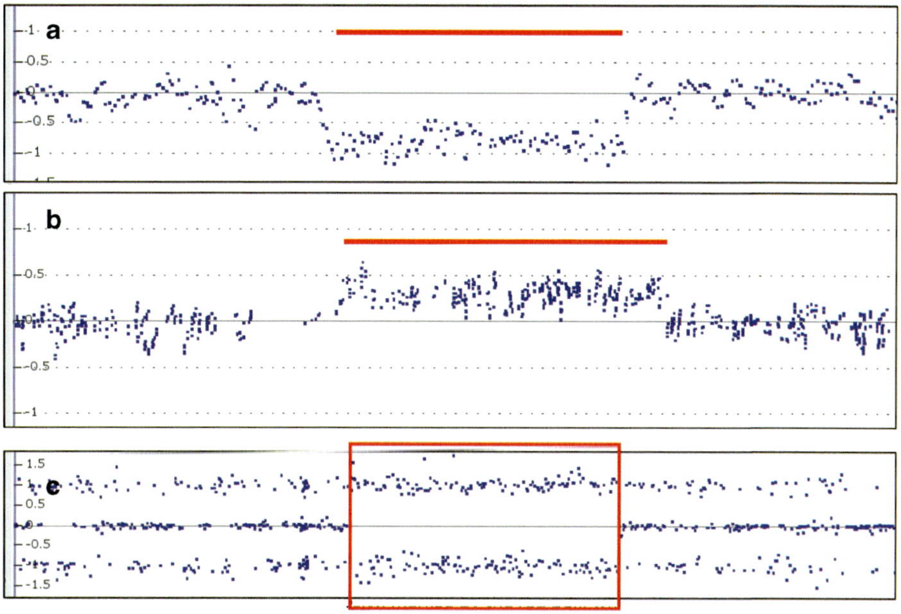

Fig. 4.2 The log2 ratio illustrates: (**a**) a region of loss, indicated by the red line, where the probes shift down within the segment; (**b**) a region of gain, where the probes shift up within the segment; and (**c**) a region demonstrating neutral loss of heterozygosity, marked by the red box, where the probes are absent at the log2 zero line

from approximately 60 base pairs to 200 kilobases (kb), and their quantity is typically several hundred thousands, depending on the specific array platform and intended application. All contemporary microarray platforms utilize probes ranging from 25 base pairs to 60 base pairs in length, with varying probe densities (examples include Agilent, ThermoFisher, and Illumina clinical-grade microarray platforms). Following hybridization, any unbound DNA is washed away, and the fluorescent dye signal intensity is measured using a scanner. The ratio of fluorescent intensity between the patient and control sample is then used to measure relative copy number differences. A decrease in intensity in the patient's sample indicates a loss of a specific chromosomal segment, while an increase in intensity is consistent with a gain (Fig. 4.2a, b).

SNP Array

SNP array contains SNP-based oligonucleotide probes designed based on regions in the genome where SNPs are present. In contrast to aCGH, the SNP array employs an in-silico control, thereby removing the necessity for a separate control sample. Enzymatically fragmented DNA sequences from the patient sample are labeled with fluorescent dyes and hybridized to the chip containing probes. After washing any unbound DNA, the chip is subjected to laser confocal scanning. Emitted fluorescence signal intensities are then measured and analyzed by a computer software to identify regions with copy number variation. Similar to aCGH, loss or gain of genomic material is visualized as a decrease or increase in intensity, respectively. Furthermore, SNP arrays can identify copy-neutral loss of heterozygosity (CN-LOH), which is visualized on the allele frequency track by a lack of probes in the central track (Fig. 4.2c).

Advantages and Limitations of Microarray Testing

Chromosomal microarray analysis (CMA) is a powerful tool that offers significant benefits compared to traditional cytogenetic methods. It allows chromosome evaluation at a significantly higher resolution than standard karyotype analysis, enabling detection of genomic imbalances throughout the whole genome in a single assay [14]. Additionally, this technology has greater sensitivity to detect low-level mosaic copy number alterations that are below the resolution of conventional karyotype or fluorescence in situ hybridization (FISH). Another advantage of CMA is that it does not require cell culture in contrast to traditional cytogenetic analysis. This allows for a faster turnaround time for results, generally within four to five days, and decreases the likelihood of receiving no results due to potential culture failure of tissue samples. reduce [15]. Furthermore, microarray requires relatively low quantities of DNA (~250 nanograms). Certain platforms employ a methodology that utilizes Molecular Inversion Probe (MIP) technology for the analysis of copy number variations in formalin-fixed, paraffin-embedded (FFPE) tissue specimens [16]. Microarrays offer high-resolution capabilities, allowing for the detection of copy number alterations as small as approximately 10 kilobases (kb). In contrast, traditional karyotyping typically identifies alterations larger than 5 to 10 megabases (Mb). [17, 18]. However, the accuracy in finding a loss or gain by microarray depends on the density and coverage of the probes in that particular region.

Both aCGH and SNP arrays are effective in detecting chromosomal aneuploidies, as well as segmental deletions and duplications. In addition to identifying copy number alterations, SNP arrays can identify regions with CN-LOH, and better characterize complex copy number changes [19]. The combination of higher resolution and enhanced genomic coverage offered by both types of platforms significantly improves diagnostic yield over traditional karyotyping. Furthermore, microarrays are utilized to enhance the detection of smaller copy number alterations in cancer, which is crucial for diagnosis, prognosis, and sometimes for determining appropriate treatment strategies [20]. CMA may also be useful to clarify the origin of derivative chromosomes, chromosomes with poor morphology, and marker chromosomes.

One limitation of microarray technology is its inability to detect balanced structural chromosomal alterations, such as Robertsonian translocations, reciprocal translocations, and inversions. In certain cancers, particularly leukemias and lymphomas where specific translocations play a critical role in disease progression, other techniques should be employed to identify these balanced structural variants.

Furthermore, microarrays lack the sensitivity required to detect low-level mosaicism, typically below 10–20% [15]. Consequently, microarray testing may not be as effective for monitoring changes during cancer treatment or during periods of remission. Lastly, it is important to note that microarrays rely on pre-defined probes to identify known genetic copy number variants. As a result, any alterations that lack corresponding probes on the microarray platform will not be detectable [2].

Consideration of Microarray Platform Choice for Detection of Acquired Genomic Aberrations

The ACMG published a set of guidelines to assist clinical laboratories in validation of microarray, proper use, and interpretation and reporting of results [6]. Identification of clinically significant chromosomal imbalances is dependent on the design and resolution (resolution varies from several thousand to several million probes) of the microarray platform utilized. Any imbalance exceeding the established minimum consecutive probe number showing a loss or a gain of genomic material is expected to be detectable by the microarray platform. The minimum number of probes required to ensure reliable detection of a gain or loss within a designated region of interest—specifically, a region with a cancer gene—should be determined by each laboratory. If the employed platform lacks adequate coverage of these regions, this limitation should be clearly indicated in the report.

In diagnostic cases, where microarray analysis is considered as a substitute for a FISH panel in copy number testing, it is essential to validate the probe density of the genomic regions targeted by the FISH panels. Additionally, the software parameters and cut-off values should be established by hybridizing positive controls whenever possible prior to offering array analysis as a clinical test. The validation set should include samples for which clinical testing will be provided. Furthermore, small aberrations involving well-characterized genes known to be important prognostic indicators, and clearly associated with the specific cancer type, must be thoroughly investigated [21].

In cancer samples, the presence of both neoplastic and non-neoplastic cells can complicate the identification of genetically abnormal neoplastic cells, particularly when detecting small genomic aberrations within mixed cell populations. Typically, the detection threshold for mosaicism or low-level clonal abnormalities via microarray analysis is approximately 10–20%. The sensitivity for detecting abnormalities is generally influenced by factors such as the level of clonality, the size of the abnormality, and the extent of probe coverage (including both oligonucleotide and SNP probes) over the affected region. Larger abnormalities are typically more readily identified at lower levels of clonality (approximately 10%) [22, 23]. Conversely, smaller copy number alterations with limited probe coverage may pose challenges for detection at a 10% clonality level. Consequently, establishing the detection sensitivity for low-level clonal changes is crucial and should be disclosed by the testing laboratory [22].

Laboratories must develop expertise in identifying low levels of clonality, data interpretation, and determining their cut-off levels by validating the array platform with appropriate positive controls through blind analysis. Positive controls should consist of representative samples with defined percentages of the targeted anomaly, for example as determined by interphase FISH analysis conducted on uncultured samples [24]. Moreover, to detect smaller size imbalances, an array platform with probes enriched in genes known to influence patient management is needed. For detection of CN-LOH, it is recommended to utilize an array platform containing SNP probes. However, the ability to detect CN-LOH may vary based on the specific type of abnormality and the blast percentage [25–27]. Therefore, it is also essential to validate the platform's performance for CN-LOH detection using samples that exhibit well-characterized regions with CN-LOH.

Furthermore, laboratories should recognize the limitations of the algorithms utilized in the software packages, which may lack sufficient sensitivity to accurately detect low-level clonal events while generating a significant number of false positives. Therefore, it is essential to conduct visual inspections and manual review of the data to identify aberrations that may be present in a clonal state.

Microarray Data Interpretation

Microarray data interpretation for acquired genetic anomalies differs from that of constitutional abnormalities. In the context of neoplasia, microarray analysis often reveals numerous genomic alterations. The interpretation of these acquired genomic alterations in a routine clinical diagnostic setting requires a solid understanding of clinically relevant abnormalities tied to the pathology diagnosis. This knowledge is essential for producing clear and comprehensible reports that highlight pertinent recurrent and prognostic genetic markers. In addition, it is essential to recognize possible constitutional abnormalities and indicate those in the final report. While utilizing a matched germline DNA sample can help differentiate acquired abnormalities from constitutional abnormalities, thereby easing interpretation, it can be challenging for many diagnostic laboratories to simultaneously obtain constitutional normal DNA from the patient along with neoplastic samples.

In 2019, the ACMG and the Cancer Genomics Consortium (CGC) proposed technical laboratory standards for the interpretation and reporting of acquired copy number abnormalities and CN-LOH in neoplastic disorders [28]. The system includes a four-tier evidence-based categorization, which is based on the level of available evidence for acquired copy number alterations and CN-LOH regarding their diagnostic, prognostic, and therapeutic relevance: Tier 1, clonal variants with strong clinical significance; Tier 2, clonal variants with some clinical significance; Tier 3, clonal variants with no documented neoplastic disease association; and Tier 4, benign or likely benign variants. The document emphasizes that the interpretation of the clinical significance of copy number alterations and CN-LOH through this tier system should be conducted in conjunction with the clinical and pathological diagnoses, as well as other laboratory assessments, including G-banded karyotyping, FISH, and any other relevant tests.

Tier 1 variants with strong diagnostic, prognostic, and/or therapeutic clinical significance are further subdivided into Tier 1A and Tier 1B. Tier 1A includes germline pathogenic variants associated with cancer predisposition or acquired variants that are either defined in the World Health Organization (WHO) classification of hematopoietic and lymphoid neoplasms [29], included in professional guidelines as clinically significant variants, and/or can be treated with a targeted Food and Drug Administration (FDA) approved drug. Tier 1B are acquired variants associated with a specific neoplasm, prognosis, or treatment response as shown by high- or good-quality evidence with expert consensus and/or confirmed and reproduced by independent groups. Tier 2 variants with some diagnostic, prognostic, and/or therapeutic clinical significance include both recurrent variants observed in different neoplasms but are not specific to a particular tumor type, and variants associated with specific neoplasm, prognosis, or treatment response with average-quality evidence with expert consensus and/or confirmed and reproduced by independent groups. Tier 3 variants with no documented neoplastic disorder association include all variants that do not meet criteria for Tier 1 or 2 and cannot be classified as constitutional benign or likely benign. Lastly, Tier 4 are constitutional benign or likely benign variants that are not listed in the ClinGen curated benign variants and/or the Database of Genomic Variants (DGV) or gnomAD database with greater than or equal to 1% population frequency [28].

The analysis of microarray data from patients with hematological malignancies necessitates a thorough examination of the entire genome to accurately call ploidy, copy number alterations, and CN-LOH across varying levels of clonality. To reliably identify clinically significant alterations, visual inspection and manual review of the data are strongly recommended [11].

To facilitate and standardize the interpretation of these complex samples, the following workflow is recommended:

1. Conduct a comprehensive review of the entire genome to evaluate the log2 ratio alongside the allele frequency track for each chromosome, with the objective of determining ploidy and identifying any specific chromosomal aneuploidies. The combined log2 ratio and allelic differentiation plots derived from arrays containing SNPs can provide valuable insights into subclonal populations and ploidy levels. To accurately identify clinically significant alterations, it is advisable to conduct visual inspections and manual review of the data.
2. Analyze each chromosome individually to identify any low-level whole or large segmental copy number gains or losses, as well as CN-LOH.
3. Analyze each chromosome individually to identify any small segmental copy number gains or losses, as well as CN-LOH. Incorporating gene tracks to highlight regions significant to leukemia development is highly advantageous.
4. Carefully review breakpoints of interstitial or terminal losses or gains involving two chromosome arms with breakpoints within genes known to be associated with a specific gene fusion because of an interchromosomal rearrangement. In

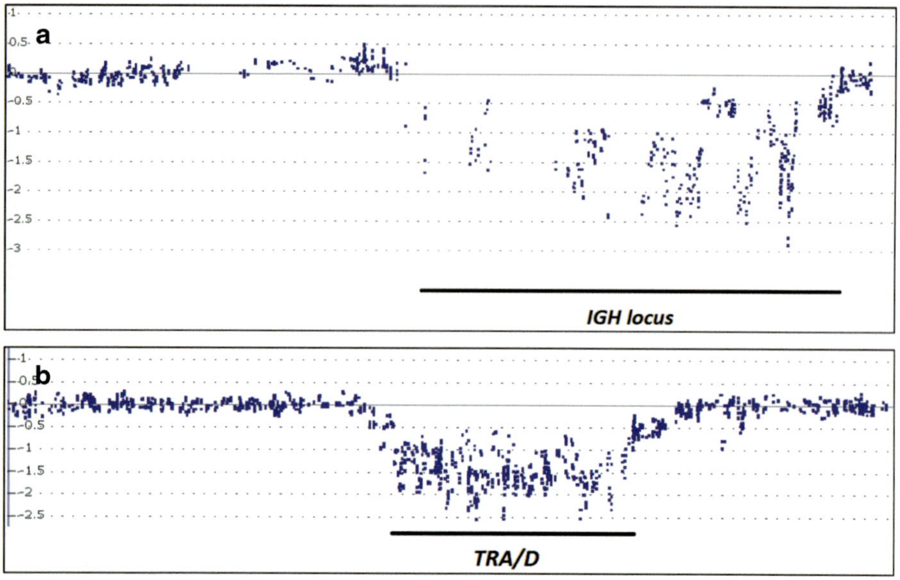

Fig. 4.3 Example of a biallelic loss (**a**) within *IGH* locus at 14q13.33, and (**b**) within *TRA/D* locus at 14q11.2. These changes are consistent with a clonal process; however, they may not necessarily indicate gene rearrangement. If these changes are to be documented in the clinical report, it is recommended to note that these losses represent clonal events

the presence of a suspected fusion, the report should describe the possibility of a gene fusion without classifying the variants using the tier system until the fusion is confirmed by other techniques.

5. Focal monoallelic copy number alterations in T-cell receptor or immunoglobulin genes need to be reviewed carefully, as these typically represent non-leukemic genomic rearrangements that occur during normal T-cell and B-cell development. However, biallelic losses in T-cell receptors and *IGH* genes indicate clonal events, although these may not be consistent with gene rearrangements (Fig. 4.3a, b).
6. Regions of CN-LOH should be manually reviewed as clonal changes may not be flagged by the analysis software. CN-LOH may have a higher level of clinical significance if they span a gain-of-function variant in an oncogene and/or loss-of-function variant in a tumor suppressor gene. This is especially important for integrated reporting of copy number alterations, regions of CN-LOH, and sequence-level variants results.

To establish microarray analysis as a standard diagnostic procedure for evaluating acquired hematological disorders, laboratories must implement a robust analytical and interpretive algorithm that accurately characterizes a broad spectrum of abnormalities identified via this modality. It is essential to develop comprehensive standard operating procedures for all stages of sample processing, based on both internal validation and established published guidelines. Additionally, laboratories must participate annually in a relevant proficiency testing or external quality assessment program.

Application of Clinical Microarray in Pediatric Leukemia: Special Considerations for Copy Number Analysis and Copy-Neutral Loss of Heterozygosity

In oncology, microarray testing serves as a reliable genome-wide technique for high-resolution chromosomal DNA analysis. Although major limitations need to be taken into consideration, microarray technology provides quick turnaround times that can facilitate timely diagnosis, subtyping, and prognostic predictions for some leukemia cases.

Pediatric Leukemia

Leukemia is the most frequently occurring cancer in children, making up 30% of all childhood cancer cases. Pediatric leukemia primarily includes four types: acute lymphoblastic leukemia (ALL), acute myelogenous leukemia (AML), chronic leukemia (chronic myelogenous leukemia (CML) and Juvenile Myelomonocytic Leukemia (JMML)), and mixed phenotype acute leukemia (MPAL). ALL is the most common, accounting for about 80% of cases, and involves abnormalities in lymphoid progenitor cells [30]. The WHO categorizes ALL into two primary subtypes based on the immunophenotyping of leukemia cells: B-cell acute lymphoblastic leukemia/lymphoma (B-ALL) and T-cell acute lymphoblastic leukemia/lymphoma (T-ALL). B-ALL is significantly more prevalent than T-ALL, representing about 80% of all ALL cases [31]. AML makes up 18% of childhood leukemia cases, while CML is very rare and typically appears in adolescents [32]. JMML is a rare, aggressive type of leukemia that accounts for about 1% to 3% of all pediatric leukemia cases and primarily found in infants or toddlers. MPAL is rare in children and is characterized by the presence of malignant blasts that express both myeloid and lymphoid antigens [33]. Identifying genetic abnormalities in leukemic cells is crucial for detecting unfavorable genetic markers and incorporating targeted therapies to lower the risk of relapse [34, 35].

In cases where a well-characterized fusion gene, indicative of a specific neoplastic disorder, serves as a prognostic indicator—common in B-ALL, T-ALL, AML, and CML—it is essential to recognize that microarray analysis should be utilized at diagnosis as an adjunct to established methodologies, such as conventional karyotyping, FISH, or reverse transcription-polymerase chain reaction (RT-PCR). This approach avoids the need for cell culture and mitigates issues related to clone selection resulting from cell proliferation. Due to 10–20% sensitivity to detect clonal events, the technique is not used to monitor minimal residual disease in a patient post treatment.

Examples of Interpretations of the Clinically Significant Copy Number Alterations and Copy-Neutral Loss of Heterozygosity Identified by Microarray in Pediatric Leukemia

B-Cell Acute Lymphoblastic Leukemia

B-ALL is the most prevalent childhood hematological cancer and is characterized by the malignant transformation of B-lymphoid progenitor cells. It is more prevalent in boys than in girls, with a male-to-female ratio of approximately 1.2:1. The peak incidence occurs between the ages of 2 and 5 years. Advances in treatment, particularly with the use of intensified chemotherapy, have significantly improved outcomes, resulting in increased overall survival for pediatric patients. However, relapse is observed in around 20% of children and is linked to a high rate of treatment failure and mortality, especially when it occurs within the first 18 months of therapy. Relapse remains the leading cause of cancer-related mortality in children and young adults [36].

Cytogenetic alterations and molecular abnormalities are commonly observed in B-ALL, and numerous molecular markers have been identified to help stratify risk and predict prognosis, as they are integral to the pathogenesis of this malignancy. These include chromosomal aneuploidy, copy number alterations, gene rearrangements, and sequence-level variants. Microarray analysis becomes an important accompanying test to detect clonal copy number alterations and ploidy changes.

High hyperdiploidy (more than 50 chromosomes) is observed in up to 30% of childhood B-ALL and is generally linked to favorable prognostic outcomes, especially in cases with double trisomy of chromosomes 4 and 10 [37] (Fig. 4.4). Low hypodiploidy (31–39 chromosomes) and near haploidy (24–30 chromosomes) are present in approximately 1% of children with B-ALL and are associated with unfavorable outcomes. The prevalence of hypodiploidy may be underestimated due to the occurrence of "masked" hypodiploidy, where hypodiploid genome undergoes duplication, resulting in a hyperdiploid modal chromosome number. Distinguishing

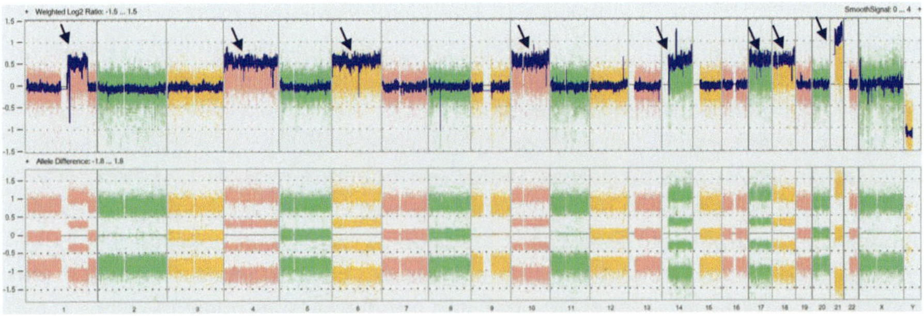

Fig. 4.4 An example of a hyperdiploid B-cell acute lymphoblastic leukemia (B-ALL) microarray profile is presented, which demonstrates an increase in chromosomal material on chromosome 1q, as well as the complete gain of chromosomes 4, 6, 10, 14, 17, 18, and 21

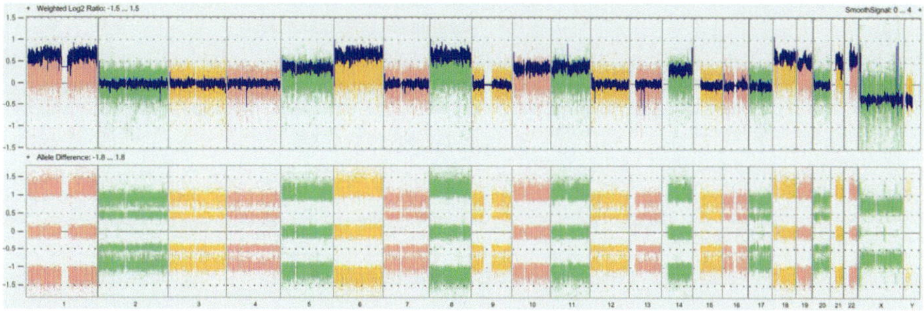

Fig. 4.5 Illustration of the copy-neutral loss of heterozygosity for chromosomes 2, 3, 4, 7, 9, 12, 13, 15, 16, 17, and 20, accompanied by a gain of the remaining chromosomes, including two copies each of chromosomes X and Y, and three to four copies of the other autosomes. This observed signal pattern is consistent with doubled low hypodiploidy

masked-hypodiploid ALL from high-hyperdiploid ALL is important in terms of the genetic and prognostic implications. Masked hypodiploidy may be indicated by specific patterns of chromosomal gain, typically showing two and four copies of chromosomes instead of three copies, as observed in high-hyperdiploid B-ALL [38]. While chromosome and FISH analysis may indicate the presence of a hypodiploid clone, only SNP microarrays can definitively confirm hypodiploid clones by detecting chromosomal LOH [39, 40] (Fig. 4.5).

While hyperdiploidy is typically associated with good outcomes, when identified concurrently with *IKZF1* loss, it is associated with poor response to treatment and higher chance of relapse [41]. Deletions of *IKZF1* can be visualized on microarray platform. The most common alterations include whole gene deletions and deletions of exons 4–7 or exons 4–8, resulting in loss of IKZF1 function [42] (Fig. 4.6a, b). Additionally, *IKZF1* losses together with homozygous *CDKN2A/CDKN2B* deletion, and/or *PAX5* deletion, have been reported to be associated with inferior outcome compared with *IKZF1* alterations alone [43] (Fig. 4.7a, b).

Similarly, the loss of *CSF2RA* and *IL3RA*, indicative of the *PPR2Y8::CRLF2* fusion, loss of *EBF1*, and loss of *RB1,* which may appear as focal deletions, have also been associated with a poor outcome [44, 45]. The *PPR2Y8::CRLF2* is typically identifiable by microarray platform as an ~300 kb intragenic deletion that increases CRLF2 expression as a result of juxtaposition of the entire coding sequence of *CRLF2* with the first non-coding exon of *P2RY8* (Fig. 4.8).

Another common B-ALL subtype includes cases with t(12;21)(p13;q22) which results in the *ETV6::RUNX1* gene fusion. When present in a balanced state, this fusion cannot be detected by microarray technology. Based on a positive molecular response to treatment and clinical outcomes, this rearrangement is generally considered to be a favorable prognostic indicator [46]. However, late relapses occur in up to 20% of patients. The other common genetic changes in the *ETV6* and *RUNX1* genes are an extra copy of *RUNX1* and/or an extra der(21)t(12;21). Approximately 20% of the t(12;21)-positive patients have more than one additional genetic change in *ETV6* or *RUNX1*. Additionally, *ETV6::RUNX1*-positive ALL patients have an

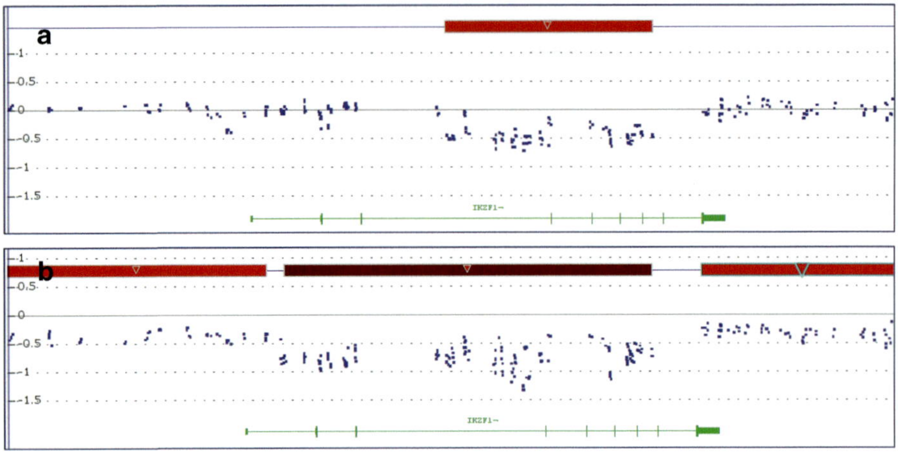

Fig. 4.6 Examples of focal *IKZF1* deletions in B-ALL cases: (**a**) an ~44 kb loss includes exons 4 through 6 of *IKZF1* (transcript NM_006060.6); (**b**) an ~78 kb loss includes exons 2 through 6 of *IKZF1*. Regions lacking probe coverage hinder the precise identification of deletion boundaries and should be taken into account when analyzing segmental losses on a microarray platform

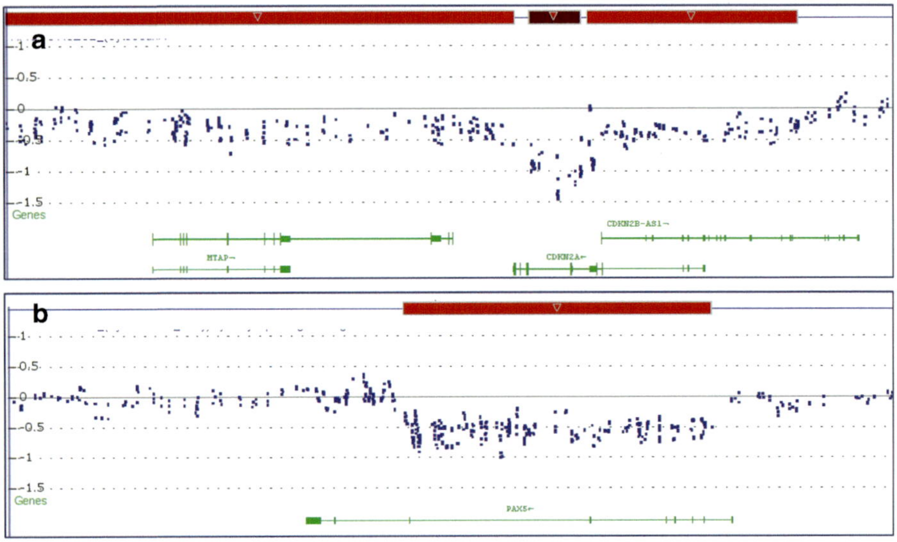

Fig. 4.7 (**a**) Example of a loss within 9p21.3 (~2 Mb) with a nested ~23 kb biallelic loss involving the *CDKN2A* gene. (**b**) Example of a loss at 9p13.2 containing exons 2–8 of *PAX5* (NM_016734.3, total 10 exons)

average of ~4 additional copy number alterations. Among these, several are recurrent deletions in genes controlling B-cell lineage differentiation, cell cycle, or nuclear hormone response. The deletion of 12p is the most common abnormality that includes the loss of wild-type *ETV6* allele. The 9p deletion can be seen in up to

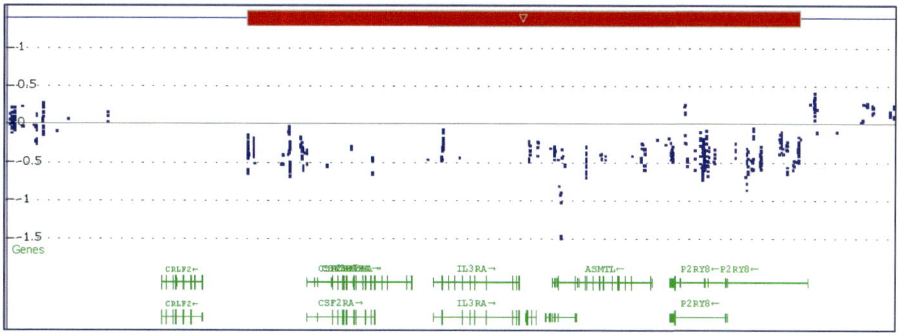

Fig. 4.8 The PR2Y8::CRLF2 rearrangement results from an interstitial microdeletion in the pseudoautosomal region 1, which is located in the short arm of both sex chromosomes. This deletion causes the CRLF2 overexpression through the juxtaposition of the entire coding sequence of *CRLF2* with the first non-coding exon of *P2RY8*, and their transcriptional control elements that are highly active in lymphoid cells. Microarray platform does notdifferentiate between the rearrangements on the X or Y chromosome

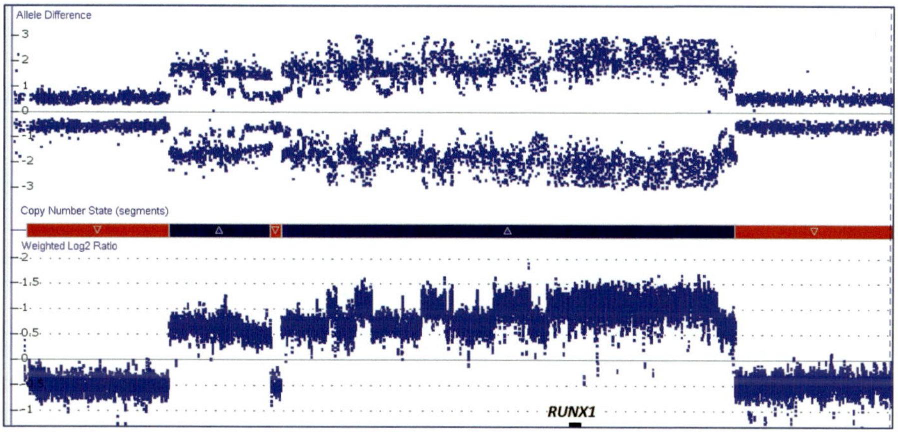

Fig. 4.9 Microarray profile for chromosome 21 showing areas of losses and gains, including amplification of a region containing *RUNX1*, a typical pattern observed in *RUNX1* amplified cases

25% of *ETV6::RUNX1*-positive patients, and it often affects the tumor suppressor *CDKN2A/CDKN2B* and the B-cell differentiation regulator *PAX5*. These changes are important to identify at diagnosis as they appear to be linked to a higher rate of disease relapse [47].

B-ALL with intrachromosomal amplification of chromosome 21 (iAMP21) is a rare abnormality, most commonly observed in older children, and is associated with poor prognosis, which has been improved with intensive treatment (Fig. 4.9). iAMP21, which is defined as the presence of five or more total copies of *RUNX1*, with three or more extra RUNX1 signals on a single abnormal chromosome 21, was first detected by FISH using the ETV6/RUNX1 probe. However, the cytogenetic heterogeneity of the iAMP21 marker chromosomes can be uncovered using microarray, particularly demonstrating that this technique is helpful for the detection of this entity when FISH results are ambiguous [48]. Similarly, B-ALL with *PAX5* amplifications, which encodes a transcription factor required for normal B-cell development, are associated with increased relapse risk in B-ALL [49]. Microarray typically detects a significant elevation in the log2 ratio consistent with high-level copy number gain of *PAX5*.

In B-ALL, many other genomic subtypes include recurrent chromosomal rearrangements, ex. involving the *KMT2A* gene. These are typically balanced and will not be identified by microarray. One of the other rearrangements, *TCF3::PBX1*, t(1;19)(p13.3;q23) may present in the balanced or unbalanced form. The unbalanced translocations resulting in 1q23qter gain and 19p13.3pter loss are associated with fewer relapses compared with those with balanced translocations [47] and are important to identify using microarray analysis adjunct to FISH testing using the TCF3 probe (Fig. 4.10).

T-Cell Acute Lymphoblastic Leukemia

Pediatric T-ALL exhibits recurrent genetic alterations in multiple pathways with no clear link to outcomes, unlike B-ALL. The three main pathways that appear to be deregulated in T-ALL include the expression of T-lineage transcription factors, *NOTCH1/MYC* signaling, and cell-cycle control pathways [50]. While many recurrent rearrangements are not detected by microarray, some alterations are detectable by this technology. Given that conventional karyotype analysis in T-ALL is often hampered by suboptimal chromosome morphology, low lymphoblast mitotic activity, and inability to detect subtle abnormalities, microarray analysis may be useful to detect several T-ALL-related recurrent changes. The most common submicroscopic deletion is observed at the 9p21.3 region, which harbors tumor suppressor genes *CDKN2A/CDKN2B*. These deletions can either be monoallelic or biallelic. *CDKN2A* losses are typically more frequent compared to *CDKN2B* losses in T-ALL patients [51].

A deletion of approximately 80 kb in the 1p33 region results in the *STIL::TAL1* fusion, which positions *TAL1* under the regulation of the *STIL* promoter, leading to its overexpression (Fig. 4.11). *PTEN* losses, typically ~500 kb in size, at 10q23.31, varying in size, have been linked to PTEN–PI3K–AKT pathway deregulation by disrupting the phosphatase domain of *PTEN* and are associated with a more adverse therapeutic consequence [52].

A recurrent gain of the 13q31.2q31.3 region (at least 5 Mb in size) involving microRNA (miRNA) cluster miR-17–92 appears to promote leukemogenesis in *NOTCH1*-induced T-ALL in vivo [53].

A cryptic deletion of 11p was initially discovered by aCGH in about 4% of pediatric patients with T-ALL [54]. The localization of genomic breakpoints in the deletion is heterogeneous. In most del(11p) cases, the oncogene *LMO2* is activated independent from other recurrent cytogenetic abnormalities that are frequently

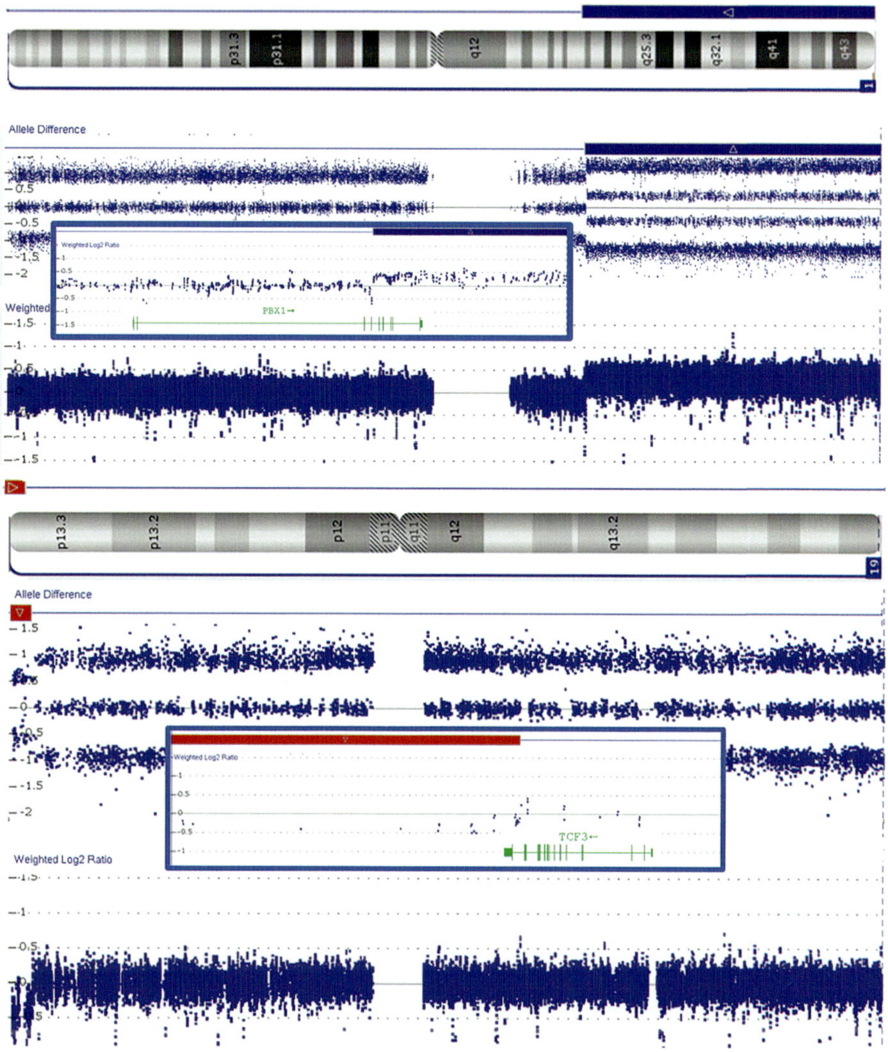

Fig. 4.10 The unbalanced translocation resulting in the *TCF3::PBX1* fusion shows gain of the 1q23 to 1qter region and loss of the 19p13.3 to 19pter region. Zoomed in boxed images show the duplication breaking in the *PBX1* gene and the deletion in the *TCF3* gene

present in T-ALL. When analyzing T-ALL microarray data, it is important to review regulatory sequences upstream of *LMO2* as their loss contributes to ectopic expression and disease pathogenesis [55].

Some T-ALL cases appear to have copy number alterations and CN-LOH that are important in T-ALL leukemogenesis; however, their exact role in disease is unclear [56, 57]. These include biallelic losses of T-cell receptor and *IGH* loci biallelic losses as well as CN-LOH of 6p involving *HLA-I* loci (Fig. 4.12).

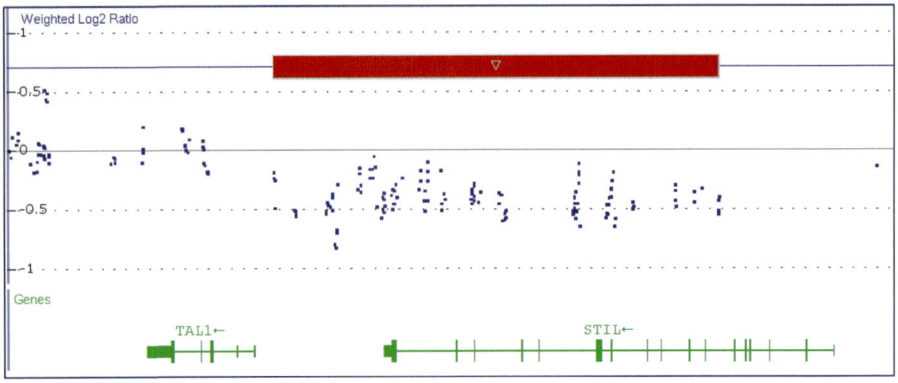

Fig. 4.11 A deletion of approximately 63 kb in the 1p33 region, resulting in the *STIL::TAL1* fusion, positions *TAL1* under the regulation of the *STIL* promoter, which in turn leads to its overexpression. While the deletion associated with this fusion appears typical on microarray, the specific breakpoints of the deletion cannot be accurately defined identified due to significant gaps at both ends of the deletion

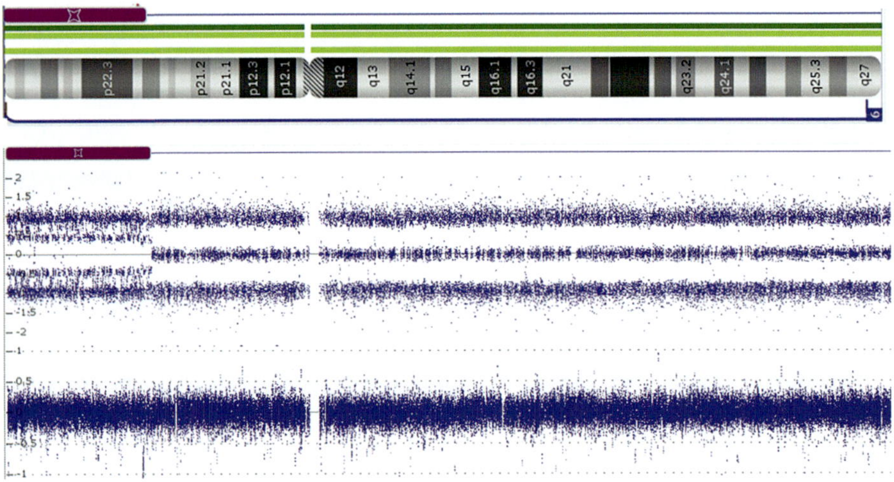

Fig. 4.12 Somatic copy-neutral loss of heterozygosity (CN-LOH) for chromosome 6p contains the *HLA-I* locus that codes for the major histocompatibility complex (MHC) class I molecule. This aberration may arise from selective pressure to escape immune surveillance through deletion of *HLA* alleles. CN-LOH of 6p involving *HLA-I* genes can cause a simultaneous loss of all three *HLA-I* genes leading to loss of HLA haplotype. This is a frequent mechanism that reduces the variety of tumor antigens presented to T-cells, which may subsequently affect the efficacy of cancer immunotherapy

Acute Myeloid Leukemia

Approximately 50–60% of newly diagnosed AML patients present with cytogenetic abnormalities. According to the WHO-2022 classification, AML can be categorized into two groups: (1) AML with defining chromosomal abnormalities and (2) AML defined by differentiation [58]. Common genetic abnormalities include translocationst(15;17)(q24.1;q21.1)), t(8;21)(q22;q22), t(9;22), t(6;9), t(1;22), t(8;16), t(7;11), t(12;22), t(16;21), inversions involving chromosome 16, inv(16)(p13.1q22), or 3, inv(3)(q21q26.2), and translocations involving *KMT2A* at 11q23 [59, 60]. These events are typically balanced in nature and are not detectable by microarray analysis. Some are unbalanced and can be easily detected by microarray. However, the detected imbalances in the absence of FISH, chromosome, or other molecular testing may not necessarily indicate a translocation or an inversion (Fig. 4.13). AML with myelodysplastic syndrome (MDS)-related changes typically harbor monosomies or deletions of part or all of chromosomes 5 or 7, trisomy 8, monosomy of chromosome 17/del 17p, and loss of 11q, 13q, or 20q [61]. These changes are detectable by microarray that can define precise breakpoints and better characterize changes in a complex karyotype. While rare, amplifications of *MYC* and *KMT2A* in the form of double minutes, ring and marker chromosomes, or homogenously staining regions have been found in AML cases in association with poor prognosis [62, 63]. In the absence of FISH probes, these abnormalities can be detected by microarray.

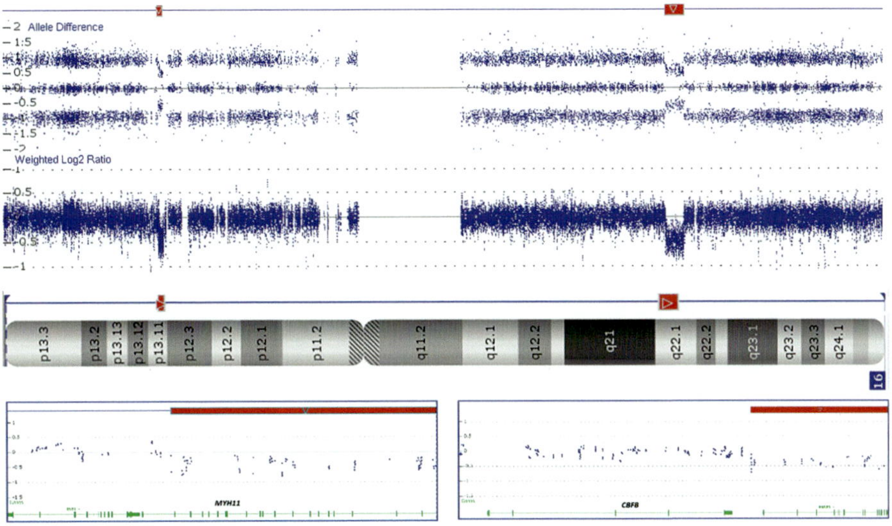

Fig. 4.13 Loss in the 16p13.11 region (~0.5 Mb), which includes the 5′ portion of the *MYH11* gene, and loss in the 16q22.1 region (~1.8 Mb), which appears to be directly downstream of the *CBFB* gene. Given the diagnosis of AML with eosinophilia, the identified losses may support a possible fusion between *CBFB* and *MYH11*; however, they do not directly show that. Additional testing is required to confirm *MYH11::CBFB* fusion

Mixed Phenotype Acute Leukemia

MPALis a rare hematological malignancy in children, accounting for less than 5% of pediatric acute leukemias. MPAL is heterogeneous and can exhibit myeloid, T-cell, and B-cell lineage markers. By integrating genotypic and phenotypic diagnostic criteria, the disease has been classified into three subgroups. This classification is based on the presence of the t(9;22)(q34.1;q11.2)/*BCR::ABL1* rearrangement, chromosomal abnormalities at band 11q23 that result in the rearrangement of the *KMT2A* gene, and the immunophenotype of the leukemic cells, which includes their combinations of myeloid, B-cell, and T-cell lineage markers [29]. The balanced *BCR::ABL1* and *KMT2A* rearrangements will not be detectable by microarray testing. Nevertheless, cytogenetic alterations are frequent and predominantly associated with complex karyotype involving chromosome 21 abnormalities [64]. In these instances, microarray analysis can significantly aid in resolving complex chromosomal changes. MPAL is typically treated with high-risk leukemia protocols [33]. Microarray analysis serves as an important adjunct to detect small copy number alterations involving B-cell and T-cell development genes as well.

Conclusion

Chromosome and FISH analyses play a crucial role in identifying abnormalities within individual cells, offering insights into clonal evolution and heterogeneity, which are significant indicators of disease progression. Unlike chromosome analysis, which depends on the mitotic index, microarray analysis examines DNA extracted from pooled cells, thus providing a comprehensive snapshot of copy number alterations and CN-LOH in a single assay. The relationship between cytogenetics and molecular analysis is continuously advancing, with microarray analysis being recognized as the standard of care in the routine evaluation of pediatric hematological cancers.

References

1. Schena M, Shalon D, Davis RW, et al. Quantitative monitoring of gene expression patterns with a complementary DNA microarray. Science. 1995;270:467–70. https://doi.org/10.1126/science.270.5235.467.
2. Bumgarner R. Overview of DNA microarrays: types, applications, and their future. Curr Protoc Mol Biol. 2013. Chapter 22:Unit 22.1. https://doi.org/10.1002/0471142727.mb2201s101.
3. Trevino V, Falciani F, Barrera-Saldaña HA. DNA microarrays: a powerful genomic tool for biomedical and clinical research. Mol Med. 2007;9–10:527–41. https://doi.org/10.2119/2006-00107.Trevino.
4. Miller DT, Adam MP, Aradhya S, et al. Consensus statement: chromosomal microarray is a first-tier clinical diagnostic test for individuals with developmental disabilities or congenital anomalies. Am J Hum Genet. 2010;86(5):749–64. https://doi.org/10.1016/j.ajhg.2010.04.006.
5. Manning M, Hudgins L, Professional Practice and Guidelines Committee. Array-based technology and recommendations for utilization in medical genetics practice for detec-

tion of chromosomal abnormalities. Genet Med. 2010;11:742–5. https://doi.org/10.1097/GIM.0b013e3181f8baad.
6. Cooley LD, Lebo M, Li MM, et al. American College of Medical Genetics and Genomics technical standards and guidelines: microarray analysis for chromosome abnormalities in neoplastic disorders. Genet Med. 2013;15(6):484–94. https://doi.org/10.1038/gim.2013.49.
7. D'Angelo G, Di Rienzo T, Ojetti V. Microarray analysis in gastric cancer: a review. World J Gastroenterol. 2014;20(34):11972–6. https://doi.org/10.3748/wjg.v20.i34.11972.
8. Virtanen C, Woodgett J. Clinical uses of microarrays in cancer research. Methods Mol Med. 2008;141:87–113. https://doi.org/10.1007/978-1-60327-148-6_6.
9. Song J, Shao H. SNP array in hematopoietic neoplasms: a review. Microarrays (Basel). 2015;5(1):1. https://doi.org/10.3390/microarrays5010001.
10. Perez-Diez A, Morgun A, Shulzhenko N. Microarrays for cancer diagnosis and classification. In: Madame Curie bioscience database [Internet]. Austin: Landes Bioscience; 2000–2013. Available from: https://www.ncbi.nlm.nih.gov/books/NBK6624/.
11. Peterson JF, Aggarwal N, Smith CA, et al. Integration of microarray analysis into the clinical diagnosis of hematological malignancies: how much can we improve cytogenetic testing? Oncotarget. 2015;6(22):18845–62. https://doi.org/10.18632/oncotarget.4586.
12. Wilson CH, Tsykin A, Wilkinson CR, et al. Experimental design and analysis of microarray data. Appl Mycol Biotechnol. 2006;6:1–36. https://doi.org/10.1016/S1874-5334(06)80004-3.
13. Chi M, Rodgers L, Brady A, et al. Representational oligonucleotide microarray analysis: a high-resolution method to detect genome copy number variation. Genome Res. 2003;10:2291–305. https://doi.org/10.1101/gr.1349003.
14. Bi W, Borgan C, Pursley AN, et al. Comparison of chromosome analysis and chromosomal microarray analysis: what is the value of chromosome analysis in today's genomic array era? Genet Med. 2013;6:450–7. https://doi.org/10.1038/gim.2012.152.
15. Shaffer LG. The principles of clinical cytogenetics. 2013. p. 441–50.
16. Wang Y, Carlton VE, Karlin-Neumann G, et al. High quality copy number and genotype data from FFPE samples using Molecular Inversion Probe (MIP) microarrays. BMC Med Genet. 2009;2:8. https://doi.org/10.1186/1755-8794-2-8.
17. Carter NP. Methods and strategies for analyzing copy number variation using DNA microarrays. Nat Genet. 2007;39(7 Suppl):S16–21. https://doi.org/10.1038/ng2028.
18. Martin CL, Warburton D. Detection of chromosomal aberrations in clinical practice: from karyotype to genome sequence. Annu Rev Genomics Hum Genet. 2015;16:309–26. https://doi.org/10.1146/annurev-genom-090413-025346.
19. Coughlin CR 2nd, Scharer GH, Shaikh TH. Clinical impact of copy number variation analysis using high-resolution microarray technologies: advantages, limitations and concerns. Genome Med. 2012;4(10):80. https://doi.org/10.1186/gm381.
20. Liu L, So A, Fan J. Analysis of cancer genomes through microarrays and next-generation sequencing. Transl Cancer Res. 2015;4(3):212–8. https://doi.org/10.3978/j.issn.2218-676X.2015.05.04.
21. Mangum DS, Meyer JA, Mason CC, et al. Association of combined focal 22q11.22 deletion and IKZF1 alterations with outcomes in childhood acute lymphoblastic leukemia. JAMA Oncol. 2021;7(10):1521–8. https://doi.org/10.1001/jamaoncol.2021.2723.
22. Schoumans J, Suela J, Hastings R, et al. Guidelines for genomic array analysis in acquired haematological neoplastic disorders. Genes Chromosom Cancer. 2016;55(5):480–91. https://doi.org/10.1002/gcc.22350.
23. Peterson JF, Van Dyke DL, Hoppman NL, et al. The utilization of chromosomal microarray technologies for hematologic neoplasms: an ACLPS critical review. Am J Clin Pathol. 2018;150(5):375–84. https://doi.org/10.1093/ajcp/aqy076.
24. Shao L, Akkari Y, Cooley LD, et al. Chromosomal microarray analysis, including constitutional and neoplastic disease applications, 2021 revision: a technical standard of the American College of Medical Genetics and Genomics (ACMG). Genet Med. 2021;23(10):1818–29. https://doi.org/10.1038/s41436-021-01214-w.

25. Yeung CCS, McElhone S, Chen XY, et al. Impact of copy neutral loss of heterozygosity and total genome aberrations on survival in myelodysplastic syndrome. Mod Pathol. 2018;31(4):569–80. https://doi.org/10.1038/modpathol.2017.157.
26. Sulong S, Moorman AV, Irving JA, et al. A comprehensive analysis of the CDKN2A gene in childhood acute lymphoblastic leukemia reveals genomic deletion, copy number neutral loss of heterozygosity, and association with specific cytogenetic subgroups. Blood. 2009;113(1):100–7. https://doi.org/10.1182/blood-2008-07-166801.
27. O'Keefe C, McDevitt MA, Maciejewski JP. Copy neutral loss of heterozygosity: a novel chromosomal lesion in myeloid malignancies. Blood. 2010;115(14):2731–9. https://doi.org/10.1182/blood-2009-10-201848.
28. Mikhail FM, Biegel JA, Cooley LD, et al. Technical laboratory standards for interpretation and reporting of acquired copy-number abnormalities and copy-neutral loss of heterozygosity in neoplastic disorders: a joint consensus recommendation from the American College of Medical Genetics and Genomics (ACMG) and the Cancer Genomics Consortium (CGC). Genet Med. 2019;21(9):1903–16. https://doi.org/10.1038/s41436-019-0545-7.
29. WHO Classification of Tumours Editorial Board, editor. World Health Organization classification of haematolymphoid tumours. 5th ed. Lyon: IARC; 2024.
30. Kaplan JA. Leukemia in children. Pediatr Rev. 2019;40(7):319–31. https://doi.org/10.1542/pir.2018-0192.
31. Inaba H, Teachey D, Annesley C, et al. Pediatric acute lymphoblastic leukemia, Version 2.2025, NCCN clinical practice guidelines in oncology. J Natl Compr Cancer Netw. 2025;23(2):41–62. https://doi.org/10.6004/jnccn.2025.0006.
32. Puumala SE, Ross JA, Aplenc R, et al. Epidemiology of childhood acute myeloid leukemia. Pediatr Blood Cancer. 2013;60(5):728–33. https://doi.org/10.1002/pbc.24464.
33. Batra S, Ross AJ. Pediatric mixed-phenotype acute leukemia: what's new? Cancers (Basel). 2021;13(18):4658. https://doi.org/10.3390/cancers13184658.
34. Lagunas-Rangel FA, Chávez-Valencia V, Gómez-Guijosa MÁ, et al. Acute myeloid leukemia-genetic alterations and their clinical prognosis. Int J Hematol Oncol Stem Cell Res. 2017;11(4):328–39.
35. Iacobucci I, Mullighan CG. Genetic basis of acute lymphoblastic leukemia. J Clin Oncol. 2017;35(9):975–83. https://doi.org/10.1200/JCO.2016.70.7836.
36. Adomako J, Jiménez-Camacho KE, Correa-Lara MVM, et al. Acute lymphoblastic leukemia relapse: biomarkers, hopes, and challenges. Trends Mol Med. 2025;S1471-4914(25):00107–8. https://doi.org/10.1016/j.molmed.2025.04.005.
37. Paulsson K, Johansson B. High hyperdiploid childhood acute lymphoblastic leukemia. Genes Chromosom Cancer. 2009;48(8):637–60. https://doi.org/10.1002/gcc.20671.
38. Zhang L, Habeebu SSM, Li W. Prognostic and predictive biomarkers in precursor B-cell acute lymphoblastic leukemia. In: Li W, editor. Leukemia [Internet]. Brisbane: Exon Publications; 2022. Chapter 10.
39. Creasey T, Enshaei A, Nebral K, et al. Single nucleotide polymorphism array-based signature of low hypodiploidy in acute lymphoblastic leukemia. Genes Chromosom Cancer. 2021;60(9):604–15. https://doi.org/10.1002/gcc.22956.
40. Choi SM, Papenhausen P, Wertheim G, et al. Near-haploid B lymphoblastic leukemia with an apparent hyperdiploid karyotype: the critical role of SNP analysis in establishing proper diagnosis. J Hematop. 2014;7:27–32. https://doi.org/10.1007/s12308-013-0189-5.
41. Mullighan CG, Su X, Zhang J, et al. Deletion of IKZF1 and prognosis in acute lymphoblastic leukemia. N Engl J Med. 2009;360(5):470–80. https://doi.org/10.1056/NEJMoa0808253.
42. Wang'ondu RW, Ashcraft E, Chang TC, et al. Heterogeneity of IKZF1 genomic alterations and risk of relapse in childhood B-cell precursor acute lymphoblastic leukemia. Leukemia. 2025. https://doi.org/10.1038/s41375-025-02633-3.
43. Stanulla M, Dagdan E, Zaliova M, et al. IKZF1plus defines a new minimal residual disease-dependent very-poor prognostic profile in pediatric B-cell precursor acute lymphoblastic leukemia. J Clin Oncol. 2018;36(12):1240–9. https://doi.org/10.1200/JCO.2017.74.3617.

44. Holmfeldt L, Wei L, Diaz-Flores E, et al. The genomic landscape of hypodiploid acute lymphoblastic leukemia. Nat Genet. 2013;45(3):242–52. https://doi.org/10.1038/ng.2532.
45. Somasundaram R, Jensen CT, Tingvall-Gustafsson J, et al. EBF1 and PAX5 control pro-B cell expansion via opposing regulation of the Myc gene. Blood. 2021;137(22):3037–49. https://doi.org/10.1182/blood.2020009564.
46. Zhang X, Rastogi P, Shah B, et al. B lymphoblastic leukemia/lymphoma: new insights into genetics, molecular aberrations, subclassification and targeted therapy. Oncotarget. 2017;8(39):66728–41. https://doi.org/10.18632/oncotarget.19271.
47. Chang TC, Chen W, Qu C, et al. Genomic determinants of outcome in acute lymphoblastic leukemia. JCO. 2024;42:3491–503. https://doi.org/10.1200/JCO.23.02238.
48. Tsuchiya KD, Davis B, Gardner RA. Is intrachromosomal amplification of chromosome 21 (iAMP21) always intrachromosomal? Cancer Genet. 2017;218–219:10–4. https://doi.org/10.1016/j.cancergen.2017.08.005.
49. Amaral TFD, Villares MD, Blunk CB, et al. Pax5 alterations in children, adolescents and young adults with B-other acute lymphoblsatic leukemia. Hematol Transfus Cell Ther. 2024;46(4):S410–1. https://doi.org/10.1016/j.htct.2024.09.690.
50. Inaba H, Mullighan CG. Pediatric acute lymphoblastic leukemia. Haematologica. 2020;105(11):2524–39. https://doi.org/10.3324/haematol.2020.247031.
51. Mitrakos A, Kattamis A, Katsibardi K, et al. High resolution Chromosomal Microarray Analysis (CMA) enhances the genetic profile of pediatric B-cell acute lymphoblastic leukemia patients. Leuk Res. 2019;83:106177. https://doi.org/10.1016/j.leukres.2019.106177.
52. Martelli AM, Paganelli F, Fazio A, et al. The key roles of PTEN in T-cell acute lymphoblastic leukemia development, progression, and therapeutic response. Cancers (Basel). 2019;11(5):629. https://doi.org/10.3390/cancers11050629.
53. Yu L, Slovak ML, Mannoor K, et al. Microarray detection of multiple recurring submicroscopic chromosomal aberrations in pediatric T-cell acute lymphoblastic leukemia. Leukemia. 2011;25(6):1042–6. https://doi.org/10.1038/leu.2011.33.
54. Van Vlierberghe P, van Grotel M, Beverloo HB, et al. The cryptic chromosomal deletion del(11)(p12p13) as a new activation mechanism of LMO2 in pediatric T-cell acute lymphoblastic leukemia. Blood. 2006;108(10):3520–9. https://doi.org/10.1182/blood-2006-04-019927.
55. Abdulla HD, Alserihi R, Flensburg C, et al. Overexpression of Lmo2 initiates T-lymphoblastic leukemia via impaired thymocyte competition. J Exp Med. 2023;220(6):e20212383. https://doi.org/10.1084/jem.20212383.
56. Lee GT, Chung YJ. Comparison of the copy-neutral loss of heterozygosity identified from whole-exome sequencing data using three different tools. Genomics Inform. 2022;20(1):e4. https://doi.org/10.5808/gi.21066.
57. Tasian SK, Loh ML, Hunger SP. Childhood acute lymphoblastic leukemia: integrating genomics into therapy. Cancer. 2015;121(20):3577–90. https://doi.org/10.1002/cncr.29573.
58. Park HS. What is new in acute myeloid leukemia classification? Blood Res. 2024;59(1):15. https://doi.org/10.1007/s44313-024-00016-8.
59. Foucar K, Anastasi J. Acute myeloid leukemia with recurrent cytogenetic abnormalities. Am J Clin Pathol. 2015;144(1):6–18. https://doi.org/10.1309/AJCPI9C8UILYQTNS.
60. Kumar CC. Genetic abnormalities and challenges in the treatment of acute myeloid leukemia. Genes Cancer. 2011;2(2):95–107. https://doi.org/10.1177/1947601911408076.
61. Snaith O, Poveda-Rogers C, Laczko D, et al. Cytogenetics and genomics of acute myeloid leukemia. Best Pract Res Clin Haematol. 2024;37(1):101533. https://doi.org/10.1016/j.beha.2023.101533.
62. Tang R, Cheng A, Guirales F, et al. c-MYC amplification in AML. J Assoc Genet Technol. 2021;47(4):202–12.
63. Mohamed A. MLL amplification in leukemia. Atlas Genet Cytogenet Oncol Haematol. 2010. Available: http://atlasgeneticsoncology.org/haematological/1547/mll-amplification-in-leukemia.
64. Chang TY, Chen SH, Jaing TH, et al. Cytogenetic aberration in mixed-phenotype acute leukemia in children: a single-center retrospective review. Pediatr Neonatol. 2021;62(1):21–5. https://doi.org/10.1016/j.pedneo.2020.07.016.

Next-Generation Sequencing in Pediatric Leukemia

5

Yang Cao, Kevin E. Fisher, and Ying-Chen Claire Hou

Introduction

Morphologic, immunophenotypic, and genetic criteria are all used to diagnose hematologic malignancies. While chromosome analysis and fluorescence in-situ hybridization (FISH) assays are widely used to detect chromosomal and structural abnormalities, assessment of sequence-based alterations is also needed to provide diagnostic, prognostic, and therapeutic information. Next-generation sequencing (NGS), or massively parallel sequencing, is an overarching term for sequencing technologies that generate enormous volumes of sequencing data by employing a combination of template preparation, sequencing and imaging, and genome alignment and assembly methods [1]. For most clinical molecular laboratories, NGS is essential for obtaining nucleotide-based diagnostic, prognostic, and therapeutic data from blood, bone marrow, and tissue samples for hematologic malignancies. This chapter will highlight established and emerging NGS applications for both myeloid and lymphoid pediatric leukemias, and the similarities and differences in DNA- and RNA-based sequencing approaches. In addition, the chapter will review

Y. Cao
Department of Pathology and Immunology, Washington University School of Medicine, St. Louis, MO, USA
e-mail: cao.yang@wustl.edu

K. E. Fisher (✉)
Department of Pathology, Texas Children's Hospital, Houston, TX, USA

Department of Pathology & Immunology, Baylor College of Medicine, Houston, TX, USA
e-mail: kevin.fisher@bcm.edu

Y.-C. C. Hou
The Steve and Cindy Rasmussen Institute for Genomic Medicine, Nationwide Children's Hospital, Columbus, OH, USA

Department of Pathology and Pediatrics, The Ohio State University, Columbus, OH, USA

W. Li (ed.), *Laboratory Assessments of Pediatric Leukemia*,
https://doi.org/10.1007/978-3-032-26557-9_5

professional guidelines for variant classification for somatic and germline findings and discuss the importance of germline correlation when interpreting sequencing data in pediatric leukemia samples.

NGS Methodology

Various NGS methods and platforms, each with unique strengths and weaknesses, are utilized for oncology applications. However, Illumina and ThermoFisher (Ion Torrent) instruments comprise the majority of sequencing platforms currently used in clinical molecular diagnostics of pediatric leukemia samples [2–5], and thus will be used as illustrative examples in this section. Regardless of the platform used, extracted nucleic acid derived from blood, bone marrow, or other specimens must be "prepared" for NGS testing. The testing process can be partitioned into four main phases: pre-analytic optimization, library preparation, sequencing and data generation, and analysis.

Pre-analytic Optimization

The purpose of the pre-analytic optimization phase is to identify and enrich for the cells of interest (i.e., optimize neoplastic cellularity) and determine the quantity, quality, and suitability of the nucleic acid for NGS. Most clinical NGS oncology assays utilize a minimum blast percentage of approximately 10–20% due to recommendations that clinical assays detect heterozygous mutations at variant allele fraction (VAF) thresholds of at least 5% [6]. In blood and bone marrow samples, neoplastic cell content estimates are typically derived from cell counts, cell differentials, or flow cytometric assessments of blast percentages. Flow cytometry can detect blast percentages at levels approaching 0.01% [7], so false-negative NGS results must be considered when such low-positive samples are tested. Neoplastic cell content estimation in lymphomas, by contrast, is typically performed by scoring a hematoxylin and eosin (H&E)-stained slide from the corresponding formalin-fixed, paraffin-embedded (FFPE) tissue sample. Thus, the College of American Pathology (CAP) recommends that for all tissue-based oncology testing, qualified personnel assess neoplastic cell content prior to nucleic acid extractions to safeguard against potential false-negative results [8]. However, morphologic estimation of tumor percentage is notoriously inconsistent as multiple factors such as admixed normal cells, tumor necrosis, and tumor heterogeneity can all influence tumor cell estimation [9]. Of note, for constitutional (i.e., germline) testing, cellular enrichment is typically not an essential component of the pre-analytic process as all cells are predicted to harbor the genetic alteration(s) of interest.

The amount of nucleic acid required for testing is variable and depends on the library preparation method and sequencing chemistry. However, most assays are optimized for nucleic acid quantities ranging from 100 nanograms for targeting DNA or RNA sequencing to 1000 nanograms for exome and transcriptome sequencing [10, 11]. Nucleic acid yields are directly correlated with the number of cells obtained. Diagnostic blood and bone marrow samples often harbor abundant nucleic acid given that leukemia, by definition, is a proliferation of abnormal leukocytes. Conversely, samples with low cellularity such as fibrotic or post-treatment bone marrows, cytologic preparations, or cerebral spinal fluid specimens may fail to yield sufficient nucleic acid. Another important pre-analytic consideration is the "useability" or "amplifiability" of the nucleic acid. Successful NGS requires intact, double-stranded DNA to amplify nucleic acid and generate library preparations needed for sequencing. Some factors that can affect DNA integrity include heavy metal fixatives, formalin-fixation, decalcification solutions, "old" samples, improper storage conditions, cellular necrosis, and various native and non-native biologic agents [12–14]. Fortunately, blood and bone marrow samples are routinely collected in lavender top (EDTA) tubes which yield high quality, intact DNA for nearly all NGS applications if processed within a reasonable timeframe [15].

Library Preparation

NGS library preparation encompasses the enrichment of the nucleic acid sequences of interest and the conversion of the desired nucleic acid templates into engineered fragments that can be sequenced on the intended sequencing system [16]. Various library preparation methods are available for both DNA and RNA templates, and the selection of the library preparation method depends on the intended sequence to be captured (e.g., targeted panel vs. exome vs. genome) and the sequencing instrument (e.g., Illumina or Ion Torrent). Nevertheless, most library preparation protocols utilize a process of fragmentation, target enrichment, and the addition of sequence-specific adapters [17]. Genes and gene regions with diagnostic, prognostic, or therapeutic significance are targeted for enrichment using amplicon-based or hybrid capture-based approaches. Amplicon-based target enrichment utilizes flanking primer pairs to target and enrich for sequence of interest via polymerase chain reaction (PCR) amplification. Extracted genomic DNA is, thus, fragmented and enriched for selected amplicons with identical start and stop coordinates (Fig. 5.1a). For pediatric leukemia, the ThermoFisher Ion Torrent Oncomine Childhood Cancer [4] and AmpliSeq for Illumina Childhood Cancer [5] assays are commercially available assays that utilize this approach. In contrast, hybrid capture-based approaches require that the nucleic acid fragmentation occurs upfront, either via enzymatic cleavage or sonication, prior to hybridization with various complementary oligonucleotide sequences that overlap the target also known as "probes" or "baits." The binding of the probes to the target allows for the enrichment of the sequence fragments of interest (Fig. 5.1b) [18]. The FoundationOne Heme assay and whole exome sequencing are examples of hybrid capture-based NGS assays used in pediatric leukemia [19, 20].

Amplicon-based target enrichment assays generate abundant sequencing coverage and are ideal for lower-quality samples (e.g., FFPE), low quantities of input DNA, low-level/subclonal variant detection, and/or MRD monitoring. Additionally,

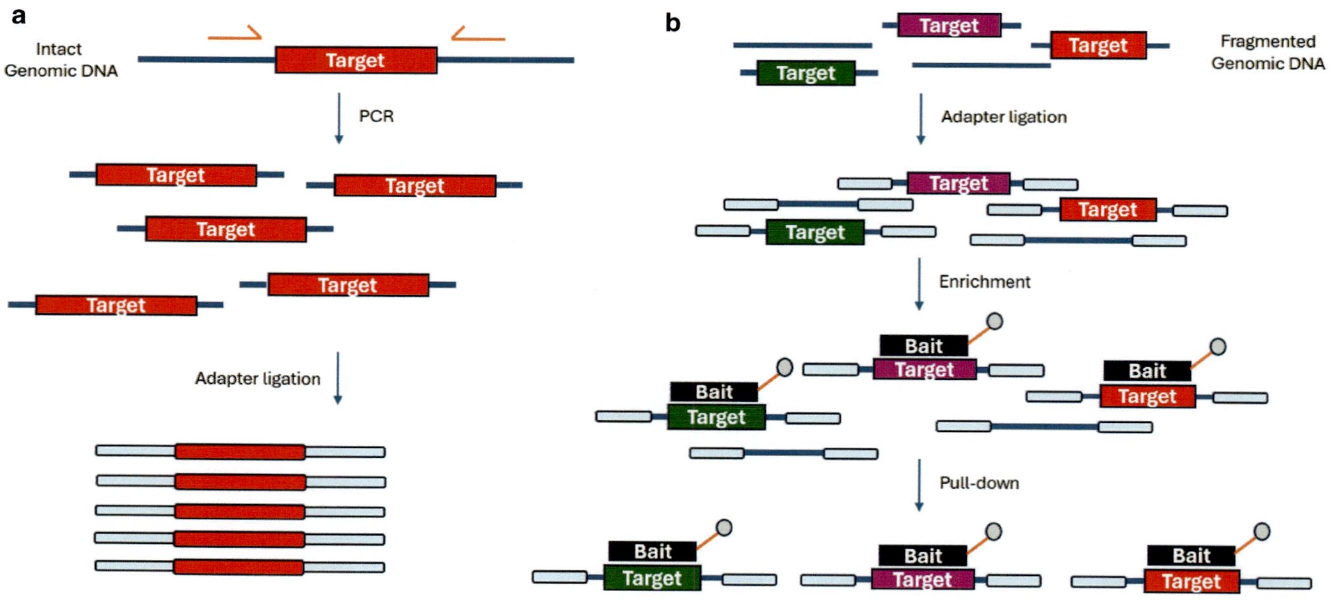

Fig. 5.1 Next-generation sequencing target enrichment approaches. (**a**) Amplicon-based target enrichment utilizes PCR (orange primers) to amplify targeted regions of interest directly from genomic DNA. Adapters are ligated after amplification to generate library fragments. This approach is optimized for fewer targets. (**b**) Capture-based approaches first require nucleic acid fragmentation and then adapter ligation. Capture of the targets of interest using tiled complementary oligonucleotide "bait" sequences are then used to enrich for fragments of interest. This approach is scalable to many targets (e.g., the exome)

amplicon-based library preparation times are typically shorter and are less susceptible to target drop-out when compared to capture-based approaches. PCR-based library preparation is a widely used approach due to its ability to amplify low-input DNA samples, making it suitable for a broad range of applications. However, PCR-free methods, which avoid amplification steps, provide the advantage of reducing potential bias introduced by PCR artifacts, resulting in a more accurate representation of the original genome, especially in regions prone to amplification errors or GC-rich areas. Capture-based enrichment allows for scalability and can handle larger gene panels (e.g., exome-wide analysis), is less susceptible to sequence artifacts introduced by PCR, and is the preferred method for copy-number calling algorithms from sequencing data [18, 21, 22]. In general, there is a direct correlation between the number of bases sequenced and copy-number calling accuracy; copy-number data from genome sequencing tends to be more accurate when compared to exome or targeted sequencing data [23]. However, copy-number calling from genome sequencing data is currently used for focused, gene-specific assessments [24], while applications for whole genome copy-number calling in pediatric leukemia continue to evolve.

After target enrichment, the selected bases must be prepared for sequencing by adding sequencing adapters [25]. An "adapter" is an inclusive term for bases that are added to the sequence of interest or "insert." All adapters contain platform-specific sequences that anchor the insert to the sequencing platform (e.g., to beads in Ion Torrent workflows and the flow cell for Illumina sequencing workflows). Additionally, the adapter may also contain sample-specific index sequences called "barcodes" or "indexes" that allow for unique sample identification when multiplexing multiple samples in a single sequencing run. Adapter molecules also contain primer binding sites that allow the molecule to be sequenced from one end (single-end sequencing) or both ends (paired-end sequencing). Additionally, some adapters incorporate short, randomly generated nucleotide sequences called unique molecular identifiers (UMIs) that tag individual molecules and help correct for artifactual errors caused during library preparation, target enrichment, or sequencing [26]. UMIs can resolve duplicate reads introduced in the amplification steps, increase the accuracy of mutation detection, and improve variant detection at low VAFs when used judiciously [27]. Schematic examples of an Illumina paired-end sequencing adapter with UMIs (Fig. 5.2a) and a single-end sequencing adapter for Ion Torrent (Fig. 5.2b) are shown.

Sequencing and Data Generation

After library preparation, the sample is ready to be sequenced. As noted, each library preparation method is tailored for the sequencing instrument, and each instrument has a fixed sequencing capacity (i.e., number of bases that can be sequenced). Generally, there is an inverse relationship between the number of bases targeted and the number of samples that can be sequenced simultaneously (multiplexed) to achieve the desired coverage for each sample. For example, the AmpliSeq

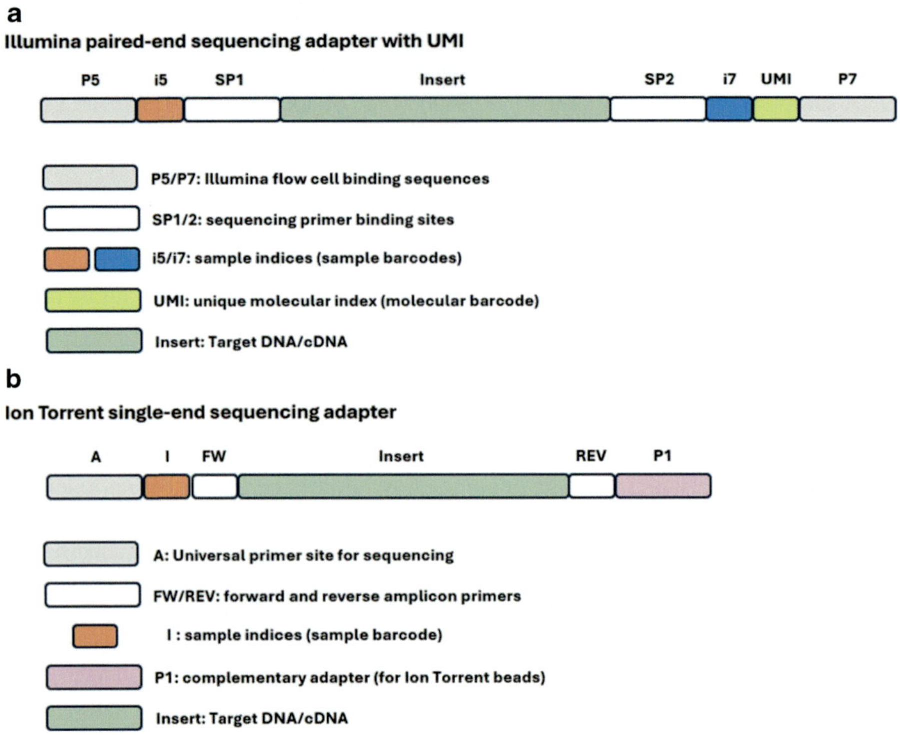

Fig. 5.2 Library adapters for Illumina and Ion Torrent chemistries. (**a**) An example of a capture-based Illumina adapter is shown. It includes dual sample barcodes (i5/i7) to uniquely identify the sample as well as adapters (P5/P7) to attach the flow cell. The optional unique molecular index (UMI) allows for molecule-level resolution. (**b**) An example of an amplicon-based Ion Torrent adapter is shown. The forward and reverse primers (FW/REV) are used during amplicon-based enrichment. The single index (I) allows for unique sample identification and the universal primer binding site (**a**) is used for signal amplification after the adapter is anchored to the bead via a complementary binding sequence (P1)

for Illumina Childhood Cancer Panel targets approximately 350,000 bases [5]; it is recommended that 5 samples be multiplexed together on an Illumina MiSeq instrument whereas on the NextSeq500 high-volume flow cell, nearly 80 libraries can be sequenced in a single run. Thus, consideration for panel size and predicted throughput is needed prior to sequencer selection.

All NGS instruments generate sequencing data from numerous DNA or RNA molecules simultaneously; hence, the term "massively parallel sequencing" is often synonymous with NGS [28]. Illumina sequencing utilizes a similar chemistry to Sanger sequencing whereby complementary fluorescently labeled dideoxynucleoside triphosphates (ddNTPs) are inserted resulting in chain termination, and the incorporated fluorescent signals are recorded using laser capture. Specifically, sequencing libraries are added to a flow cell (a hollow glass slide coated with oligonucleotides), and the library fragments anneal to the complementary

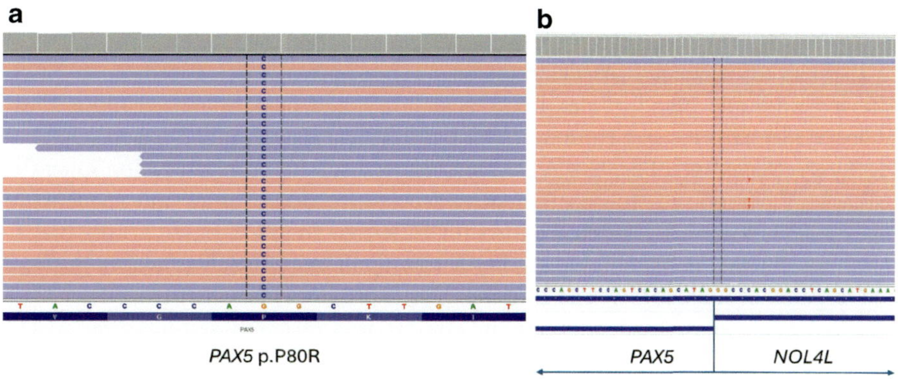

Fig. 5.3 Detection of WHO-defined B-ALL entities using DNA and RNA NGS (**a**) DNA NGS reads highlighting the *PAX5* c.239C>G single nucleotide variant that results in the p.Pro80Arg (p.R80R) missense mutation using Integrative Genomics Viewer (IGV). (**b**) The IGV split-read sequence of RNA NGS reads spanning *PAX5* exon 4 and *NOL4L* exon 8 consistent with the *PAX5::NOL4L* fusion reported in the B-ALL with *PAX5*-alt. *PAX5*: NM_016734.3; *NOL4L*: NM_080616.4

oligonucleotides on the surface of a flow cell (Figs. 5.1c and 5.2). The anchored library fragments then undergo a PCR amplification process called "bridge amplification" to generate "clusters" of the same nucleotide sequence; cluster generation is required to amplify the fluorescent signal for detection on the instrument. Once the sequencing cycle is completed, the ddNTPs are then enzymatically converted to deoxynucleoside triphosphates (dNTPs) in a process called cyclic reversible termination (CRT), and another round of fluorescently-labeled dNTPs are incorporated. The process repeats for the number of sequencing cycles needed to cover the insert in one or both directions (paired-end sequencing) [1]. Once completed, millions of sequence fragments from all areas of the flow cell are ready for the bioinformatics workflow.

CRT is widely considered the most accurate NGS methodology but requires costly instrumentation and technical expertise, and the sequencing process is time-consuming [28]. ThermoFisher Ion Torrent employs a process of bead-based emulsion PCR signal amplification and detection of hydrogen ion release (pH change) after nucleotide incorporation [29]. This approach often requires less nucleic acid input, less capital investment, and affords shorter sequencing times [30, 31]. In the ThermoFisher Ion Torrent workflow (Fig. 5.3), library adapters hybridize to complementary oligonucleotides affixed to beads. Each bead is encapsulated in a single oil droplet such that PCR amplification can occur inside the bead, and each bead contains a clonally amplified template from a single library molecule. The beads are then distributed on a microwell plate with one bead in each well. Nucleotides are added to the beads and nucleotide incorporation is detected by a change in the pH. The cycles are repeated until the sequence has been constructed [32]. This approach is widely utilized, but it is prone to errors, particularly in homopolymer regions, and there is literature cautioning against the use of Ion Torrent NGS technology when assessing for the important NM_015338.6(ASXL1):c.1934dup p.(Gly646Trpfs*12) variant in myeloid malignancies [33, 34].

Element Biosciences' AVITI sequencer represents a novel approach to NGS, offering a unique blend of flexibility, scalability, and performance. Unlike traditional NGS platforms like Illumina, which primarily rely on optical-based sequencing-by-synthesis methods, the AVITI sequencer uses its proprietary IonSphere™ technology, enabling a more efficient and cost-effective capture and sequencing process. This innovative method allows for PCR-free and PCR-based library preparation workflows, enhancing versatility across applications such as whole-genome and targeted sequencing. While Illumina platforms are widely recognized for their high accuracy and broad adoption in clinical and research settings, the AVITI sequencer is designed to offer a comparable level of data quality, with the added benefit of potentially lower costs and faster turnaround times, making it an appealing alternative for diverse genomic projects.

Bioinformatic Workflow

A classical bioinformatic workflow for whole genome sequencing (WGS), whole exome sequencing (WES), and targeted gene sequencing data analysis comprises three main phases: sequence alignment, variant calling, and filtered annotation. In the alignment step, each of the short NGS reads is mapped to positions on the human reference genome using various alignment methods [35], resulting in a sequence alignment file stored as a sequence alignment/map (SAM) or binary alignment/map (BAM) file. Routine quality control of BAMs should be performed by evaluating sequence metrics to verify if sufficient sequencing coverage has been achieved and to evaluate. Variant calling is then performed by which the aligned sequences are compared with reference sequences to find the positions that deviate from the reference, producing a list of calls detailed in a variant call format (VCF) file. A paired tumor-matched normal sample (e.g., blood, buccal, or skin) from the same patient allows the pipeline to distinguish true somatic alterations from constitutional ones. Tumor-only sequencing also has been employed as a cost-effective approach, but the downside of this approach is that it cannot distinguish true somatic mutations and sometimes follow-up testing is required. Benchmarking of somatic mutation callers using a reference truth set of somatic mutations is recommended for the validation of any somatic variant calling pipeline [36].

Variant filtering and annotation are the last steps of the bioinformatic workflow. Through filtering with population databases such as gnomAD or TopMed, the number of variants is reduced by removing potential germline variants. This step should be performed with caution to prevent filtering potentially significant recurrent mutations from human tumors. Internal data generated from a set of normal germline specimens and compilation of these data into a "panel of normals" has been employed to filter out germline variants or recurrent sequencing artifacts as well [37]. However, in healthy individuals, clonal hematopoiesis generating somatic mutations in myeloid malignancy-associated genes, such as *DNMT3A, TET2,* and

ASXL1, is well-established and can potentially confound this method [38]. Thus, the "panel of normal" approach needs to be carefully evaluated prior to the implementation. For annotation, several programs can be applied such as ANNOVAR, which consults various annotation databases, including RefSeq, CADD, SIFT, and PolyPhen, as well as the Ensembl Variant Effect Predictor (VEP) [39–41].

Variant Nomenclature

The Human Genome Variation Society (HGVS) standard nomenclature provides transcript reference sequences to annotate all variants and is used for clinical interpretation and reporting [42]. HGVS has collaborated with the International System for Human Cytogenomic Nomenclature (ISCN) [43] to provide recommendations and rules for complex alterations, including translocations, inversions, deletions, insertions, and supernumerary chromosomes, and these rules are provided on the HGVS website (Table 5.1). The HUGO Gene Nomenclature Committee (HGNC) has also published recommendations for the designation of gene fusions [44] and has recommended the use of the "::" symbol to separate genes instead of slashes or hyphens (e.g., *BCR::ABL1* replaces *BCR/ABL1* and *BCR-ABL1*). Furthermore, the Variant Interpretation for Cancer Consortium (VICC) has developed gene fusion specification through consensus among stakeholders with expertise in clinical diagnostics and informatics.

Various web-based variant validation tools including Mutalyzer 3, ClinGen Allele Registry, or VariantValidator [45–47] allow users to examine if the nomenclature of the sequence level variations is compliant with the HGVS recommendations for clinical reports. Clinical laboratories utilize different reference genomes

Table 5.1 Resources for variant nomenclature and genome annotations

Variant nomenclature resources and validation tools	Website
Human Genome Variation Society	https://hgvs-nomenclature.org/stable/
International System for Human Cytogenomic Nomenclature	https://iscn.karger.com/
HUGO Gene Nomenclature Committee	https://www.genenames.org/
Variant Interpretation for Cancer Consortium	https://fusions.cancervariants.org/
Mutalyzer 3	https://mutalyzer.nl/
ClinGen Allele Registry	https://reg.clinicalgenome.org/redmine/projects/registry/genboree_registry/landing
VariantValidator	https://variantvalidator.org/
Conversion of genome coordinates and annotations	
UCSC LiftOver	https://genome.ucsc.edu/cgi-bin/hgLiftOver
Ensembl Assembly Converters	https://grch37.ensembl.org/Homo_sapiens/Tools/AssemblyConverter?db=core
Liftover	https://liftover.broadinstitute.org/

typically either the Genome Reference Consortium Human Build 37 (GRCh37), also known as hg19, or GRCh38/hg38. Web-based tools including UCSC LiftOver, Ensembl Assembly Converters, or Liftover, are useful for converting variants, positions, or intervals from one reference genome to another (Table 5.1). Of note, several scientific organizations provide additional background about molecular methods and practice resources, including the introduction of NGS bioinformatics and file types or how to use Integrative Genomics Viewer (IGV) to manually review variant calls, for the analysis and reporting of molecular results. These resources are instrumental in the accurate reporting and analysis of molecular results, ensuring that clinicians can reliably detect genetic alterations associated with pediatric leukemia. Additionally, organizations such as the American Association for Cancer Research (AACR) and the Global Alliance for Genomics and Health (GA4GH) provide guidelines on best practices for data sharing, integration of multi-omics approaches, and maintaining data quality. The NCI's Cancer Data Science program also offers training materials and tools to help with advanced analysis techniques, including the use of machine learning in genomic data interpretation. Access to these resources is critical for fostering collaboration and ensuring consistency in the interpretation of complex genomic data, ultimately improving patient outcomes in precision medicine.

Variant Classification and Interpretation

Germline Variants

In 2015, The American College of Medical Genetics and Genomics (ACMG) and the Association for Molecular Pathology (AMP) released a landmark publication providing standards and guidelines for the interpretation of germline sequence variants in genes associated with inherited disorders [48]. These ACMG-AMP guidelines defined 28 criteria (including population data, case-control studies, *de novo* observations, segregation studies, functional data, and computational algorithms), whereby each line of evidence receives an assigned weight that results in a score and the final categorical classification of each variant. Subsequently, many gene- and disease-specific refinements of the ACMG/AMP have been developed, which has been largely spearheaded by the Clinical Genome Resource (ClinGen) via the formation of ClinGen expert panels [49]. Of particular interest to the genetic predisposition to leukemias, is the establishment of the ClinGen Myeloid Malignancy Variant Curation Expert Panel which has published specifications for interpreting germline *RUNX1* variants in association with hereditary thrombocytopenia and/or hematologic cancer predisposition syndrome (OMIM: 601399, 601626) [50]. Furthermore, since the publication of the initial ACMG-AMP guidelines, the ClinGen Sequence Variant Interpretation Working Group has further refined the scoring. These updated recommendations can be found on the ClinGen Sequence Variant Interpretation website (https://clinicalgenome.org/working-groups/

sequence-variant-interpretation/). A list of databases that are useful for the interpretation of germline variants is provided (Table 5.2).

Table 5.2 Databases for gene and disease associations and disease-associated germline/somatic variants

Gene and disease association for constitutional disorders	Website	Summary
OMIM	https://www.omim.org/	A database of human genes and genetic conditions
ClinGen Gene Curation	https://search.clinicalgenome.org/kb/genes/	Expert curation of gene and disease association
Germline variant database		
ClinVar	http://www.ncbi.nlm.nih.gov/clinvar	A database of human variations classified for diseases and drug responses, with supporting evidence.
HGMD	http://www.hgmd.org	A database of variant annotations published in the literature.
LOVD	https://www.lovd.nl/	A database of curated gene variant
Population database		
gnomAD	https://gnomad.broadinstitute.org/	A database of variants found in exome and genome sequences from around the world
All of Us	https://databrowser.researchallofus.org/snvsindels	A database of SNVs/Indels variants found in the National Institutes of Health's All of Us Research Program
In silico prediction		
REVEL	https://sites.google.com/site/revelgenomics/	A meta-predictor that combines 13 individual tools with high sensitivity and specificity
CADD	http://cadd.gs.washington.edu	A prediction tool that integrates diverse genomic features derived from surrounding sequence context, gene model annotations, evolutionary constraint, epigenetic measurements, and functional predictions
SpliceAI	https://spliceailookup.broadinstitute.org/	A deep learning based tool for the predicted effect on splicing
Variant Effect Predictor	https://useast.ensembl.org/info/docs/tools/vep/script/vep_plugins.html	The Ensembl toolset to provide annotations for sequence alterations and access to various *in silico* prediction tools
Cancer-specific variant database		
OncoKB	https://www.oncokb.org/	An FDA recognized precision oncology knowledge database

(continued)

Table 5.2 (continued)

Gene and disease association for constitutional disorders	Website	Summary
Cancer hotspot	https://www.cancerhotspots.org/#/home	A resource for statistically significant mutations in cancer
Catalog of Somatic Mutations in Cancer	https://cancer.sanger.ac.uk/cosmic	A comprehensive resource for exploring somatic mutations in cancer
My Cancer Genome	https://www.mycancergenome.org/	A database with assertions derived from FDA drug labels, NCCN and other professional society guidelines and clinical trials on the clinical impact of somatic mutation in cancer
cBioPortal	https://www.cbioportal.org/	An open-access resources for interactive exploration of cancer genomics data sets
CIViC	https://civicdb.org/welcome	An open-source, expert-curated resource for somatic mutations
The Clinical Knowledgebase	https://ckbhome.genomenon.com/	A curated database of gene/variant annotations
ClinGen Somatic Expert Group	https://clinicalgenome.org/curation-activities/somatic/	Expert curation and guidelines of somatic mutations

Somatic Variants

With the recognition of the urgent need for standardization of interpretation and reporting sequence variants in cancer, the Association for Molecular Pathology (AMP), College of American Pathologists (CAP), American Society of Clinical Oncology (ASCO), and American College of Medical Genetics and Genomics (ACMG) published the guidelines in 2017 [51]. The guidelines recommend a four-tiered classification and reporting system centered on clinical and experimental evidence in cancer diagnosis, prognosis, and/or therapeutics [52]. In addition, in 2022 the ClinGen Somatic Cancer Clinical Domain Working Group and ClinGen Germline/Somatic Variant Subcommittee, the Cancer Genomics Consortium (CGC), and the Variant Interpretation for Cancer Consortium (VICC) have developed a standard operating procedure for the classification of oncogenicity of somatic variants [53]. Finally, the Somatic Working Group of ClinGen has published several documents and included resources for cancer variant interpretation. A list of databases that are useful for the interpretation of somatic variants is provided (Table 5.2).

Notably, it is reported that nearly 5% of pediatric leukemia patients may harbor a germline cancer predisposition variant [54], and that these germline variants may be unmasked during somatic testing [55, 56]. There is an extensive list of genes with established or emerging associations with myeloid malignancies such as *RUNX1*, *GATA2*, *SAMD9/9L*, *ANKRD26*, *CEBPA*, *DDX41*, *ETV6*, and many others. The World Health Organization has acknowledged this association in the recently released 5th edition of the *Classification of Hematolymphoid Tumours* which includes a diagnostic category called "myeloid neoplasms with genetic predisposition" [57]. In the absence of matched tumor-normal sequencing that can distinguish the origin of mutation, it is recommended to maintain a high index of suspicion for germline origin and employ testing platforms that are comprehensive for the genes and mutation types that confer germline risk [58].

NGS Applications

Targeted DNA Panels

High-sensitivity detection methods are needed to detect somatic variants with low variant allele fraction/frequency (VAF); thus, gene panel testing is often employed for hematological cancer clinical workups. Targeted panel tests allow the detection of genetic alterations in dozens to hundreds of genes. However, the composition of these panels is not standardized and despite recommendations regarding minimum targets for interrogation of adult leukemias [59], there is limited literature in pediatric leukemias [60]. Regardless, the minimum required regions to ensure sequencing coverage for the detection of recurrent variants associated with hematological cancer needs to be evaluated prior to the gene panel design. The WHO guidelines, National Comprehensive Cancer Network (NCCN) guidelines, Cancer Gene Census in the Catalogues of Somatic Mutations in Cancer (COSMIC), and cancer genes list in OncoKB are valuable resources for users to evaluate gene list and recurrent hotspot variants [61–64]. Sequencing depth and a minimum number of variant reads can be empirically determined and a detection threshold at a VAF $\geq 5\%$ is commonly established in clinical tests.

WES and WGS

The efforts of consortia, including The Cancer Genome Atlas (TCGA) project, the Pediatric Cancer Genome Project, the International Cancer Genome Consortium, and the Children's Oncology Group–National Cancer Institute (COG-NCI) Therapeutically Applicable Research to Generate Effective Treatments (TARGET) project used comprehensive genomic approaches, including whole exome sequencing (WES), whole genome sequencing (WGS), and RNA-seq, and have advanced the knowledge of cancer genomic landscapes and discovered novel driver mutations [20, 65, 66]. These efforts also provide valuable data that subsequently promotes the development of tools and resources facilitating analysis and somatic mutation interpretation. WES and analysis of protein-coding regions have discovered new cancer-driver genes and pathways [67–69]. The pivotal publication by Ley et al. performed paired tumor-normal sequencing of a cytogenetically normal AML using WGS and identified ten genes with tumor-specific mutations and discovered the genes involved in myeloid cancer progression [70]. WGS is also an efficient method to detect structural rearrangements, fusions, and copy-number alterations commonly observed in myeloid malignancies [71]. Currently, several clinically validated WGS tests for hematological malignancies are available and have recently been summarized in recent publications [71–75]. Similarly, WGS has been employed for childhood B-cell acute lymphoblastic leukemia and detected subtype-defining genetic abnormalities [76, 77].

RNA-Based NGS

Although NGS is primarily utilized for the detection, annotation, and interpretation of DNA-based sequence variants, RNA-based NGS testing has emerged as a powerful tool to assess for fusion genes and gene rearrangements in pediatric leukemias. RNA-based NGS can complement FISH and cytogenetic assays to resolve cryptic fusions and delineate fusion partners. In pediatric acute myeloid leukemia, many of the diagnostic gene fusions produce chimeric fusion transcripts (e.g., *RUNX1::RUNX1T1*, *PML::RARA,* or *CBFB::MYH11*) which can be detected by targeted NGS testing. RNA-based targeted NGS can improve diagnostic accuracy by revealing karyotypically cryptic fusions (e.g., *NUP98::NSD1*, *KMT2A::MLLT10,* and *CBFA2T3::GLIS2*) when compared to conventional methods [78]. Also, current COG AML research treatment protocols require confirmation of the *KMT2A* fusion partner to appropriately risk-stratify patients; this information is difficult to obtain without RNA-based NGS given the number of known *KMT2A* fusion partners [79, 80]. In pediatric B-acute lymphoblastic leukemia/lymphoma (B-ALL), fusion gene detection is also helpful to diagnose the high-risk *BCR::ABL1*-like B-ALL (Philadelphia-like [Ph-like] B-ALL), and detection of the diagnostic kinase fusion can assist in targeted therapy selection [77, 81, 82]. RNA-based NGS can also assess gene expression; gene expression can be used to subclassify pediatric B-ALLs into *BCR::ABL1*-like (Philadelphia-like) B-ALL as well as other established and emerging (e.g., *ETV6::RUNX1*-like) molecular subtypes [83]. Lastly, RNA transcriptome sequencing has been used extensively in T-acute lymphoblastic leukemia/lymphoma (T-ALL) to identify biomarkers and distinct expression profiles in this heterogeneous disease [84].

As pediatric leukemia classifications continue to evolve, NGS approaches are needed to provide diagnostic, prognostic, and therapeutic information in the clinical management of these patients. Per the *WHO Classification of Haematolymphoid Tumours, 5th edition*, NGS methods are recommended to diagnose B-ALL with other defined genetic alterations [64]. The diagnosis of B-ALL with *PAX5* p.P80R requires DNA sequencing to detect the underlying single nucleotide variant resulting in the missense mutation and the diagnosis of B-ALL with *PAX5*-alt requires RNA sequencing to assess for the various *PAX5* fusions (Fig. 5.3b) [85, 86]. Additionally, both DNA and NGS approaches are widely utilized to determine eligibility for FDA-approved therapeutics [87] or potential clinical-trial enrollment [88].

Minimal Residual Disease (MRD) Detection

Minimal Residual Disease (MRD) detection by NGS is a powerful approach to monitoring leukemia at a molecular level, offering significantly higher sensitivity than traditional methods like flow cytometry or cytogenetics. MRD refers to the small number of leukemia cells that may remain in a patient after treatment, which is often undetectable by conventional imaging or clinical assessment but can lead to relapse. NGS-based MRD testing involves identifying specific genetic mutations, fusion genes, or unique DNA/RNA sequences that are present in the leukemic cells but absent in normal cells, allowing for precise quantification of residual disease.

NGS offers several advantages over other MRD detection methods. Its high sensitivity allows it to detect single leukemia cells among millions of normal cells, enabling earlier detection of relapse before clinical symptoms appear. Additionally, NGS can be tailored to a patient's unique genetic alterations, providing personalized, highly sensitive MRD detection that is more accurate than generic marker-based methods. This is particularly useful in diseases like pediatric leukemia, where genetic heterogeneity can be significant. The ability to monitor MRD with NGS not only improves the detection of relapse but also helps guide treatment decisions, allowing for timely interventions and potentially improving overall survival.

Summary and Future Directions

NGS has revolutionized the diagnosis, treatment, and understanding of pediatric leukemia. By providing high-throughput, detailed insights into genetic, transcriptomic, and epigenetic alterations, NGS has enabled the identification of novel genetic mutations, fusion genes, and pathways implicated in leukemogenesis to allow more precise classification of leukemia subtypes, enhance risk stratification, and inform personalized treatment strategies. Notably, NGS has advanced the detection of minimal residual disease (MRD), offering higher sensitivity compared to traditional methods, which helps guide therapeutic decisions and monitor for relapse. Moreover, the identification of actionable mutations has facilitated the development of targeted therapies, such as tyrosine kinase inhibitors in Philadelphia chromosome-positive acute lymphoblastic leukemia (Ph+ ALL) and FLT3 inhibitors in acute myeloid leukemia (AML), improving survival rates for certain high-risk groups. In addition, NGS has shed light on epigenetic dysregulation, including DNA methylation and histone modification patterns, contributing to the development of therapies targeting epigenetic regulators.

Long-read sequencing, which captures longer fragments of DNA and RNA, represents a promising frontier for further enhancing leukemia testing. This approach has the potential to more accurately identify structural variations, such as large gene fusions, translocations, and complex genomic rearrangements that can be challenging to detect with short-read sequencing. In particular, long-read RNA sequencing could provide deeper insights into the transcriptomic landscape of pediatric leukemia, allowing for the detection of novel fusion transcripts, alternative splicing events, and complex gene expression patterns that may play a critical role in disease progression and response to therapy. By overcoming limitations in short-read sequencing, long-read technologies could contribute to more comprehensive genetic profiling, ultimately improving diagnostic accuracy and personalized treatment strategies. Please see more information regarding long-read sequencing in Chap. 7.

Despite these advancements, challenges remain, including the interpretation of variants of uncertain significance (VUS), integration of multi-omics data, and ensuring equitable access to NGS technologies. Looking ahead, one promising direction to further unravel the complexity of pediatric leukemia is the incorporation of multi-omics, combining genomic, transcriptomic, proteomic, and epigenomic data to create a comprehensive understanding of leukemogenesis. This holistic perspective will facilitate the discovery of novel biomarkers and therapeutic targets, enhancing both diagnostics and treatment strategies. Advances in single-cell sequencing technology will also enable a deeper exploration of tumor heterogeneity and clonal dynamics, shedding light on mechanisms of treatment resistance and disease relapse. Another key area of development is the broader application of liquid biopsy techniques, such as the use of circulating tumor DNA (ctDNA) for non-invasive monitoring of minimal residual disease (MRD) and early relapse detection. These approaches could provide real-time insights into disease progression with minimal patient burden. The integration of artificial intelligence (AI) and machine learning into NGS workflows is expected to revolutionize data analysis, improving the interpretation of complex datasets and enabling the prediction of treatment outcomes with greater precision.

Furthermore, efforts to make NGS more accessible and cost-effective are essential for ensuring equitable application in diverse healthcare settings. This includes developing scalable NGS technologies and training clinicians to interpret and act on sequencing data. As these advancements unfold, NGS will continue to push the boundaries of precision medicine in pediatric leukemia, improving survival rates and long-term outcomes for children worldwide.

References

1. Metzker ML. Sequencing technologies—the next generation. Nat Rev Genet. 2010;11(1):31–46.
2. Chang F, Lin F, Cao K, Surrey LF, Aplenc R, Bagatell R, et al. Development and clinical validation of a large fusion gene panel for pediatric cancers. J Mol Diagn JMD. 2019;21(5):873–83.
3. Goodwin S, McPherson JD, McCombie WR. Coming of age: ten years of next-generation sequencing technologies. Nat Rev Genet. 2016;17(6):333–51.
4. Hiemenz MC, Ostrow DG, Busse TM, Buckley J, Maglinte DT, Bootwalla M, et al. OncoKids: a comprehensive next-generation sequencing panel for pediatric malignancies. J Mol Diagn JMD. 2018;20(6):765–76.
5. Vicente-Garcés C, Esperanza-Cebollada E, Montesdeoca S, Torrebadell M, Rives S, Dapena JL, et al. Technical validation and clinical utility of an NGS targeted panel to improve molecular characterization of pediatric acute leukemia. Front Mol Biosci. 2022;9:854098.
6. Petrackova A, Vasinek M, Sedlarikova L, Dyskova T, Schneiderova P, Novosad T, et al. Standardization of sequencing coverage depth in NGS: recommendation for detection of clonal and subclonal mutations in cancer diagnostics. Front Oncol. 2019;9:851.
7. Gupta S, Devidas M, Loh ML, Raetz EA, Chen S, Wang C, et al. Flow-cytometric vs. -morphologic assessment of remission in childhood acute lymphoblastic leukemia: a report from the Children's Oncology Group (COG). Leukemia. 2018;32(6):1370–9.

8. Jennings LJ, Arcila ME, Corless C, Kamel-Reid S, Lubin IM, Pfeifer J, et al. Guidelines for validation of next-generation sequencing-based oncology panels: a joint consensus recommendation of the Association for Molecular Pathology and College of American Pathologists. J Mol Diagn JMD. 2017;19(3):341–65.
9. Smits AJ, Kummer JA, de Bruin PC, Bol M, van den Tweel JG, Seldenrijk KA, et al. The estimation of tumor cell percentage for molecular testing by pathologists is not accurate. Mod Pathol. 2014;27(2):168–74.
10. Kofanova O, Bellora C, Garcia Frasquilho S, Antunes L, Hamot G, Mathay C, et al. Standardization of the preanalytical phase of DNA extraction from fixed tissue for next-generation sequencing analyses. New Biotechnol. 2020;54:52–61.
11. Zhu Q, Hu Q, Shepherd L, Wang J, Wei L, Morrison CD, et al. The impact of DNA input amount and DNA source on the performance of whole-exome sequencing in cancer epidemiology. Cancer Epidemiol Biomarkers Prev. 2015;24(8):1207–13.
12. Chen H, Luthra R, Goswami RS, Singh RR, Roy-Chowdhuri S. Analysis of pre-analytic factors affecting the success of clinical next-generation sequencing of solid organ malignancies. Cancer. 2015;7(3):1699–715.
13. Goswami RS, Luthra R, Singh RR, Patel KP, Routbort MJ, Aldape KD, et al. Identification of factors affecting the success of next-generation sequencing testing in solid tumors. Am J Clin Pathol. 2016;145(2):222–37.
14. Ascierto PA, Bifulco C, Palmieri G, Peters S, Sidiropoulos N. Preanalytic variables and tissue stewardship for reliable next-generation sequencing (NGS) clinical analysis. J Mol Diagn JMD. 2019;21(5):756–67.
15. Permenter J, Ishwar A, Rounsavall A, Smith M, Faske J, Sailey CJ, et al. Quantitative analysis of genomic DNA degradation in whole blood under various storage conditions for molecular diagnostic testing. Mol Cell Probes. 2015;29(6):449–53.
16. Head SR, Komori HK, LaMere SA, Whisenant T, Van Nieuwerburgh F, Salomon DR, et al. Library construction for next-generation sequencing: overviews and challenges. BioTechniques. 2014;56(2):61–4, 6, 8, passim.
17. Hess JF, Kohl TA, Kotrová M, Rönsch K, Paprotka T, Mohr V, et al. Library preparation for next generation sequencing: a review of automation strategies. Biotechnol Adv. 2020;41:107537.
18. Singh RR. Target enrichment approaches for next-generation sequencing applications in oncology. Diagnostics (Basel, Switzerland). 2022;12(7).
19. Chmielecki J, Bailey M, He J, Elvin J, Vergilio JA, Ramkissoon S, et al. Genomic profiling of a large set of diverse pediatric cancers identifies known and novel mutations across tumor spectra. Cancer Res. 2017;77(2):509–19.
20. Farrar JE, Schuback HL, Ries RE, Wai D, Hampton OA, Trevino LR, et al. Genomic profiling of pediatric acute myeloid leukemia reveals a changing mutational landscape from disease diagnosis to relapse. Cancer Res. 2016;76(8):2197–205.
21. Samorodnitsky E, Jewell BM, Hagopian R, Miya J, Wing MR, Lyon E, et al. Evaluation of hybridization capture versus amplicon-based methods for whole-exome sequencing. Hum Mutat. 2015;36(9):903–14.
22. Pritchard CC, Salipante SJ, Koehler K, Smith C, Scroggins S, Wood B, et al. Validation and implementation of targeted capture and sequencing for the detection of actionable mutation, copy number variation, and gene rearrangement in clinical cancer specimens. J Mol Diagn JMD. 2014;16(1):56–67.
23. Gabrielaite M, Torp MH, Rasmussen MS, Andreu-Sánchez S, Vieira FG, Pedersen CB, et al. A comparison of tools for copy-number variation detection in germline whole exome and whole genome sequencing data. Cancers. 2021;13(24).
24. Garcia-Heras J. The confirmatory diagnostic value of whole genome sequencing (WGS) as a standalone test for childhood B-cell ALL: the results of a NOPHO trials cohort. J Assoc Genet Technol. 2023;49(4):162–6.
25. Yohe S, Thyagarajan B. Review of clinical next-generation sequencing. Arch Pathol Lab Med. 2017;141(11):1544–57.
26. Smith T, Heger A, Sudbery I. UMI-tools: modeling sequencing errors in Unique Molecular Identifiers to improve quantification accuracy. Genome Res. 2017;27(3):491–9.

27. Bieler J, Kubik S, Macheret M, Pozzorini C, Willig A, Xu Z. Benefits of applying molecular barcoding systems are not uniform across different genomic applications. J Transl Med. 2023;21(1):305.
28. McCombie WR, McPherson JD, Mardis ER. Next-generation sequencing technologies. Cold Spring Harb Perspect Med. 2019;9(11).
29. Rothberg JM, Hinz W, Rearick TM, Schultz J, Mileski W, Davey M, et al. An integrated semiconductor device enabling non-optical genome sequencing. Nature. 2011;475(7356):348–52.
30. Li X, Buckton AJ, Wilkinson SL, John S, Walsh R, Novotny T, et al. Towards clinical molecular diagnosis of inherited cardiac conditions: a comparison of bench-top genome DNA sequencers. PLoS One. 2013;8(7):e67744.
31. Quail MA, Smith M, Coupland P, Otto TD, Harris SR, Connor TR, et al. A tale of three next generation sequencing platforms: comparison of Ion Torrent, Pacific Biosciences and Illumina MiSeq sequencers. BMC Genomics. 2012;13:341.
32. Golan D, Medvedev P. Using state machines to model the Ion Torrent sequencing process and to improve read error rates. Bioinformatics (Oxford, England). 2013;29(13):i344–51.
33. Alberti MO, Srivatsan SN, Shao J, McNulty SN, Chang GS, Miller CA, et al. Discriminating a common somatic ASXL1 mutation (c.1934dup; p.G646Wfs*12) from artifact in myeloid malignancies using NGS. Leukemia. 2018;32(8):1874–8.
34. Yannakou CK, Jones K, McBean M, Thompson ER, Ryland GL, Doig K, et al. ASXL1 c.1934dup;p.Gly646Trpfs*12-a true somatic alteration requiring a new approach. Blood Cancer J. 2017;7(12):656.
35. Alser M, Rotman J, Deshpande D, Taraszka K, Shi H, Baykal PI, et al. Technology dictates algorithms: recent developments in read alignment. Genome Biol. 2021;22(1):249.
36. Xu C. A review of somatic single nucleotide variant calling algorithms for next-generation sequencing data. Comput Struct Biotechnol J. 2018;16:15–24.
37. Gerstung M, Beisel C, Rechsteiner M, Wild P, Schraml P, Moch H, et al. Reliable detection of subclonal single-nucleotide variants in tumour cell populations. Nat Commun. 2012;3:811.
38. Genovese G, Kähler AK, Handsaker RE, Lindberg J, Rose SA, Bakhoum SF, et al. Clonal hematopoiesis and blood-cancer risk inferred from blood DNA sequence. N Engl J Med. 2014;371(26):2477–87.
39. Hunt SE, Moore B, Amode RM, Armean IM, Lemos D, Mushtaq A, et al. Annotating and prioritizing genomic variants using the Ensembl Variant Effect Predictor-A tutorial. Hum Mutat. 2022;43(8):986–97.
40. McLaren W, Gil L, Hunt SE, Riat HS, Ritchie GR, Thormann A, et al. The Ensembl variant effect predictor. Genome Biol. 2016;17(1):122.
41. Wang K, Li M, Hakonarson H. ANNOVAR: functional annotation of genetic variants from high-throughput sequencing data. Nucleic Acids Res. 2010;38(16):e164.
42. den Dunnen JT, Dalgleish R, Maglott DR, Hart RK, Greenblatt MS, McGowan-Jordan J, et al. HGVS recommendations for the description of sequence variants: 2016 update. Hum Mutat. 2016;37(6):564–9.
43. ISCN. 2024—An International System for Human Cytogenomic Nomenclature (2024). Cytogenet Genome Res. 2024;164(Suppl 1):1–224.
44. Bruford EA, Antonescu CR, Carroll AJ, Chinnaiyan A, Cree IA, Cross NCP, et al. HUGO Gene Nomenclature Committee (HGNC) recommendations for the designation of gene fusions. Leukemia. 2021;35(11):3040–3.
45. Lefter M, Vis JK, Vermaat M, den Dunnen JT, Taschner PEM, Laros JFJ. Mutalyzer 2: next generation HGVS nomenclature checker. Bioinformatics (Oxford, England). 2021;37(18):2811–7.
46. Pawliczek P, Patel RY, Ashmore LR, Jackson AR, Bizon C, Nelson T, et al. ClinGen Allele Registry links information about genetic variants. Hum Mutat. 2018;39(11):1690–701.
47. Freeman PJ, Hart RK, Gretton LJ, Brookes AJ, Dalgleish R. VariantValidator: accurate validation, mapping, and formatting of sequence variation descriptions. Hum Mutat. 2018;39(1):61–8.
48. Richards S, Aziz N, Bale S, Bick D, Das S, Gastier-Foster J, et al. Standards and guidelines for the interpretation of sequence variants: a joint consensus recommendation of the American College of Medical Genetics and Genomics and the Association for Molecular Pathology. Genet Med. 2015;17(5):405–24.

49. Rehm HL, Berg JS, Brooks LD, Bustamante CD, Evans JP, Landrum MJ, et al. ClinGen—the clinical genome resource. N Engl J Med. 2015;372(23):2235–42.
50. Luo X, Feurstein S, Mohan S, Porter CC, Jackson SA, Keel S, et al. ClinGen Myeloid Malignancy Variant Curation Expert Panel recommendations for germline RUNX1 variants. Blood Adv. 2019;3(20):2962–79.
51. Li MM, Datto M, Duncavage EJ, Kulkarni S, Lindeman NI, Roy S, et al. Standards and Guidelines for the Interpretation and Reporting of Sequence Variants in Cancer: a Joint Consensus Recommendation of the Association for Molecular Pathology, American Society of Clinical Oncology, and College of American Pathologists. J Mol Diagn JMD. 2017;19(1):4–23.
52. Mikhail FM, Biegel JA, Cooley LD, Dubuc AM, Hirsch B, Horner VL, et al. Technical laboratory standards for interpretation and reporting of acquired copy-number abnormalities and copy-neutral loss of heterozygosity in neoplastic disorders: a joint consensus recommendation from the American College of Medical Genetics and Genomics (ACMG) and the Cancer Genomics Consortium (CGC). Genet Med. 2019;21(9):1903–16.
53. Horak P, Griffith M, Danos AM, Pitel BA, Madhavan S, Liu X, et al. Standards for the classification of pathogenicity of somatic variants in cancer (oncogenicity): Joint recommendations of Clinical Genome Resource (ClinGen), Cancer Genomics Consortium (CGC), and Variant Interpretation for Cancer Consortium (VICC). Genet Med. 2022;24(9):1991.
54. Bloom M, Maciaszek JL, Clark ME, Pui CH, Nichols KE. Recent advances in genetic predisposition to pediatric acute lymphoblastic leukemia. Expert Rev Hematol. 2020;13(1):55–70.
55. Churpek JE, Pyrtel K, Kanchi KL, Shao J, Koboldt D, Miller CA, et al. Genomic analysis of germ line and somatic variants in familial myelodysplasia/acute myeloid leukemia. Blood. 2015;126(22):2484–90.
56. Douglas SPM, Lahtinen AK, Koski JR, Leimi L, Keränen MAI, Koskenvuo M, et al. Enrichment of cancer-predisposing germline variants in adult and pediatric patients with acute lymphoblastic leukemia. Sci Rep. 2022;12(1):10670.
57. Liu YC, Eldomery MK, Maciaszek JL, Klco JM. Inherited predispositions to myeloid neoplasms: pathogenesis and clinical implications. Annual Rev Pathol. 2024.
58. Roloff GW, Godley LA, Drazer MW. Assessment of technical heterogeneity among diagnostic tests to detect germline risk variants for hematopoietic malignancies. Genet Med. 2021;23(1):211–4.
59. Song JS. Clinically relevant core genes for hematologic malignancies in clinical NGS panel testing. Blood Res. 2023;58(4):224–8.
60. Kolekar P, Balagopal V, Dong L, Liu Y, Foy S, Tran Q, et al. SJPedPanel: a pan-cancer gene panel for childhood malignancies to enhance cancer monitoring and early detection. Clin Cancer Res. 2024;30(18):4100–14.
61. Tate JG, Bamford S, Jubb HC, Sondka Z, Beare DM, Bindal N, et al. COSMIC: the catalogue of somatic mutations in cancer. Nucleic Acids Res. 2019;47(D1):D941–d7.
62. Chakravarty D, Gao J, Phillips SM, Kundra R, Zhang H, Wang J, et al. OncoKB: a precision oncology knowledge base. JCO Precis Oncol. 2017;2017.
63. Inaba H, Teachey D, Annesley C, Batra S, Beck J, Colace S, et al. Pediatric acute lymphoblastic leukemia, version 2.2025, NCCN clinical practice guidelines in oncology. J Natl Comprehens Cancer Netw JNCCN. 2025;23(2):41–62.
64. Cree IA, The WHO. Classification of Haematolymphoid Tumours. Leukemia. 2022;36(7):1701–2.
65. Bolouri H, Farrar JE, Triche T Jr, Ries RE, Lim EL, Alonzo TA, et al. The molecular landscape of pediatric acute myeloid leukemia reveals recurrent structural alterations and age-specific mutational interactions. Nat Med. 2018;24(1):103–12.
66. Ley TJ, Miller C, Ding L, Raphael BJ, Mungall AJ, Robertson A, et al. Genomic and epigenomic landscapes of adult de novo acute myeloid leukemia. N Engl J Med. 2013;368(22):2059–74.
67. Lawrence MS, Stojanov P, Mermel CH, Robinson JT, Garraway LA, Golub TR, et al. Discovery and saturation analysis of cancer genes across 21 tumour types. Nature. 2014;505(7484):495–501.
68. Ptashkin RN, Ewalt MD, Jayakumaran G, Kiecka I, Bowman AS, Yao J, et al. Enhanced clinical assessment of hematologic malignancies through routine paired tumor and normal sequencing. Nat Commun. 2023;14(1):6895.

69. Vogelstein B, Papadopoulos N, Velculescu VE, Zhou S, Diaz LA Jr, Kinzler KW. Cancer genome landscapes. Science (New York, NY). 2013;339(6127):1546–58.
70. Ley TJ, Mardis ER, Ding L, Fulton B, McLellan MD, Chen K, et al. DNA sequencing of a cytogenetically normal acute myeloid leukaemia genome. Nature. 2008;456(7218):66–72.
71. Duncavage EJ, Schroeder MC, O'Laughlin M, Wilson R, MacMillan S, Bohannon A, et al. Genome sequencing as an alternative to cytogenetic analysis in myeloid cancers. N Engl J Med. 2021;384(10):924–35.
72. Hou YC, Neidich JA, Duncavage EJ, Spencer DH, Schroeder MC. Clinical whole-genome sequencing in cancer diagnosis. Hum Mutat. 2022;43(11):1519–30.
73. Newman S, Nakitandwe J, Kesserwan CA, Azzato EM, Wheeler DA, Rusch M, et al. Genomes for kids: the scope of pathogenic mutations in pediatric cancer revealed by comprehensive DNA and RNA sequencing. Cancer Discov. 2021;11(12):3008–27.
74. Sosinsky A, Ambrose J, Cross W, Turnbull C, Henderson S, Jones L, et al. Insights for precision oncology from the integration of genomic and clinical data of 13,880 tumors from the 100,000 Genomes Cancer Programme. Nat Med. 2024;30(1):279–89.
75. Wrzeszczynski KO, Felice V, Abhyankar A, Kozon L, Geiger H, Manaa D, et al. Analytical validation of clinical whole-genome and transcriptome sequencing of patient-derived tumors for reporting targetable variants in cancer. J Mol Diagn JMD. 2018;20(6):822–35.
76. Ryan SL, Peden JF, Kingsbury Z, Schwab CJ, James T, Polonen P, et al. Whole genome sequencing provides comprehensive genetic testing in childhood B-cell acute lymphoblastic leukaemia. Leukemia. 2023;37(3):518–28.
77. Brady SW, Roberts KG, Gu Z, Shi L, Pounds S, Pei D, et al. The genomic landscape of pediatric acute lymphoblastic leukemia. Nat Genet. 2022;54(9):1376–89.
78. Hoffmeister LM, Suttorp J, Walter C, Antoniou E, Behrens YL, Göhring G, et al. Panel-based RNA fusion sequencing improves diagnostics of pediatric acute myeloid leukemia. Leukemia. 2024;38(3):538–44.
79. Meyer C, Larghero P, Almeida Lopes B, Burmeister T, Gröger D, Sutton R, et al. The KMT2A recombinome of acute leukemias in 2023. Leukemia. 2023;37(5):988–1005.
80. Tomizawa D, Tsujimoto SI. Risk-stratified therapy for pediatric acute myeloid leukemia. Cancers. 2023;15(16).
81. Reshmi SC, Harvey RC, Roberts KG, Stonerock E, Smith A, Jenkins H, et al. Targetable kinase gene fusions in high-risk B-ALL: a study from the Children's Oncology Group. Blood. 2017;129(25):3352–61.
82. Roberts KG, Li Y, Payne-Turner D, Harvey RC, Yang YL, Pei D, et al. Targetable kinase-activating lesions in Ph-like acute lymphoblastic leukemia. N Engl J Med. 2014;371(11):1005–15.
83. Hu Z, Kovach AE, Yellapantula V, Ostrow D, Doan A, Ji J, et al. Transcriptome sequencing allows comprehensive genomic characterization of pediatric B-acute lymphoblastic leukemia in an academic clinical laboratory. J Mol Diagn JMD. 2024;26(1):49–60.
84. Pölönen P, Di Giacomo D, Seffernick AE, Elsayed A, Kimura S, Benini F, et al. The genomic basis of childhood T-lineage acute lymphoblastic leukaemia. Nature. 2024;632(8027):1082–91.
85. Gu Z, Churchman ML, Roberts KG, Moore I, Zhou X, Nakitandwe J, et al. PAX5-driven subtypes of B-progenitor acute lymphoblastic leukemia. Nat Genet. 2019;51(2):296–307.
86. Passet M, Boissel N, Sigaux F, Saillard C, Bargetzi M, Ba I, et al. PAX5 P80R mutation identifies a novel subtype of B-cell precursor acute lymphoblastic leukemia with favorable outcome. Blood. 2019;133(3):280–4.
87. Zhao X, Kotch C, Fox E, Surrey LF, Wertheim GB, Baloch ZW, et al. NTRK fusions identified in pediatric tumors: the frequency, fusion partners, and clinical outcome. JCO Precis Oncol. 2021;1.
88. Schwab C, Cranston RE, Ryan SL, Butler E, Winterman E, Hawking Z, et al. Integrative genomic analysis of childhood acute lymphoblastic leukaemia lacking a genetic biomarker in the UKALL2003 clinical trial. Leukemia. 2023;37(3):529–38.

Optical Genome Mapping and Its Application in Hematological Malignancies

6

John Herriges and Lei Zhang

Introduction

Pediatric leukemias are classified into diagnostic subtypes and prognostic categories based on the presence of genetic abnormalities [1]. Typical genetic workup for pediatric leukemia patients includes molecular testing to look for sequence-level variants and cytogenetic testing to look for chromosome-level changes and gene rearrangements. The initial link between chromosome abnormalities and leukemias was made in 1960 with the discovery of the "Philadelphia" chromosome, which was later shown to be derived from a translocation between chromosomes 9 and 22 [2, 3]. Chromosome banding techniques (e.g., G-banding) were developed in the 1970s, which identified unique banding patterns along each chromosome, allowing for a better characterization of clonal genomic changes in leukemia samples [4]. Fluorescence in situ hybridization (FISH) was initially incorporated into clinical cytogenetic laboratories in the 1980s to enable reliable detection of clonal rearrangements and segmental copy number variants (CNVs) that may be missed by chromosome analysis [5–7]. More recently, labs have started to incorporate chromosomal microarray (CMA) into their analysis of hematologic malignancies, which allows for the detection of previously cryptic CNVs and copy-neutral loss of heterozygosity (CN-LOH) [8, 9].

Each of the aforementioned techniques provides valuable information about clonal genetic changes within leukemias and has its strengths and weaknesses (Table 6.1). Chromosome analysis can identify both structural (balanced and unbalanced) and numerical chromosomal alterations as well as changes in ploidy. It is a single cell genome wide analysis that can assess for the presence of clonal changes;

J. Herriges (✉) · L. Zhang
Department of Pathology and Laboratory Medicine, Children's Mercy Kansas City, University of Missouri Kansas City—School of Medicine, Kansas City, MO, USA
e-mail: jherriges@cmh.edu; lzhang@cmh.edu

W. Li (ed.), *Laboratory Assessments of Pediatric Leukemia*,
https://doi.org/10.1007/978-3-032-26557-9_6

Table 6.1 Comparison of current genetic testing with OGM

	Chromosomes	FISH	Microarray	OGM	Next generation sequencing	RNA-seq
Samples	Viable cells	Viable/fresh cells, fixed cells/tissue	Viable/fresh/frozen cells, fixed cells/tissue	Viable/fresh/frozen cells and tissue/	Viable/fresh/frozen cells, fixed cells/tissue	Viable/fresh/frozen cells, Fixed cells/tissue
Level of assessment	Single cell	Single cell	Whole sample/multi cell	Whole sample/multi cell	Whole sample/multi cell	Whole sample/multi cell
Coverage	Whole genome	Targeted	Whole genome	Whole genome	Whole genome	Whole transcriptome or targeted
Variants detected	SV, CNV, Ploidy	SV, CNV	CNV, LOH	SV, CNV, LOH	SV, CNV, LOH, SNV	SV, CNV, LOH, SNV
Resolution	~5–10 Mb	>~70 kb	>~5–25 kb	>~500 bp–5 kb	Single nucleotide	Single nucleotide
Sensitivity	~10%	~1–5%	~10–15%	~5–10%	<5% ~ 15%[a]	~5–10%
Processing time	~5–10 days	1–2 days	~5–10 days	~5–10 days	~5–28 days	~14–28 days

SV structural variant, *CNV* copy number variant, *LOH* loss of heterozygosity, *SNV* single nucleotide variant, [a]dependent on coverage and pipeline however, the overall resolution of these studies is typically ~5–10 Mb, meaning the precise genomic content involved is not always known. Additionally, chromosome banding pattern recognition can be very difficult in leukemia samples and can take years to master, with some considering the analysis to be akin to an art form. FISH testing has a higher resolution than chromosomes with probes that are designed to detect balanced and unbalanced structural rearrangements as well as deletions, duplications, and aneuploidies (Table 6.1). FISH studies also have a quicker turnaround time, with certain studies (e.g., PML/RARA probes) being run in less than a day. Moreover, FISH has a superior lower limit of detection, making it a better test to genetically follow patients for minimal residual disease. The primary disadvantage of the FISH technique is that it is targeted, and it is not feasible to run FISH probes for all genes or rearrangements, so targeted FISH panels are developed to examine common and therapeutically relevant cytogenetic changes. This means that FISH is less suited for the discovery of rare or atypical gene fusions. CMA has a much higher resolution than both chromosome and FISH studies and gives information on CN-LOH (Table 6.1). However, CMA cannot detect balanced structural variants, which are a hallmark of pediatric hematologic malignancies.

Optical Genomic Mapping (OGM)—General Principles

Optical mapping of the genome is a technique that has been around since the mid-1990s and was first used to map the genomes of model organisms like Saccharomyces cerevisiae [10, 11]. It was later used to look at the structural variation within the human genome, and more recently has been incorporated into the genomic workup of both hematologic and solid tumors to better understand the genomic drivers of tumor development [12–15].

OGM can be performed on blood and bone marrow samples as well as solid tumors. It utilizes ultra-high molecular weight (UHMW) DNA and requires that the samples undergo a special isolation procedure using commercial kits that allow long strands of DNA (>150 kb) to remain intact. After isolation, these long strands of DNA are fluorescently labeled with a direct labeling enzyme (DLE1) that recognizes the hexamer CTTAAG (Fig. 6.1). On average, this hexamer occurs every ~5 kb throughout the genome, though the labeling patterns of long strands of DNA can vary considerably. This labeling method does not involve nicking the UHMW DNA and maintains the integrity of these long strands. After labeling, samples are loaded on a chip composed of a series of nanochannels that individual linearized molecules of labeled DNA can travel through without tangling or folding back on themselves (Fig. 6.1). Each chip contains thousands of nanochannels, which allow for high-throughput imaging of a genome at high coverage (>300×). The labeled DNA molecules are brought through these channels using electrophoresis and are imaged (Fig. 6.1). Images of labeled DNA are then converted into digitalized DNA molecules that are assembled through three different pipelines. The first pipeline is the rare variant (RV) assembly pipeline, which is generally used in cancer samples. In the RV pipeline, molecules are aligned directly to the reference genome, with

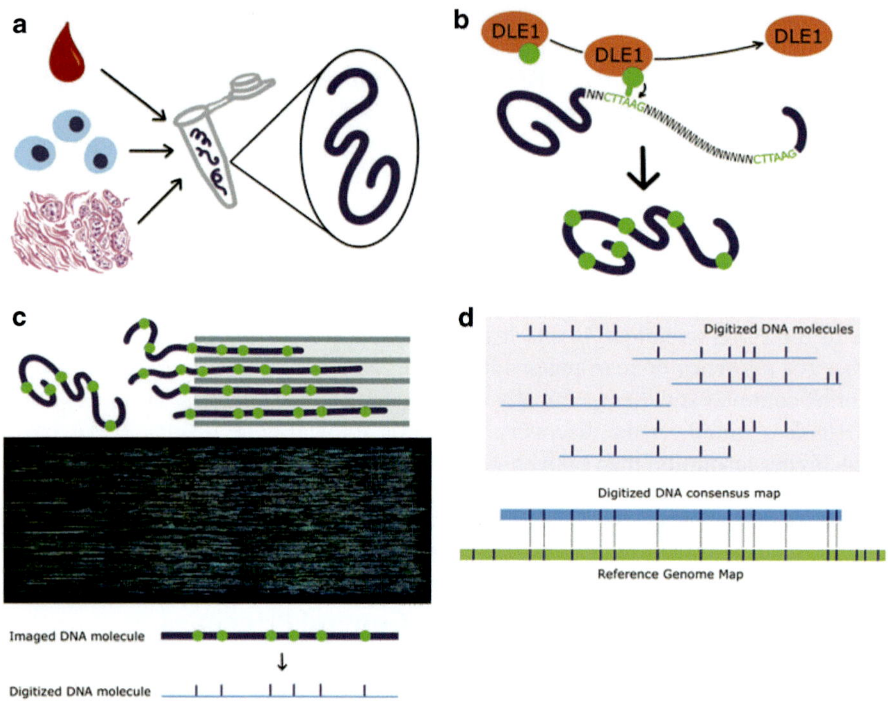

Fig. 6.1 OGM processing. Ultra-high molecular weight DNA is isolated from blood/bone marrow, solid tissues, or cell lines (**a**). DNA is then labeled using DLE1 (**b**). Labeled DNA is then run through a series of nanochannels, and the DNA molecules are imaged (**c**). Digitized DNA molecules are then processed and compared to a reference genome map (**d**)

misalignments representing potential structural variants (SV). A consensus map is then built using clusters of molecules that show the same SV and are realigned to the reference genome. The RV pipeline is used for cancer samples because it looks at molecules with low variant allele frequencies (VAF), making it ideal for detecting low-level clonal findings. The de novo (DN) assembly pipeline is generally used for constitutional analysis but has been shown to help with the detection of certain rearrangements in tumors [13]. This pipeline pairwise aligns all molecules to each other to create a consensus map that is then compared to the reference genome map. The DN pipeline has a higher resolution than the RV pipeline and can detect structural variants down to 500 bp but may miss variants with low VAFs (e.g., low-level clonal findings) [16]. The third pipeline is the Guided Assembly (GA). The initial processing of the GA is similar to the DN assembly pipeline, but instead of creating a consensus map through pairwise alignment of molecules, it uses a reference genome for refinement and haplotype splitting [17]. The generated GA consensus maps are then refined like the DN pipeline, and structural variants are identified through comparison of the refined maps to the reference genome. The GA has a similar lower limit of detection to the RV pipeline and is reported to have more accurate VAF calculations for low-level clonal findings [17]. Additionally, the GA is reported to be able to detect smaller insertions, deletions, and duplications at lower VAFs. Of note, the GA represents the newest available pipeline, so it is not as well represented in the published literature as the RV and DN analysis pipelines.

Visualization of OGM data is platform specific. Currently, the most prominent commercially available OGM platform is offered by Bionano Genomics. Their data can be visualized on two programs, Bionano Access and VIA. Importantly, both programs allow users to filter variants based on data quality and the presence of similar calls within control databases. This significantly reduces the amount of noise that a user may encounter when analyzing a case. Bionano Access displays the genome through circos plots and linearized genome-wide copy number profiles (Fig. 6.2a, b). For SVs, Bionano Access allows users to visualize the location of labeled hexamers within a patient sample and align them to the reference genome. Deletions and duplications are called when labels are lost and gained, respectively (Fig. 6.2c, d). Balanced structural abnormalities like inversions and translocations will show DNA maps with rearranged labels that map to one or more chromosomes (Fig. 6.2e, f). Breakpoints assigned to SVs represent the last correctly mapping label. This means that there is a level of ambiguity regarding where the precise breakpoints lie, which can impact the affected gene content.

The VIA software utilizes the same data as Bionano Access but has a separate algorithm for CNV detection. Unlike Bionano Access, VIA allows users to add calls and adjust breakpoints of copy number changes, making it better suited for detecting and reporting large segmental CNVs and aneuploidies. VIA also allows users to check for copy-neutral loss of heterozygosity (LOH) in samples run on all pipelines; whereas, this cannot be done on samples run through the RV pipeline in Bionano Access. While VIA does display structural variants detected by OGM, it does not allow users to visualize labels within structural variants, so Bionano Access remains an important data visualization tool for labs doing their primary analysis through VIA, similar to how IGV is used to visualize sequence-level variants in NGS. VIA software also allows users to create a database of calls and save variant interpretation annotations, which can help improve case interpretation times as well as consistency of variant interpretation over time. These features are absent from Bionano Access.

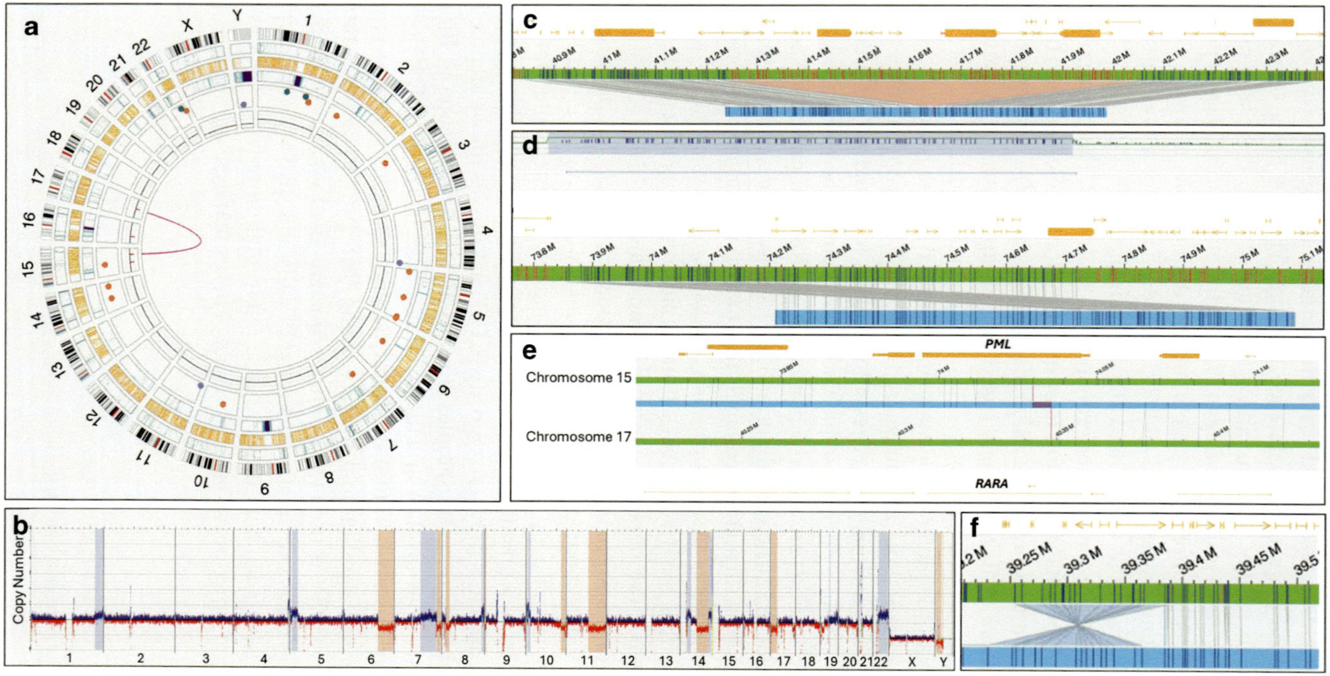

Fig. 6.2 Visualization of OGM data. OGM data can be visualized in a circos plot (**a**) or a linearized genome (**b**). Structural variants detectable by OGM include deletions (**c**), duplications (**d**), translocations (**e**), and inversions (**f**). For structural variants, the reference genome is represented by the green bar and the patient's molecule is denoted by the blue bar. The gray lines between the patient and reference (c-f) represent the corresponding probes, with translocations showing probes that map to two chromosomes (**e**) and inversions showing probes that map to different parts of the same chromosome (f)

Optical Genomic Mapping (OGM)—Compared to Standard Cytogenetic Technologies

Compared to standard cytogenetic technologies, OGM has a significantly higher resolution, with a processing time that is in line with chromosome analysis and CMA (Table 6.1) [18]. FISH testing is still faster than OGM, with STAT probes being completed within 24 hours. This means that OGM should not be used as a primary detection method for rearrangements requiring a rapid turnaround time, such as *PML*::*RARA* fusion, but for most rearrangements, the turnaround time associated with OGM should not significantly impact treatment. An additional point to consider with OGM is the throughput of the currently available instruments. This is not a major consideration for traditional cytogenetic testing methodologies because they can all be run as individual samples. For OGM, the Saphyr system allows users to run six total samples (on two different chips) at a time, with a minimum of three samples per run. This lower throughput may not be suitable for larger labs with higher volumes. While for smaller labs, with lower volumes, the minimum threshold of three samples per run may prolong turnaround times because they need to wait for samples to fill up the chip [19]. The newer Stratys system for OGM allows for up to 12 single-sample chips to be run at a time, with the option to prioritize up to three samples [20]. This may be more scalable for larger labs and removes the need for batching by smaller labs.

OGM can detect structural and copy number variants at the gene level, including balanced and unbalanced translocations, inversions, insertions, duplications, and deletions [21, 22]. Furthermore, for gained material, such as a duplication, OGM can show orientation (e.g., tandem versus inverted), which cannot be seen by CMA. Therefore, OGM can help to clarify complex karyotypes, which often have added material of unknown origin or complex structural rearrangements such as chromoplexy. Structural variants detectable by OGM can involve protein-coding elements like the t(12;21) that results in an *ETV6*::*RUNX1* fusion, or non-protein-coding elements like the IGH locus or T-cell receptor loci that can alter gene expression [23, 24]. This means that promoter or enhancer hijacking fusions, which may be missed by RNA-fusion panel testing, can be detected by OGM [25, 26]. However, changes in gene expression are not detectable by OGM and would have to be confirmed by an orthogonal method. OGM represents a whole genome test like CMA and karyotyping, but has reduced ability to detect variants near telomeres and centromeres, as well as other regions of the genome that have high levels of repetitive sequences (e.g., segmental duplications). Thus, rearrangements and copy number variants involving telomeres and repetitive elements may require orthogonal confirmation by another technology, such as FISH. Additionally, because OGM is not a single-cell analysis, detection of clonal evolution can be more difficult, and unlike chromosomes, changes in ploidy caused by endoreduplication (e.g., tetraploidy) cannot be detected. CN-LOH can be detected by OGM; however, the overall resolution is ~25 Mb, as compared to the ~3 Mb that is detectable by CMA [27].

OGM is unbiased in its ability to detect structural variants, so unlike FISH, it can detect both well-established gene fusions that are typically tested for in leukemia

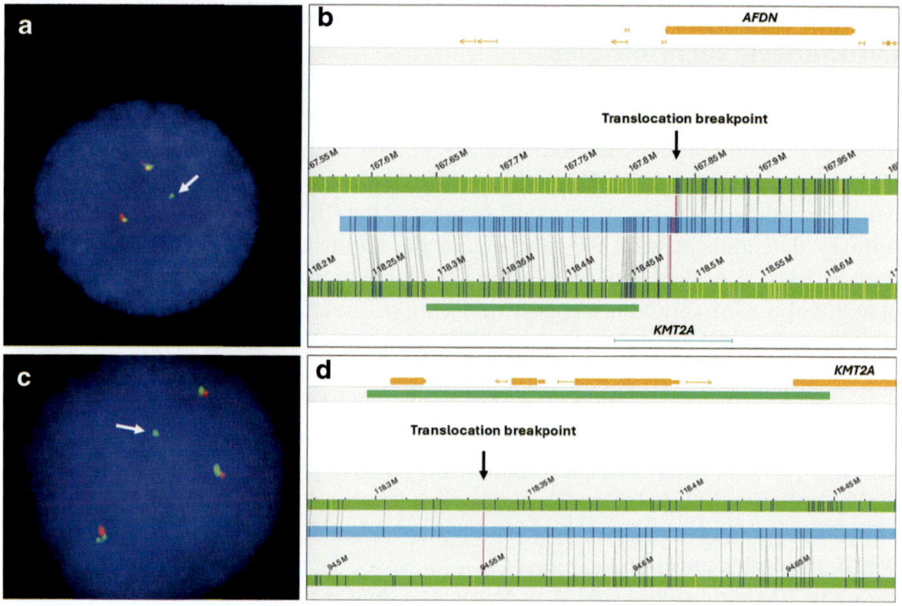

Fig. 6.3 OGM refining FISH breakpoints. Case 1 shows the gain of the 5′ portion (green; arrow) of the KMT2A FISH probe (**a**), and OGM shows fusion of *KMT2A* with *AFDN* (**b**). Case 2 shows gain of the 5′ portion (green; arrow) of the KMT2A FISH probe (**c**) but OGM shows that the rearrangement happened 5′ of KMT2A (**d**; arrow) and does not result in a rearrangement of the *KMT2A* gene. The green bar in **c** and **d** represents the location of the 5′ KMT2A FISH probe

patients as well as rare or novel fusions that have not been previously reported. Some well-established fusions involve genes with many fusion partners (e.g., *KMT2A*), and historically, cytogenetic labs have tested for these using break-apart FISH probes, which means that the fusion partner is not always known. OGM can identify those partner genes that can impact risk stratification and treatment (Fig. 6.3) [1, 28]. The higher resolution of OGM also leads to more precise breakpoints when compared to FISH, which can impact tumor classification. For example, the gain of a portion of the 5′ KMT2A break apart FISH probe in one case can result in the recurrent *KMT2A*::*AFDN* fusion (Fig. 6.3). In a second case, gain of that same segment of the KMT2A probe can result from a translocation near *KMT2A* that does not actually result in a *KMT2A* rearrangement (Fig. 6.3). By FISH, both cases are consistent with *KMT2A* rearranged leukemia, but OGM clarifies that *KMT2A* is only rearranged in the first case. Although OGM has higher resolution than FISH, one of its weaknesses is that the breakpoints for translocations/fusions are not as well defined as molecular assays (e.g., RNA sequencing assays or genome sequencing), which can often provide the exact exons and sequences involved and can also provide CNV and CN-LOH information (Table 6.1) [26, 29, 30]. The imprecise nature of OGM's breakpoints can be especially important when trying to determine the best assays to genetically track minimal residual disease (MRD), as

OGM's lower limit of detection has been reported to be a VAF of ~5–10% [31, 32]. This is too high to accurately track low-level MRD seen by flow cytometry, which is currently the gold standard for following disease, and is higher than the lower limit of detection of most FISH probes (Table 6.1). The higher lower limit of detection for OGM also means that it may miss certain subclonal findings even when there is a high tumor burden.

While OGM has most frequently been compared to traditional cytogenetic technologies, recent advances in molecular techniques have allowed techniques like whole genome sequencing of DNA and RNA-sequencing to screen for gene fusions and copy number events [26, 29, 30, 33]. These assays are more precise in their ability to map breakpoints, and they can also detect LOH and single-nucleotide variants (SNVs) that are prognostically significant. A recent study has even proposed that genome sequencing could serve as an alternative to cytogenetic analysis in myeloid malignancies, as it can have similar turnaround times to chromosomes and FISH, while providing additional relevant information that can adjust patient risk stratification [30]. RNA sequencing also allows labs to perform whole transcriptome analysis, which can classify tumors based on gene expression profiles [33]. This can be especially important when traditional testing is not able to identify a clear driver. However, these assays are often higher cost to implement and run, and typically require significant local bioinformatic support, which is not true of OGM [26, 29]. Additionally, while these genome-wide molecular techniques can have similar processing times, for many labs, it will not be feasible to rapidly process these cases, which can lead to longer turnaround times.

OGM Nomenclature

Nomenclature describing OGM results is included in the recently released 2024 version of the International System of Cytogenomic Nomenclature (ISCN) and aligns with other cytogenetic testing while using the prefix "ogm" (Table 6.2) [34]. The overall nomenclature for aneuploidies, losses, and gains called by the copy number algorithm is similar to the array ISCN nomenclature. Smaller copy number variants (deletions and duplications) are called using the structural variant algorithm in OGM. The reported breakpoints associated with deletions will often not align with the size of the reported CNV because the listed ISCN breakpoints represent the last correctly mapped label flanking the deletion, and there will often be a variable region between these labels that is unaffected (Fig. 6.4). For duplications, the reported breakpoints will represent the affected labels, so the actual duplication can be slightly larger than the reported breakpoints. Other structural variants, including insertions (intrachromosomal or interchromosomal), inversions, and translocations, follow the same basic rules that apply to chromosome study nomenclature; however, the nucleotide breakpoints are included, and gene fusions can be indicated at the end of the string (e.g., "(ETV6::RUNX1)") [34, 35]. The reported breakpoints for translocations and other fusions are listed as a range instead of a single breakpoint (Table 6.2). For insertions, the region that genomic material is

Table 6.2 OGM ISCN nomenclature

OGM finding	ISCN nomenclature example
Aneuploidy	ogm(7)x1[0.5]
Deletion	ogm[GRCh38] 9p13.2(36,955,993_37,031,741)x1[VAF0.4] or ogm[GRCh38] del(9)(p13.2p13.2)(36,955,993_37,031,741)[VAF0.4]
Duplication	ogm[GRCh38] 21q22.12(34878048_35049381)x3[VAF0.3] or ogm[GRCh38] dup(21)(21q22.12q22.12)(34878048_35049381)[VAF0.3]
Insertion	ogm[GRCh38] ins(11;5)(p11.12;q32q35.1)(50133920~50139496;150,061,615_171,410,278)[VAF0.2]
Inversion	ogm[GRCh38] inv(5)(q32q35.1)(150,061,615~150,072,384_171,405,034~171,410,278)[VAF0.2]
Translocation	ogm[GRCh38] t(12;21)(p13.2;q22.12)(11,861,581~11,864,402;34,981,504~34,998,849)(ETV6::RUNX1)[VAF0.5]

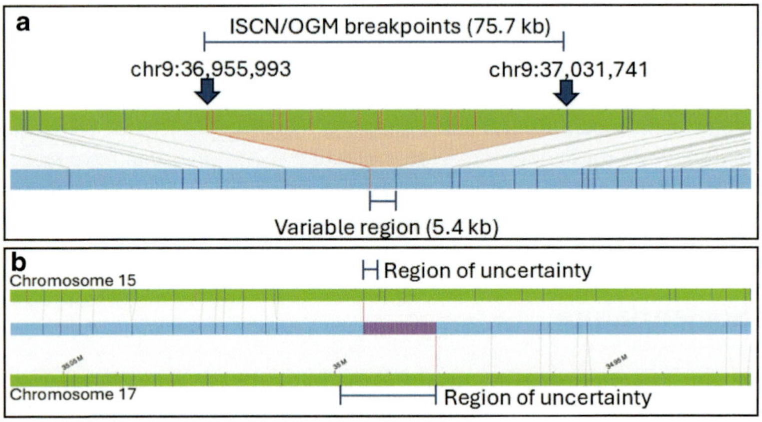

Fig. 6.4 An example of a deletion with an ISCN nomenclature of OGM[GRCh38] 9p13.2(36,955,993_37,031,741)x1[VAF0.4] (**a**). The deletion contains a ~5.4 kb variable region that is retained. An example of a translocation with an ISCN nomenclature of OGM[GRCh38] t(15;17) (p15q24.1;q21.2)(74,029,809~74,039,430;40,335,716~40,348,183)(PML::RARA) [VAF0.5] (**b**). The regions of uncertainty of the breakpoint are denoted by a tilde "~"

being inserted into is listed as a range. The use of a breakpoint range for these different types of variants is meant to account for the uncertainty associated with OGM breakpoints and may affect the associated gene content. Additionally, OGM results are often complex due to the high resolution of the platform and the ability to detect both copy number changes and structural variants. The 2020 version of ISCN had developed nomenclature strings to address complex findings on the array [36]. These symbols are used when it is not feasible to describe a finding with other nomenclature symbols. Similar prefixes are used for OGM, including "cx" for complex, "cha" for chromoanasynthesis, "cth" for chromothripsis, and "cpx" for chromoplexy. When appropriate, these prefixes can be applied to specific regions of the genome (e.g., ogm[GRCh38] 5p15.3p15.3(656,103_3,663,154)cx[VAF0.5]) or, in the case of cx, it can be applied to the entire genome (e.g., ogm (X, Y,1-22)cx). Additionally, the most recent version of the ISCN allows for variants to be reported in a tabular format that includes cytogenetic bands, breakpoints, size, variant type, VAF, and other key components such as the genes involved [34, 35]. This can make it easier to report nomenclature for complex genomes with multiple structural and copy number variants and to highlight critical genes involved.

OGM in B-Cell Acute Lymphoblastic Leukemia

B-cell acute lymphoblastic leukemia (B-ALL) represents 85% of pediatric ALL patients and is the most common leukemia in the pediatric population [1]. Classification of B-ALL patients is based on the presence of cytogenetic and molecular genetic abnormalities that are constantly evolving, including *BCR*::*ABL1*, *ETV6*::*RUNX1*, and *TCF3*::*PBX1* fusions, hyperdiploidy, hypodiploidy, and *KMT2A* rearrangements. Traditional testing for *KMT2A* rearrangement in a cytogenetics lab includes a break-apart FISH probe that can identify a rearrangement of the gene, but will not identify its partner. This strategy has been implemented because it is not feasible to test for the more than 100 gene fusion partners of *KMT2A* by FISH [37]. However, it is important to identify the *KMT2A* partner gene because it can impact overall prognosis in leukemias [1, 28]. The subtype of BCR/ABL1-like (Ph-like) B-ALL is genetically complex and defined by the presence of rearrangements that result in increased kinase activity through fusions of genes like *CRLF2*, *ABL1*, *ABL2*, *JAK2*, and *PDGFRB* [38]. This subtype is typically associated with a poorer prognosis and may benefit from targeted therapies using tyrosine kinase inhibitors like ruxolitinib and dasatinib [39]. Due to the numerous gene fusions that are driving the development of B-ALL and the feasibility of OGM to detect genome-wide fusions, several studies have investigated the potential use of OGM in B-ALL patients.

The initial studies looking at the utility of OGM in pediatric B-ALL were relatively small. Lestringant et al. and Luhmann et al. correlated OGM results with standard techniques, including chromosome analysis, FISH, CMA, and MLPA, as well as RNA-seq fusion in a handful of B-ALL patients [40, 41]. Both studies found that OGM showed high concordance with traditional testing methodologies and also identified novel rearrangements, including *IGH*::*CEBPB* fusion, a *JAK2* rearrangement, and an *ETV6*::*ABL1* fusion, that were missed by traditional testing methodologies. Additionally, both studies found that OGM missed some subclonal findings, the most critical of which was the recurrent deletion within the pseudoautosomal region of the X chromosome, which results in a *P2RY8*::*CRLF2* fusion, which can help define a leukemia as BCR/ABL1-like [1]. Of note, in two of those patients, the VAF of the *P2RY8*::*CRLF2* fusion was not reported, so it is unclear whether this was missed because it was below the limit of detection for OGM [41]. Other findings missed by OGM were below its lower limit of detection or were missed due to filtering issues.

Subsequent larger studies involving B-ALL patients have shown similar results. Rack et al. compared the results of OGM with conventional chromosome analysis, FISH, MLPA, and RT-PCR [42]. Standard technologies identified clonal abnormalities in 93% of B-ALL cases, while OGM identified clonal abnormalities in 100% of cases. However, OGM did not recognize some subclonal aberrations, with the authors stating that OGM could reliably detect aberrations present in at least 15% of cells [42]. All disease-defining structural variants identified through traditional testing methodologies were also identified by OGM in their B-ALL cohort, with OGM identifying additional recurrent chromosomal abnormalities in 7 cases, including rearrangements of *TCF3*, *JAK2*, *PAX5*, *EP300*, and *CSF1R*. Additionally, this study found that OGM showed concordance for aneuploidy with standard testing methods in ~93% of cases [42]. OGM did miss the classification of a single low hypodiploid ALL, which is associated with a poor prognosis. In this case, chromosomal aneuploidies were observed, but it was interpreted as hyperdiploidy instead of hypodiploidy. Interestingly, traditional testing methodologies were also discordant for the missed low hypodiploid ALL case, and missing this call was attributed to a low blast percentage in the tested sample. Of note, this study was performed prior to LOH detection being available by OGM, which is often a key indicator of low hypodiploidy [27].

Gao et al. compared OGM to traditional cytogenetic testing techniques (FISH and chromosomes) in 46 newly diagnosed pediatric B-ALL patients [43]. This study found that OGM had 100% concordance with standard cytogenetic techniques for known aberrations, with the exception of the recurrent deletion resulting in the *P2RY8*::*CRLF2* fusion, which was missed in 3 cases. Seventeen cases from their cohort had OGM findings that either refined the cytogenetic breakpoints or identified novel fusions, like *JAK2*::*TEK* and *FLI1*::*EWSR1*.

Several additional studies have also been published that focus on utilizing OGM in certain B-ALL subtypes. Amplification of exons 2-5 of *PAX5* (PAX5-ITM) is a recurrent finding in ~1% of pediatric B-ALL patients [44]. This finding is not detectable by traditional cytogenetic techniques and has been associated with a higher incidence of relapse. Although CMA can detect copy number gains involving *PAX5*, it will not provide information on genomic structure to definitively prove the *PAX5*-ITM is present. Jean et al. demonstrated that OGM can detect the gain of *PAX5* exons associated with the *PAX5*-ITM, visualize their structure to prove they are in tandem, and provide a more accurate assessment of the number of extra copies of exons 2–5 that are present [45]. Another study examined results from OGM run on *ETV6*::*RUNX1* fusion and hyperdiploid B-ALL patients and found that OGM was able to detect 100% of *ETV6*::*RUNX1* fusions and chromosomal gains in hyperdiploidy cases, as well as 95% of SVs identified by traditional cytogenetic testing methods overall [23]. This was further broken down based on technique, with OGM detecting 100% of findings detected by FISH, 96% of findings detected by chromosome analysis, and 96% of findings detected by CMA. The missed calls from this study highlight one of the shortcomings of OGM in that many of the missed translocations have at least one breakpoint localizing near a centromere. Of note, this study also found that OGM detected 677 additional SVs missed by conventional testing methodologies, including deletions involving *IKZF1*, and was also able to resolve complex structural rearrangements in ~30% of *ETV6*::*RUNX1* fusion-positive cases [23].

OGM in T-Cell Acute Lymphoblastic Leukemia

T-Cell acute lymphoblastic leukemia (T-ALL) represents approximately 15% of pediatric ALL patients [1]. There are no genetically defined subtypes for T-ALL in the WHO; however, a recent large cohort study identified 15 subtypes with specific genomic drivers [46]. Recurrent cytogenetic findings in T-ALL include rearrangements involving T-cell receptor loci at 14q (TRA/D) and 7q34 (TRB) and transcription factors including *TAL1*, *TLX1*, *TLX3*, *NKX2-1*, and *HOXA* genes. To date, there have been limited studies on the utilization of OGM in pediatric T-ALL patients. Rack et al. compared OGM results in 12 T-ALL patients to conventional chromosome analysis, FISH, MLPA, and RT-PCR [42]. While FISH was able to identify *TRA/D*, *TRB*, and *TLX3* rearrangements in 7 of the cases, the specific partner gene was not known. OGM was able to identify the partner gene in all cases and also identified *IGH::TAL1*, *TRB::TLX1*, and *TRB*::*HIBADH* fusions that were missed by the other testing modalities. Luhamann et al. reported a single patient with co-existing *STIL*::*TAL1* fusion and a *TRA*::*CAPRIN1* fusion, both of which were identified by conventional testing and OGM [41]. Lestringant et al. compared OGM to traditional cytogenetic testing methodologies in four T-ALL patients (2 pediatric and 2 adult), with OGM showing high correlation with traditional methods, while also identifying novel fusions including *TRA*::*LMO2* and *TRB*::*MYC* [40]. More recently, a large cohort study looking at the utilization of OGM in hematological malignancies found that OGM had the highest utility in T-ALL patients, with OGM identifying additional Tier 1 variants in 52% of cases and additional Tier 2 variants in 38% of cases [24]. Most of the additional Tier 1 variants were translocations. Of note, this study did not specifically state whether their T-ALL cohort consisted of pediatric patients.

OGM in Acute Myeloid Leukemia

Pediatric Acute Myeloid Leukemia (AML) is classified into diagnostic subtypes and prognostic categories based on the presence of specific genetic abnormalities. There are currently 14 different pediatric AML subtypes that are defined by a genetic abnormality, with two of these being sequence-level variants in *CEBPA* and *NPM1*, and the remainder being gene rearrangements/fusions [1]. The most common cytogenetic abnormalities found in pediatric AML are *KMT2A* rearrangements, *RUNX1*::*RUNXT1* fusion, and *CBFB*::*MYH11* fusion. Similar to *KMT2A* rearrangements in B-ALL, *KMT2A* has many different partner genes in AML, with the partner gene impacting risk stratification [1, 37]. Additional cytogenetic findings include *NUP98* rearrangements and *CBFA2T3*::*GLIS2* fusion, which are both cytogenetically cryptic and associated with a poor prognosis.

There have been limited studies on OGM in pediatric AML, with the lone study coming from Suttorp et al., which involved 24 patients [47]. They compared OGM results to chromosome analysis and FISH testing, with only 6 cases having OGM results that were identical to conventional testing methods. Three of the discrepant cases had calls detected by chromosome analysis and not OGM; however, two of these calls were deemed to be artifacts. Nine of the discrepant cases had additional calls identified by OGM that were missed by conventional testing methods. Six patients had abnormalities identified by OGM and conventional testing methods that were missed by the others, including one patient who was found to have a *CBFA2T3*::*GLIS2* fusion by OGM but not conventional testing methods. Patient risk stratification using conventional testing methods and OGM was the same for all but one case, with the lone exception being the patient with a *CBFA2T3*::*GLIS2* fusion, who had been classified as intermediate risk based on conventional testing and high risk based on OGM results [47].

There have been several studies on the utilization of OGM in the adult AML population [32, 48–50]. Levy et al. compared the results for OGM in 100 adult patients with conventional cytogenetic testing (chromosome analysis, FISH, and microarray testing) [48]. They found that OGM had a 98.4% sensitivity for the sentinel chromosomal abnormalities, with the single missed finding being a *BCR*::*ABL1* fusion that was present below OGM's limit of detection. Their calculated specificity was 100%, and the accuracy for all results was 99.6% [48]. Thirteen of their cases were found to have additional findings on OGM that were clinically significant, including 5 patients with altered risk stratification based on OGM results and 8 patients with OGM findings that could make them eligible for trials [48]. One limitation of this study was that only 19% of their patients had FISH testing in addition to chromosome analysis, with many of the novel OGM findings representing recurrent AML rearrangements (e.g., *KMT2A* and *NUP98* rearrangements) that would have been caught with a standard pediatric AML FISH panel. The authors also note discrepancies between OGM results and FISH results for probes that were abnormal in <20% of nuclei, suggesting that OGM may not be suitable to look for low level clones or minimal residual disease. Similar results were noted by smaller studies on adult AML patients, which showed a high concordance of OGM with chromosome and FISH results, with the only abnormalities missed by OGM being low level subclonal findings near OGM's lower limit of detection, ploidy changes, and structural variants with breakpoints in regions with low coverage (e.g., telomeres and centromeres) [49, 50]. These smaller studies also showed additional findings by OGM that were clinically relevant, including *KMT2A* partial tandem duplications (PTDs), *NUP98* rearrangements, and an *ETV6* rearrangement that was missed by traditional testing. Overall, OGM results from these studies adjusted risk stratification for 3 (5%) patients, with 2 having a better European Leukemia Net (ELN) risk stratification score and 1 having a worse score [49, 50].

More recently, a large cohort study from Loghavi et al. involving 159 AML patients found that 39% of patients showed completely concordant results with OGM and traditional testing methodologies; 11% of patients had concordant results between OGM and traditional testing, with OGM clarifying a fusion gene partner; 37% had partially concordant results; and 11% had entirely discordant results [32]. Similar to previous studies, most abnormalities missed by OGM were below the assay's lower limit of detection. Additionally, OGM was able to detect class-defining gene rearrangements involving *MECOM*, *NUP98*, and *KMT2A*; *KMT2A-PTD*; chromoanagenesis; and gene amplifications that were missed by traditional testing. Overall, Loghavi et al. showed that ~5% of newly diagnosed AML patients had an altered ELN risk stratification based on OGM results, and ~6% had a change in diagnosis [32]. Finally, the most recent study on OGM in AML found that OGM identified additional Tier 1 aberrations in 13% of cases [24].

Summary

For decades, cytogenetic workup of new leukemia patients has involved chromosome analysis and FISH studies. More recently, labs have incorporated microarray testing into their clinical workup to look for cytogenetically cryptic clonal CNVs. These studies have identified recurrent genome abnormalities that define leukemias and help guide therapy decisions, which impact patient outcomes. OGM represents a novel technology that has recently been incorporated into the workup of hematologic malignancies [13]. Most studies to date have focused on the utility of this technology in adult patients; however, there have been several smaller studies using pediatric populations.

Limitations of OGM include a reduced ability to detect low-level clonal events, reduced detection of variants involving repetitive regions of the genome (e.g., centromeres and telomeres), and reduced CN-LOH detection. Among these, the reduced detection of variants overlapping repetitive elements is of particular importance, as some recurrent findings in pediatric leukemias (e.g., *P2RY8*::*CRLF2* and *IGH*::*CRLF2*) overlap these regions. The *P2RY8*::*CRLF2* fusion was shown to be particularly difficult for OGM to detect, with multiple studies citing missed fusions [40, 43]. This fusion is of specific importance because it helps define a genetic subtype in B-ALL and has potential therapeutic implications [1]. Not detecting low-level clonal abnormalities by OGM was noted in several studies [51]. This limits the utilization of OGM to diagnostic samples or relapsed samples with a higher blast count (>20%). Genetic testing of samples with low-level minimal residual disease (MRD) would require an alternative method such as FISH or a molecular fusion assay, which typically have lower limits of detection.

The strengths of OGM include it being a single assay that can detect almost everything traditional cytogenetic methods test for. It is also higher resolution than traditional cytogenetic testing methodologies and provides a genome-wide view of structural rearrangements. Although certain regions of the genome do pose a problem for OGM, concordance studies have shown that it has a high sensitivity, specificity, positive predictive value, and accuracy when compared to traditional cytogenetic testing methodologies [31, 48]. Additionally, all large cohort comparison studies on hematologic malignancies to date have demonstrated that OGM is able to detect genetic abnormalities that were missed by traditional testing modalities or provide additional information that helped to further genetically define the malignancy [24, 31, 48, 51]. For some cases, this was defining the fusion partners of a gene/locus already known to be rearranged, while in others it was identifying novel fusions that were missed by traditional testing methodologies. Importantly, multiple studies showed that incorporating OGM results led to altered risk stratification for patients, demonstrating the clinical benefit of OGM testing [32, 47, 48].

In summary, OGM represents a novel technology that can be used to detect clonal abnormalities traditionally tested for using chromosome analysis, FISH, and CMA methodologies. Although there are limitations associated with this technology, studies have repeatedly demonstrated that the increased resolution and genome-wide structural variation detection provide additional clinical utility, suggesting that incorporation of OGM into clinical testing algorithms for newly diagnosed pediatric leukemias results in better genetic classification.

References

1. WHO Classification of Tumours Editorial Board. Paediatric tumours [Internet]. Lyon: International Agency for Research on Cancer; 2022 [(WHO classification of tumours series, 5th ed.; vol. 7). Available from: https://tumourclassification.iarc.who.int/chapters/44.
2. Rowley JD. Letter: A new consistent chromosomal abnormality in chronic myelogenous leukaemia identified by quinacrine fluorescence and Giemsa staining. Nature. 1973;243(5405):290–3.
3. Nowell PCHDA. A minute chromosome in human chronic granulocytic leukemia. Science. 1960;132:1497.
4. Seabright M. A rapid banding technique for human chromosomes. Lancet. 1971;2(7731):971–2.
5. Levsky JM, Singer RH. Fluorescence in situ hybridization: past, present and future. J Cell Sci. 2003;116(Pt 14):2833–8.
6. Pinkel D, Gray JW, Trask B, van den Engh G, Fuscoe J, van Dekken H. Cytogenetic analysis by in situ hybridization with fluorescently labeled nucleic acid probes. Cold Spring Harb Symp Quant Biol. 1986;51(Pt 1):151–7.
7. Spathas DH, Stewart J, Singer IO, Theriault A, Bovey M, Connor JM. Detection of t(12;21) in childhood acute lymphoblastic leukemia by fluorescence in situ hybridization. Cancer Genet Cytogenet. 1999;110(1):7–13.
8. Wang Y, Miller S, Roulston D, Bixby D, Shao L. Genome-wide single-nucleotide polymorphism array analysis improves prognostication of acute lymphoblastic leukemia/lymphoma. J Mol Diagn. 2016;18(4):595–603.
9. Xu X, Bryke C, Sukhanova M, Huxley E, Dash DP, Dixon-Mciver A, et al. Assessing copy number abnormalities and copy-neutral loss-of-heterozygosity across the genome as best practice in diagnostic evaluation of acute myeloid leukemia: an evidence-based review from the cancer genomics consortium (CGC) myeloid neoplasms working group. Cancer Genet. 2018;228–229:218–35.
10. Schwartz DC, Li X, Hernandez LI, Ramnarain SP, Huff EJ, Wang YK. Ordered restriction maps of Saccharomyces cerevisiae chromosomes constructed by optical mapping. Science. 1993;262(5130):110–4.
11. Zhou S, Wei F, Nguyen J, Bechner M, Potamousis K, Goldstein S, et al. A single molecule scaffold for the maize genome. PLoS Genet. 2009;5(11):e1000711.
12. Teague B, Waterman MS, Goldstein S, Potamousis K, Zhou S, Reslewic S, et al. High-resolution human genome structure by single-molecule analysis. Proc Natl Acad Sci USA. 2010;107(24):10848–53.

13. Smith AC, Neveling K, Kanagal-Shamanna R. Optical genome mapping for structural variation analysis in hematologic malignancies. Am J Hematol. 2022;97(7):975–82.
14. Levy B, Kanagal-Shamanna R, Sahajpal NS, Neveling K, Rack K, Dewaele B, et al. A framework for the clinical implementation of optical genome mapping in hematologic malignancies. Am J Hematol. 2024;99(4):642–61.
15. Goldrich DY, LaBarge B, Chartrand S, Zhang L, Sadowski HB, Zhang Y, et al. Identification of somatic structural variants in solid tumors by optical genome mapping. J Pers Med. 2021;11(2).
16. Bionano. Bionano System Application Specifications. Document number CG-00008, Sep 6, 2024. https://Bionano.com/wp-content/uploads/2023/08/CG-00008-Bionano-Saphyr-System-Application-Specifications.pdf.
17. Bionano. Bionano Solve Theory of Operation: structural variant calling. Document Number: 30110. 2021. https://Bionano.com/wp-content/uploads/2025/08/CG-30110-Bionano-Solve-Theory-of-Operation-Structural-Variant-Calling.pdf. 2025.
18. Brody F, Dubuc A, Kim A. Optical genome mapping: a 'tool' with significant potential from discovery to diagnostics. CAP Article.
19. Bionano. Reveal more genomic variation that matters with optical genome mapping. Bionano document. https://bionano.com/wp-content/uploads/BNG-23-064-Saphyr-Brochure-Update-2023_6.0_DIGITAL.pdf.
20. Bionano. Elevate the OGM Sample-to-Report Workflow with the Stratys™ System. Bionano document. https://bionano.com/wp-content/uploads/2024/01/Stratys-Brochure.pdf.
21. Smith AC, Hoischen A, Raca G. Cytogenetics is a science, not a technique! Why optical genome mapping is so important to clinical genetic laboratories. Cancers (Basel). 2023;15(22)
22. Lu S, Liu K, Wang D, Ye Y, Jiang Z, Gao Y. Genomic structural variants analysis in leukemia by a novel cytogenetic technique: optical genome mapping. Cancer Sci. 2024;115(11):3543–51.
23. Brandes D, Yasin L, Nebral K, Ebler J, Schinnerl D, Picard D, et al. Optical genome mapping identifies novel recurrent structural alterations in childhood ETV6::RUNX1+ and high hyperdiploid acute lymphoblastic leukemia. Hemasphere. 2023;7(8):e925.
24. Toruner GA, Hu S, Loghavi S, Ok CY, Tang Z, Wei Q, et al. Clinical utility of optical genome mapping as an additional tool in a standard cytogenetic workup in hematological malignancies. Cancers (Basel). 2025;17(9).
25. Brown LM, Lonsdale A, Zhu A, Davidson NM, Schmidt B, Hawkins A, et al. The application of RNA sequencing for the diagnosis and genomic classification of pediatric acute lymphoblastic leukemia. Blood Adv. 2020;4(5):930–42.
26. Lestringant V, Guermouche-Flament H, Jimenez-Pocquet M, Gaillard JB, Penther D. Cytogenetics in the management of hematological malignancies: an overview of alternative technologies for cytogenetic characterization. Curr Res Transl Med. 2024;72(3):103440.
27. Barseghyan H, Pang AWC, Clifford B, Serrano MA, Chaubey A, Hastie AR. Comparative benchmarking of optical genome mapping and chromosomal microarray reveals high technological concordance in CNV identification and additional structural variant refinement. Genes (Basel). 2023;14(10).
28. Gorecki M, Koziol I, Kopystecka A, Budzynska J, Zawitkowska J, Lejman M. Updates in KMT2A gene rearrangement in pediatric acute lymphoblastic leukemia. Biomedicines. 2023;11(3).
29. Balciuniene J, Ning Y, Lazarus HM, Aikawa V, Sherpa S, Zhang Y, et al. Cancer cytogenetics in a genomics world: Wedding the old with the new. Blood Rev. 2024;66:101209.
30. Duncavage EJ, Schroeder MC, O'Laughlin M, Wilson R, MacMillan S, Bohannon A, et al. Genome sequencing as an alternative to cytogenetic analysis in myeloid cancers. N Engl J Med. 2021;384(10):924–35.
31. Sahajpal NS, Mondal AK, Tvrdik T, Hauenstein J, Shi H, Deeb KK, et al. Clinical validation and diagnostic utility of optical genome mapping for enhanced cytogenomic analysis of hematological neoplasms. J Mol Diagn. 2022;24(12):1279–91.

32. Loghavi S, Wei Q, Ravandi F, Quesada AE, Routbort MJ, Hu S, et al. Optical genome mapping improves the accuracy of classification, risk stratification, and personalized treatment strategies for patients with acute myeloid leukemia. Am J Hematol. 2024;99(10):1959–68.
33. Hu Z, Kovach AE, Yellapantula V, Ostrow D, Doan A, Ji J, et al. Transcriptome sequencing allows comprehensive genomic characterization of pediatric B-acute lymphoblastic leukemia in an academic clinical laboratory. J Mol Diagn. 2024;26(1):49–60.
34. ISCN 2024: an International System for Human Cytogenomic Nomenclature (2024). Hastings RJ, Moore S, Chia N, editors. S.Karger AG; 2024.
35. Moore S, McGowan-Jordan J, Smith AC, Rack K, Koehler U, Stevens-Kroef M, et al. Genome mapping nomenclature. Cytogenet Genome Res. 2023;163(5-6):236–46.
36. ISCN 2020: an International System for Human Cytogenomic Nomenclature (2020) Reprint of 'Cytogenetic and Genome Research 2020, Vol. 160, No. 7–8'. McGowan-Jordan J, Hastings RJ, Moore S, editors. S.Karger AG; 2020.
37. Meyer C, Burmeister T, Groger D, Tsaur G, Fechina L, Renneville A, et al. The MLL recombinome of acute leukemias in 2017. Leukemia. 2018;32(2):273–84.
38. Roberts KG, Li Y, Payne-Turner D, Harvey RC, Yang YL, Pei D, et al. Targetable kinase-activating lesions in Ph-like acute lymphoblastic leukemia. N Engl J Med. 2014;371(11):1005–15.
39. Harvey RC, Tasian SK. Clinical diagnostics and treatment strategies for Philadelphia chromosome-like acute lymphoblastic leukemia. Blood Adv. 2020;4(1):218–28.
40. Lestringant V, Duployez N, Penther D, Luquet I, Derrieux C, Lutun A, et al. Optical genome mapping, a promising alternative to gold standard cytogenetic approaches in a series of acute lymphoblastic leukemias. Genes Chromosom Cancer. 2021;60(10):657–67.
41. Luhmann JL, Stelter M, Wolter M, Kater J, Lentes J, Bergmann AK, et al. The clinical utility of optical genome mapping for the assessment of genomic aberrations in acute lymphoblastic leukemia. Cancers (Basel). 2021;13(17).
42. Rack K, De Bie J, Ameye G, Gielen O, Demeyer S, Cools J, et al. Optimizing the diagnostic workflow for acute lymphoblastic leukemia by optical genome mapping. Am J Hematol. 2022;97(5):548–61.
43. Gao H, Xu H, Wang C, Cui L, Huang X, Li W, et al. Optical genome mapping for comprehensive assessment of chromosomal aberrations and discovery of new fusion genes in pediatric B-acute lymphoblastic leukemia. Cancers (Basel). 2022;15(1).
44. Schwab C, Nebral K, Chilton L, Leschi C, Waanders E, Boer JM, et al. Intragenic amplification of PAX5: a novel subgroup in B-cell precursor acute lymphoblastic leukemia? Blood Adv. 2017;1(19):1473–7.
45. Jean J, Kovach AE, Doan A, Oberley M, Ji J, Schmidt RJ, et al. Characterization of PAX5 intragenic tandem multiplication in pediatric B-lymphoblastic leukemia by optical genome mapping. Blood Adv. 2022;6(11):3343–6.
46. Polonen P, Di Giacomo D, Seffernick AE, Elsayed A, Kimura S, Benini F, et al. The genomic basis of childhood T-lineage acute lymphoblastic leukaemia. Nature. 2024;632(8027):1082–91.
47. Suttorp J, Luhmann JL, Behrens YL, Gohring G, Steinemann D, Reinhardt D, et al. Optical genome mapping as a diagnostic tool in pediatric acute myeloid leukemia. Cancers (Basel). 2022;14(9).
48. Levy B, Baughn LB, Akkari Y, Chartrand S, LaBarge B, Claxton D, et al. Optical genome mapping in acute myeloid leukemia: a multicenter evaluation. Blood Adv. 2023;7(7):1297–307.
49. Balducci E, Kaltenbach S, Villarese P, Duroyon E, Zalmai L, Friedrich C, et al. Optical genome mapping refines cytogenetic diagnostics, prognostic stratification and provides new molecular insights in adult MDS/AML patients. Blood Cancer J. 2022;12(9):126.
50. Gerding WM, Tembrink M, Nilius-Eliliwi V, Mika T, Dimopoulos F, Ladigan-Badura S, et al. Optical genome mapping reveals additional prognostic information compared to conventional cytogenetics in AML/MDS patients. Int J Cancer. 2022;150(12):1998–2011.
51. Coccaro N, Anelli L, Zagaria A, Tarantini F, Cumbo C, Tota G, et al. Feasibility of optical genome mapping in cytogenetic diagnostics of hematological neoplasms: a new way to look at DNA. Diagnostics (Basel). 2023;13(11).

Long-Read Sequencing for the Diagnosis of Pediatric Leukemia

7

Josephine B. Oehler, Bahareh A. Mojarad, Yang Cao, and Ulf Schmitz

J. B. Oehler
Computational Biomedicine Lab, College of Science and Engineering, James Cook University, Townsville, QLD, Australia

College of Medicine and Dentistry, James Cook University, Cairns, QLD, Australia
e-mail: josephine.oehler@my.jcu.edu.au

B. A. Mojarad
Cancer Genetics & Genomics Laboratory, BC Cancer, Vancouver, BC, Canada

Department of Pathology & Laboratory Medicine, Faculty of Medicine, University of British Columbia, Vancouver, BC, Canada
e-mail: bahareh@bccancer.bc.ca

Y. Cao
Department of Pathology and Immunology, Washington University School of Medicine, St. Louis, MO, USA
e-mail: cao.yang@wustl.edu

U. Schmitz (✉)
Computational Biomedicine Lab, College of Science and Engineering, James Cook University, Townsville, QLD, Australia

Centre for Tropical Bioinformatics and Molecular Biology, Australian Institute of Tropical Health and Medicine, James Cook University, Cairns, Australia

Centenary Institute, The University of Sydney, Camperdown, Australia
e-mail: ulf.schmitz@jcu.edu.au

W. Li (ed.), *Laboratory Assessments of Pediatric Leukemia*,
https://doi.org/10.1007/978-3-032-26557-9_7

Introduction

Leukemia is the most common childhood cancer, representing approximately 25% of cancer cases in children under the age of 15 [1, 2]. With an incidence rate of roughly 3.4 per 100,000 children annually, pediatric leukemia remains a critical focus of pediatric oncology. Although treatment advancements have elevated survival rates above 85%, leukemia continues to be the leading cause of cancer-related deaths among children and adolescents, highlighting the necessity for innovative diagnostic tools.

Long-read sequencing (LRS) represents a significant advancement in genomic technologies, offering unparalleled insights into the genetic underpinnings of diseases and has opened new avenues in the diagnosis and treatment of pediatric leukemia. Unlike short-read sequencing (SRS), which has been the conventional method for genomic analysis, LRS can generate reads spanning tens of thousands to even hundreds of thousands of bases [3]. This capability allows for a more comprehensive and accurate analysis of the genome, overcoming many limitations associated with SRS, such as difficulty in reconstructing lengthy sequence contigs, identifying complex structural variants, and avoiding polymerase chain reaction (PCR)-induced biases. The precision and depth provided by LRS facilitate a holistic understanding of the genetic landscape, which is particularly crucial for complex diseases like leukemia.

In pediatric leukemia, where genetic mutations and rearrangements are highly heterogeneous, the application of LRS offers a transformative approach to diagnosis, prognosis, and treatment. The technology's ability to detect novel genetic markers and mutations that were previously obscured by the limitations of SRS has led to a reclassification of leukemia subtypes based on genetic profiles [4]. This is instrumental in developing more precise and personalized treatment approaches, ultimately improving patient outcomes.

Table 7.1 Features of PacBio and Oxford Nanopore Technologies (ONT) long-read sequencing

	PacBio	ONT
Read length	Long, up to >1M bp (typically 10–30 kb)	Long, up to >1M bp (typically 10–50 kb)
Accuracy	High with HiFi reads (99.9% accuracy)	High with R10.4 chemistry (99.3% accuracy)
Throughput	High (depending on the platform, e.g., ~100 Gb per SMRT-cell on Revio)	Variable, depending on platform (from 5 Gb to 200 Gb per flowcell)
Real-time sequencing	Yes	Yes
PCR amplification	Not required	Not required

(continued)

Table 7.1 (continued)

	PacBio	ONT
Portability	Limited	High (portable devices like MinION, PromethION)
Application in cancer research	Precise SNP detection, haplotype phasing, structural variant analysis	Real-time analysis, characterization of complex genomic variants, and low input material requirement

Background of Long-Read Sequencing

Features of the Two Dominant Long-Read Sequencing Platforms

In the realm of genomic analysis, SRS has long been the relied-upon method due to its precision, scalability, and cost-efficiency [5]. However, the inherent limitations of SRS have posed significant obstacles in deciphering the intricacies of the genome, particularly in the context of cancer research [1, 2].

LRS, or third-generation sequencing, has now emerged as a transformative technology that overcomes some of the constraints of SRS, allowing a more in-depth analysis of the genome (Table 7.1). The two principal players in the LRS arena, Pacific Biosciences' (PacBio) single-molecule real-time (SMRT) sequencing and Oxford Nanopore Technologies' (ONT) nanopore sequencing, have provided new insights into genetics [6]. Both approaches not only preserve DNA integrity but also facilitate the direct detection of base modifications such as methylation, providing invaluable insights into epigenetic regulation [7].

PacBio's SMRT sequencing harnesses parallel polymerase systems bound to circularized DNA with hairpin sequencing adaptors, enabling the incorporation of labeled bases that fluoresce during sequencing (Fig. 7.1a) [8, 9]. The circular consensus sequencing (CCS) approach employed by PacBio generates HiFi reads that have substantially lower error rates compared to traditional SMRT sequencing [10]. Thus, despite initial challenges with higher error rates, PacBio has overcome this hurdle with HiFi reads, achieving error rates akin to SRS, thereby setting the bar for the accuracy of LRS [10]. PacBio's Revio System claims exceptional throughput (1300 human HiFi genomes per year) and read accuracy (≥Q30), empowering comprehensive genomic coverage and precise methylation profiling [11]. Long reads with high accuracy are particularly well-suited for applications requiring precise variant detection and haplotype phasing. Moreover, the ability to detect base modifications directly enables the elucidation of epigenetic alterations, for example, those underlying cancer progression and therapy response.

ONT's nanopore sequencing leverages the unique signal generated via disruption in ionic current flow as DNA fragments traverse nanopores embedded in a membrane [12, 13]. During base calling, this "squiggle" signal is interpreted via machine learning-based DNA or RNA models that help determine the accurate nucleic acid sequence. Since its commercial release in 2014, ONT's technology has undergone significant advancements, including adaptive sampling, which

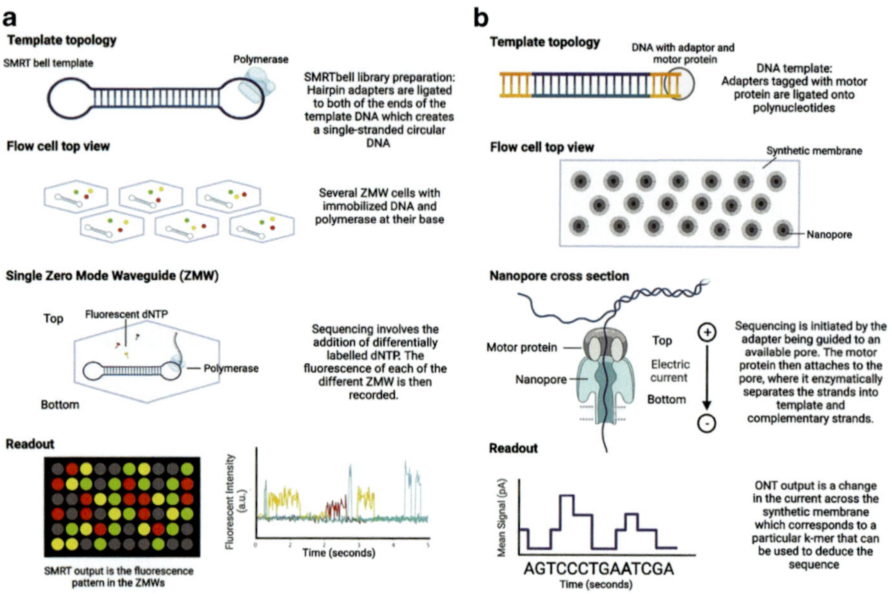

Fig. 7.1 Schematic diagram of (**a**) PacBio SMRT sequencing and (**b**) ONT. (Created with BioRender.com [1])

dynamically adjusts sequencing parameters to target regions of interest, enhancing efficiency and accuracy [14, 15]. With the introduction of V14 chemistry kits, higher sequencing accuracies (Q20) are achieved [16, 17]. ONT's nanopore sequencing offers portability and lower input material requirements, making it a compelling choice for field-based applications and scenarios where rapid turnaround times are critical. Nanopore sequencers such as the MinION and PromethION provide flexibility and versatility, enabling researchers to conduct sequencing experiments in diverse environments with minimal infrastructure requirements [18, 19].

Applications of Long-Read Sequencing in Oncology

Various methodologies are routinely used in the field of cancer genetics and diagnostics, including karyotyping and fluorescence in-situ hybridization (FISH), chromosomal microarray analysis (CMA), next-generation sequencing (NGS), and optical genome mapping (OGM), each with its own advantages and drawbacks. The main advantage that LRS offers in cancer genetics is the ability to combine the benefits of all these methodologies into a nearly 'all-in-one' assay.

The transformative potential of LRS in oncology has been underscored by its recognition as the "Method of the Year 2022" by *Nature Methods*, reflecting its profound impact on medical and biological research [20]. In cancer research, LRS holds immense promise for unraveling the complexities of tumorigenesis, tumor

Table 7.2 Applications of long-read sequencing in oncology

Application	Description
Structural variant detection	Comprehensive detection and characterization of large-scale genomic rearrangements
Haplotype phasing	Precise determination of allele-specific variations and haplotype reconstruction
Epigenetic profiling	Direct detection of DNA methylation patterns and other epigenetic modifications
Liquid biopsy analysis	Non-invasive detection and monitoring of circulating tumor DNA for cancer diagnosis and treatment monitoring
Transcriptome analysis	Accurate identification of alternative splicing events, isoform diversity, and fusion transcripts
Tumor evolution dynamics	Tracking clonal evolution, mutational signatures, and metastatic progression
Mutational signature analysis	Identification and characterization of mutational processes shaping cancer genomes
Genome structural complexity	Deciphering complex genomic rearrangements and repetitive regions

heterogeneity, and therapeutic resistance mechanisms. By providing comprehensive genomic coverage and precise characterization of structural variants, LRS facilitates the identification of driver mutations, oncogenic fusion events, and clonal evolution dynamics (Table 7.2).

Moreover, the ability to detect base modifications directly enables the elucidation of epigenetic alterations underlying cancer progression and therapy response. For example, aberrant DNA methylation patterns are associated with tumor initiation, progression, and metastasis, making them valuable biomarkers for cancer diagnosis and prognosis [21]. LRS allows for the precise mapping of DNA methylation patterns across the genome, enabling the identification of novel regulatory elements and the characterization of epigenetic landscapes in cancer cells [21].

Furthermore, LRS has the potential to transform liquid biopsy approaches for cancer detection and monitoring. Liquid biopsies, which involve analytes, such as circulating tumor DNA (ctDNA) or other biomarkers in bodily fluids, offer a minimally invasive alternative to traditional tissue biopsies and hold promise for early cancer detection, treatment monitoring, and personalized therapy selection [22]. LRS technologies can provide comprehensive genomic profiling of ctDNA, enabling the detection of structural rearrangements and complex genomic alterations that may be missed by conventional SRS methods [22, 23].

In addition to its applications in cancer research, LRS has revolutionized the understanding of structural variation and genome architecture. Large-scale genomic rearrangements, such as chromosomal translocations, inversions, and duplications, play a crucial role in cancer development and evolution [24]. LRS technologies enable the precise detection and characterization of these structural variants, providing insights into their impact on gene expression, regulatory networks, and cancer phenotypes.

Moreover, LRS facilitates the assembly of complex genomic regions, including repetitive sequences, segmental duplications, and transposable elements, which are often challenging to resolve with SRS approaches [25]. These genomic features are frequently associated with genetic disorders, cancer susceptibility loci, and evolutionary dynamics, highlighting the importance of comprehensive genome analysis in understanding health and disease [24].

Applications of Long-Read Sequencing in Leukemia

Leukemias are genetically heterogeneous diseases with various types of driver mutations identified to date. These include fusions detectable by karyotype or FISH analysis, cytogenetically cryptic fusions that require higher resolution assays such as PCR, NGS, or OGM, sequence-level variants detectable only by NGS, copy number variants, and SVs identifiable with NGS or OGM, and some complex SVs that may not be detectable by NGS (Table 7.3).

Table 7.3 Comparison of essential metrics and limitations between methods used for genetic testing of pediatric leukemia in clinical labs

Method	Resolution	Variants typically detected	TAT in the clinic	Select limitations
FISH	~100 Kb	Translocations and fusions, deletions	Few days	Requires knowledge of the target region, may miss small deletions
Karyotype analysis	~5–10 Mb	Translocations and fusions, large deletions	1–2 weeks	Misses small CNVs, requires culturing cells cannot detect low-level mosaicism
CMA	~20–200 Kb	Unbalanced rearrangements, large gains and losses, LOH	2–4 weeks	Cannot detect balanced rearrangements, inversions, independent clones, or low VAF variants
NGS	Single base	SNVs, indels, CNVs, SVs	1–3 weeks	Bioinformatically challenging, cannot identify independent clones[b], or routinely detect ploidy changes[c], cannot sequence through repetitive elements
LRS	Single base	SNVs, indels, CNVs, SVs, STRs, phasing of variants, triple repeat expansion	1–3 weeks[a]	Bioinformatically challenging, cannot identify independent clones[b] or routinely detect ploidy changes[c]
OGM	~0.5–5 Kb	Translocations and fusions, insertions, inversions, deletions and duplications	1–2 weeks	Cannot detect independent clones, ploidy changes, or whole-arm translocations

[a]Expected TAT based on emerging evidence, [b]Single-cell sequencing technologies may overcome this limitation, [c]Advanced bioinformatic tools may be used to estimate ploidy. *LOH* loss of heterozygosity, *STR* short tandem repeats, *TAT* turnaround time, *VAF* variant allele frequency

The journey of LRS in the realm of leukemia diagnostics began in the early 2010s, a period marked by rapid technological advancements in genomic sequencing. Initially, the application of LRS was primarily experimental and used within the confines of research laboratories with the aim of pushing the boundaries of what could be seen within the human genome. Early studies focused on understanding the broad spectrum of genetic diversity in leukemia, characterized by complex genetic rearrangements and mutation patterns that vary significantly across patients [26]. Over time, the insights gained from LRS have led to a reclassification of leukemia subtypes based on genetic profiles, facilitating more precise and personalized treatment approaches.

Several studies have been conducted to compare the performance of LRS to NGS in different cancer types, including leukemias. For example, LRS was used to identify resistance mutations in the kinase domain of *BCR::ABL1* in patients with chronic myeloid leukemia (CML) [27]. LRS correctly identified mutations originally detected by Sanger sequencing, which is routinely used in clinical labs to detect resistance mutations in the TKI domain. Moreover, LRS identified mutations that were not detectable by Sanger sequencing due to their low frequency, which was below the limit of detection of this assay [27].

Wang et al. used transcriptional data from nanopore long-read mRNA sequencing with shallow depth on 134 specimens from a pediatric cohort with acute myeloid leukemia (AML) and B-cell acute lymphoblastic leukemia (B-ALL) to demonstrate that the lineage of acute leukemia can be accurately interpreted from the gene expression profiles [28]. Furthermore, this data was used to identify major molecular subtypes based on the presence of driver mutations or fusions in B-ALL and AML patients.

Enhanced Genetic Profiling

LRS has resulted in a paradigm shift in the genetic profiling of leukemia, providing an unprecedented level of detail and accuracy in understanding genetic mutations and variants.

Comprehensive Analysis of Genetic Mutations and Variants

LRS technology excels in sequencing extended DNA fragments, capturing detailed information about genetic mutations and variants critical for understanding and treating leukemia. The ability to sequence long DNA fragments without the need for PCR amplification reduces the risk of errors and artifacts, resulting in more accurate genetic profiles.

A seminal study by Au et al. highlighted the application of nanopore LRS in rapidly detecting DNA translocations with exact breakpoints in AML [29]. This study demonstrated that LRS could identify novel insertions, deletions, and complex structural variants that were undetectable by SRS. For example, in a newly diagnosed AML patient, nanopore whole-genome sequencing revealed the exact breakpoints of translocations t(10;12) and t(5;11), which conventional methods could not precisely identify. This comprehensive genetic profiling allowed for a more nuanced understanding of the genetic underpinnings of AML and informed the development of targeted therapies [29].

Another study conducted by Cumbo et al. implemented and validated a nanopore sequencing-based assay targeting six frequently mutated genes in AML [30]. LRS on the MinION sequencer detected all but one variant within 24 h in the genomes of 22 AML patients, including SNVs and indels, validated via S5 or Sanger sequencing. This demonstrated that rapid long-read nanopore sequencing for gene mutation analysis in AML is feasible, reducing the turnaround time and guiding clinical decisions [30].

LRS allows for the high-resolution analysis of copy number variations (CNVs) and single-nucleotide polymorphisms (SNPs), which are often implicated in leukemia [31]. By providing detailed genetic profiles, LRS helps identify novel mutations and genetic alterations critical for understanding the disease's progression and response to treatment. A recent study utilized optical genome mapping (OGM) and whole exome sequencing (WES) to analyze somatic alterations in pediatric B-cell precursor acute lymphoblastic leukemia (BCP-ALL). PacBio LRS was then used to validate selected structural variants (SVs) that were newly detected by OGM. This combined approach helped identify novel SVs and single-nucleotide variants (SNVs) that were previously undetectable with traditional methods [32].

Clonal Tracking

LRS has shown potential in advancing clonal tracking in pediatric leukemia by providing detailed insights into genetic variations associated with disease progression and therapeutic responses [33]. Clonal evolution, a hallmark of cancer progression and relapse, is particularly critical in pediatric leukemia, where understanding the genetic dynamics of the disease can directly impact treatment strategies.

A recent study focused on the integration of single-cell RNA-seq, DNA-seq, ATAC-seq, and long-read Oxford Nanopore sequencing to analyze clonal evolution in pediatric AML [33]. Single-cell LRS enabled the detection of novel links between genetic, transcriptomic, and epigenetic changes in distinct (sub)clones, previously not identifiable through traditional SRS [33].

Another study demonstrated the significant capability of LRS to detect and track clonal dynamics in pediatric ALL. Using nanopore sequencing of clonal immunoglobulin heavy chain (IGH) rearrangements in cell-free DNA (cfDNA), researchers were able to monitor clonal heterogeneity and track the response of individual B-ALL clones throughout treatment [34]. This approach provided critical insights into the presence of leukemic clones even when diagnostic cell-count thresholds for minimal residual disease (MRD) were not met, highlighting the potential of LRS for early detection and monitoring of relapse [34].

The impact of LRS on clonal tracking in pediatric leukemia is profound, offering a high-resolution view of the genetic and epigenetic landscapes of the disease. This technology significantly improves the accuracy of monitoring disease progression and understanding clonal evolution. By detecting sub-clonal variations that may drive relapse, LRS provides a comprehensive picture of how leukemia evolves during treatment. Integrating LRS into clinical settings offers substantial benefits for managing pediatric leukemia. It enables continuous monitoring of clonal dynamics, crucial for early relapse detection and real-time adaptation of treatment strategies.

Liquid Biopsy and ctDNA Analysis

Liquid biopsies, which include the analysis of ctDNA from bodily fluids such as blood, offer a minimally invasive alternative to traditional tissue biopsies. This approach holds significant promise for the early detection, monitoring, and treatment of pediatric leukemia [35, 36].

For instance, a study by Peneder et al. showed the application of multimodal analysis of cell-free DNA for pediatric cancers [37]. This study introduced an integrated genetic and epigenetic analysis method that achieved sensitive detection and classification of ctDNA in peripheral blood, independent of genetic alterations, demonstrating the potential of LRS in pediatric cancer diagnostics [37].

The use of LRS for ctDNA analysis also offers significant advantages in identifying structural variants and complex genomic rearrangements [38]. Traditional SRS methods often struggle with accurately mapping these alterations due to their limited read length. However, LRS can generate reads spanning tens of thousands of bases, enabling the comprehensive characterization of structural variants [7]. This capability is particularly valuable in leukemia, where chromosomal translocations and other large-scale rearrangements play a critical role in disease progression and treatment resistance.

Moreover, the direct detection of epigenetic modifications in ctDNA, such as DNA methylation patterns, is now possible and will provide crucial clues for understanding tumor behavior and response to therapy [39]. Traditional methods often require bisulfite conversion, which can introduce biases and reduce sequence complexity. LRS has the unique capability to directly sequence native DNA without the need for bisulfite treatment, thereby preserving the full epigenetic landscape. This approach could provide a more accurate and detailed methylation profile, enhancing our understanding of tumor biology and enabling the development of more precise therapeutic interventions [40, 41].

In conclusion, the use of LRS for ctDNA analysis has the potential to revolutionize the field of pediatric leukemia diagnosis. By providing high-resolution, comprehensive insights into the genetic and epigenetic landscape of leukemia, LRS enhances the sensitivity and specificity of ctDNA analysis, enabling early detection, precise monitoring, and personalized treatment strategies. These advancements hold significant promise for improving clinical outcomes and reducing the burden of leukemia in pediatric patients.

Potential Application in the Clinical Setting

Given that multiple assays are currently the standard of care for understanding the genetic heterogeneity involved in leukemia, LRS, with its ability to detect all these types of variants in a single assay, has emerged as a promising alternative (Table 7.3).

Implementing LRS in a clinical cancer genetics laboratory to replace multiple assays reduces turnaround time and lowers the costs associated with performing multiple tests. Furthermore, an all-in-one assay is particularly valuable in cancer genetics, where there is often limited tumor material (e.g., hemodilute bone marrow aspirate) available. Due to these advances, the field has begun to adopt LRS, with many studies demonstrating its superior performance.

OGM has recently been incorporated into the clinical workflow of many labs to complement conventional cytogenetics by providing genome-level information on structural and copy number variants at a resolution unattainable by karyotyping (Table 7.3). However, the resolution is limited by the distance between labels in specific regions of the genome, meaning that smaller CNVs or SVs may not be identified, and accurate breakpoints cannot always be defined. To compare the resolution and accuracy of LRS to OGM, de Boer et al. used 18 bone marrow aspirate specimens from patients diagnosed with leukemia and performed OGM alongside LRS using ONT. This study demonstrated that the higher resolution of LRS relative to OGM provides more accurate breakpoints, which are necessary to define the regions impacted by CNVs or SVs. In three samples, for instance, the improved accuracy of the breakpoints resulted in redefining the extent of deletions that were presumed by OGM to encompass the *TP53* locus and were therefore classified as clinically relevant. In fact, data from LRS showed that *TP53* was not affected by these deletions [42]. The precise identification of the genes involved in SVs and CNVs is indispensable for the accurate classification of leukemias, as it informs diagnosis, prognosis, and treatment.

Efforts are underway to implement LRS in the clinic, and some centers have begun to clinically utilize LRS in various cancer types, including leukemias. A recent study performed at Children's Mercy Hospital in Kansas City investigated the results of LRS on 11 pediatric leukemia cases with corresponding normal (remission) samples, including seven cases of pediatric B-ALL and four cases of pediatric AML [43]. Five of these samples had known driver mutations identified through clinical genetic testing, including *ETV6::RUNX1*, *KMT2A::AFF1*, *RUNX1::RUNX1T1*, *KMT2A::AFDN* fusions, and one case with a fusion in *NUP98* detected by FISH with an unknown fusion partner. In contrast, the driver mutation for the remaining six cases was unknown despite routine clinical genetic profiling using karyotyping, FISH, microarray, and molecular testing.

PacBio HiFi LRS (Revio) with 30× coverage correctly identified the fusions in the five cases with known driver mutations and provided precise breakpoints. This method also helped identify the fusion partner in a case where the partner could not be determined due to the limitations of the FISH assay [44]. Specifically, it identified a *NUP98*::*NSD1* fusion, which is cytogenetically cryptic and cannot be identified using karyotyping. Furthermore, two of the six cases with unknown driver mutations were resolved using the LRS approach, identifying *KMT2A::MLLT10* and *ZNF384::TCF3* cytogenetically cryptic translocations in an AML and B-ALL case, respectively. This finding is significant because *KMT2A* rearranged AML is a genetically defined disease subtype according to the WHO classification and is also prognostically significant, indicating a higher risk [43]. Additionally, identification of this translocation could qualify the patient for treatment with Gemtuzumab [45].

In pediatric patients, this finding may indicate the need for a bone marrow transplant. Rearrangements involving *ZNF384* may be detected in 3-5% of pediatric ALL, where *TCF3* is one of the fusion partners identified for this gene to date. Precise detection of such fusions will facilitate studies investigating appropriate targeted treatment strategies. Overall, this pilot study demonstrates the improved performance of LRS as a single test, reducing the need for additional tests, decreasing turnaround time, and providing valuable diagnostic and treatment information, particularly in cases with negative genetic profiles [45].

Aberrant methylation patterns and the corresponding gene-expression signatures have also been observed in relapsed and therapy-resistant samples across various cancer types and have been linked to mechanisms of resistance to therapy [43]. Therefore, studying DNA methylation patterns is one of the major focus areas in cancer research. The main methodology to investigate methylation patterns has been bisulfite conversion of cytosine to thymine followed by NGS [43]. However, this technique comes with limitations, including DNA degradation, CpG artifacts introduced during PCR-based library preparation, and the inability to distinguish 5-methylcytosine from 5-hydroxymethylcytosine. LRS provides improved resolution of the methylome and, as such, has been utilized recently in cancer research. In one study, Magi et al. used nanopore LRS to analyze the methylomes of samples at diagnosis and relapse from three patients with AML, who had received standard chemotherapy and had relapsed with chemo-resistant leukemia [46]. Differential methylation analysis between samples at diagnosis and relapse demonstrated that transcription factors, genes associated with drug-resistance, oncogenes, tumor suppressor genes, as well as several cancer-related pathways (e.g., mTOR and MAPK) are overrepresented in relapse AML samples [46]. While further studies are required to confirm these findings, this initial observation demonstrates the application of LRS in better understanding mechanisms of chemoresistance in AML.

Current Challenges and Considerations and Future Directions

While LRS has many potential clinical applications in leukemia, its implementation in daily practice still faces limitations and challenges. The high cost of LRS instrumentation and validation for clinical applications is a significant challenge. Conventional cytogenetics, FISH, targeted sequencing, PCR-based assays, and NGS remain the standard in leukemia genetic testing. Therefore, any clinical lab pursuing LRS implementation would need to incur additional costs to validate this assay, likely starting as a research-use-only tool to support the genetic diagnosis of the disease.

These challenges are exacerbated by the lower sample throughput as care-providing physicians gradually build trust in this assay, and issues with insurance and reimbursement are resolved. The initial phase of launching LRS-based assays in the clinical lab is further complicated by poor scalability, longer turnaround times, and the need to allocate limited resources between maintaining current workflows that provide the standard of care and implementing this new, complex assay.

Another significant challenge in the clinical application of LRS is the training of staff. This includes technicians setting up the wet lab, data analysts and bioinformatics teams responsible for cleaning and analyzing the data, and genome analysts and lab geneticists interpreting the results. Implementing this complex assay requires significant time and resources, not only for the initial setup but also for ongoing staff training throughout the entire process.

This challenge is further compounded by the limited resources currently available for bioinformatic workflows, variant calling (particularly for fusions, SVs, and long indels), and the interpretation of such complex data. For instance, population databases, like those available for NGS data, are still underdeveloped for LRS. Nevertheless, there is growing interest and investment in developing these resources. For example, "long-read-tools.org", developed by Amarasinghe et al., offers a comprehensive catalogue of downstream analysis tools for long-read technologies [47]. The objective of this database is to provide researchers globally with a gateway to access existing tools for their long-read-based research.

Minimal Residual Disease Detection

Minimal residual disease (MRD) detection is crucial for the management of pediatric leukemia, particularly in ALL, where the presence of even a small number of leukemia cells post-treatment can indicate a higher risk of relapse [48]. While LRS offers theoretical benefits such as heightened sensitivity and specificity, its application in MRD monitoring is currently limited, with most evidence coming from other methodologies. Future research may elucidate whether LRS can contribute meaningfully to MRD detection and its integration into clinical workflows, but current data suggest its impact may be less significant than initially anticipated in this context.

The Need for Novel Pipelines to Generate New Insights into Leukemia

As the capabilities of LRS in leukemia research continue to expand, the horizon for future possibilities broadens significantly. The integration of LRS with advanced computational tools and interdisciplinary approaches is poised to transform the understanding of leukemia at a genetic and systemic level, paving the way for ground-breaking advancements in personalized medicine.

Enhancing Predictive Analytics

LRS holds transformative potential in the realm of predictive analytics for leukemia research, particularly when integrated with artificial intelligence (AI) or machine learning (ML). The comprehensive and detailed genomic data generated by LRS offers a unique opportunity to refine AI/ML models, enabling the identification of intricate genetic patterns and structural variations that may escape detection by traditional sequencing methods.

By leveraging the depth of information provided by LRS, predictive models can achieve unprecedented accuracy in forecasting disease progression, assessing patient responses to treatment, and identifying individuals at higher risk of relapse. This synergy between LRS and AI/ML could revolutionize personalized medicine, providing clinicians with actionable insights to develop tailored therapeutic strategies that maximize efficacy while minimizing unnecessary interventions.

Interdisciplinary Approaches to Genetic Research

The future of leukemia research is moving toward an interdisciplinary model that integrates data from other molecular layers, such as epigenetics, proteomics, and metabolomics [49]. This multi-omics approach allows for a holistic view of the disease mechanisms at play, contributing to the identification of novel therapeutic targets and enhancing the precision of existing treatments [50, 51]. This method is already being explored in studies where LRS data is combined with epigenetic markers to uncover underlying mechanisms of drug resistance and disease progression in leukemia cells [50, 52].

Additionally, the future of leukemia research also hinges on enhancing collaborations across different scientific disciplines and technology sectors. By fostering partnerships between genomic researchers, bioinformaticians, clinical oncologists, and technology developers, the integration of LRS into research and clinical practice can be optimized [53–55]. These collaborations will not only speed up the translation of LRS insights from the laboratory to the clinic but also ensure that the technology adapts to the changing landscape of healthcare and biomedical research [54, 56]. Through such synergistic efforts, the full potential of LRS to revolutionize leukemia diagnosis and treatment can be realized, marking a new era in the fight against this complex disease.

Collaborative efforts can also drive the development of standardized protocols and guidelines for the clinical implementation of LRS, ensuring that the technology is accessible and beneficial to a broader patient population [56]. Through collaboration, researchers and clinicians can overcome the technical and logistical challenges associated with LRS, ultimately improving patient outcomes and advancing the field of leukemia research.

Innovative Therapeutic Development and Clinical Trials

LRS holds promise for advancing therapeutic development and optimizing clinical trial design in leukemia research. By providing comprehensive genomic and molecular insights, LRS can aid in identifying critical pathways and genetic mutations that drive various leukemia subtypes. These insights enable the design of targeted therapies that address specific disease mechanisms, paving the way for more effective treatments.

In clinical trials, LRS can facilitate patient stratification based on detailed genetic profiles, ensuring that treatments are tested in well-defined groups likely to benefit the most. This precision medicine approach not only enhances the relevance and statistical power of trials but also streamlines the development process by focusing resources on high-potential therapies. Ultimately, LRS has the potential to accelerate the path from discovery to implementation, contributing to the development of tailored treatments that improve patient outcomes.

By continually advancing LRS technologies and integrating them with other scientific disciplines, the research community can significantly improve the understanding, diagnosis, and treatment of leukemia, ultimately leading to better patient outcomes and personalized care strategies. This ongoing evolution in leukemia research underscores the transformative potential of LRS in modern oncology, setting the stage for the next generation of medical breakthroughs.

Conclusions

The integration of LRS into cancer genetics represents a significant advancement in the genetic analysis of pediatric leukemias. LRS offers a comprehensive approach to detecting a wide array of genetic variants, including fusions, sequence-level mutations, CNVs, and SVs, in a single assay, and with higher resolution and accuracy than traditional methods like karyotyping, NGS, and OGM. This capability is crucial for the precise classification, diagnosis, and treatment of leukemia, as demonstrated by studies identifying previously undetectable mutations and redefining clinically relevant deletions. Moreover, LRS has shown promise in identifying lineage and molecular subtypes of leukemia, which are essential for tailoring treatment strategies. Additionally, LRS's ability to provide detailed methylome analyses highlights its potential to uncover mechanisms of chemoresistance, particularly in relapsed and therapy-resistant cases. Overall, the adoption of LRS in clinical settings could streamline diagnostic processes, reduce the need for multiple tests, and enhance our understanding of leukemia's genetics, ultimately improving patient outcomes.

References

1. Oehler JB, Wright H, Stark Z, Mallett AJ, Schmitz U. The application of long-read sequencing in clinical settings. Human Genomics. 2023;17(1):73. https://doi.org/10.1186/s40246-023-00522-3.
2. Amarasinghe SL, Su S, Dong X, Zappia L, Ritchie ME, Gouil Q. Opportunities and challenges in long-read sequencing data analysis. Genome Biol. 2020;21(1):30. https://doi.org/10.1186/s13059-020-1935-5.

3. Marwaha S, Knowles JW, Ashley EA. A guide for the diagnosis of rare and undiagnosed disease: beyond the exome. Genome Med. 2022;14(1):23. https://doi.org/10.1186/s13073-022-01026-w.
4. Labrador J, Martínez-Cuadrón D, Boluda B, et al. Evolving patterns and clinical outcome of genetic studies performed at diagnosis in acute myeloid leukemia patients: real life data from the PETHEMA Registry. Cancer. 2024;130(20):3436–51. https://doi.org/10.1002/cncr.35431.
5. Logsdon GA, Vollger MR, Eichler EE. Long-read human genome sequencing and its applications. Nat Rev Genet. 2020;21(10):597–614. https://doi.org/10.1038/s41576-020-0236-x.
6. Yu SCY, Deng J, Qiao R, et al. Comparison of single molecule, real-time sequencing and nanopore sequencing for analysis of the size, end-motif, and tissue-of-origin of long cell-free DNA in plasma. Clin Chem. 2023;69(2):168–79. https://doi.org/10.1093/clinchem/hvac180.
7. Ermini L, Driguez P. The application of long-read sequencing to cancer. Cancers (Basel). 2024;16(7). https://doi.org/10.3390/cancers16071275.
8. Eid J, Fehr A, Gray J, et al. Real-time DNA sequencing from single polymerase molecules. Science. 2009;323(5910):133–8. https://doi.org/10.1126/science.1162986.
9. Rhoads A, Au KF. PacBio sequencing and its applications. Genomics Proteomics Bioinf. 2015;13(5):278–89. https://doi.org/10.1016/j.gpb.2015.08.002.
10. Gil-Gil T, Berryhill BA, Manuel JA, et al. The evolution of heteroresistance via small colony variants in Escherichia coli following long term exposure to bacteriostatic antibiotics. bioRxiv. 2023. https://doi.org/10.1101/2023.10.30.564761.
11. Manuel JG, Heins HB, Crocker S, et al. High coverage highly accurate long-read sequencing of a mouse neuronal cell line using the PacBio Revio sequencer. bioRxiv. 2023. https://doi.org/10.1101/2023.06.06.543940.
12. Kasianowicz JJ, Brandin E, Branton D, Deamer DW. Characterization of individual polynucleotide molecules using a membrane channel. Proc Natl Acad Sci USA. 1996;93(24):13770–3. https://doi.org/10.1073/pnas.93.24.13770.
13. Wang Y, Yang Q, Wang Z. The evolution of nanopore sequencing. Front Genet. 2014;5:449. https://doi.org/10.3389/fgene.2014.00449.
14. Deamer D, Akeson M, Branton D. Three decades of nanopore sequencing. Nat Biotechnol. 2016;34(5):518–24. https://doi.org/10.1038/nbt.3423.
15. Geyer J, Opoku KB, Lin J, et al. Real-time genomic characterization of pediatric acute leukemia using adaptive sampling. Leukemia. 2025:1–9.
16. Xu L, Seki M. Recent advances in the detection of base modifications using the Nanopore sequencer. J Hum Genet. 2020;65(1):25–33. https://doi.org/10.1038/s10038-019-0679-0.
17. Loose M, Malla S, Stout M. Real-time selective sequencing using nanopore technology. Nat Methods. 2016;13(9):751–4. https://doi.org/10.1038/nmeth.3930.
18. Jain M, Olsen HE, Paten B, Akeson M. The Oxford Nanopore MinION: delivery of nanopore sequencing to the genomics community. Genome Biol. 2016;17(1):239. https://doi.org/10.1186/s13059-016-1103-0.
19. Wang Y, Zhao Y, Bollas A, Wang Y, Au KF. Nanopore sequencing technology, bioinformatics and applications. Nat Biotechnol. 2021;39(11):1348–65. https://doi.org/10.1038/s41587-021-01108-x.
20. Marx V. Method of the year: long-read sequencing. Nat Methods. 2023;20(1):6–11. https://doi.org/10.1038/s41592-022-01730-w.
21. Ni Y, Liu X, Simeneh ZM, Yang M, Li R. Benchmarking of Nanopore R10.4 and R9.4.1 flow cells in single-cell whole-genome amplification and whole-genome shotgun sequencing. Comput Struct Biotechnol J. 2023;21:2352–64. https://doi.org/10.1016/j.csbj.2023.03.038.
22. Yu SCY, Choy LYL, Lo YMD. 'Longing' for the next generation of liquid biopsy: the diagnostic potential of long cell-free DNA in oncology and prenatal testing. Mol Diagn Ther. 2023;27(5):563–71. https://doi.org/10.1007/s40291-023-00661-2.
23. Brockley LJ, Souza VGP, Forder A, et al. Sequence-based platforms for discovering biomarkers in liquid biopsy of non-small-cell lung cancer. Cancers (Basel). 2023;15(8). https://doi.org/10.3390/cancers15082275.

24. Warburton PE, Sebra RP. Long-read DNA sequencing: recent advances and remaining challenges. Annu Rev Genomics Hum Genet. 2023;24:109–32. https://doi.org/10.1146/annurev-genom-101722-103045.
25. Balachandran P, Walawalkar IA, Flores JI, Dayton JN, Audano PA, Beck CR. Transposable element-mediated rearrangements are prevalent in human genomes. Nat Commun. 2022;13(1):7115. https://doi.org/10.1038/s41467-022-34810-8.
26. Penter L, Borji M, Nagler A, et al. Integrative genotyping of cancer and immune phenotypes by long-read sequencing. Nat Commun. 2024;15(1):32. https://doi.org/10.1038/s41467-023-44137-7.
27. Schaal W, Ameur A, Olsson-Strömberg U, Hermanson M, Cavelier L, Spjuth O. Migrating to long-read sequencing for clinical routine BCR-ABL1 TKI resistance mutation screening. Cancer Informat. 2022;21:11769351221110872. https://doi.org/10.1177/11769351221110872.
28. Wang J, Bhakta N, Ayer Miller V, et al. Acute leukemia classification using transcriptional profiles from low-cost nanopore mRNA sequencing. JCO Precis Oncol. 2022;6:e2100326.
29. Au CH, Ho DN, Ip BBK, et al. Rapid detection of chromosomal translocation and precise breakpoint characterization in acute myeloid leukemia by nanopore long-read sequencing. Cancer Genet. 2019;239:22–5. https://doi.org/10.1016/j.cancergen.2019.08.005.
30. Cumbo C, Minervini CF, Orsini P, et al. Nanopore targeted sequencing for rapid gene mutations detection in acute myeloid leukemia. Gene. 2019;10(12):1026.
31. Olivucci G, Iovino E, Innella G, Turchetti D, Pippucci T, Magini P. Long read sequencing on its way to the routine diagnostics of genetic diseases. Front Genet. 2024;15:1374860. https://doi.org/10.3389/fgene.2024.1374860.
32. Brandes D, Yasin L, Nebral K, et al. Optical genome mapping identifies novel recurrent structural alterations in childhood ETV6::RUNX1+ and high hyperdiploid acute lymphoblastic leukemia. Hemasphere. 2023;7(8):e925. https://doi.org/10.1097/hs9.0000000000000925.
33. Grasso C, Brazda P, te Pas BM, et al. Transcriptional heterogeneity and clonal evolution between diagnosis and relapse in pediatric acute myeloid leukemia. Blood. 2023;142(Supplement 1):2746. https://doi.org/10.1182/blood-2023-182852.
34. Sampathi S, Chernyavskaya Y, Haney MG, et al. Nanopore sequencing of clonal IGH rearrangements in cell-free DNA as a biomarker for acute lymphoblastic leukemia. Front Oncol. 2022;12:958673. https://doi.org/10.3389/fonc.2022.958673.
35. Talotta D, Almasri M, Cosentino C, Gaidano G, Moia R. Liquid biopsy in hematological malignancies: current and future applications. Front Oncol. 2023;13:1164517. https://doi.org/10.3389/fonc.2023.1164517.
36. Sundby RT, Pan A, Shern JF. Liquid biopsies in pediatric oncology: opportunities and obstacles. Curr Opin Pediatr. 2022;34(1):39–47. https://doi.org/10.1097/mop.0000000000001088.
37. Peneder P, Stütz AM, Surdez D, et al. Multimodal analysis of cell-free DNA whole-genome sequencing for pediatric cancers with low mutational burden. Nat Commun. 2021;12(1):3230. https://doi.org/10.1038/s41467-021-23445-w.
38. Conlin LK, Aref-Eshghi E, McEldrew DA, Luo M, Rajagopalan R. Long-read sequencing for molecular diagnostics in constitutional genetic disorders. Hum Mutat. 2022;43(11):1531–44. https://doi.org/10.1002/humu.24465.
39. Koval AP, Blagodatskikh KA, Kushlinskii NE, Shcherbo DS. The detection of cancer epigenetic traces in cell-free DNA. Front Oncol. 2021;11:662094. https://doi.org/10.3389/fonc.2021.662094.
40. Gouil Q, Keniry A. Latest techniques to study DNA methylation. Essays Biochem. 2019;63(6):639–48. https://doi.org/10.1042/ebc20190027.
41. Jiang N, Pan J, Fang S, et al. Liquid biopsy: circulating exosomal long noncoding RNAs in cancer. Clin Chim Acta. 2019;495:331–7. https://doi.org/10.1016/j.cca.2019.04.082.
42. de Boer EN, Vroom V, Scheper AJ, et al. Cas9-directed long-read sequencing to resolve optical genome mapping findings in leukemia diagnostics. Sci Rep. 2024;14(1):8508. https://doi.org/10.1038/s41598-024-59092-6.

43. Abla O, Ries RE, Triche T, Jr., et al. Structural variants involving MLLT10 fusion are associated with adverse outcomes in pediatric acute myeloid leukemia. Blood Adv. 2024;8(8):2005–17. https://doi.org/10.1182/bloodadvances.2023010805.
44. Lansdon LA, Yoo B, Keskus A, et al. Successful classification of clinical pediatric leukemia genetic subtypes via structural variant detection using HiFi long-read sequencing. medRxiv. 2024. https://doi.org/10.1101/2024.11.05.24316078.
45. Pollard JA, Guest E, Alonzo TA, et al. Gemtuzumab ozogamicin improves event-free survival and reduces relapse in pediatric KMT2A-rearranged AML: results from the phase III Children's Oncology Group Trial AAML0531. J Clin Oncol. 2021;39(28):3149–60. https://doi.org/10.1200/jco.20.03048.
46. Magi A, Mattei G, Mingrino A, et al. High-resolution Nanopore methylome-maps reveal random hyper-methylation at CpG-poor regions as driver of chemoresistance in leukemias. Commun Biol. 2023;6(1):382. https://doi.org/10.1038/s42003-023-04756-8.
47. Amarasinghe SL, Ritchie ME, Gouil Q. Long-Read-Tools.Org: an interactive catalogue of analysis methods for long-read sequencing data. GigaScience. 2021;10(2). https://doi.org/10.1093/gigascience/giab003.
48. Hayashi H, Makimoto A, Yuza Y. Treatment of pediatric acute lymphoblastic leukemia: a historical perspective. Cancer. 2024;16(4):723.
49. Tsagiopoulou M, Gut IG. Machine learning and multi-omics data in chronic lymphocytic leukemia: the future of precision medicine? Mini review. Front Genet. 2024;14. https://doi.org/10.3389/fgene.2023.1304661.
50. Pettini F, Visibelli A, Cicaloni V, Iovinelli D, Spiga O. Multi-omics model applied to cancer genetics. Int J Mol Sci. 2021;22(11):5751.
51. Mavridou D, Psatha K, Aivaliotis M. Proteomics and drug repurposing in CLL towards precision medicine. Cancer. 2021;13(14):3391.
52. Barrow TM, Nakjang S, Lafta F, et al. Epigenome-wide analysis reveals functional modulators of drug sensitivity and post-treatment survival in chronic lymphocytic leukaemia. Br J Cancer. 2021;124(2):474–83. https://doi.org/10.1038/s41416-020-01117-8.
53. Rahman B, Lamb A, Protheroe A, et al. Genomic sequencing in oncology: considerations for integration in routine cancer care. Eur J Cancer Care (Engl). 2022;31(3):e13584. https://doi.org/10.1111/ecc.13584.
54. Boehm JS, Jacks T. Radical collaboration: reimagining cancer team science. Cancer Discov. 2024;14(4):563–8. https://doi.org/10.1158/2159-8290.Cd-23-1496.
55. Broes S, Saesen R, Lacombe D, Huys I. Past, current, and future cancer clinical research collaborations: the case of the european organisation for research and treatment of cancer. Clin Transl Sci. 2021;14(1):47–53. https://doi.org/10.1111/cts.12863.
56. Knoppers T, Haley CE, Bouhouita-Guermech S, et al. From code to care: clinician and researcher perspectives on an optimal therapeutic web portal for acute myeloid leukemia. PLoS ONE. 2024;19(4):e0302156. https://doi.org/10.1371/journal.pone.0302156.

Flow Cytometric Measurable Residual Disease Assessment in Acute Leukemia

8

Prashant R. Tembhare, Gaurav Chatterjee, Sweta Rajpal, and Anumeha Chaturvedi

Definition of MRD

Measurable residual disease (MRD), previously referred to as minimal residual disease, is defined as the small population of residual leukemic cells that persist during or following treatment at levels undetectable by conventional morphological assessment [1–4] (Fig. 8.1). In acute leukemias, traditional response criteria rely on morphological complete remission (CR), characterized by fewer than 5% blasts in bone marrow aspirates [5–9]. However, numerous studies have demonstrated that morphological CR lacks the sensitivity required for accurate prognostication, as it fails to detect submicroscopic disease burden [3, 4, 9–12]. This limitation is further compounded by the presence of benign hematopoietic precursors—such as regenerating myeloid blasts and B-cell progenitors (hematogones)—which may mimic residual leukemia, leading to diagnostic ambiguity. Conversely, highly sensitive techniques, including multiparametric flow cytometry (MFC) and molecular assays (e.g., quantitative polymerase chain reactions (qPCR) or next-generation sequencing (NGS)), frequently identify clinically significant residual disease even in bone marrow in morphological remission [13]. The transition in terminology from minimal to measurable underscores the importance of assay sensitivity and standardization, reflecting the ability of modern techniques to quantify residual disease with precision, thereby enabling more accurate risk stratification and therapeutic decision-making [7, 13].

P. R. Tembhare (✉) · G. Chatterjee · S. Rajpal
Hematopathology Department, ACTREC, Tata Memorial Center, HBNI University, Navi Mumbai, Maharashtra, India

A. Chaturvedi
Hematopathology Department, Homi Bhabha Cancer Hospital and Research Centre, Visakhapatnam, Andhra Pradesh, India

W. Li (ed.), *Laboratory Assessments of Pediatric Leukemia*, https://doi.org/10.1007/978-3-032-26557-9_8

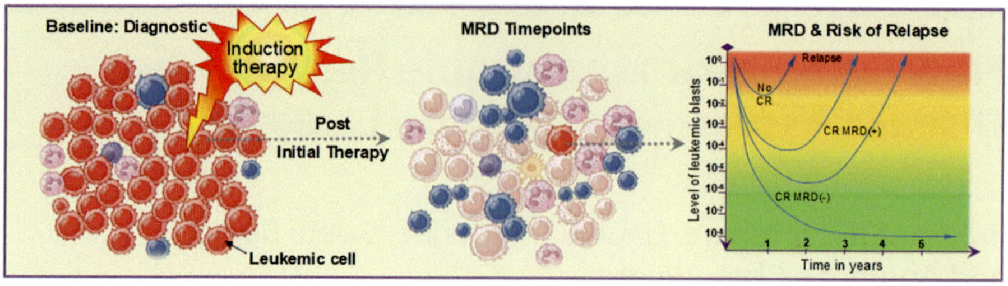

Fig. 8.1 The image explains the concept of measurable residual disease (MRD) dynamics in acute leukemia. The figure is divided into three panels. The left panel represents the diagnostic bone marrow, predominantly infiltrated by leukemic blasts (depicted in red cells), indicating high disease burden at presentation. The middle panel illustrates the post-induction marrow, where leukemic burden has significantly decreased. Although morphologically in remission, a small population of residual leukemic cells persists—undetectable by conventional microscopy but identifiable by sensitive techniques such as flow cytometry or molecular assays. The right panel presents a conceptual graph correlating MRD levels with relapse risk over time, demonstrating that higher MRD levels following initial therapy are associated with shorter relapse-free intervals, underscoring the prognostic value of MRD assessment

Clinical Significance of MRD in Acute Leukemia

The achievement of negative MRD status has emerged as one of the most relevant independent predictors of favorable prognosis and prolonged disease-free survival in patients with acute leukemia [3–6, 12, 14–22]. This correlation holds true across multiple treatment protocols, leukemia subtypes, and baseline risk-category, establishing MRD status as a critical biomarker for therapeutic decision-making. The MRD status prior to hematopoietic stem cell transplantation (HSCT) has also been correlated with post-transplant outcomes [23–28].

The clinical utility of MRD monitoring extends beyond initial response assessment, as serial evaluation enables detection of relapse through conversion from MRD-negative to MRD-positive status, often weeks to months before hematologic recurrence [1, 6, 29–32]. This early warning provides a crucial window for preemptive therapeutic intervention, including treatment intensification, alternative targeted therapies, or timely HSCT. Furthermore, MRD levels serve as a key parameter for dynamic risk stratification, guiding the escalation or de-escalation of therapy based on individual disease biology and response patterns [17, 33–40]. The prognostic validity and reproducibility of MRD assessment have led to its widespread adoption as a surrogate endpoint in clinical trials, where it frequently serves as a more sensitive and earlier indicator of treatment efficacy than traditional morphological complete remission criteria [6, 41–45]. This paradigm shift toward MRD-driven response assessment has fundamentally transformed clinical trial design and therapeutic algorithms in modern leukemia management. Thus, MRD status is considered a surrogate or secondary end point in various clinical trials [6].

Historical Evolution and Technological Advancements in MRD Detection

The scientific investigation of MRD detection in human leukemias originated in the early 1980s, building upon pivotal preclinical studies that demonstrated an inverse correlation between leukemic cell burden and survival outcomes in rodent models [46–49]. Initial clinical methodologies employed two to three color immunofluorescence microscopy, which provided the first evidence that T-cell acute lymphoblastic leukemia (T-ALL) could be monitored at submicroscopic levels [46–49]. This era witnessed parallel development of two transformative technologies: allele-specific oligonucleotide PCR (ASO-PCR) and multiparametric flow cytometry. The subsequent advent of real-time quantitative PCR (RQ-PCR) significantly enhanced the sensitivity and reproducibility of molecular detection methods, while flow cytometric approaches capitalized on the identification of aberrant immunophenotypic patterns through multidimensional analysis of "empty spaces" in cellular distribution plots—a strategy that offered both rapid turnaround and reduced technical complexity compared to molecular techniques [50, 51].

The field has since progressed exponentially, transitioning from the 3–4 color to 12–16 color flow cytometry panels and from conventional (0.01%) to highly sensitive (0.0002%) or next-generation flow (NGF) assays, improving the accuracy and sensitivity of MRD assays. Modern detection platforms now incorporate [52–55]:

- High-sensitivity or next-generation flow cytometry (NGF) with increased sensitivity and standardization
- RQ-PCR with improved dynamic range
- Droplet Digital PCR (ddPCR) enabling absolute quantification
- NGS for sensitive tracking of clones/variants

While conventional cytogenetic techniques such as karyotyping and fluorescence in situ hybridization (FISH) retain diagnostic utility, their limited sensitivity (typically 1–5%) renders them inadequate for comprehensive MRD assessment in the modern therapeutic context [56, 57]. This technological evolution has fundamentally transformed MRD monitoring from a research tool to a clinically indispensable component of leukemia management. Table 8.1 highlights the commonly used MRD detection techniques with their sensitivities, advantages and limitations [1, 3, 41, 53, 54, 58–60].

Advantages and Limitations of MFC MRD

Among these techniques, MFC stands out as one of the most sensitive and specific techniques for MRD assessment. This technology can identify minute populations of residual leukemic cells (as rare as 2 in 100,000 hematopoietic cells) by detecting aberrant immunophenotypes that distinguish them from normal progenitors. MFC offers several practical advantages, including broad applicability (>90% of cases),

Table 8.1 Comparison of techniques for MRD evaluation in acute leukemia

Technique	Sensitivity	Advantages	Limitations	Applicability [1, 2, 13]
MFC	10^{-3} to 10^{-5}	Rapid and sensitive; relatively cost-effective; enables simultaneous assessment of sample quality and immune profiling; capable of detecting lineage switches based on emerging clones	Operator-dependent; requires significant expertise and methodological standardization	Highly applicable across all leukemia subtypes, regardless of genomic characteristics B-ALL: >90% T-ALL: >90% AML: 85–90%
RQ-PCR	10^{-3} to 10^{-5}	Rapid, sensitive, and standardized with established guidelines	Requires pre-treatment baseline evaluation; prone to cross-contamination; cannot identify new clonal populations; depends on standard curve-based quantification	Limited applicability—only relevant in cases with a known gene fusion or mutation at diagnosis B-ALL: 25–40% (age-dependent) T-ALL: 10–15% AML: 40–50%
dPCR	10^{-3} to 10^{-5}	High sensitivity; allows absolute quantification without standard curves	Requires pre-treatment baseline; risk of cross-contamination; limited ability to detect new clones; lacks procedural standardization	Limited applicability—relevant only in patients with detectable gene fusions or mutations at diagnosis
NGS	10^{-6}	Exceptionally sensitive; detects novel clonal populations and their evolution; applicable in a broad range of cases	Expensive, longer turnaround times, requires baseline genomic profiling and extensive bioinformatics infrastructure	Broad applicability when baseline genomic data is available B-ALL: >90% T-ALL: >90% AML: ~90%
NGF or HS-MFC	10^{-6}	Highly sensitive; reduced inter-observer variability; good concordance with NGS	Comparatively high cost; requires large event acquisition (~10 million cells); demands high-quality samples and methodological standardization	Widely applicable regardless of genomic profile

Applicability of RQ-PCR for IG/TR genes for MRD evaluation in B-ALL and T-ALL is >95% [12]
MFC Multiparametric flow cytometry, *qPCR* quantitative polymerase chain reaction, *dPCR* digital PCR, *NGS* next-generation sequencing, *NGF or HS-MFC* next-generation flow or high-sensitivity MFC

cost-effectiveness, rapid turnaround time, simple infrastructure, and widespread availability [3, 58–60]. While NGS and RQ-PCR theoretically offer greater analytical sensitivity, their practical implementation is often constrained by higher costs, prolonged processing times, and dependence on pre-identified genetic targets [52–55].

In practice, MFC demonstrates robust MRD detection across most acute leukemia subtypes, except in scenarios where RQ-PCR can leverage highly specific genetic markers (e.g., *NPM1* mutations in acute myeloid leukemia (AML) or *PML::RARA* in APL) [41, 61]. With well-defined immunophenotypic aberrancies, MFC can reliably detect MRD at sensitivity levels beyond 0.01–0.001%. Importantly, the "different-from-normal" approach in MFC enables not only tracking of the founding leukemic clone but also detection of immunophenotypically divergent subclones—a critical advantage over targeted molecular assays that may miss emerging populations if not predefined [1, 41, 62]. Furthermore, MFC provides an intrinsic quality control mechanism by assessing hemodilution in bone marrow aspirates, a feature currently not evaluable in molecular methods [63].

Despite these strengths, MFC-MRD has notable limitations. Its accuracy is highly operator-dependent, requiring rigorous standardization (e.g., EuroFlow protocols) to mitigate interlaboratory variability [1, 3, 41, 53–55]. It may also fail to detect mature myeloid cells carrying certain genetic abnormalities, such as *BCR::ABL1* in CML chronic phase or *NPM1*-mutated mature myeloid cells/*PML::RARA*-positive mature cells in APL. Recent studies underscore the complementary role of integrating MFC with molecular techniques (e.g., NGS or ddPCR), demonstrating that combined approaches enhance prognostic stratification and refine relapse risk prediction [1, 53, 54, 64–66]. Thus, while MFC remains a cornerstone of MRD assessment, its optimal clinical application often necessitates a multimodal diagnostic framework.

Clinically Significant Level of MRD and Time Points

B-ALL MRD

Measurement of MRD levels, as a tool to guide therapy at response assessment time points, has now been established in various contemporary ALL treatment protocols. MRD is typically evaluated at standardized time points, with the most critical assessment occurring at the end of induction (EOI) therapy (day 28–35) followed by end of consolidation (EOC) therapy (day 78–82) [4, 6, 14, 53, 54, 67]. Other time points for therapeutic response assessment using MRD include "Day-8 peripheral blood MRD" in COG protocols, "day-15 bone marrow MRD" evaluations in St. Jude and European cooperative groups protocols, etc. [68]. EOI bone marrow MRD (day 28–35) has been used for response-adapted therapeutic modifications in the Indian Collaborative Childhood Leukaemia (ICiCLe) and other pediatric and adult protocols [59, 69–72]. The most commonly used clinically actionable cut-off of MRD in these early time points is 0.01%. The preferred specimen for MRD analysis at EOI and subsequent intervals is bone marrow, owing to its significantly enhanced sensitivity (1–3 logs greater) compared to peripheral blood assessments [73]. Pretransplant and post-transplant MRD status further provides powerful prognostic information, especially when present at a higher level (≥0.01%) [74, 75]. The presence of such a higher level of MRD may further direct additional therapy pretransplant. In addition to patients being treated with conventional chemotherapy, MRD status has proven useful for providing crucial prognostic information in patients treated with anti-CD19 bispecific antibody (Blinatumomab) or anti-CD19-CAR-T cells therapies [76, 77]. Interestingly, a lower level of cut-off may be clinically important in these patients. Pulsipher and colleagues have demonstrated that any level of NGS-MRD > 0 (but not any cut-off even as low as 10^{-6}) in BM at day-28, 3, and 6 months was associated with inferior event-free and overall survival in patients with B-ALL treated with Tisagenlecleucel therapy [58, 77–80]. A recent effort from Litzow et al. further showed that adding Blinatumomab during consolidation improved outcomes in adult patients with *BCR::ABL1*-negative B-ALL who were MFC-MRD<0.01% after induction and intensification chemotherapy [81].

T-ALL MRD

For T-ALL, MRD thresholds and testing time points may vary across different protocols. However, similar to B-ALL MRD, a cut-off of ≥0.01% is widely used for risk stratification in T-ALL too, particularly at the EOI and EOC phases, though some protocols adopt higher thresholds (≥0.1%) for EOI or later time points [82–89]. Testing typically occurs at EOI and EOC, with some groups extending monitoring to weeks 10–16 or beyond. Certain protocols, such as those in India (ICiCLe-ALL) and Germany (GMALL), emphasize EOC evaluation, while others, like the Modified BFM approach, incorporate sequential testing if initial results are positive. Variations in MRD significance—such as any positivity at week 22 (GIMEMA, Italy) or distinct EOI/EOC thresholds (PALG-Poland, PATHEMA-Spain)—highlight the need for protocol-specific interpretation [83–85, 88]. These differences underscore the importance of standardized yet adaptable MRD monitoring to guide treatment decisions in T-ALL.

AML MRD

The European LeukemiaNet (ELN) working group has established ≥0.1% of CD45+ cells as the standard threshold for defining MFC-MRD positivity in clinical decision-making [41]. However, multiple studies demonstrate that MRD levels <0.1% (down to 0.001% or any detectable levels) retain prognostic significance for disease-free survival (DFS), cumulative incidence of relapse and overall survival (OS) [5, 7, 10, 17, 19, 21, 24, 30, 41, 52, 64]. One of the technical considerations for detecting MRD with lower thresholds (0.01–0.001%) is a requirement of acquisition of ≥2 million events and adequately validated AML MRD assay.

Optimal MRD Assessment Time Points:

Consensus recommendations for bone marrow sampling [5, 21, 24, 41]:

- Post-induction: (Predicts chemosensitivity; guides consolidation intensity)
  - After 1st induction cycle (day 14–21)
  - After 2nd induction cycle (day 28–42)
- Post-consolidation: Before maintenance therapy (Identifies patients needing alternative strategies)
- Transplant settings: (Guides relapse prevention interventions)
  - Pre-transplant (defines baseline risk)
  - Day +30, +60, +100 post-transplant

MFC-Based MRD Approach, and Challenges

The success of an MFC-MRD depends on providing a reliable n-dimensional resolution and separation (n = number of markers used in the panel) of leukemic blasts from the immunophenotypically closest possible normal cells (usually normal progenitors, and a few other low-frequency hematopoietic cells in bone marrow sharing immunophenotypic features) in the context of the particular gating strategy used. To achieve the highest resolution of residual leukemic cells from other bone marrow elements, the following two approaches are recommended [41, 90–95]:

Different from Normal approach (DfN): DfN Approach refers to identification of tumor cells based on deviation from the normal expression or maturation pattern of reference normal cells of respective lineage. The application of this approach requires extensive knowledge and expertise regarding the normal maturation patterns and immunophenotypic shifts associated with chemotherapy.

Identification of Leukemia-Associated Immunophenotypes (LAIPs): LAIP refers to aberrant expression or downregulation of an antigen in tumor cells when compared to the reference normal cells of respective lineage.

Establishing MRD assays by MFC includes the following major steps:

- Designing an antibody panel for distinguishing MRD from other BM cells,
- Standardizing sample processing to achieve the required sensitivity,
- Designing software-based data analysis approaches:
  - Fixing the gating strategy for identifying target cells and
  - Mapping the normal maturation sequences of precursor cells to mature cells,

- Evaluation of abnormalities or "deviation-from-normal" in each sample,
- Calculation and reporting of MRD.

Designing an Antibody Panel

B-ALL MRD

Antibody Panel: B-ALL MRD

Contemporary MFC-BMRD panels typically consist of ≥8 color panels that incorporate

- Lineage markers for gating (typically, CD19 and CD22),
- Markers to map B-cell precursor (BCP) maturation such as CD10, CD20, CD22, CD34, CD38, and CD45,
- Additional leukemia-specific markers that helps in establishing LAIPs.

The sensitivity of such panels is typically tuned to reach at least 0.01% [6]. The expression levels of different backbone markers used for mapping maturation patterns of various stages of BPCs have been shown in Fig. 8.2.

Deviations from normal immunophenotypic maturation patterns enable the detection of residual leukemic blasts with high sensitivity. Incorporation of leukemia-associated immunophenotypes (LAIPs) further enhances MRD detection accuracy, exceeding 90% in clinical applications [96, 97]. Systematic studies by Coustan-Smith et al., subsequently validated by multiple groups, have identified >20 differentially expressed markers distinguishing leukemic blasts from normal B-cell precursors [98]. Clinically validated markers for MRD monitoring include:

- CD73, CD86, and CD304, overexpressed in 60–77%, 50–60%, and 42–59% of diagnostic samples, respectively, with higher prevalence at MRD time points (CD73: 90–95%; CD86: 65–71%; CD304: 40–41%) [99, 100].
- CD123, CD58, and CD66c, differentially expressed in 65–85%, 55–94%, and 36–46% of diagnostic samples [100], with CD123, CD304, and CD66c linked to *BCR::ABL1*.
- Other markers that have been reported in various studies include CD13, CD33, CD44, CD45RA, CD49f, CD81, and CD200.

Caution: Some "leukemia-associated" markers (e.g., CD73, CD86) exhibit weak physiological expression in specific BCP subsets (e.g., CD10+CD34− BCP2 vs. CD10+CD34+ BCP1). Thus, interpretation must rely on composite immunophenotypic patterns rather than isolated markers [59].

Generally, a sensitivity of 10^{-4} can be achieved using a standardized MFC-BMRD panel with acquisition and analysis of 0.5-1 million cells. However, Stow et al. demonstrated that MRD levels between 10^{-4} and 10^{-5} (considered below the clinically actionable cut off) at the end of induction therapy were associated with higher cumulative risk of relapse as compared to MRD negative/$<10^{-5}$ [101].

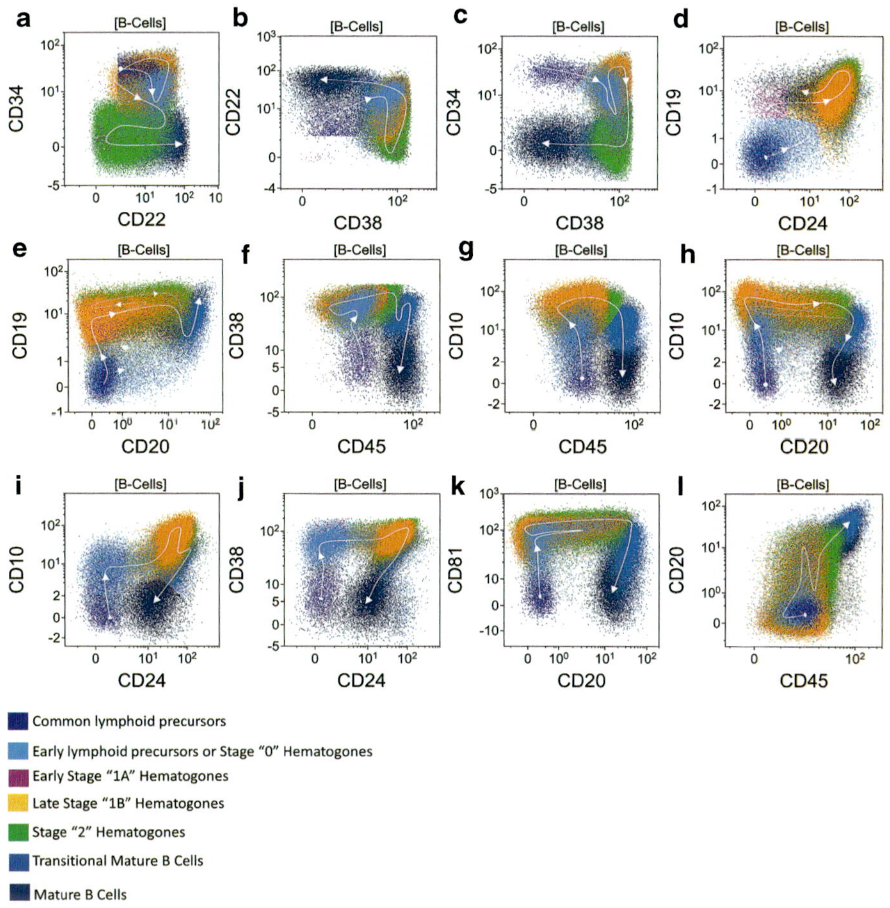

Fig. 8.2 Immunophenotypic trajectory of B-cell lineage maturation in normal bone marrow. This figure illustrates the sequential immunophenotypic stages of B-cell development as visualized by flow cytometry using a standard B-cell ALL MRD panel. Each maturation stage is color-coded and defined by characteristic expression patterns of surface markers including: common lymphoid progenitors (CLPs)—bright CD34+, dim CD38+, dim CD81+, dim CD45+, dim CD22+, negative for CD10, CD19, CD24, and CD20 (bright blue dots); Earliest B-cell precursors/ Pro-B/stage "0" hematogones—CD34+, moderate CD38+, moderate CD81+, CD22+, heterogeneous CD10, heterogeneous CD20, negative for CD19 and CD24 (cyan-blue dots); Pre–B I cells/stage "1" hematogones (BCP1)—dim CD45, dim CD19+, bright CD10, CD22+, moderate CD38+, moderate CD81+, heterogeneous CD20+ (further subdivided into: Stage 1A (early)—CD24− (pink dots), Stage 1B (late)—CD24+ (amber dots)); Pre–B II cells/stage "2" hematogones (BCP2)—moderate CD45+, moderate CD19+, bright CD10+, CD22+, bright CD24+, moderate CD38+, moderate CD81+, and heterogeneous CD20, (green dots) but CD34−; Immature/transitional B-cells—bright CD45, moderate CD19+, dim CD10, dim CD38, dim CD81. CD22+, moderate CD24+, CD34−, and bright CD20 (steel blue dots); mature B-cells—bright CD45, moderate CD19+, bright CD22, moderate CD24+, CD34−, and bright CD20 but CD10−, CD38−, and CD81 (deep navy blue dots)White arrowed curves illustrate the directionality and continuity of B-cell maturation across developmental stages. This detailed trajectory aids in distinguishing physiological hematogones from aberrant B-cell precursors during measurable residual disease assessment

Moreover, in routine practice, a lower limit of detection (LOD)/lower limit of quantification (LLOQ) is desirable as a subset of the bone marrow aspirate samples may be hemodiluted with underrepresentation of residual leukemic blasts. In this context, the Euroflow consortium and we (at TMC) have established highly sensitive MFC-BMRD assays capable of reaching <10^{-4} comparable to PCR-based methods, once adequate events (4–5 million cells) are acquired [59, 102] A key factor for achieving this is standardized processing, including bulk erythrocyte lysis and instrument settings. "First-pull" of 0.5–1 ml of BM is preferred for MRD evaluation. Using such well-standardized assays, a LOD of 2×10^{-6} and LLOQ of 1×10^{-5} can be achieved with acquisition of ~4–5 million events. The Euroflow consortium has documented a concordance of 98% with PCR-based methods using such a highly sensitive MFC-BMRD assay.

Antibody Panel: T-ALL MRD

Unlike B-ALL, where MRD assessment often relies on deviation from maturation patterns of normal BCPs and the identification of LAIPs, the evaluation of MRD in T-ALL predominantly involves the exclusion of normal cell populations, making it inherently more challenging. Accurate interpretation, therefore, necessitates a clear understanding of antigen expression variations of normal T cells.

Contemporary MFC-based T-ALL MRD panels typically employ ≥8-color antibody combinations that incorporate:

- Core T-lineage markers: CD7, intracytoplasmic CD3 (cyCD3), and surface CD3 (sCD3) for T-cell lineage gating.
- Set of maturation and differentiation markers: CD1a, CD2, CD4, CD5, CD6, CD8, CD38, CD48 and CD45, which help delineate normal T-cell ontogeny.
- Immaturity markers: TdT, CD1a, CD99, CD34, and CD10.
- Exclusion of NK cell markers: CD16, CD56 and NKp80.

Early stages of T-cell development occur predominantly in the thymus. Figure 8.3 schematically illustrated antigen expression patterns of immature T-cell in thymus. Since immature T-cells are not normally found in bone marrow or peripheral blood, rendering immaturity-associated markers such as TdT, CD99, CD34, and CD10 are valuable for diagnostic immunophenotyping. However, these markers are variably expressed across T-ALL cases and may be downregulated or lost following treatment [103], limiting their reliability for longitudinal MRD assessment. Among them, TdT presents technical limitations due to challenges in standardizing nuclear staining and is negative in up to 10% of T-ALL cases [60, 104, 105]. Immature T-cells shows a unique pattern of cytoplasmic CD3 expression in the absence of surface CD3 expression. A major challenge in T-ALL MRD detection lies in its nature as a diagnosis of exclusion—requiring precise separation of residual leukemic blasts from normal T/NK-lineage cells as a subset of these cells also has cytoplasmic CD3 expression in the absence of surface CD3 expression. This becomes particularly difficult when phenotypic overlap exists, potentially compromising both the sensitivity and specificity of MRD detection. Therefore, the antibody panel

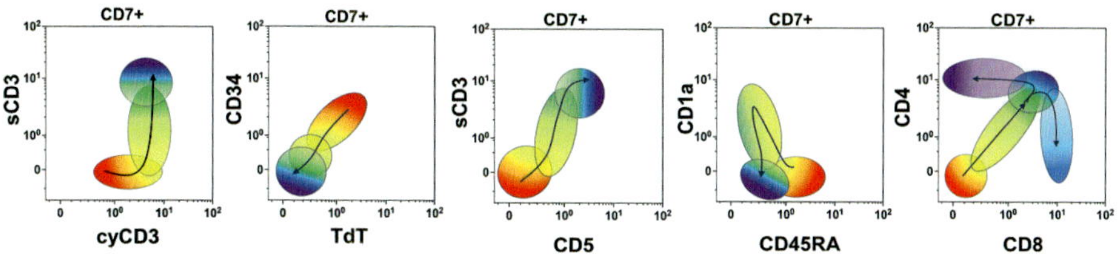

Fig. 8.3 Schematic representation of thymic T-cell maturation integrated with flow cytometric immunophenotyping. This figure illustrates key stages of intrathymic T-cell development using cartoon depictions of maturing thymocytes overlaid on background flow cytometry dot plots. The immunophenotypic progression is defined by sequential acquisition and downregulation of surface and intracellular markers including CD7, CD5, CD1a, CD3, CD4, CD8, and TdT. Early thymic progenitors with cytoplasmic -CD3+/nuclear TdT+/surface CD7+/surface CD5+ phenotype; Intermediate cortical thymocytes expressing CD1a and dual CD4+/CD8+ (double-positive) stages; Late stages characterized by acquisition of surface CD3 and loss of TdT, culminating in mature CD4+ or CD8+ single-positive T cells. This integrated approach provides a visual reference for normal T-lineage maturation, aiding in the identification of immunophenotypic deviations associated with T-lymphoblastic leukemias during diagnostic and MRD assessments

for T-MRD needs careful designing and optimization with thoughtful integration of both surface and intracellular markers to improve discriminatory power in post-therapy settings.

Several groups have developed high-dimensional, multiparametric flow cytometry panels tailored to address the challenges posed by post-therapy T-ALL MRD monitoring in bone marrow samples. The COG employs a 2-tube, 12-antigen panel comprising both surface and intracellular markers—CD2, CD3, CD4, CD5, CD7, CD8, CD34, CD45, and CD99 [60]. The EuroFlow consortium utilizes a 12-color, 2-tube panel, consisting of 15 and 13 markers, respectively [106]. A shared backbone of eight markers—CD16+NKp80, cyCD3, sCD3, CD5, CD7, CD34, CD45, and CD45RA—is complemented by CD6, CD38, and TdT in both tubes. Tube-1 includes a single-fluorochrome cocktail for CD117, CD13, and CD33, while Tube-2 incorporates CD2, CD4, CD8, and CD99 [106]. At TMC, we use a 13-color, 14-antibody single-tube panel incorporating surface CD3, cytoplasmic CD3, CD4, CD5, CD7, CD8, CD16+CD56, CD34, CD38, CD45, CD94, CD161, and CD48. Collectively, these panels are designed to detect residual disease based on detection of CD7+ immature T-cells and exclusion of CD7 expressing other hematopoietic cells including pDCs, myeloid precursors, normal T and NK-cells with strategies that prioritize sensitivity, reproducibility, and accurate distinction from normal hematopoietic cells.

Antibody Panel AML MRD

In contrast to ALL MRD, AML MRD assessment is a complex and challenging assay. Contrary to B-ALL MRD, where residual leukemic cells need to be distinguished from normal BCP, AML MRD requires discrimination from a heterogeneous population of normal myeloid progenitor compartment cells that eventually differentiates into granulocytic, monocytic, erythroid, dendritic cell, basophil, and mast cell lineages. To identify MRD in AML, residual leukemic cells must be differentiated from these six to seven subsets of myeloid progenitor cells [41, 92, 93, 95]. Therefore, in addition to the backbone markers recommended by the ELN working group for AML MRD (e.g., CD45, CD34, CD38, CD117, HLA-DR), the antibody panel should include various markers to identify myeloid progenitors differentiating towards different hematopoietic cells [92, 95, 107]. These include:

- Granulocytic precursors: CD13, CD15, CD33
- Monocytic precursors: CD64, CD33, CD14, CD36
- Erythroid precursors: CD36, CD71
- Plasmacytoid dendritic cells, basophils, and mast cell precursors: HLA-DR, CD123, CD203c.

Figure 8.4 illustrates the normal maturation stages of hematopoietic progenitors, their differentiation into various sub-lineages, and corresponding antigen expression patterns. Deviations from these patterns—such as abnormal antigen intensities or asynchronous marker expression—allow the detection of aberrancies using the DfN approach.

The antibody panel also needs to incorporate lymphoid markers frequently expressed on leukemic cells (e.g., CD7, CD19, CD56) to detect LAIPs. Additional rarely expressed lymphoid markers (e.g., CD2, CD4, CD5, CD11b, CD25) can further enhance the assay's sensitivity. A combination of CD34 and CD38 (CD34+ CD38+/−) helps evaluate the earliest hematopoietic precursors, including hematopoietic stem cells (HSCs). Overexpression of CD33 and CD123, along with aberrant expression of CD7 or CD56, can aid in identifying leukemic stem cells (LSCs) [108–110]. Additional markers—such as CD45RA, CD52, CD54, CD96, CD97, CD366 (Tim-3), and CD371 (CLL-1)—can be included to detect further aberrancies in committed progenitors and stem cells [110–114]. A minimum 8-color antibody panel has been recommended by ELN working group for AML MRD [41, 95]. The utilization of AMLMRD panels with more than 8-color allows simultaneous evaluation of more markers, improving the detection of deviation from normal antigen expression and thereby increasing sensitivity and accuracy. Furthermore, the additional use of a customized antibody combination tuned to the diagnostic immunophenotype can also help.

Sample Preparation, Processing, and Acquisition

BM Versus PB

In ALL, MRD assessment can be performed in peripheral blood (PB) or bone marrow (BM), with BM being the gold standard due to higher sensitivity and better disease representation [18, 69, 70, 115–121]. PB typically exhibits MRD levels one log or more lower than in BM, increasing the risk of false-negative results. However, PB MRD monitoring offers a less invasive alternative, with lower concordance rates (~70–80%) compared to BM [122, 123]. Studies suggest that PB MRD may miss

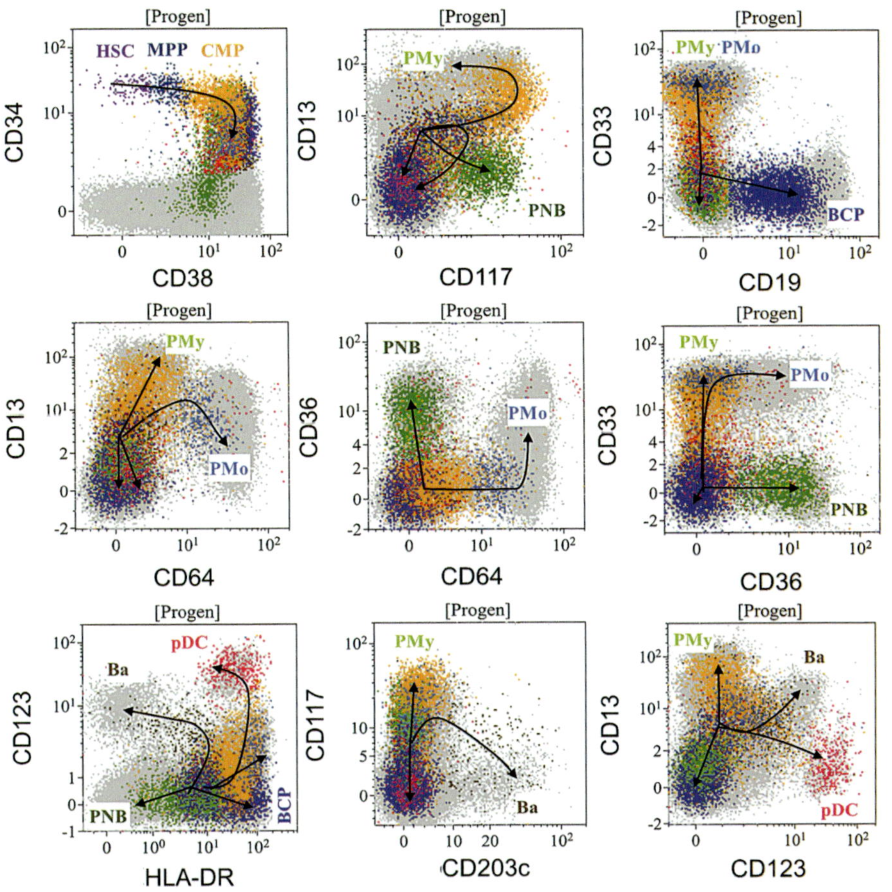

Fig. 8.4 Normal immunophenotypic maturation patterns of CD34⁺ hematopoietic progenitors into lineage-committed precursors. The figure illustrates the differentiation trajectories of hematopoietic stem cells (HSCs), visualized using flow cytometric dot plots and commonly applied antibody combinations. Each plot shows the progression of hematopoietic stem cells (dark purple dots) into specific lineage-restricted precursors, with black arrows indicating the direction of maturation. Lineage assignments are color-coded as follows: orange dots- Granulocytic precursors; light blue dots- Monocytic precursors; green dots- Erythroid precursors; dark blue dots- B-cell precursors; Pink dots- Plasmacytoid dendritic cell (pDC) precursors; dark brown dots- Basophil precursors. Gray-colored dots represent background mature mononuclear cells derived from the CD45 versus SSC progenitor gate. This figure serves as a reference map for assessing deviations in progenitor maturation, which may occur in leukemic or dysplastic states. Abbreviations: *Ba* Basophils, *BCP* B-cell precursors, *CMP* Common myeloid progenitors, *HSC* Hematopoietic stem cells, *MPP* Multipotent progenitors, *PMy* Precursor myeloid cells, *PMo* Precursor monocytes, *PNB* Precursor normoblasts, *pDC* Plasmacytoid dendritic cells

low-level disease, particularly in B-ALL, whereas BM MRD correlates more strongly with relapse risk [18, 115, 119, 120, 122]. However, the concordance between PB and BM is higher in T-ALL MRD [73, 124].

Similarly, bone marrow (BM) aspirates remain the ideal sample for AML MRD evaluation, and some studies have explored the use of PB in AML [18, 116, 125, 126]. Another critical consideration in BM sampling is hemodilution, which can also lead to false negatives. To minimize this risk, the first-pull BM aspirate (0.5–1 mL) is strongly recommended for MRD monitoring. It is recommended to collect the BM samples in ethylenediaminetetraacetic acid (EDTA) or heparin anticoagulants, transported at 8–20°C, and processed within 48–72 h of collection [3, 41, 59, 95]. The EuroFlow Consortium's bulk-lysis-stain method is the preferred processing technique for MRD assays, though some centers still use the stain-lyse-wash method [127].

For optimal sensitivity, a minimum acquisition of 1,000,000 viable events per tube is recommended. However, the goal should be to collect the highest possible number of relevant events to achieve higher sensitivity. In ALL, recent studies have demonstrated the sensitivity <0.001% using high-sensitivity or next-generation flow cytometry techniques. Acquiring at least 4–5 million cells enhances MRD assay sensitivity, while a minimum of 40 abnormal blast events ensures reliable MRD detection [3, 58–60].

MRD Analysis Approach

B-ALL MRD

Gating Strategy and Mapping the Normal Maturation of BCP

Approach to B-ALL MRD primarily depends on the evaluation of immunophenotypic maturation patterns. The key concept is that normal BCPs follow well-conserved and predictable sequences of antigen modulation during maturation. Abnormal leukemic B-blasts in some ways deviate from this preserved maturational pattern in all cases. Therefore, the critical steps to MFC-BMRD assessment depend on (a) focusing on the target population (primarily BCPs) using gating, and (b) charting the pattern of BCP maturation as faithfully as possible, with respect to the markers present in the panel.

The primary B-cell-specific gating using pan-B cell makers such as CD19 or CD22 forms the basis of the gating strategy following conventional chemotherapy. The approach of gating and mapping the normal maturation used at TMC is represented in Fig. 8.5i. After initial common gating steps that include exclusion of doublets using FSC height versus area and debris using SSC versus FSC, the first step towards MRD analysis is separating mononuclear cells (MNC) with the help of CD45/SSC or CD38/SSC followed by the B-cell isolation with CD19 and or CD22. At this stage, one can add a few additional dot plots to remove unwanted artefacts to get a clean B-cell population. For example, the CD10/CD38 plot is used to exclude CD38bright/CD10- plasma cells and the CD20/CD45 plot is used to exclude CD45bright non-B lymphocytes (predominantly NK-cells with CD19-trogocytosis)

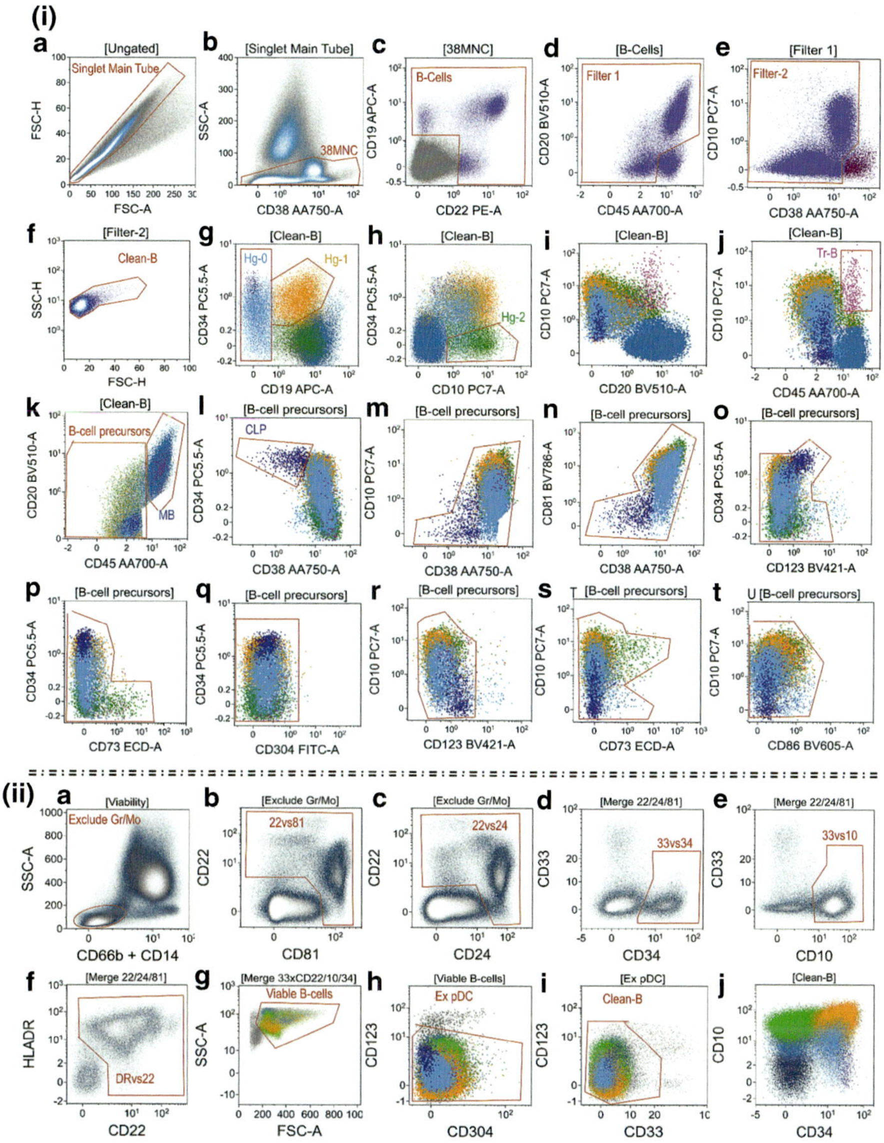

Fig. 8.5 Gating strategy for measurable residual disease (MRD) detection in B-acute lymphoblastic leukemia (B-ALL) at TMC. This figure illustrates the stepwise flow cytometric approach for identifying residual leukemic cells in B-ALL using immunophenotypic deviation from normal B-cell maturation, as shown in Fig. 8.2. The approach includes two panels corresponding to different treatment contexts: Part I—Post-Conventional Chemotherapy MRD Strategy: Mononuclear cells (MNCs) are identified using CD38 versus SSC to exclude granulocytes and debris. The initial B-lineage gate is created using CD19 versus CD22. Subsequent gating steps are applied to exclude normal hematopoietic components, such as plasma cells (CD38-bright/CD10−) and non-B lymphocytes (CD45-bright), along with common artifacts. The resulting "clean B cells" are subjected to template-based analysis to detect aberrant immunophenotypes indicating residual leukemic

populations, based on deviation from normal B-cell maturation. Part II—Post Anti-CD19 Targeted Immunotherapy MRD Strategy: Given potential CD19 downregulation, MNCs are gated after excluding granulocytes and monocytes using CD66b/CD14 versus SSC. A Boolean gate "Merge 22/24/81" is constructed using "OR" logic from CD22 versus CD24 and CD22 versus CD81 plots. A secondary Boolean gate "Merge 33xCD22/10/34" includes events from CD34 versus CD33, CD10 versus CD33, and CD22 versus HLA-DR plots. Additional steps remove debris, plasmacytoid dendritic cells, and basophils, yielding a refined "clean B-cell" population. These cells are then assessed for MRD through deviation-from-normal patterns using a standardized B-lineage maturation template

resulting in a yield of clean B-cells for further downstream analysis. One important point here is that the exclusion gates should be used in a context-specific manner. For example, the CD10/CD38 plot to exclude plasma cells should not inadvertently exclude CD10 negative MRD as typically seen in B-ALL with *KMT2A*/*ZNF384* rearrangements.

Thus, isolated "clean B cells" are then analyzed using combinations of various markers demonstrating normal maturation patterns of BCP. The BCPs in BM typically mature through reproducibly recognizable stages (illustrated in Fig. 8.2). Briefly, immature markers such as CD34, CD10, TdT, and CD38 are gradually lost during B-cell maturation with simultaneous gain in maturity-associated markers such as CD20 and CD45. However, integrated highly multiplexed multi-omics studies have started to demonstrate that the BM B-cell differentiation is more complex and involves a higher number of well-conserved, reproducible stages than traditionally appreciated and possible non-linear parallel pathways of differentiation (Fig. 8.2) [128]. The MFC-BMRD strategy involves drawing gates/boundaries on the normal maturing B-cells in control samples (staging control or regenerative non-B-ALL patient samples). A combination of such well-charted gates/boundaries of normal is then used as template/semi-automates algorithms to analyze a given sample.

Common Aberrancies and Challenges

Having established the boundaries of normal, typical MFC-BMRD approach assesses the deviation from it in a given patient sample. Generally, two aberrations in a cluster of 10–20 cells are needed to convincingly call MRD. The common abnormalities in leukemic B-blasts in comparison to normal BCPs include asynchronous expression of CD10/CD34 with CD38 (CD10+/CD38− and CD34+/CD38−); aberrant overexpression of CD73, CD304, CD86 in CD10+/CD34+ precursors; negative expression of CD45 (dimmer than normal BCP1); asynchronous overexpression of CD20 (CD20 moderate/bright positivity in CD34+ or CD45dim precursors), etc. Figure 8.6 illustrates a few examples of B-ALL MRD with various immunophenotypic aberrancies differentiating from background BCPs. A knowledge of the diagnostic immunophenotype is preferred but not necessary while applying the deviation-from-normal strategy. An important point while considering diagnostic phenotype is that therapy-induced immunophenotypic shifts (CD10/CD34 loss and upregulation of CD20/CD45) have been reported in leukemic B-blasts [129, 130]. After identification, MRD is calculated using nucleated cells (stained with Syto dyes) or viable cells as a denominator.

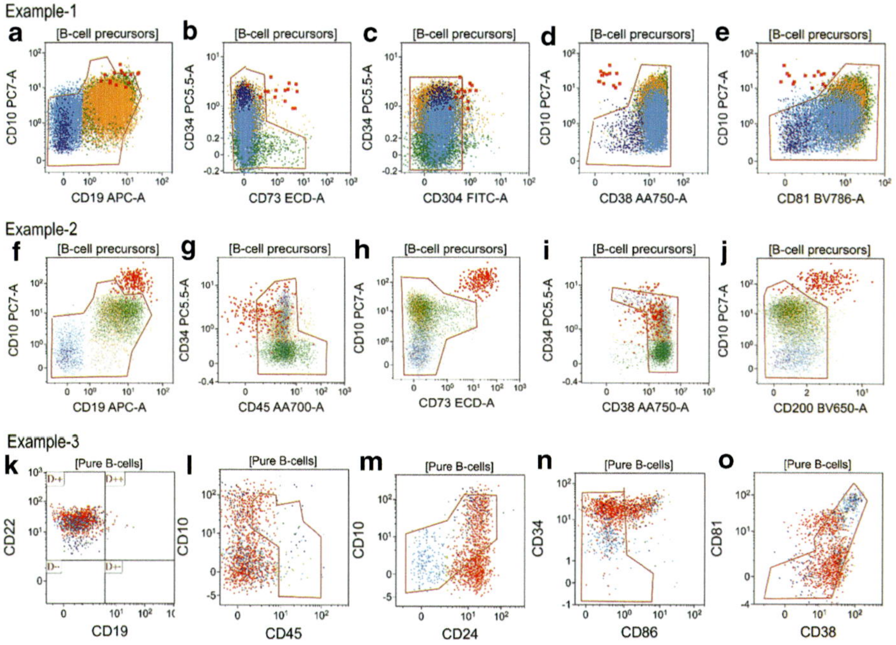

Fig. 8.6 Illustrative examples of residual leukemic B-blasts detected using a standardized flow cytometry-based B-lineage MRD (MFC-BMRD) panel. The figure demonstrates MRD-positive examples with representative dot plots, where red-colored dots highlight residual leukemic B-cell populations exhibiting immunophenotypic deviation from normal maturation patterns, as defined by standardized templates. Example 1: Detection of very low-level MRD (0.0002%) characterized by CD10+/CD34+/CD38−/CD81−/CD73+/dim CD304+ immunophenotype. This case was identified through acquisition of over 6 million events, underscoring the high sensitivity of the MFC-BMRD panel. Example 2: MRD population with a distinct bright CD10+/CD34+/CD200+/ bright CD73+ immunophenotype. Example 3: An MRD population identified in a patient undergoing anti-CD19 therapy (blinatumomab), using a CD19-agnostic gating approach. The abnormal cells exhibited a CD22+/CD24+/CD19−/CD45−/ heterogeneous CD10/heterogeneous CD86 profile, highlighting CD19-negative MRD in the post-immunotherapy setting

The MFC-BMRD strategy depends heavily on "deviation-from-normal" analysis and hence, it is imperative to be aware of all possible normal variations of BCP maturation and other low-level recurrently occurring cells that immunophenotypically mimic leukemic B-blasts. This is especially relevant in high-sensitivity settings as increased event acquisition can make the low-level immunophenotypic mimics more prominent. We have demonstrated that normal BCPs show a considerable immunophenotypic shift, most apparent in CD34 and CD10 downregulation and CD20 upregulation in regenerative BCP1 (pre-B/hematogone stage-1) compared to treatment-naïve bone marrow. This regenerative immunophenotypic shift is most prominent after intensive therapy and gradually reduces after consolidation and subsequent follow-up time points. Figure 8.7 additionally depicts a catalog of low-level common immunophenotypic mimics and Table 8.2 provides their

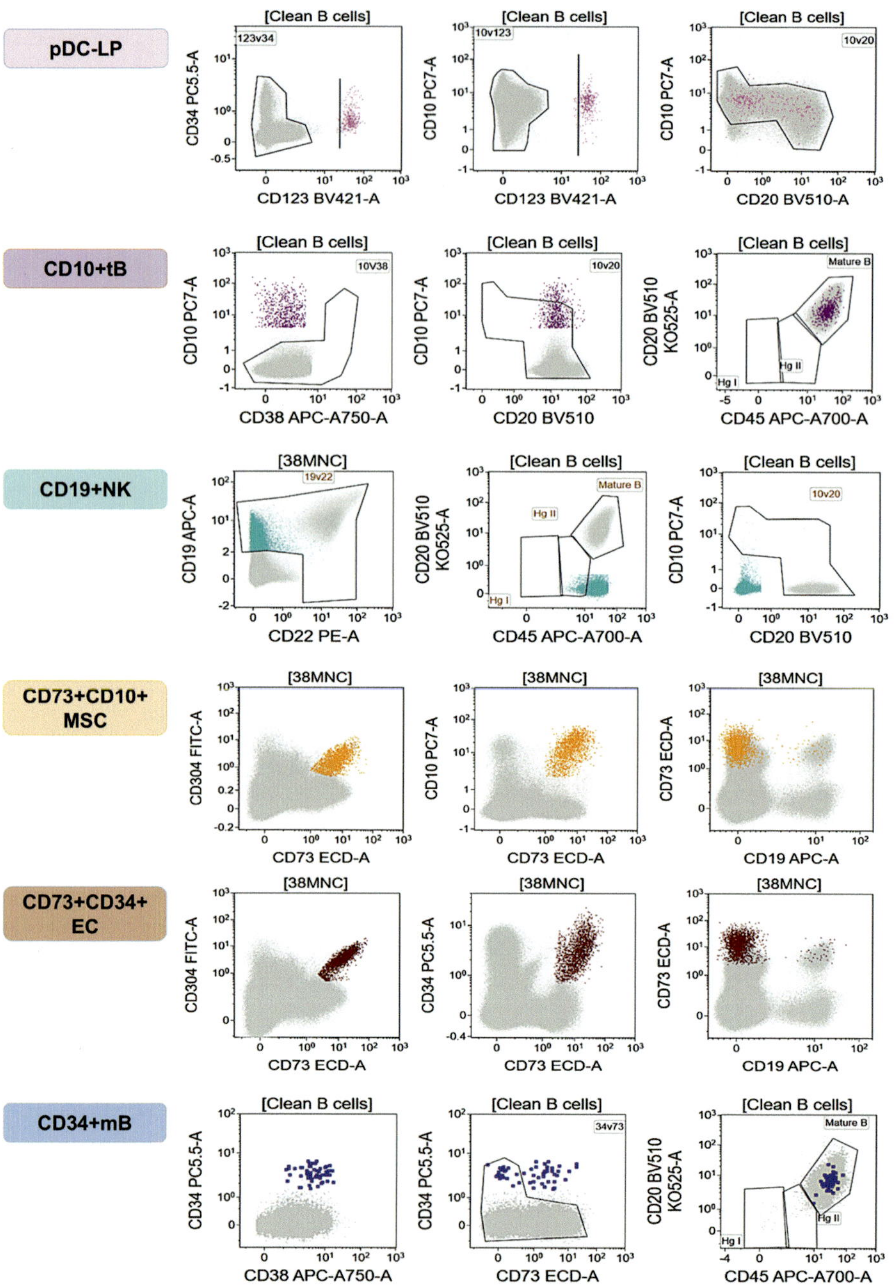

Fig. 8.7 Immunophenotypic mimics of B-lymphoid blasts in flow cytometric MRD (B-MRD) analysis. This figure presents representative dot plots of recurrently encountered low-level cellular populations that can mimic residual leukemic B-blasts during high-sensitivity flow cytometric MRD evaluation, particularly when large event counts are acquired. These immunophenotypically distinct, yet potentially confounding, populations are color-coded and annotated for reference.

These include: pDC-LP (pink dots): Plasmacytoid dendritic cell-like precursors showing partial B-lineage features; CD10+ tB cells (deep purple dots): Transitional B-cells with strong CD10 expression, sometimes overlapping with B-lymphoblast phenotype; CD19+ NK cells (cyan dots): Natural killer cells aberrantly expressing CD19, potentially misclassified as B-lineage events; MSC (orange dots): Mesenchymal stromal/stem cells occasionally detected in bone marrow aspirates; EC (deep brown dots): Endothelial cells with distinct immunophenotypic signatures; CD34+ mB cells (bright blue dots): CD34-positive mature B-cells, a rare but recognized subset with potential overlap in blast gate regions. This reference aids in distinguishing true residual leukemic blasts from benign immunophenotypic mimics, thereby reducing false-positive MRD interpretations in B-ALL

Table 8.2 Immunophenotypic profiling of low-level immunophenotypic mimics in high-sensitivity MFC-BMRD analysis [131]

Population	Immunophenotypic characteristics
pDC-LP	Mimics MRD: Bright CD123 in CD34+CD10+CD19+ cells Identification clues: Distinctly bright CD123 (usually brighter than what is seen in leukemic B-blasts and at the same level with other pDC) and no other LAIP
CD10+tB	Mimics MRD: CD10bright CD38dim-to-negative B cells Identification clues: Bright CD45/CD20 (equivalent to mature B cells), CD34−
CD19+NK	Mimics MRD: CD19+CD38+CD20-CD10-CD86+ phenotype, especially in CD10-negative B-ALL Identification clues: CD45 bright, CD19 weak
CD73+CD10+ MSC	Mimics MRD: CD73+CD10+CD304+CD19-phenotype, especially in a post anti-CD19 therapy setting Identification clues: Negative expression of CD45/CD20/CD19, distinctly bright CD73/CD304
CD73+CD34+ EC	Mimics MRD: CD73+CD34+CD304+CD19-phenotype, especially in a post anti-CD19 therapy setting Identification clues: Negative expression of CD45/CD20/CD19, distinctly bright CD73/CD304
CD34+mB	Mimics MRD: CD34+CD38dim-to-negative B cells Identification clues: Bright CD45/CD20 (equivalent to mature B cells), CD10−

Abbreviations: *pDC-LP* plasmacytoid dendritic cell (pDC) precursors differentiating from B-lymphoid cells, *CD10+ tB* transitional B-cells with overexpression of CD10, *MSC* mesenchymal stromal/stem cells, *EC* endothelial cells, *CD34+mB* CD34+ mature B cells

immunophenotypic characteristics and clues to identify them. Taken together, these data strongly argue in favor of creating immunophenotypic mimics-aware templates/algorithms on regenerative marrows (e.g., negative T-ALL/AML MRD samples) for *error-free* BMRD analysis.

Modifications of Panel and Gating Strategy for CD19-Targeted Therapy
Modern MFC-MRD assays face the unique challenge of needing to be flexible and nimble to improvise for specific targeted therapies used. In the context of B-ALL, the adoption of anti-CD19 therapies such as Blinatumomab and anti-CD19

CAR-T-cells necessitates a CD19-agnostic gating approach, as loss/downregulation of CD19 expression in the leukemic B-blasts can be seen commonly following these therapies. The basic principle of designing such MFC-assays is the following:

Incorporation of additional B-cell gating markers: A combination of CD22 and CD24 has been most commonly used to gate B-cells following anti-CD19 therapy. Cherian and colleagues first proposed such an approach of designing a rough B-cell gate to include all cells that express either CD22 or CD24 [132]. Our approach at TMC includes using CD81 along with CD22/CD24. Other markers that have been used for this purpose include cytoplasmic CD79a and HLADR [58].

Incorporation of markers of exclusion: A challenge of using non-CD19 B-cell markers as a gating strategy is that none of these markers are specific to the B-cell lineage. For instance, CD22 is expressed in basophils, mast cells, and pDCs, while CD24 is expressed in myeloid cells, monocytes, and immune cells. Therefore, the B-ALL MRD panels following anti-CD19 therapy include markers of exclusion, such as CD66b or CD33 to exclude myeloid/monocytic cells, CD3/CD7 to exclude T/NK cells, etc. A sequential/Boolean gating strategy is used, combining the expression of CD22/CD24 or other B cell markers while excluding CD66b/CD33-positive cells.

Recalibration of "normal": A complete recalibration of the mapping of normal BCPs and low-level recurrently occurring immunophenotypic mimics is necessary while using a CD19-agnostic gating approach. Recognition of two CD19-negative normal precursors is specifically important in this context (Fig. 8.2). These include (1) *early lymphoid progenitor cells* (or common lymphoid progenitors) characterized by bright-CD34, dim-CD38, dim-CD22, dim-CD81, but negative CD10, CD19, and CD24 expression; and (2) *pro-BCPs or stage-0 hematogones* characterized by CD22+, CD34+, moderate CD38+, heterogeneous CD10, moderate CD81, but negative CD19 and CD24 expression.

Target sensitivity: Growing evidences suggest that a lower cut-off level may be clinically more relevant for patients following anti-CD19 therapy [76, 77]. Contemporary post-antiCD19 MFC-BMRD protocols reach a sensitivity of 0.001%. A comparison of various described protocols can be seen in Table 8.3. Our approach of a modified gating strategy for post-antiCD19 MRD assay is illustrated in Fig. 8.5b.

T-MRD

T-MRD detection fundamentally relies on a thorough understanding of normal T-cell ontogeny and an "approach of exclusion of normal T/NK cells with immunophenotypic overlap with T-ALL leukemic cells,". In brief, the earliest T-cell progenitors—termed early T-cell precursors or double-negative T cells—express CD2, cytoCD3, CD7, CD34, CD99, and TdT, while lacking surface expression of CD4, CD5, CD8, and CD48. This is followed by a stage characterized by co-expression of CD4 and CD8 (double-positive) and the acquisition of CD1a, marking cortical thymocytes. In the final stages of maturation, T cells undergo lineage commitment

Table 8.3 A comparison between various contemporary MFC-BMRD protocols for patients receiving anti-CD19 therapy

Study	Panel design & markers	Gating strategy	Events collected	Sensitivity
Cherian et al. (2016) [132]	8-color panel including CD22, CD24, CD10, CD20, CD34, CD38, CD45, and CD66b	CD19-independent gating based on CD22 or CD24 expression, excluding CD66b-positive cells	>500,000	Reaches ≤0.01% (10^{-4}), formal LOD/LLOQ testing not done
Mikhailova et al. (2022) [133]	11-color panel including CD22, cytoplasmic CD79a, CD24, CD10, CD34, CD38, CD45, CD20, CD58, CD19, SYTO41	Sequential gating using CD22 and iCD79a, supplemented by CD10/CD24. No markers to exclude myeloid/monocytic cells	>300,000	Reaches 0.01% (10^{-4}); formal LOD/LLOQ testing not done
Gao et al. (2023) [134]	14-color panel including CD22, CD24, CD10, CD34, CD38, CD45, CD58, CD81, CD86, CD123, CD66c, CD73, CD304, CD66b	Gating based on CD19, CD22 or CD24 expression, excluding CD66b-positive cells	~2 million	LOD 0.0004 (4×10^{-6}), LLOQ 0.001% (10^{-5})
Chatterjee et al. (2024), TMC [58]	15-color panel including CD22, CD24, CD81, CD33, HLADR, CD10, CD34, CD38, CD19, CD20, CD45, CD123, CD304, CD73, CD86	CD19-independent gating using CD22 or CD24 or CD81, with CD33 as an exclusion marker	~5 million	LOD 0.0004 (4×10^{-6}), LLOQ 0.001% (10^{-5})
Roy et al. (Abstract published in 2024), COG [135]	10-color 2-tube panel includes CD20, CD10, CD38, CD19, CD58, CD45, CD9, etc. supplemented by CD22, CD24, CD73, CD81, CD123, and CD304	Using a combination of CD19, CD22, CD24, the detailed strategy not specified	4 million	Reaches 0.001% (10^{-5})
Verbeek et al. (2025), EuroFlow Consortium [80]	2-tube 12-color panel including CD22, CD24, CD81, HLADR, CD34, CD38, CD19, CD10, CD20, CD45, CD123, CD66c, CD73, CD304, CD3, CD7	CD22, CD24, and HLADR were additional B cell gating markers. CD3/CD7 was used to exclude T cells. This is followed by a semi-automated analysis strategy supplemented by expert evaluation	>4 million events	Sensitivity: 0.001% (10^{-5})

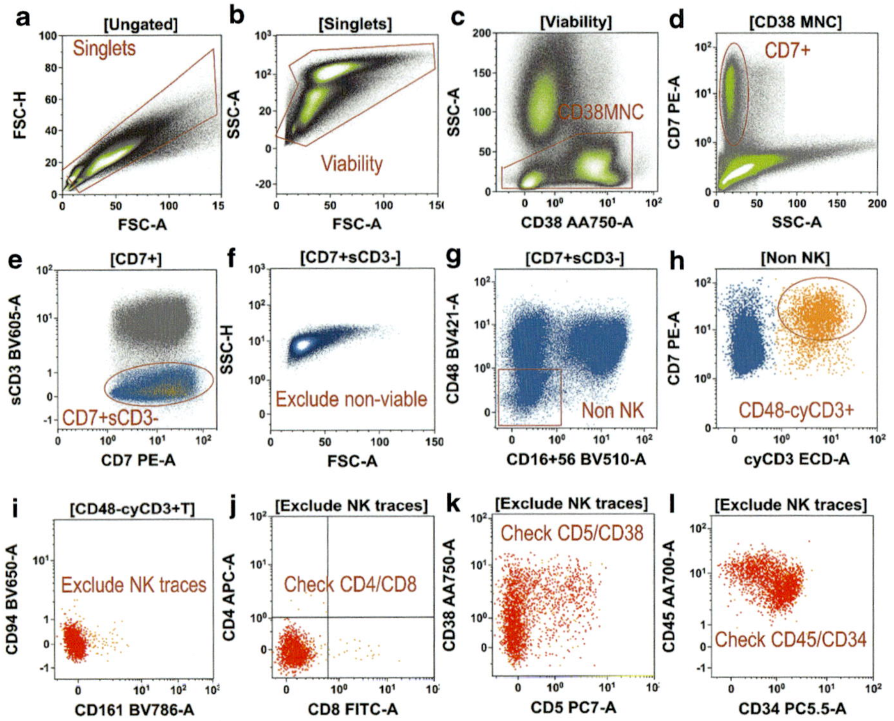

Fig. 8.8 Gating strategy for T-lymphoblastic leukemia (T-ALL) measurable residual disease (MRD). This figure illustrates the sequential flow cytometric gating approach used for identifying residual T-lymphoblasts in T-ALL MRD assessment: Flow cytometric gating begins with singlets (**a**) and viable cells (**b**), followed by selection of mononuclear cells based on CD38/SSC (**c**). CD7+/SSC^low cells are gated to enrich for T-lineage cells (**d**), and immature T cells are identified as $CD7^+$/surface $CD3^-$ (**e**). A secondary viability gate is applied (**f**), and NK cells are excluded using CD16/CD56 and CD48 (**g**). Residual cells are refined as CD48−/cytoCD3+ (**h**) with further NK exclusion via CD94 and CD161 (**i**). Final confirmation of MRD confirmed with expression of CD4 versus CD8 (**j**), CD5 versus CD38 (**k**), and CD45 versus CD34 (**l**) to assess maturation and detect aberrant phenotypes. This comprehensive gating strategy is designed to distinguish residual leukemic blasts from normal or reactive T-lineage cells and NK-cell contaminants, ensuring accurate MRD detection

and exhibit single positivity for either CD4 or CD8, along with sCD3 expression Fig. 8.3 [136–141]. Importantly, the presence of cells with a thymic (immature) immunophenotype in peripheral blood or bone marrow is considered abnormal.

The analytical strategy for T-MRD detection primarily involves following major steps (illustrated in Fig. 8.8). Doublets and debris are excluded using FSC-A versus FSC-H and SSC-A versus FSC-A dot plots initially. T-cells are isolated with pan-T cell markers, usually with CD7. The CD7+ cells typically include mature T-cells, NK-cells, a subset of regenerating myeloid precursor cells with weak CD7 expression, a subset of CD7+ plasmacytoid dendritic cells (pDCs), and residual leukemic blasts in MRD-positive samples. Hence, the next step involves exclusion of these

CD7+ other hematopoietic cells. For example, mature T-cells are excluded based on sCD3+ expression, NK-cells with CD16+/CD56+, and weak-CD7+ myeloid blasts and pDCs are excluded by further isolating only cytoplasmic CD3+$^{+}$ events (as these two populations are cytoCD3 negative) [60]. Further, expression of immaturity markers such as CD1a, CD99, TdT, and CD34 can be useful to identify MRD [34, 105]. However, CD1a and CD34 are helpful only in a subset of samples and CD99 and TdT usually shows post-therapeutic loss of expression and thus may not be helpful in significant number of samples [60, 103]. Recently, CD48 has been shown to be a useful marker as it is positive in mature T-cells and NK-cells but is typically negative in T-ALL blasts [34]. Additionally, a few subsets of cells that can interfere with T-ALL MRD approach based on exclusion of normal cells include a subset of mature T cells with loss of sCD3 and CD56/CD16 negative precursor NK-cells, both of which express CD7 and cyCD3. sCD3-negative mature T-cells (possibly resulting from cytoplasmic processing steps) are excluded based on strong CD45 expression, moderate CD48, and presence of mutually exclusive CD4+ or CD8+ subsets similar to sCD3+ mature T-cells. Similarly, the subset of CD56/CD16 immature NK-cells can be excluded using moderate CD38, weak/heterogeneous CD8, strong CD45, moderate CD48, and absence of CD4 and CD5 expression. The addition of other NK cell markers such as NKp80 or CD94 can be useful to remove these NK cells. In such samples, the diagnostic immunophenotype of T-ALL blasts is very useful for making decisions. We have published the detailed gating strategy that involves the utilization of a combination of CD5/CD38 and CD4/CD8, along with other T/NK cell markers [60].

A few cases, especially with ETPALL immunophenotype, have partial or heterogeneous CD56 expression. In such cases, precaution must be taken not to exclude CD56+ cells and carefully evaluate the expression of CD8 and CD48. Similarly, in rare cases, T-ALL cells can present with sCD3 expression; usually, it is weak in intensity. In such cases, sCD3+ events cannot be excluded directly. Instead, sCD3 expression is used in combination with negative CD48 and aberrant loss or co-expression of CD4/CD8 for MRD detection. Figure 8.9 illustrates a few examples of T-ALL MRD.

AML MRD

The immunophenotype of AML blasts at diagnosis is critical in AML MRD monitoring. MFC-MRD analysis in AML integrates two principal methodologies: LAIP and DfN Approach [41, 92, 94, 95, 142].

LAIP-Based Approach: LAIPs can be broadly classified into two groups based on aberrancies:

- Group-1: Aberrant lymphoid markers (e.g., CD2, CD7, CD19, and CD56).
- Group-2: Altered progenitor markers (e.g., CD34, CD38, CD117, HLA-DR).

Key considerations: LAIPs identified at diagnosis enable MRD tracking, but immunophenotypic shifts post-therapy (due to clonal selection or plasticity) may lead to false negatives [95, 142]. Tracking ≥2 LAIPs to improve sensitivity from the

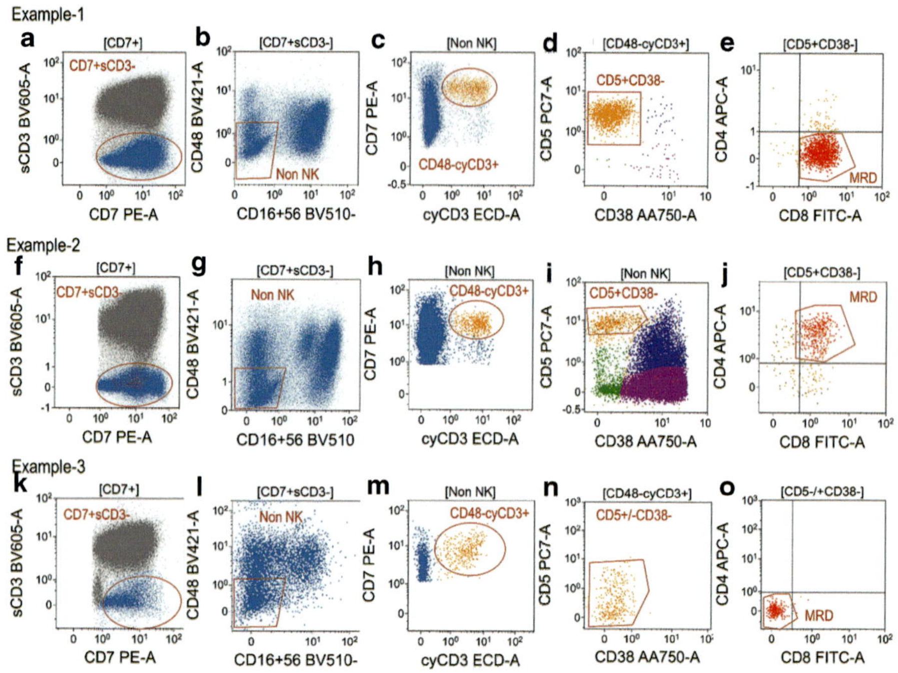

Fig. 8.9 Illustrative examples of T-ALL measurable residual disease (MRD) detected by flow cytometry. [**a**–**e**] Example 1: CD8+/CD5+ MRD population with uniform CD8 expression and absent or dim CD4. [**f**–**j**] Example 2: CD4+/CD8+ double-positive MRD population, consistent with a cortical thymic immunophenotype. [**k**–**o**] Example 3: CD4⁻/CD8⁻ double-negative MRD population, reflecting an early immature T-cell phenotype

diagnostic sample is recommended to avoid false-positive or negative results due to the shift or absence of one [95, 142, 143].

Pitfalls LAIP-based approach:

- Regenerating CD34+ progenitors may express CD7/CD56 weakly (false positives) [95, 142, 143].
- LAIP requires diagnostic samples, which may be unavailable for referral cases.
- May miss secondary clones or therapy-resistant subclones with divergent immunophenotypes.

DfN Approach: Advantages and Requirements

The DfN approach detects MRD by identifying deviations from normal antigenic patterns in hematopoietic progenitors and do not require diagnostic immunophenotype. However, it needs a comprehensive antibody panel that cover common maturation patterns of myeloid precursors towards various lineages. Normal myeloid progenitors also follow a strict maturation pattern as shown in Fig. 8.4.

Immunophenotypic maturation sequences of myeloid precursors begin with early-stage hematopoietic stem cells (HSC) defined with weak to negative CD38, strong CD34, relatively higher CD45, weak HLADR, variable CD117, and weak CD13/CD33 expression. HSC are usually negative for lymphoid markers such as CD2, CD5, CD7, and CD56, and other lineage-associated markers such as CD11b, CD15, CD36, CD64, CD45RA, and CD371. These cells prominently differentiate into precursor cells of granulocytic, monocytic, dendritic, erythroid, B-lymphoid, basophil/mast cell lineages, which can be elaborated using the combination of various markers. These maturation sequences or patterns of early myeloid progenitor cells differentiate towards the committed progenitors. Deviation from these normal patterns can be considered aberrant maturation and designated as residual disease.

The usual deviations include [92, 107, 142]:

- Loss of antigen expression leading to deviation from normal maturation patterns of myeloid precursors. For example, myeloid blasts with CD34+ but CD117 and or HLADR and or CD38-negative expression.
- Increased intensity (overexpression) of common myelomonocytic makers compared to normal myeloid progenitors such as CD11b, CD13, CD33, CD36, CD64, CD71, and CD123.
- Decreased intensity (underexpression) of common myelomonocytic makers such as CD13, CD33, CD117, and CD71, and other markers such as CD34, CD38, CD45, and HLADR, compared to normal myeloid progenitors.

Gating Strategy

The initial gating strategy for AML MRD analysis (Fig. 8.10) also follows the same principles involving doublet exclusion using FSC-H versus FSC-A properties, removal of debris with FSC versus SSC properties, isolation of mononuclear cells using CD45 versus SSC or CD38 versus SSC, and identification of myeloid precursor cells and their maturation sequences as described below.

- Blast/Progenitor Identification: Leukemic blasts typically show:
  - Weak CD45 expression + low SSC
  - Expression of immature markers (CD34, CD117)
  - Absence of maturation markers (CD11b, CD14, strong CD15)
- Lineage-Specific Subpopulation Analysis:
  - Granulocytic progenitors: CD13+CD33+
  - Monocytic progenitors: CD33+CD64+CD36+
  - Erythroid progenitors: CD36+ (with absent myeloid/monocytic markers) and strong CD71 expression
  - Plasmacytoid dendritic/basophil progenitors: CD123+HLA-DR+/−
- Progenitor Compartmentalization: The MNC progenitor pool is stratified into three immunophenotypically distinct subsets using CD34 and CD117 expression patterns:
  - CD34+ hematopoietic stem/progenitor cells (HSPCs)

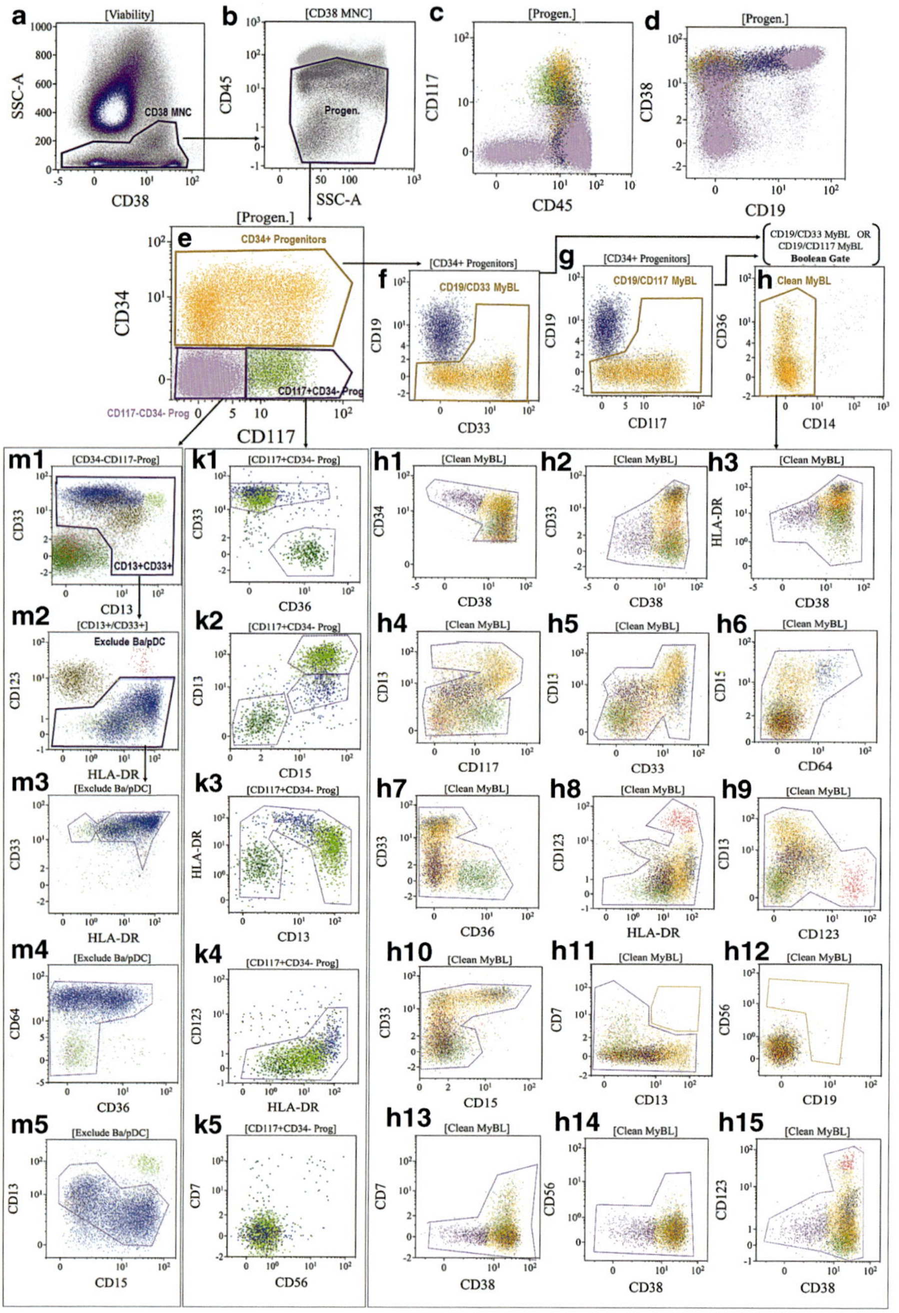

Fig. 8.10 Gating strategy for AML measurable residual disease (MRD) analysis. Mononuclear cells (MNCs) were identified by excluding granulocytes (CD38 vs. SSC, plot [**a**]) and then gated to enrich for progenitor cells by excluding CD45-bright lymphocytes and monocytes (Progen gate,

- CD117+CD34− early committed myeloid and/or erythroid progenitors
- CD34-CD117− more differentiated progenitor populations
- Identification of aberrant antigen expression patterns through:
- LAIP analysis (including lymphoid marker expression: CD7, CD19, CD56)
- Different-from-normal (DfN) approach evaluating asynchronous antigen expression

This compartmentalized strategy enables the targeted evaluation of progenitor subsets based on diagnostic leukemia-associated immunophenotypes (LAIPs) such as the AML blasts were CD34 negative or CD117 negative. It further allows the focused analysis of relevant populations (e.g., preferential assessment of CD117+CD34− compartment in CD34-negative AML cases) and parallel assessment of differentiation patterns through established maturation trajectories (Fig. 8.10, Table 8.4). (Representative MRD cases across all compartments are illustrated in Fig. 8.11).

Critical Analytical Considerations

There are certain critical considerations that need to be kept in mind during MFC-MRD analysis.

- The post intensive chemotherapy regenerating marrow can show some unusual antigen expression patterns; such as CD34+ progenitors in regeneration may show transient CD7 or CD56 expression, requiring careful distinction from true MRD. Regenerating erythroid progenitors usually have more CD7 expression than myeloid progenitors. Similarly, restricted expression of CD13 or CD33 results in clustered maturation patterns during hematopoietic recovery [55, 92, 95, 142, 143].
- Sensitivity optimization: Acquisition of ≥1 million cells is recommended for reliable 0.01% sensitivity [41, 95].
- Panel design: ≥8-color panels are now standard, with EuroFlow recommendations providing harmonized approaches [41, 95].
- Data analysis: Use of reference databases or predefined templates for normal regeneration patterns improves DfN accuracy

Fig. 8.10 (continued) plot [**b**]). Progenitor subsets were classified into: (1) CD34+, (2) CD117+/CD34−, and (3) CD34−/CD117− compartments (plot [**e**]). CD34+ B-cell precursors were excluded using Boolean gates combining CD19/CD33 ([**f**]) or CD19/CD117 ([**g**]) to isolate non-lymphoid CD34$^+$ progenitors. A "Clean MyBL" gate was created by removing CD14$^+$CD36$^+$ monocytes (plot [**h**]), and these cells were analyzed for abnormal maturation patterns across panels [h1–h15] based on normal reference profiles (Fig. 8.4). CD117+/CD34− progenitors were further assessed for aberrancies using deviation from normal maturation patterns indicated with gates inside plots (plots [k1–k5]), while CD117−/CD34− progenitors were gated after excluding CD13−/CD33− cells ([m1]) and basophils/plasmacytoid dendritic cells ([m2]), with analysis shown in plots [m3–m5]

Table 8.4 Immunophenotype of various normal precursor populations commonly seen in bone marrow samples for AML MRD analysis

CD45vSSC progenitor compartment	Sub-populations	Immunophenotype of sub-populations (Based on the markers commonly used in AML MRD panel)																
		Backbone markers					Myeloid markers			Monocytic, pDC, basophil, mast cell markers					Lymphoid markers			
		CD 34	CD 38	CD 45	CD 117	HLA -DR	CD 13	CD 33	CD 15	CD 36	CD 64	CD 14	CD 123	CD 203c	CD 7	CD 56	CD 19	CD 22
CD34+	HSC & MPP	++	−/+	++	V+	+	+	+	−	−	−	−	−/+	−	−	−	−	−
	GMP	++	++	+	V+	++	V+	++	S+	−	S+	−	−/+	−	S−/+	S+*	−	−
	pDCP	+	++	++	−	++	−/+	+	−	+	+	−	+++	−	P+	P+	−	−/+
	BaP	+	++	++	−/+	−/+	++	+	−	−/+	−	−	++	+	−	−	−	−
	MEP	+	++	+	++	−/+	−	−	−	−/+	−	−	−	−	S−/+	−	−	−
	CLP	++	+	+	−	++	−	−	−	−	−	−	−	−	−	−	−	+
	BCP (Hg1)	++	++	+	−	++	−	−	−	−	−	−	−	−	−	−	+	++
	MCP	+	++	++	++	−	+	++	−	−/+	−/+	−	−/+	+	−	−	−	−
CD34-CD117+	PMy	−	−/+	+	+	−/+	+++	++	+++	−/+	+	−	−	−	−	−*	−	−
	PMo	−	+	++	−/+	++	−	++	+	+	++	−	+	−	−	−*	−	−
	PNB	−	+	−/+	++	−/+	−	−	−	++	−	−	−	−	S−/+	−	−	−
	MC	−	++	++	+++	−		++	−		−/+	−	−/+	++	−	−	−	−
CD34-CD117−	imMo	−	−	++	−	++	−/+	++	+	++	++	−/+	+	−	−	−*	−	−
	NRBC	−	−	−/+	−	−	−	−	−	+++	−	−	−	−	−	−	−	−
	pDC	−	+	++	−	++	−	++	−	+	−	−	+++	−	P+	P+	−	−/+
	Ba	−	+	++	−	−	++	+	−	+	−	−	+++	−	−	−	−	−/+
	PCs	−	+++	V+	−	−	−	−	−	−	−	−	−	−	−	−	+	−
	BCP	−	++	+	−	++	−	−	−	−	−	−	−	−	−	−	++	++
	NK	−	+	++	−	−	−	−	−	−	−	−	−	−	++	++	−	−

*CD56 can be weakly positive in a subset of these populations in regenerative bone marrow samples submitted for MRD evaluation.***Note:*** (−) negative, (−/+) dim positive to negative, (+) dim positive, (++) moderate positive, (+++) strong positive, *p* partial, *S* subset, *V* variable

Abbreviations. *BaP* basophils precursors, *BCP* B-cell precursors, *CLP* common lymphoid progenitors, *GMP* granulocyte-macrophage (monocyte) progenitors, *Hg1* hematogones stage-1, *HSC* hematopoietic stem cells, *imMo* immature monocytes, *MCP* Mast cell precursors, *MPP* multipotent progenitors, *MEP* megakaryocyte erythrocyte progenitors, *NK* Natural Killer cells, *NRBC* nucleated RBCs, *PCs* plasma cells, *pDCP* Plasmacytoid dendritic cell precursors, *PMy* Precursor myeloid cells (promyelocytes), *PMo* Precursor monocytes (promonocytes), *PNB* Precursor normoblasts (pronormoblasts)

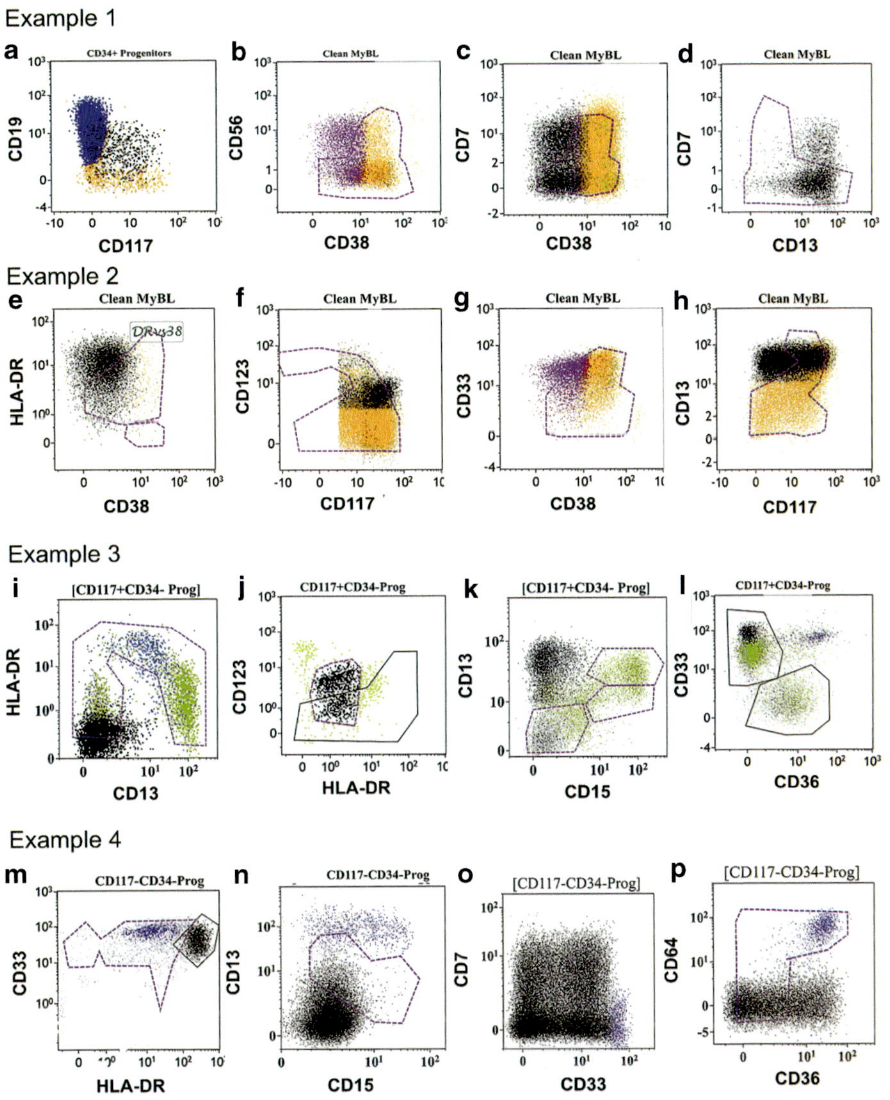

Fig. 8.11 Illustrative examples of AML measurable residual disease (MRD) detection across progenitor compartments. MRD populations (black dots) are shown from three compartments in different patients: CD34$^+$ progenitors (**a**–**h**), CD117+/CD34− progenitors (**i**–**l**), and CD117−/CD34− progenitors (**m**–**p**). Residual leukemic cells are marked with black dots in all plots, except in **b** and **g**, where MRD is highlighted in purple color to indicate aberrant CD56 expression (**b**) and CD33 overexpression (**g**) in CD38$^-$ stem cell populations

Quality Control (QC)

Quality Control in Flow Cytometry-Based MRD Assessment should include the following areas [95, 143–145].

Instrument Quality Control: It should be performed with daily calibration beads such as CS&T beads, Rainbow beads, and flow check beads as per manufacturer's recommendations.

Reagent Quality Assurance: It includes validation of new reagent lots against established controls and use of pre-validated antibody cocktails to minimize pipetting variability, ensure lot-to-lot consistency, and reduce inter-operator variability.

MRD Analysis Template Development, Verification, and Maintenance [2, 94, 95, 142, 143]

Template Establishment: Minimum 20 control bone marrow samples are required to design the template, which should preferably include 10 normal non-leukemic samples and 10 post-chemotherapy regenerating samples, possibly samples spanning relevant age groups

- Template verification: Demonstration of ≤10% coefficient of variation for marker expression intensities and verification of sensitivity to 0.01% (10^{-4}) aberrant populations [76].
- Template maintenance/revalidation: It includes monthly re-evaluation of templates using control samples, quarterly template updates using control samples, and updated regeneration patterns [84].
- Competency assurance: It is done through personnel training, regular participation in MRD-specific workshops, and continuing medical education (CME) programs, and annual inter/intra-laboratory competency assessments [146–149].
- External quality assessment: It includes enrollment in international EQA programs (e.g., UK NEQAS) or regular performance review with peer laboratories [146–151].

Additional QC Measures

Sample Processing Controls can be performed through:

- Assessment of cell viability using viability dyes (e.g., 7-AAD, DAPI), especially in transported samples [95, 143].
- Hemodilution assessment via either marrow representing cellular elements such as mast cells, erythroid precursors, and myeloid/lymphoid precursors, or monitoring cells predominant in blood and scant in marrow, for example, mature granulocytes (CD16+) [63, 95, 152–154].

Data analysis QC can be performed by monitoring the following parameters [147–149]

- Blind re-analysis of 10% random cases
- Quarterly review of false positive/negative rates
- Maintenance of an internal MRD case registry for longitudinal follow-up

Limit of Detection (LOD)/Lower Limit of Quantitation (LLOQ)

The limit of detection (LOD) and lower limit of quantitation (LLOQ) are critical parameters in MRD detection, defining the assay's sensitivity and precision [155]. The LOD represents the lowest level at which MRD can be reliably distinguished from background noise, typically requiring a signal significantly above negative control [94, 156, 157]. In flow cytometry, this is often determined by the number of abnormal cells detected within a large population of normal cells, usually ranging between 10^{-5} and 10^{-6} (1 in 100,000 to 1 in 1,000,000 cells) [2, 58–60, 94, 142]. The LLOQ, on the other hand, is the lowest MRD level that can be quantified with acceptable accuracy and precision (CV < 25%), often requiring higher cell counts than the LOD to ensure reproducibility [3, 156, 157]. Factors influencing these limits include sample quality, antibody panel specificity, instrument sensitivity, and data analysis techniques.

In B-ALL, flow cytometry-based MRD assays typically demonstrated to achieve a LOD of "10–20" MRD events with sensitivity of 1×10^{-4} to 10^{-5} (1 in 10,000 to 1 in 100,000 cells), and a LLOQ around "40–50" MRD events with sensitivity of 10^{-3} to 10^{-4} due to the high immunophenotypic distinction between leukemic and normal B-cell precursors [143, 145]. For T-ALL, MRD detection is more challenging due to overlapping markers with normal T-cell maturation, resulting in a slightly higher LOD (20 MRD events, sensitivity ~10^{-4}) and LLOQ (50 MRD events; ~10^{-3} to 10^{-4}) [34, 158]. Recently, the Euroflow consortium and we have established an LOD of 2×10^{-6} with 10 MRD events and LLOQ of 1×10^{-5} with 40-44 MRD events after the acquisition of ~4–5 million events in B-ALL MRD [3, 59]. We also have established a LOD of 5×10^{-6} with 20 MRD events and LLOQ of 1×10^{-5} with 50 MRD events after acquisition of ~5 million events in T-ALL MRD [60].

In contrast to ALL MRD, it is challenging to establish and implement the LOD and LLOQ for AML MRD due to the high immunophenotypic heterogeneity of AML leukemic blasts [2, 94, 95]. The ELN working group of AML MRD has recommended determining LOD and LLOQ for each antibody combination whenever feasible, especially when regulatory authorities require such validation for clinical decision-making [41, 95]. In contrast to ALL and multiple myeloma, residual leukemic cells in AML often exhibit significant immunophenotypic overlap with normal myeloid progenitor cells. This overlap is influenced by the degree of LAIPs distinguishing residual leukemic cells from normal progenitors. Consequently, the LOD and LLOQ established for one specific immunophenotype may not be applicable to AML cases with differing LAIPs. The reliability of LOD and LLOQ in AML is largely dependent on the antibody panel used, including the markers and their combinations defining LAIPs and DfN immunophenotypes. Although establishing immunophenotype-specific LOD and LLOQ is under consideration, it remains a technically complex and demanding process. A technical guideline issued by the ELN working group on AML-MRD recommends defining the LOD as a cluster of 20 events involving more than one LAIP and the LLOQ as a cluster of 100 events for MFC-MRD assays [95]. Future research focused on immunophenotype-specific LOD and LLOQ could provide valuable insights into their practical utility.

Future Directions

Advancements in Database-Guided MFC-MRD Detection Methodologies

Recent investigations have demonstrated the potential of computational approaches for flow cytometry-based MRD detection. Several studies have pioneered a database-guided analytical method utilizing Infinicyt software, which incorporates "*Integrated Analytical Framework*" based on simultaneous application of LAIP and DfN principles, automated pattern recognition through principal component analysis (PCA), and systematic comparison against reference databases containing comprehensive immunophenotypic profiles or machine learning based MRD analysis [159–167]. It has technical advantages such as enhanced reproducibility through reduced observer-dependent variability and quantitative documentation of aberration frequencies across populations. However, such approach presents several technical challenges too that includes requirement for strict adherence to the predefined antibody panel used for database generation, sensitivity to technical variations in instrument configuration or sample processing protocols, and dependence on proprietary software infrastructure.

Recent Technological Advances in MFC-MRD for AML

Current conventional flow cytometry has limitations. Standard 8–10 color flow cytometry panels, while clinically validated, present several constraints such as restricted marker combinations that limit simultaneous evaluation of multiple LAIPs/DfN aberrancies, suboptimal detection of immunophenotypically heterogeneous subclones, and a lower sensitivity threshold. Recently available high-parameter flow cytometry innovations, such as full-spectrum flow cytometry (FSFC) and mass cytometry (CyTOF), enable comprehensive immunophenotypic profiling through simultaneous assessment of ≥18 markers per tube and improved fluorochrome separation, allowing enhanced detection of rare aberrant populations and improved resolution of normal versus malignant progenitors due to minimal spectral overlap [168–171].

Additionally, the sensitivity of the MRD assay can be achieved as high as 2×10^{-6} (0.0002%) level by acquiring a higher number of cells up to 10 million cells [3, 59]. Thus, standardization of high-parameter panels through multicentric collaborations, development of automated analysis pipelines for complex datasets, and prospective trials validating the clinical utility of ultra-sensitive detection can provide more sensitive and accurate MRD assays.

The integration of these novel computational approaches with conventional template-based analysis may yield significant improvements in analytical sensitivity, interlaboratory reproducibility, and clinical applicability. The particular promise lies in hybrid methodologies that combine database-driven pattern recognition, quantitative deviation analysis, and expert-guided template evaluation.

References

1. Dekker SE, Rea D, Cayuela J-M, Arnhardt I, Leonard J, Heuser M. Using measurable residual disease to optimize management of AML, ALL, and chronic myeloid leukemia. Am Soc Clin Oncol Educ Book. 2023;43:e390010.
2. Tembhare PR. Monitoring measurable/minimal residual disease in acute myeloid leukemia: multiparametric flow cytometry-based approach. Indian J Med Paediatr Oncol. 2023;44(6):554–65.
3. van Dongen JJ, van der Velden VH, Brüggemann M, Orfao A. Minimal residual disease diagnostics in acute lymphoblastic leukemia: need for sensitive, fast, and standardized technologies. Blood. 2015;125(26):3996–4009.
4. Borowitz MJ, Devidas M, Hunger SP, Bowman WP, Carroll AJ, Carroll WL, et al. Clinical significance of minimal residual disease in childhood acute lymphoblastic leukemia and its relationship to other prognostic factors: a Children's Oncology Group study. Blood. 2008;111(12):5477–85.
5. Short NJ, Zhou S, Fu C, Berry DA, Walter RB, Freeman SD, et al. Association of measurable residual disease with survival outcomes in patients with acute myeloid leukemia: a systematic review and meta-analysis. JAMA Oncol. 2020;6(12):1890–9.
6. Berry DA, Zhou S, Higley H, Mukundan L, Fu S, Reaman GH, et al. Association of minimal residual disease with clinical outcome in pediatric and adult acute lymphoblastic leukemia: a meta-analysis. JAMA Oncol. 2017;3(7):e170580.
7. Hourigan CS, Gale RP, Gormley NJ, Ossenkoppele GJ, Walter RB. Measurable residual disease testing in acute myeloid leukaemia. Leukemia. 2017;31(7):1482–90.
8. Moors I, Vandepoele K, Philippé J, Deeren D, Selleslag D, Breems D, et al. Clinical implications of measurable residual disease in AML: review of current evidence. Crit Rev Oncol Hematol. 2019;133:142–8.
9. Döhner H, Wei AH, Appelbaum FR, Craddock C, DiNardo CD, Dombret H, et al. Diagnosis and management of AML in adults: 2022 recommendations from an international expert panel on behalf of the ELN. Blood. 2022;140(12):1345–77.
10. Inaba H, Coustan-Smith E, Cao X, Pounds SB, Shurtleff SA, Wang KY, et al. Comparative analysis of different approaches to measure treatment response in acute myeloid leukemia. J Clin Oncol. 2012;30(29):3625–32.
11. Loken MR, Alonzo TA, Pardo L, Gerbing RB, Raimondi SC, Hirsch BA, et al. Residual disease detected by multidimensional flow cytometry signifies high relapse risk in patients with de novo acute myeloid leukemia: a report from Children's Oncology Group. Blood. 2012;120(8):1581–8.
12. Brodersen LE, Gerbing RB, Pardo ML, Alonzo TA, Paine D, Fritschle W, et al. Morphologic remission status is limited compared to ΔN flow cytometry: a Children's Oncology Group AAML0531 report. Blood Adv. 2020;4(20):5050–61.
13. Schuurhuis GJ, Heuser M, Freeman S, Bene MC, Buccisano F, Cloos J, et al. Minimal/measurable residual disease in AML: a consensus document from the European LeukemiaNet MRD Working Party. Blood. 2018;131(12):1275–91.

14. Pui CH, Pei D, Raimondi SC, Coustan-Smith E, Jeha S, Cheng C, et al. Clinical impact of minimal residual disease in children with different subtypes of acute lymphoblastic leukemia treated with Response-Adapted therapy. Leukemia. 2017;31(2):333–9.
15. Tembhare PR, Narula G, Khanka T, Ghogale S, Chatterjee G, Patkar NV, et al. Post-induction measurable residual disease using multicolor flow cytometry is strongly predictive of inferior clinical outcome in the real-life management of childhood T-cell acute lymphoblastic leukemia: a study of 256 patients. Front Oncol. 2020;10:577.
16. Winter SS, Dunsmore KP, Devidas M, Wood BL, Esiashvili N, Chen Z, et al. Improved survival for children and young adults with T-lineage acute lymphoblastic leukemia: results from the Children's Oncology Group AALL0434 methotrexate randomization. J Clin Oncol. 2018;36(29):2926–34.
17. Freeman SD, Virgo P, Couzens S, Grimwade D, Russell N, Hills RK, et al. Prognostic relevance of treatment response measured by flow cytometric residual disease detection in older patients with acute myeloid leukemia. J Clin Oncol. 2013;31(32):4123–31.
18. Karol SE, Coustan-Smith E, Pounds S, Wang L, Inaba H, Ribeiro RC, et al. Clinical impact of minimal residual disease in blood and bone marrow of children with acute myeloid leukemia. Blood Adv. 2023;7(14):3651–7.
19. Langebrake C, Creutzig U, Dworzak M, Hrusak O, Mejstrikova E, Griesinger F, et al. Residual disease monitoring in childhood acute myeloid leukemia by multiparameter flow cytometry: the MRD-AML-BFM Study Group. J Clin Oncol. 2006;24(22):3686–92.
20. Borowitz MJ, Wood BL, Devidas M, Loh ML, Raetz EA, Salzer WL, et al. Prognostic significance of minimal residual disease in high risk B-ALL: a report from Children's Oncology Group study AALL0232. Blood. 2015;126(8):964–71.
21. Buldini B, Rizzati F, Masetti R, Fagioli F, Menna G, Micalizzi C, et al. Prognostic significance of flow-cytometry evaluation of minimal residual disease in children with acute myeloid leukaemia treated according to the AIEOP-AML 2002/01 study protocol. Br J Haematol. 2017;177(1):116–26.
22. Weng XQ, Shen Y, Sheng Y, Chen B, Wang JH, Li JM, et al. Prognostic significance of monitoring leukemia-associated immunophenotypes by eight-color flow cytometry in adult B-acute lymphoblastic leukemia. Blood Cancer J. 2013;3(8):e133.
23. Appelbaum FR. Measurement of minimal residual disease before and after myeloablative hematopoietic cell transplantation for acute leukemia. Best Pract Res Clin Haematol. 2013;26(3):279–84.
24. Buckley SA, Wood BL, Othus M, Hourigan CS, Ustun C, Linden MA, et al. Minimal residual disease prior to allogeneic hematopoietic cell transplantation in acute myeloid leukemia: a meta-analysis. Haematologica. 2017;102(5):865–73.
25. Chang YJ, Zhao XS, Wang Y, Liu YR, Xu LP, Zhang XH, et al. Effects of pre- and post-transplantation minimal residual disease on outcomes in pediatric patients with acute myeloid leukemia receiving human leukocyte antigen-matched or mismatched related donor allografts. Am J Hematol. 2017;92(12):E659–e61.
26. Cloos J, Ossenkoppele GJ, Dillon R. Minimal residual disease and stem cell transplantation outcomes. Hematology Am Soc Hematol Educ Program. 2019;2019(1):617–25.
27. Milano F, Gooley T, Wood B, Woolfrey A, Flowers ME, Doney K, et al. Cord-blood transplantation in patients with minimal residual disease. N Engl J Med. 2016;375(10):944–53.
28. Paras G, Morsink LM, Othus M, Milano F, Sandmaier BM, Zarling LC, et al. Conditioning intensity and peritransplant flow cytometric MRD dynamics in adult AML. Blood. 2022;139(11):1694–706.
29. Chen X, Cherian S. Role of minimal residual disease testing in acute myeloid leukemia. Clin Lab Med. 2021;41(3):467–83.
30. Vedula RS, Lindsley RC. Measurement of residual disease in acute myeloid leukemia. Curr Hematol Malig Rep. 2017;12(6):574–81.
31. Ribera JM, Oriol A, Morgades M, Montesinos P, Sarrà J, González-Campos J, et al. Treatment of high-risk Philadelphia chromosome-negative acute lymphoblastic leukemia in adolescents and adults according to early cytologic response and minimal residual disease after consoli-

dation assessed by flow cytometry: final results of the PETHEMA ALL-AR-03 trial. J Clin Oncol. 2014;32(15):1595–604.

32. Popov A, Henze G, Roumiantseva J, Budanov O, Belevtsev M, Verzhbitskaya T, et al. A simple procedure to identify children with B-lineage acute lymphoblastic leukemia who can be successfully treated with low or moderate intensity: sequential versus single-point minimal residual disease measurement. Pediatr Blood Cancer. 2023;70(6):e30295.
33. Platzbecker U, Middeke JM, Sockel K, Herbst R, Wolf D, Baldus CD, et al. Measurable residual disease-guided treatment with azacitidine to prevent haematological relapse in patients with myelodysplastic syndrome and acute myeloid leukaemia (RELAZA2): an open-label, multicentre, phase 2 trial. Lancet Oncol. 2018;19(12):1668–79.
34. Reiterová M, Kohlscheen S, Maglia O, Sala S, Schumich A, Maurer-Granofszky M, et al. Flow-cytometric MRD detection in pediatric T-ALL: a multicenter AIEOP-BFM consensus-based guided standardized approach. Clin Chem Lab Med. 2025.
35. Zhang W, Cai J, Wang X, Ma Y, Zhu X, Yu J, et al. Prognostic and therapeutic implications of measurable residual disease levels during remission induction of childhood ALL. Blood. 2025;145(17):1890–902.
36. Appelbaum FR. Hematopoietic cell transplantation as treatment of patients with acute myeloid leukemia with measurable residual disease after consolidation therapy. Best Pract Res Clin Haematol. 2018;31(4):405–9.
37. Ceppi F, Rizzati F, Colombini A, Conter V, Cazzaniga G. Utilizing the prognostic impact of minimal residual disease in treatment decisions for pediatric acute lymphoblastic leukemia. Expert Rev Hematol. 2021;14(9):795–807.
38. Pettit K, Stock W, Walter RB. Incorporating measurable ('minimal') residual disease-directed treatment strategies to optimize outcomes in adults with acute myeloid leukemia. Leuk Lymphoma. 2016;57(7):1527–33.
39. Scrideli CA, Assumpção JG, Ganazza MA, Araújo M, Toledo SR, Lee ML, et al. A simplified minimal residual disease polymerase chain reaction method at early treatment points can stratify children with acute lymphoblastic leukemia into good and poor outcome groups. Haematologica. 2009;94(6):781–9.
40. Vega-García N, Perez-Jaume S, Esperanza-Cebollada E, Vicente-Garcés C, Torrebadell M, Jiménez-Velasco A, et al. Measurable residual disease assessed by flow-cytometry is a stable prognostic factor for pediatric T-cell acute lymphoblastic leukemia in consecutive SEHOP protocols whereas the impact of oncogenetics depends on treatment. Front Pediatr. 2020;8:614521.
41. Heuser M, Freeman SD, Ossenkoppele GJ, Buccisano F, Hourigan CS, Ngai LL, et al. 2021 Update on MRD in acute myeloid leukemia: a consensus document from the European LeukemiaNet MRD Working Party. Blood. 2021;138(26):2753–67.
42. Xu D, Yang Y, Yin Z, Tu S, Nie D, Li Y, et al. Risk-directed therapy based on genetics and MRD improves the outcomes of AML1-ETO-positive AML patients, a multi-center prospective cohort study. Blood Cancer J. 2023;13(1):168.
43. Gui G, Hourigan CS. Measurable residual disease assessment as a surrogate marker in new drug development in acute myeloid leukemia. Cancer J (Sudbury, Mass). 2022;28(1):73–7.
44. Meddi E, Savi A, Moretti F, Mallegni F, Palmieri R, Paterno G, et al. Measurable residual disease (MRD) as a surrogate efficacy-response biomarker in AML. Int J Mol Sci. 2023;24(4).
45. Minimal residual disease evaluation in childhood acute lymphoblastic leukemia: a clinical evidence review. Ontario Health Technol Assess Ser. 2016;16(7):1–52.
46. Bradstock KF, Janossy G, Tidman N, Papageorgiou ES, Prentice HG, Willoughby M, et al. Immunological monitoring of residual disease in treated thymic acute lymphoblastic leukaemia. Leuk Res. 1981;5(4-5):301–9.
47. van Dongen JJ, Hooijkaas H, Comans-Bitter M, Hählen K, de Klein A, van Zanen GE, et al. Human bone marrow cells positive for terminal deoxynucleotidyl transferase (TdT), HLA-DR, and a T cell marker may represent prothymocytes. J Immunol. 1985;135(5):3144–50.

48. Cheson BD, Cassileth PA, Head DR, Schiffer CA, Bennett JM, Bloomfield CD, et al. Report of the National Cancer Institute-sponsored workshop on definitions of diagnosis and response in acute myeloid leukemia. J Clin Oncol. 1990;8(5):813–9.
49. Hagenbeek A, Martens AC. Minimal residual disease in acute leukaemia: preclinical studies in a relevant rat model (BNML). Baillieres Clin Haematol. 1991;4(3):609–35.
50. Beckman RJ, Salzman GC, Stewart CC. Classification and regression trees for bone marrow immunophenotyping. Cytometry. 1995;20(3):210–7.
51. Bashashati A, Brinkman RR. A survey of flow cytometry data analysis methods. Adv Bioinforma. 2009;2009:584603.
52. Zhao Z, Lan J. Detection methods and prognosis implications of measurable residual disease in acute myeloid leukemia. Ann Hematol. 2024;103(12):4869–81.
53. Ramos Elbal E, Fuster JL, Campillo JA, Galera AM, Cortés MB, Llinares ME, et al. Measurable residual disease study through three different methods can anticipate relapse and guide early interventions in childhood acute lymphoblastic leukemia. Clin Transl Oncol. 2024;26(1):278–87.
54. Saygin C, Cannova J, Stock W, Muffly L. Measurable residual disease in acute lymphoblastic leukemia: methods and clinical context in adult patients. Haematologica. 2022;107(12):2783–93.
55. Zhou Y, Wood BL. Methods of detection of measurable residual disease in AML. Curr Hematol Malig Rep. 2017;12(6):557–67.
56. Kasprzyk A, Secker-Walker LM. Increased sensitivity of minimal residual disease detection by interphase FISH in acute lymphoblastic leukemia with hyperdiploidy. Leukemia. 1997;11(3):429–35.
57. Zwick D, Cooley L, Hetherington M. Minimal residual disease testing of acute leukemia by flow cytometry immunophenotyping: a retrospective comparison of detection rates with flow cytometry DNA ploidy or FISH-based methods. Lab Hematol. 2006;12(2):75–81.
58. Chatterjee G, Dhende P, Raj S, Shetty V, Ghogale S, Deshpande N, et al. 15-color highly sensitive flow cytometry assay for post anti-CD19 targeted therapy (anti-CD19-CAR-T and blinatumomab) measurable residual disease assessment in B-lymphoblastic leukemia/lymphoma: real-world applicability and challenges. Eur J Haematol. 2024;112(1):122–36.
59. Tembhare PR, Subramanian Pg PG, Ghogale S, Chatterjee G, Patkar NV, Gupta A, et al. A high-sensitivity 10-color flow cytometric minimal residual disease assay in B-lymphoblastic leukemia/lymphoma can easily achieve the sensitivity of 2-in-10(6) and is superior to standard minimal residual disease assay: a study of 622 patients. Cytometry B Clin Cytom. 2020;98(1):57–67.
60. Tembhare PR, Chatterjee G, Khanka T, Ghogale S, Badrinath Y, Deshpande N, et al. Eleven-marker 10-color flow cytometric assessment of measurable residual disease for T-cell acute lymphoblastic leukemia using an approach of exclusion. Cytometry B Clin Cytom. 2021;100(4):421–33.
61. Dillon R, Hills R, Freeman S, Potter N, Jovanovic J, Ivey A, et al. Molecular MRD status and outcome after transplantation in NPM1-mutated AML. Blood. 2020;135(9):680–8.
62. Jacobsohn DA, Loken MR, Fei M, Adams A, Brodersen LE, Logan BR, et al. Outcomes of measurable residual disease in pediatric acute myeloid leukemia before and after hematopoietic stem cell transplant: validation of difference from normal flow cytometry with Chimerism studies and Wilms tumor 1 gene expression. Biol Blood Marrow Transplant. 2018;24(10):2040–6.
63. Óskarsson J, Rögnvaldsson S, Thorsteinsdottir S, Aspelund T, Gunnarsson SB, Hákonardóttir GK, et al. Determining hemodilution in diagnostic bone marrow aspirated samples in plasma cell disorders by next-generation flow cytometry: proposal for a bone marrow quality index. Blood Cancer J. 2023;13(1):177.
64. Patkar N, Kakirde C, Shaikh AF, Salve R, Bhanshe P, Chatterjee G, et al. Clinical impact of panel-based error-corrected next generation sequencing versus flow cytometry to detect measurable residual disease (MRD) in acute myeloid leukemia (AML). Leukemia. 2021;35(5):1392–404.

65. Singh J, Gorniak M, Grigoriadis G, Westerman D, McBean M, Venn N, et al. Correlation between a 10-color flow cytometric measurable residual disease (MRD) analysis and molecular MRD in adult B-acute lymphoblastic leukemia. Cytometry B Clin Cytom. 2022;102(2):115–22.
66. van der Linde R, Gatt PN, Smith S, Fernandez MA, Vaughan L, Blyth E, et al. Measurable residual disease (MRD) by flow cytometry in adult B-acute lymphoblastic leukaemia (B-ALL) and acute myeloid leukaemia (AML): correlation with molecular MRD testing and clinical outcome at one year. Cancers. 2023;15(20).
67. Bassan R, Brüggemann M, Radcliffe HS, Hartfield E, Kreuzbauer G, Wetten S. A systematic literature review and meta-analysis of minimal residual disease as a prognostic indicator in adult B-cell acute lymphoblastic leukemia. Haematologica. 2019;104(10):2028–39.
68. Campana D, Pui CH. Minimal residual disease-guided therapy in childhood acute lymphoblastic leukemia. Blood. 2017;129(14):1913–8.
69. Loosveld M, Nivaggioni V, Arnoux I, Bernot D, Michel G, Béné MC, et al. Early (Day 15 post diagnosis) peripheral blood assessment of measurable residual disease in flow cytometry is a strong predictor of outcome in childhood B-lineage lymphoblastic leukemia. Cytometry B Clin Cytom. 2019;96(2):128–33.
70. Salina TD, Ferreira YA, Alves EB, Ferreira CM, De Paula EV, Mira MT, et al. Role of peripheral blood minimum residual disease at day 8 of induction therapy in high-risk pediatric patients with acute lymphocytic leukemia. Sci Rep. 2016;6:31179.
71. Basso G, Veltroni M, Valsecchi MG, Dworzak MN, Ratei R, Silvestri D, et al. Risk of relapse of childhood acute lymphoblastic leukemia is predicted by flow cytometric measurement of residual disease on day 15 bone marrow. J Clin Oncol. 2009;27(31):5168–74.
72. Radu LE, Colita A, Pasca S, Tomuleasa C, Popa C, Serban C, et al. Day 15 and day 33 minimal residual disease assessment for acute lymphoblastic leukemia patients treated according to the BFM ALL IC 2009 protocol: single-center experience of 133 cases. Front Oncol. 2020;10:923.
73. Kotrova M, Volland A, Kehden B, Trautmann H, Ritgen M, Wäsch R, et al. Comparison of minimal residual disease levels in bone marrow and peripheral blood in adult acute lymphoblastic leukemia. Leukemia. 2020;34(4):1154–7.
74. Short NJ, Jabbour E, Albitar M, de Lima M, Gore L, Jorgensen J, et al. Recommendations for the assessment and management of measurable residual disease in adults with acute lymphoblastic leukemia: a consensus of North American experts. Am J Hematol. 2019;94(2):257–65.
75. Bader P, Salzmann-Manrique E, Balduzzi A, Dalle JH, Woolfrey AE, Bar M, et al. More precisely defining risk peri-HCT in pediatric ALL: pre- vs post-MRD measures, serial positivity, and risk modeling. Blood Adv. 2019;3(21):3393–405.
76. Nguyen D, Jabbour E, Jain N, Karrar O, Nasnas C, Haddad FG, et al. Clearance of very low levels of measurable residual disease with blinatumomab significantly improves outcomes in B-cell acute lymphoblastic leukemia. Blood. 2024;144(Supplement 1):1465.
77. Pulsipher MA, Han X, Maude SL, Laetsch TW, Qayed M, Rives S, et al. Next-generation sequencing of minimal residual disease for predicting relapse after tisagenlecleucel in children and young adults with acute lymphoblastic leukemia. Blood Cancer Discov. 2022;3(1):66–81.
78. Maude SL, Laetsch TW, Buechner J, Rives S, Boyer M, Bittencourt H, et al. Tisagenlecleucel in children and young adults with B-cell lymphoblastic leukemia. N Engl J Med. 2018;378(5):439–48.
79. Verbeek MWC, Buracchi C, Laqua A, Nierkens S, Sedek L, Flores-Montero J, et al. Flow cytometric minimal residual disease assessment in B-cell precursor acute lymphoblastic leukaemia patients treated with CD19-targeted therapies—a EuroFlow study. Br J Haematol. 2022;197(1):76–81.
80. Verbeek MWC, Reiterová M, Laqua A, Rodríguez BS, Sedek L, Buracchi C, et al. Minimal residual disease assessment following CD19-targeted therapy in B-cell precursor acute lymphoblastic leukemia using standardized 12-color flow cytometry: a EuroFlow study. HemaSphere. 2025;9(4):e70125.

81. Litzow MR, Sun Z, Mattison RJ, Paietta EM, Roberts KG, Zhang Y, et al. Blinatumomab for MRD-negative acute lymphoblastic leukemia in adults. N Engl J Med. 2024;391(4):320–33.
82. Dunsmore KP, Winter SS, Devidas M, Wood BL, Esiashvili N, Chen Z, et al. Children's Oncology Group AALL0434: a phase III randomized clinical trial testing nelarabine in newly diagnosed T-cell acute lymphoblastic leukemia. J Clin Oncol. 2020;38(28):3282–93.
83. Das N, Banavali S, Bakhshi S, Trehan A, Radhakrishnan V, Seth R, et al. Protocol for ICiCLe-ALL-14 (InPOG-ALL-15-01): a prospective, risk stratified, randomised, multicentre, open label, controlled therapeutic trial for newly diagnosed childhood acute lymphoblastic leukaemia in India. Trials. 2022;23(1):102.
84. Aziz Z, Zahid M, Mahmood R, Maqbool S. Modified BFM protocol for childhood acute lymphoblastic leukemia: a retrospective analysis. Med Pediatr Oncol. 1997;28(1):48–53.
85. Gökbuget N, Hoelzer D, Arnold R, Böhme A, Bartram CR, Freund M, et al. Treatment of Adult ALL according to protocols of the German Multicenter Study Group for Adult ALL (GMALL). Hematol Oncol Clin North Am. 2000;14(6):1307–25. ix
86. Rijneveld AW, van der Holt B, de Weerdt O, Biemond BJ, van de Loosdrecht AA, van der Wagen LE, et al. Clofarabine added to intensive treatment in adult patients with newly diagnosed ALL: the HOVON-100 trial. Blood Adv. 2022;6(4):1115–25.
87. Teachey DT, O'Connor D. How I treat newly diagnosed T-cell acute lymphoblastic leukemia and T-cell lymphoblastic lymphoma in children. Blood. 2020;135(3):159–66.
88. Ribera JM, Ortega JJ, Oriol A, Bastida P, Calvo C, Pérez-Hurtado JM, et al. Comparison of intensive chemotherapy, allogeneic, or autologous stem-cell transplantation as postremission treatment for children with very high risk acute lymphoblastic leukemia: PETHEMA ALL-93 Trial. J Clin Oncol. 2007;25(1):16–24.
89. Huguet F, Chevret S, Leguay T, Thomas X, Boissel N, Escoffre-Barbe M, et al. Intensified therapy of acute lymphoblastic leukemia in adults: report of the randomized GRAALL-2005 clinical trial. J Clin Oncol. 2018;36(24):2514–23.
90. Buccisano F, Palmieri R, Piciocchi A, Arena V, Maurillo L, Del Principe MI, et al. Clinical relevance of an objective flow cytometry approach based on limit of detection and limit of quantification for measurable residual disease assessment in acute myeloid leukemia. A post-hoc analysis of the GIMEMA AML1310 trial. Haematologica. 2022;107(12):2823–33.
91. Paiva B, Vidriales MB, Sempere A, Tarín F, Colado E, Benavente C, et al. Impact of measurable residual disease by decentralized flow cytometry: a PETHEMA real-world study in 1076 patients with acute myeloid leukemia. Leukemia. 2021;35(8):2358–70.
92. PR T. Monitoring measurable/minimal residual disease in acute myeloid leukemia: multiparametric flow cytometry-based approach. Ind J Med Paediatr Oncol. 2023;44(6):554–65.
93. Roshal M, Gao Q. Flow cytometry evaluation of acute myeloid leukemia minimal residual disease based on an understanding of the normal maturation patterns in the blast compartments. Am J Clin Pathol. 2025.
94. Tettero JM, Dakappagari N, Heidinga ME, Oussoren-Brockhoff Y, Hanekamp D, Pahuja A, et al. Analytical assay validation for acute myeloid leukemia measurable residual disease assessment by multiparametric flow cytometry. Cytometry B Clin Cytom. 2023;104(6):426–39.
95. Tettero JM, Freeman S, Buecklein V, Venditti A, Maurillo L, Kern W, et al. Technical aspects of flow cytometry-based measurable residual disease quantification in acute myeloid leukemia: experience of the European LeukemiaNet MRD Working Party. HemaSphere. 2022;6(1):e676.
96. Cherian S, Soma LA. How I diagnose minimal/measurable residual disease in B lymphoblastic leukemia/lymphoma by flow cytometry. Am J Clin Pathol. 2021;155(1):38–54.
97. Verbeek MWC, van der Velden VHJ. The evolving landscape of flowcytometric minimal residual disease monitoring in B-cell precursor acute lymphoblastic leukemia. Int J Mol Sci. 2024;25(9).
98. Coustan-Smith E, Song G, Clark C, Key L, Liu P, Mehrpooya M, et al. New markers for minimal residual disease detection in acute lymphoblastic leukemia. Blood. 2011;117(23):6267–76.

99. Sędek Ł, Theunissen P, Sobral da Costa E, van der Sluijs-Gelling A, Mejstrikova E, Gaipa G, et al. Differential expression of CD73, CD86 and CD304 in normal vs. leukemic B-cell precursors and their utility as stable minimal residual disease markers in childhood B-cell precursor acute lymphoblastic leukemia. J Immunol Methods. 2019;475:112429.
100. Tembhare PR, Ghogale S, Ghatwai N, Badrinath Y, Kunder N, Patkar NV, et al. Evaluation of new markers for minimal residual disease monitoring in B-cell precursor acute lymphoblastic leukemia: CD73 and CD86 are the most relevant new markers to increase the efficacy of MRD 2016; 00B: 000-000. Cytometry B Clin Cytom. 2018;94(1):100–11.
101. Stow P, Key L, Chen X, Pan Q, Neale GA, Coustan-Smith E, et al. Clinical significance of low levels of minimal residual disease at the end of remission induction therapy in childhood acute lymphoblastic leukemia. Blood. 2010;115(23):4657–63.
102. Theunissen P, Mejstrikova E, Sedek L, van der Sluijs-Gelling AJ, Gaipa G, Bartels M, et al. Standardized flow cytometry for highly sensitive MRD measurements in B-cell acute lymphoblastic leukemia. Blood. 2017;129(3):347–57.
103. Roshal M, Fromm JR, Winter S, Dunsmore K, Wood BL. Immaturity associated antigens are lost during induction for T cell lymphoblastic leukemia: implications for minimal residual disease detection. Cytometry B Clin Cytom. 2010;78(3):139–46.
104. Zhou Y, Fan X, Routbort M, Cameron Yin C, Singh R, Bueso-Ramos C, et al. Absence of terminal deoxynucleotidyl transferase expression identifies a subset of high-risk adult T-lymphoblastic leukemia/lymphoma. Mod Pathol. 2013;26(10):1338–45.
105. Dworzak MN, Fröschl G, Printz D, Zen LD, Gaipa G, Ratei R, et al. CD99 expression in T-lineage ALL: implications for flow cytometric detection of minimal residual disease. Leukemia. 2004;18(4):703–8.
106. Sedek L, Soriano B, Słota Ł, Brüggemann M, Lasia A, Kohlscheen S, et al. A novel 12-color 2-tube next generation flow approach enables sensitive detection of measurable residual disease in virtually all T-cell acute lymphoblastic leukemia patients. Blood. 2024;144(Supplement 1):4218.
107. Grimwade D, Freeman SD. Defining minimal residual disease in acute myeloid leukemia: which platforms are ready for "prime time"? Blood. 2014;124(23):3345–55.
108. Bruserud Ø, Aasebø E, Hernandez-Valladares M, Tsykunova G, Reikvam H. Therapeutic targeting of leukemic stem cells in acute myeloid leukemia—the biological background for possible strategies. Expert Opin Drug Discov. 2017;12(10):1053–65.
109. Cloos J, Harris JR, Janssen J, Kelder A, Huang F, Sijm G, et al. Comprehensive protocol to sample and process bone marrow for measuring measurable residual disease and leukemic stem cells in acute myeloid leukemia. J Visualiz Exp JoVE. 2018:133.
110. Wouters R, Cucchi D, Kaspers GJ, Schuurhuis GJ, Cloos J. Relevance of leukemic stem cells in acute myeloid leukemia: heterogeneity and influence on disease monitoring, prognosis and treatment design. Expert Rev Hematol. 2014;7(6):791–805.
111. Heo SK, Noh EK, Ju LJ, Sung JY, Jeong YK, Cheon J, et al. CD45(dim)CD34(+)CD38(-) CD133(+) cells have the potential as leukemic stem cells in acute myeloid leukemia. BMC Cancer. 2020;20(1):285.
112. Das N, Panda D, Gajendra S, Gupta R, Thakral D, Kaur G, et al. Immunophenotypic characterization of leukemic stem cells in acute myeloid leukemia using single tube 10-colour panel by multiparametric flow cytometry: deciphering the spectrum, complexity and immunophenotypic heterogeneity. Int J Lab Hematol. 2024;46(4):646–56.
113. Al-Mawali A, Gillis D, Lewis I. Immunoprofiling of leukemic stem cells CD34+/CD38-/CD123+ delineate FLT3/ITD-positive clones. J Hematol Oncol. 2016;9(1):61.
114. Khaldoyanidi SK, Hindoyan A, Stein A, Subklewe M. Leukemic stem cells as a target for eliminating acute myeloid leukemia: gaps in translational research. Crit Rev Oncol Hematol. 2022;175:103710.
115. Guénot C, Lacombe F, Allou K, Dumezy F, Feuillard J, Geneviève F, et al. Peripheral blood minimal/measurable residual disease assessed in flow cytometry in acute myeloblastic leukemia. Leukemia. 2019;33(7):1814–6.

116. Jackson JM, Taylor JB, Witek MA, Hunsucker SA, Waugh JP, Fedoriw Y, et al. Microfluidics for the detection of minimal residual disease in acute myeloid leukemia patients using circulating leukemic cells selected from blood. Analyst. 2016;141(2):640–51.
117. Juul-Dam KL, Ommen HB, Nyvold CG, Walter C, Vålerhaugen H, Kairisto V, et al. Measurable residual disease assessment by qPCR in peripheral blood is an informative tool for disease surveillance in childhood acute myeloid leukaemia. Br J Haematol. 2020;190(2):198–208.
118. Keegan A, Charest K, Schmidt R, Briggs D, Deangelo DJ, Li B, et al. Flow cytometric minimal residual disease assessment of peripheral blood in acute lymphoblastic leukaemia patients has potential for early detection of relapsed extramedullary disease. J Clin Pathol. 2018;71(7):653–8.
119. Li W, Morgan R, Nieder R, Truong S, Habeebu SSM, Ahmed AA. Normal or reactive minor cell populations in bone marrow and peripheral blood mimic minimal residual leukemia by flow cytometry. Cytometry B Clin Cytom. 2021;100(5):590–601.
120. Schumich A, Maurer-Granofszky M, Attarbaschi A, Pötschger U, Buldini B, Gaipa G, et al. Flow-cytometric minimal residual disease monitoring in blood predicts relapse risk in pediatric B-cell precursor acute lymphoblastic leukemia in trial AIEOP-BFM-ALL 2000. Pediatr Blood Cancer. 2019;66(5):e27590.
121. Setiadi A, Owen D, Tsang A, Milner R, Vercauteren S. The significance of peripheral blood minimal residual disease to predict early disease response in patients with B-cell acute lymphoblastic leukemia. Int J Lab Hematol. 2016;38(5):527–34.
122. Muffly L, Sundaram V, Chen C, Yurkiewicz I, Kuo E, Burnash S, et al. Concordance of peripheral blood and bone marrow measurable residual disease in adult acute lymphoblastic leukemia. Blood Adv. 2021;5(16):3147–51.
123. Tembhare PR, Sriram H, Khanka T, Gawai S, Bagal B, Ghogale SG, et al. Circulating tumor plasma cells and peripheral blood measurable residual disease assessment in multiple myeloma patients not planned for upfront transplant. HemaSphere. 2024;8(4):e63.
124. Trka J, Fronkova E. Minimal residual disease detection for acute lymphoblastic leukaemia in peripheral blood-are we there yet? Br J Haematol. 2025;206(1):397–8.
125. Godwin CD, Zhou Y, Othus M, Asmuth MM, Shaw CM, Gardner KM, et al. Acute myeloid leukemia measurable residual disease detection by flow cytometry in peripheral blood vs bone marrow. Blood. 2021;137(4):569–72.
126. Sefland Ø, Gullaksen SE, Omsland M, Reikvam H, Galteland E, Tran HTT, et al. Mass cytometric single cell immune profiles of peripheral blood from acute myeloid leukemia patients in complete remission with measurable residual disease. Cytometry B Clin Cytom. 2024;106(6):485–96.
127. Kalina T, Flores-Montero J, van der Velden VHJ, Martin-Ayuso M, Böttcher S, Ritgen M, et al. EuroFlow standardization of flow cytometer instrument settings and immunophenotyping protocols. Leukemia. 2012;26(9):1986–2010.
128. Bendall SC, Davis KL, Amir el AD, Tadmor MD, Simonds EF, Chen TJ, et al. Single-cell trajectory detection uncovers progression and regulatory coordination in human B cell development. Cell. 2014;157(3):714–25.
129. Gaipa G, Basso G, Maglia O, Leoni V, Faini A, Cazzaniga G, et al. Drug-induced immunophenotypic modulation in childhood ALL: implications for minimal residual disease detection. Leukemia. 2005;19(1):49–56.
130. Dworzak MN, Gaipa G, Schumich A, Maglia O, Ratei R, Veltroni M, et al. Modulation of antigen expression in B-cell precursor acute lymphoblastic leukemia during induction therapy is partly transient: evidence for a drug-induced regulatory phenomenon. Results of the AIEOP-BFM-ALL-FLOW-MRD-Study Group. Cytometry B Clin Cytom. 2010;78(3):147–53.
131. Chatterjee G, Sriram H, Ghogale S, Deshpande N, Khanka T, Girase K, et al. Mimics and artefacts of measurable residual disease in a highly sensitive multicolour flow cytometry assay for B-lymphoblastic leukaemia/lymphoma: critical consideration for analysis of measurable residual disease. Br J Haematol. 2022;196(2):374–9.

132. Cherian S, Miller V, McCullouch V, Dougherty K, Fromm JR, Wood BL. A novel flow cytometric assay for detection of residual disease in patients with B-lymphoblastic leukemia/lymphoma post anti-CD19 therapy. Cytometry B Clin Cytom. 2018;94(1):112–20.
133. Mikhailova E, Illarionova O, Komkov A, Zerkalenkova E, Mamedov I, Shelikhova L, et al. Reliable flow-cytometric approach for minimal residual disease monitoring in patients with B-cell precursor acute lymphoblastic leukemia after CD19-targeted therapy. Cancers. 2022;14(21).
134. Gao Q, Liu Y, Aypar U, Baik J, Londono D, Sun X, et al. Highly sensitive single tube B-lymphoblastic leukemia/lymphoma minimal/measurable residual disease test robust to surface antigen directed therapy. Cytometry B Clin Cytom. 2023;104(4):279–93.
135. Roy N, Kovach AE, Wood BL. Enhanced flow cytometry and next generation sequencing assays for residual B lymphoblastic leukemia (B-ALL) reveal a subset with discordant results due to leukemic changes post-therapy. Blood. 2024;144(Supplement 1):2837.
136. Bene MC, Castoldi G, Knapp W, Ludwig WD, Matutes E, Orfao A, et al. Proposals for the immunological classification of acute leukemias. European Group for the Immunological Characterization of Leukemias (EGIL). Leukemia. 1995;9(10):1783–6.
137. Bhandoola A, von Boehmer H, Petrie HT, Zúñiga-Pflücker JC. Commitment and developmental potential of extrathymic and intrathymic T cell precursors: plenty to choose from. Immunity. 2007;26(6):678–89.
138. Levelt CN, Carsetti R, Eichmann K. Regulation of thymocyte development through CD3. II. Expression of T cell receptor beta CD3 epsilon and maturation to the CD4+8+ stage are highly correlated in individual thymocytes. J Exp Med. 1993;178(6):1867–75.
139. Shah DK, Zúñiga-Pflücker JC. An overview of the intrathymic intricacies of T cell development. J Immunol. 2014;192(9):4017–23.
140. Wu L. T lineage progenitors: the earliest steps en route to T lymphocytes. Curr Opin Immunol. 2006;18(2):121–6.
141. Zúñiga-Pflücker JC. T-cell development made simple. Nat Rev Immunol. 2004;4(1):67–72.
142. Wood BL. Acute myeloid leukemia minimal residual disease detection: the difference from normal approach. Curr Protocols Cytometry. 2020;93(1):e73.
143. Chen X, Wood BL. Monitoring minimal residual disease in acute leukemia: technical challenges and interpretive complexities. Blood Rev. 2017;31(2):63–75.
144. DiGiuseppe JA, Wood BL. Applications of flow cytometric immunophenotyping in the diagnosis and posttreatment monitoring of B and T lymphoblastic leukemia/lymphoma. Cytometry B Clin Cytom. 2019;96(4):256–65.
145. Wood BL. Flow cytometric monitoring of residual disease in acute leukemia. Methods Mol Biol (Clifton, NJ). 2013;999:123–36.
146. Scott SD, Fletcher M, Whitehouse H, Whitby L, Yuan C, Mazzucchelli S, et al. Assessment of plasma cell myeloma minimal residual disease testing by flow cytometry in an international inter-laboratory study: is it ready for primetime use? Cytometry B Clin Cytom. 2019;96(3):201–8.
147. Björklund E, Matinlauri I, Tierens A, Axelsson S, Forestier E, Jacobsson S, et al. Quality control of flow cytometry data analysis for evaluation of minimal residual disease in bone marrow from acute leukemia patients during treatment. J Pediatr Hematol Oncol. 2009;31(6):406–15.
148. Greig B. Quality control of immunophenotyping. Methods Mol Biol (Clifton, NJ). 2019;2032:227–79.
149. Maurer-Granofszky M, Schumich A, Buldini B, Gaipa G, Kappelmayer J, Mejstrikova E, et al. An extensive quality control and quality assurance (QC/QA) program significantly improves inter-laboratory concordance rates of flow-cytometric minimal residual disease assessment in acute lymphoblastic leukemia: an I-BFM-FLOW-network report. Cancers. 2021;13(23).
150. Bras AE, Matarraz S, Nierkens S, Fernández P, Philippé J, Aanei CM, et al. Quality assessment of a large multi-center flow cytometric dataset of acute myeloid leukemia patients-a EuroFlow study. Cancers. 2022;14(8).

151. Kalina T, Flores-Montero J, Lecrevisse Q, Pedreira CE, van der Velden VH, Novakova M, et al. Quality assessment program for EuroFlow protocols: summary results of four-year (2010–2013) quality assurance rounds. Cytometry Part A. 2015;87(2):145–56.
152. Hoffmann J, Thrun MC, Röhnert MA, von Bonin M, Oelschlägel U, Neubauer A, et al. Identification of critical hemodilution by artificial intelligence in bone marrow assessed for minimal residual disease analysis in acute myeloid leukemia: the Cinderella method. Cytometry Part A. 2023;103(4):304–12.
153. Tettero JM, Heidinga ME, Mocking TR, Fransen G, Kelder A, Scholten WJ, et al. Impact of hemodilution on flow cytometry based measurable residual disease assessment in acute myeloid leukemia. Leukemia. 2024;38(3):630–9.
154. Vigliotta I, Armuzzi S, Barone M, Solli V, Pistis I, Borsi E, et al. The ALLgorithMM: how to define the hemodilution of bone marrow samples in lymphoproliferative diseases. Front Oncol. 2022;12:1001048.
155. Armbruster DA, Pry T. Limit of blank, limit of detection and limit of quantitation. Clin Biochem Rev. 2008;29(Suppl 1):S49–52.
156. https://www.cytometry.org/web/modules/Module_25.pdf.
157. Clinical and Laboratory Standards Institute. Protocols for determination of limits of detection and limits of quantitation AGW, PA USA: CLSI; CLSI document EP17. 2004.
158. Dworzak MN, Gaipa G, Ratei R, Veltroni M, Schumich A, Maglia O, et al. Standardization of flow cytometric minimal residual disease evaluation in acute lymphoblastic leukemia: multicentric assessment is feasible. Cytometry B Clin Cytom. 2008;74(6):331–40.
159. Aanei CM, Veyrat-Masson R, Selicean C, Marian M, Rigollet L, Trifa AP, et al. Database-guided analysis for immunophenotypic diagnosis and follow-up of acute myeloid leukemia with recurrent genetic abnormalities. Front Oncol. 2021;11:746951.
160. Piñero P, Morillas M, Gutierrez N, Barragán E, Such E, Breña J, et al. Identification of leukemia-associated immunophenotypes by databaseguided flow cytometry provides a highly sensitive and reproducible strategy for the study of measurable residual disease in acute myeloblastic leukemia. Cancers. 2022;14(16).
161. Reiter M, Diem M, Schumich A, Maurer-Granofszky M, Karawajew L, Rossi JG, et al. Automated flow cytometric MRD assessment in childhood acute B- lymphoblastic leukemia using supervised machine learning. Cytometry Part A. 2019;95(9):966–75.
162. Wödlinger M, Reiter M, Weijler L, Maurer-Granofszky M, Schumich A, Sajaroff EO, et al. Automated identification of cell populations in flow cytometry data with transformers. Comput Biol Med. 2022;144:105314.
163. Verbeek MWC, Rodríguez BS, Sedek L, Laqua A, Buracchi C, Buysse M, et al. Minimal residual disease assessment in B-cell precursor acute lymphoblastic leukemia by semi-automated identification of normal hematopoietic cells: a EuroFlow study. Cytometry B Clin Cytom. 2024;106(4):252–63.
164. Nguyen PC, Nguyen V, Baldwin K, Kankanige Y, Blombery P, Came N, et al. Computational flow cytometry provides accurate assessment of measurable residual disease in chronic lymphocytic leukaemia. Br J Haematol. 2023;202(4):760–70.
165. Duetz C, Bachas C, Westers TM, van de Loosdrecht AA. Computational analysis of flow cytometry data in hematological malignancies: future clinical practice? Curr Opin Oncol. 2020;32(2):162–9.
166. Ko BS, Wang YF, Li JL, Li CC, Weng PF, Hsu SC, et al. Clinically validated machine learning algorithm for detecting residual diseases with multicolor flow cytometry analysis in acute myeloid leukemia and myelodysplastic syndrome. EBioMedicine. 2018;37:91–100.
167. Shopsowitz KE, Liu L, Setiadi A, Al-Bakri M, Vercauteren S. Machine learning optimized multiparameter radar plots for B-cell acute lymphoblastic leukemia minimal residual disease analysis. Cytometry B Clin Cytom. 2022;102(5):342–52.
168. Soh KT, Conway A, Liu X, Wallace PK. Development of a 27-color panel for the detection of measurable residual disease in patients diagnosed with acute myeloid leukemia. Cytometry Part A. 2022;101(11):970–83.

169. Maag AH, Swanton H, Kull M, Vegi NM, Feuring M. Immunophenotypical profiling of myeloid neoplasms with erythroid predominance using mass cytometry (CyTOF). Cytometry Part A. 2023.
170. Fokken H, Waclawski J, Kattre N, Kloos A, Müller S, Ettinger M, et al. A 19-color single-tube full spectrum flow cytometry assay for the detection of measurable residual disease in acute myeloid leukemia. Cytometry Part A. 2024;105(3):181–95.
171. Matthes T. Phenotypic analysis of hematopoietic stem and progenitor cell populations in acute myeloid leukemia based on spectral flow cytometry, a 20-color panel, and unsupervised learning algorithms. Int J Mol Sci. 2024;25(5).

Molecular Measurable Residual Disease Testing in Acute Lymphoblastic Leukemia

9

Jessica Krugman, Danielle W. Cohen, Elizabeth A. Raetz, William L. Carroll, and Gloria Paz Contreras Yametti

Introduction

Acute lymphoblastic leukemia (ALL) is the most common childhood cancer. In newly diagnosed pediatric ALL, approximately 85% of cases have a B-cell phenotype (B-ALL) and 15% have a T-cell phenotype (T-ALL). The cure rate for pediatric ALL has improved dramatically over the past five decades due to combination chemotherapy, intensification of treatment blocks, incorporation of prophylactic intrathecal therapy, and, more recently, immunotherapy. Another significant advance has been the implementation of risk stratification, tailoring treatment intensity to the predicted risk of relapse. Prognostic factors used for risk allocation in childhood ALL include clinical and laboratory features such as age, white blood cell count, the presence of central nervous system (CNS) disease at diagnosis, immunophenotype, and leukemia cytogenetic and molecular subtype.

Historically, disease burden was assessed by morphology in the peripheral blood and/or bone marrow during the first month of therapy [1, 2]. However, much greater

Authors Jessica Krugman and Danielle W. Cohen have equally contributed to this chapter.

J. Krugman · D. W. Cohen · E. A. Raetz · G. P. Contreras Yametti (✉)
Division of Pediatric Hematology/Oncology, Department of Pediatrics, NYU Grossman School of Medicine, New York, NY, USA
e-mail: Elizabeth.Raetz@nyulangone.org; Gloria.Contrerasyametti@nyulangone.org

W. L. Carroll (✉)
Division of Pediatric Hematology/Oncology, Department of Pediatrics, NYU Grossman School of Medicine, New York, NY, USA

Perlmutter Cancer Center, NYU Langone Medical Center, New York, NY, USA
e-mail: William.Carroll@nyulangone.org

W. Li (ed.), *Laboratory Assessments of Pediatric Leukemia*,
https://doi.org/10.1007/978-3-032-26557-9_9

precision has been achieved through assessment of minimal or measurable residual disease (MRD) through detection of aberrant phenotype using flow cytometry as well as molecular approaches to detect clonal markers. While most patients with ALL achieve remission (<5% blasts) at the end of induction (EOI) therapy, one third of B-ALL and two-thirds of T-ALL patients have detectable MRD using multiparameter flow cytometric or molecular methods [3]. In multivariate analyses, MRD has emerged as the most significant prognostic factor both at diagnosis and in the relapse setting, and it plays a fundamental role in risk stratification and treatment allocation. MRD methods differ in their sensitivity, resources needed, cost, and turnaround times, and can be customized to disease subtypes. This chapter describes different techniques for MRD detection with an emphasis on molecular methods and their contemporary clinical applications.

Technology

There are several techniques available for the detection of leukemic cells. Each technique relies on identifying cellular targets unique to the blast population, including DNA (i.e., immunoglobulin heavy chain [IGH], light chain [IGL], and T-cell receptor [TCR] gene rearrangements), RNA (fusion transcripts), or surface proteins (cluster of differentiation [CD] antigens). Each technique has unique advantages and disadvantages (Table 9.1), and several consortia have developed standardized

Table 9.1 Comparison of techniques for the detection of minimal residual disease in acute lymphoblastic leukemia

Method	Sensitivity	Advantages	Disadvantages
MFC	10^{-3} to 10^{-5}	Fast (hours) Relatively inexpensive Does not require a pre-treatment sample	Requires fresh sample Requires a high level of technical expertise
NGF	10^{-6}	Eliminates inter-operator variability Fast Cost-effective Widely applicable	Requires a large number of cells
RQ-PCR	10^{-4} to 10^{-5}	Uses DNA substrate (stable) Sensitive Well-standardized Widely applicable Fast turnaround for follow-up	Slow at diagnosis (weeks) Requires a high level of technical expertise Requires access to pre-treatment tissue Requires patient-specific primers

(continued)

Table 9.1 (continued)

Method	Sensitivity	Advantages	Disadvantages
RT-qPCR	10^{-4} to 10^{-5}	Sensitive Fast (hours) Patient-specific primers not required Relatively simple	Uses RNA substrate (unstable) Limited availability Low applicability Unable to detect small subclones for clonal evolution
ddPCR	10^{-3} to 10^{-5}	Sensitive Fast (hours) Absolute quantification Does not require a standard curve Requires patient-specific primers	Lack of standardization More expensive Unable to detect small subclones for clonal evolution
NGS	10^{-6}	Highly sensitive Fast (~1 week) Patient-specific primers not required Widely applicable Able to track small subclones for clonal evolution	Requires pre-treatment specimen Requires high degree of informatics expertise Expensive

MFC: multiparameter flow cytometry, *NGF*: next generation flow cytometry, *RQ-PCR*: real-time quantitative polymerase chain reaction, *RT-qPCR*: quantitative reverse transcription polymerase chain reaction, *ddPCR*: digital droplet polymerase chain reaction, *NGS*: next generation sequencing

protocols to validate and assure reproducible MRD detection for clinical application, especially in the context of clinical trials [4, 5].

Multiparametric Flow Cytometry

Multiparametric flow cytometry (MFC) is used to identify leukemic blasts via immunophenotype or surface protein expression. As discussed in Chap. 2, at diagnosis, flow cytometry can be used to establish specific antigen profiles for each individual patient, or leukemia-associated immunophenotypes (LAIPs). An additional approach, named "different from normal," is to identify leukemic cells by how they deviate from normal hematopoietic populations using a defined set of antigens as opposed to using the diagnostic sample to determine the antigens of interest [3, 6]. This assay sensitivity (10^{-4} to 10^{-5}) depends on the number of cells measured. MFC requires immediate processing; however, it is overall cost-effective, and associated with rapid turnaround times, allowing for immediate interventions that can be applicable to most patients with leukemia. The EuroFlow Consortium recently developed next generation flow cytometry (NGF), an approach that uses two tubes with seven identical backbone markers and two additional distinct markers in each tube, which further confirms the identity of low-frequency cell types. It can reach a sensitivity of 10^{-6}, comparable to molecular approaches. However, many cells (>4 million) are needed to reach this level of sensitivity. It is fast, reproducible, and cost-effective [7–9]. Please refer to Chap. 8 for more details on MRD assessment by flow cytometry.

Polymerase Chain Reaction Amplification of Antigen Receptor Rearrangements and Fusion Gene Transcripts

Real-time quantitative (RQ)-PCR-based methods commonly use IG and TCR genes to track rearrangements for MRD detection. During early stages of B- and T-lymphocyte maturation, IG and TCR genes undergo different V(D)J rearrangements, allowing for a diverse repertoire of antigen-specific lymphocytes. Since leukemic blasts originate from a common lymphoid progenitor cell, they will share the same V(D)J rearrangements, including the addition of nucleotides at junctions. Thus, this is a highly reliable method of detecting clonality. Both clonal IGH as well as TCR gene rearrangements, including TCR-delta, TCR-beta, TCR-alpha, and TCR-gamma, can be detected in >90% of B- and T-cell ALL [10, 11]. Although IG rearrangements are mostly found in B-cells, and TCR rearrangements in T-lymphocytes, both B-lineage and T-lineage leukemic cells can display either rearrangement. The detection limit of RQ-PCR is 1 in 100,000 cells (10^{-5}), but it is dependent on DNA input [12, 13].

To achieve additional sensitivity, allele-specific oligonucleotide (ASO) primers can be designed once the specific IG or TCR gene rearrangements are sequenced. Subsequently, quantification of MRD is performed by comparing the amplified product to a standard curve. RQ-PCR, which is the most widely used MRD methodology, has been standardized by the EuroMRD Consortium. The European Study Group on MRD detection in ALL (ESG-MRD-ALL) was established in 2001 and now consists of 71 MRD-PCR laboratories across 26 countries in Europe, Asia, Australia, North and South America, which aim to standardize MRD testing throughout and provide guidelines for uniform interpretation. This method does have limitations, including the time-consuming nature and additional skill required to interpret these results. Additionally, cases can have oligoclonal rearrangements leading to false-negative MRD results [14, 15].

Another method of RQ-PCR MRD detection focuses on subtype-specific translocations that lead to fusion transcripts. In many cases, RNA is used as a substrate since intron breakpoints can vary among patients with the same translocation. Reverse transcriptase PCR (RT-qPCR) generates a complementary DNA (cDNA) copy for subsequent amplification (Fig. 9.1). [17]. Known chromosomal translocations that are leukemia-specific targets and are stable during disease evolution, include *BCR::ABL1*, *TCF3::PBX1*, *EVT6::RUNX1*, and *KMT2A* and *CRLF2* rearrangements, among others. These fusion genes are prognostic at diagnosis, and the persistence of these fusions can help assess response to therapy. A major advantage of this technique is that standardized universal primers specific for each fusion

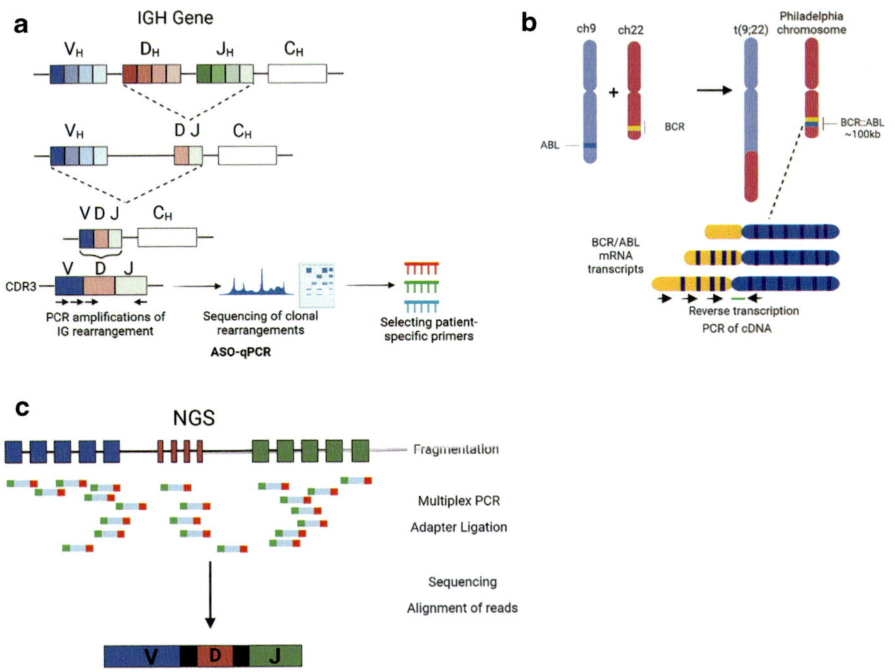

Fig. 9.1 Targets of detection for minimal residual disease (MRD) in acute lymphoblastic leukemia, adapted from Contreras Yametti et al. (2021) and Saygin et al. (2022). (**a**) Allele-specific oligonucleotide qPCR (ASO-qPCR) uses immunoglobulin (IG) and T-cell receptor (TCR) gene rearrangements to detect MRD in ALL. This method relies on the identification of V(D)J sequences from a sample at diagnosis, followed by the design of patient-specific primers for the sequencing of clonal rearrangements. (**b**) RNA is used as a substrate to track chromosomal translocations in B-ALL, such as the *BCR::ABL* fusion as a result of t(9;22)(q34;q11) translocation between chromosome 9 (ch9) and chromosome 22 (ch22). (**c**) Next-generation sequencing also targets V(D)J rearrangements using DNA as the substrate. IG and TCR rearrangements are amplified using universal primers (red, green) designed against conserved regions within the V(D)J region. [3, 16]

transcript are widely available. RT-qPCR has a sensitivity up to 10^{-5} but requires a high level of technical expertise and access to pretreatment tissue (Table 9.1).

Digital-Droplet PCR

Digital droplet PCR (ddPCR) is an additional type of PCR where a sample is partitioned into thousands of droplets and then a target fragment is amplified within each droplet. Most notably, this method differs from others as it does not require a reference standard curve because the number of amplified droplets is divided by the total number of droplets, resulting in an absolute quantification of MRD. ddPCR offers an advantage as it is more precise (detection to 10^{-5} level), does not require a standard curve, and is reproducible while reliably only requiring a small sample size.

This method is more expensive and requires specific equipment. Compared to next-generation sequencing (NGS), it is less costly and time-consuming when known target mutations are desired, such as tracking *p190* for *BCR::ABL+* ALL and *TP53* mutations [16, 18]. Although there are no standardized or established guidelines, this method is useful for MRD, donor chimerism, and quantifying *BCR::ABL1* fusion genes. Della Starza et al. compared ddPCR (by analyzing 1.5 μg DNA) to RQ-PCR, focusing on a subset of 45 slow early responders on the AIEOP-BFM ALL 200 trial [day 33 high MRD and day 78 positive not-quantifiable (PNQ) RQ-PCR MRD] [19]. Among these 45 patients, they identified 13 patients with quantifiable MRD by ddPCR at day +78, whose 5-year EFS was 36% compared to 32 patients with neg/PNQ day 78 MRD by ddPCR with a 5-year EFS of 77% ($P < 0.001$). In examining patients who had high MRD levels at day 33 by RQ-PCR but who were negative at day 78, there were too few patients with quantifiable MRD by ddPCR to determine the impact on outcome. These data demonstrated that ddPCR is more specific than RQ-PCR and can provide a potentially more accurate prognostic stratification at day +78 for cases defined as PNQ MRD by RQ-PCR. However, prospective studies with larger sample sizes are needed to define ddPCR potential impact.

Next-Generation Sequencing

The application of next-generation sequencing (NGS)-MRD has emerged as a more specific and potentially more sensitive approach, depending on input. This method requires high levels of DNA input, upwards of 2 million cells, and commonly relies on IG and TCR rearrangements as targets. Thus, NGS-MRD can detect the presence of lymphoblasts at a level of 10^{-6} nucleated cells, in comparison to existing methods such as MFC or RQ-PCR with usual thresholds of detection ranging from 10^{-4} to 10^{-5}. Universal multiplex primers are used in this technique to simultaneously amplify all combinations of rearranged IG or TCR loci. Amplified products are ligated to adapters for subsequent cluster generation and sequencing. NGS has the advantage that the original antigen receptor sequence does not have to be identified due to the multiplex initial amplification, and the method can identify additional clonal rearrangements during disease evolution. The minimum input for NGS-MRD testing is 500 nanograms of DNA [20]. NGS has been compared to MFC MRD. In an analysis of 139 samples from 54 B-ALL patients, there was a 79.9% concordance between the two methods [18]. However, 18% of samples were NGS MRD positive only, and 2.2% were MFC-MRD+/NGS MRD− [16]. Commercial assays such as ClonoSEQ (Adaptive Biotechnologies, Seattle, WA) and LymphoTrack (Invivoscribe, Inc., San Diego, CA) are available as well as "in-house" NGS MRD assays, making this approach widely accessible.

Clinical Applications of Molecular MRD in B-Cell Acute Lymphoblastic Leukemia

Monitoring MRD in Patients at Diagnosis

Both PCR-MRD and MFC-MRD have been incorporated into clinical practice, and many studies have validated their critical role in disease stratification. Both the end of induction (EOI) and end of consolidation (EOC) MRD have been shown to be the single most important prognostic factors for children with ALL receiving multiagent chemotherapy[2, 21–29] RQ-PCR-MRD has been utilized by the European and other groups, while MFC-MRD is widely used in North America.

Conter et al reported the impact of MRD by RQ-PCR at EOI (TP1) and end of consolidation (TP2) using RQ-PCR with ASO primers (two antigen receptor targets per patient) in 3184 patients enrolled on the AIEOP-BFM ALL 2000 study (NCT00430118 for BFM and NCT00613457 for AIEOP). Patients were grouped into standard risk (negative at TP1 and TP2; 42% of patients), intermediate risk (TP1+, TP2−; 52% of patients), and high risk (TP2+; 6% of patients). The 5-year EFS for these groups were 92.3%, 77.6%, and 50.1% ($p < 0.001$) [24].

Stutterheim recently reported the prognostic value of MRD detection at TP2 in a cohort of patients treated on DCOG-ALL-10 ($n = 271$) and DCOG-ALL-9 ($n = 122$) [30]. Among patients found to be MRD+ at TP2, those who achieved MRD- status at later timepoints had a 6-year cumulative incidence of relapse (CIR) of 7%. In contrast, patients who were TP2+ and positive at later timepoints had a 6-year CIR of 29.4% ($p < 0.001$). Interestingly, about 15% of patients negative at TP2 showed positive results at later timepoints, but this was not associated with an inferior prognosis, suggesting that subsequent detection was due to false positive results. Overall, these results indicate that there is little value in measuring MRD beyond this time point if EOC MRD is negative, but positive EOC MRD with persistently detectable MRD is prognostic and informs the need for incorporation of additional therapeutic interventions such as blinatumomab, inotuzumab, and CAR T-cell therapy [30].

With the goal of improving risk stratification and further refining therapy assignments by MRD, NGS-MRD has been compared to other MRD methodologies. Most experience with NGS approaches still relies on the detection of clonal antigen receptor rearrangements. Wu and colleagues examined paired pretreatment and day 29 post-treatment samples from an unselected subset of patients enrolled on the COG National Cancer Institute (NCI) standard risk (SR) B-ALL study AALL0932 (NCT01190930). MFC MRD was available in all patients. A unique IGH sequence was detected in 91 of 98 analyzable patient samples at diagnosis. At EOI, 40 samples had negative MRD by MFC and NGS, 28 samples were negative by MFC but positive by NGS, and there were 23 cases where MRD was detected by both techniques [31]. There were no false negative results by NGS-MRD. Thus, NGS detected more patients (51 of 91) with MRD compared to MFC (23 of 91). Note that many NGS-positive samples had MRD within the expected range of detection by MFC. In these cases, phenotypic maturation may have contributed to the lack of detection by MFC. Further analysis comparing MFC vs NGS MRD at the EOI was performed on a larger cohort of 619 patients enrolled on COG NCI SR (AALL0331; NCT00103285) and high-risk (HR) (AALL0232; NCT00075725) trials. Using both IGH and TCR as NGS targets, 95% of patients displayed a pretreatment clonal index sequence suitable for tracking. Using a threshold of 10^{-4}, both MFC and NGS showed an inferior outcome for patients who were MRD positive. However, there were 55 patients who were MRD negative by MFC at this level, but positive by NGS, and they had poorer 5-year EFS ($P = 0.036$). While any level of MRD by NGS was associated with an inferior outcome, the data suggested that the optimal cutoff for risk stratification remained at 10^{-4} and identified up to one-third of patients who are missed at the same threshold by MFC. Additionally, this study identified 19.9% of SR patients with undetectable NGS-MRD who had outstanding outcomes (5-year EFS of 98.1%, $p = 0.0226$) [28]. Overall, this study showed that NGS was feasible for most patients, that NGS MRD was a better risk stratifier even when using a threshold of 10^{-4}, and that NGS may identify a subgroup who have an exceptional prognosis and would be candidates for therapy de-escalation.

Kotrova et al compared RQ-PCR vs NGS MRD and sequenced samples from 76 patients treated by Berlin-Frankfurt-Munster (BFM) protocols and found that 15% of patients who were RQ-PCR MRD negative were NGS positive [32]. Patients had reassigned risk stratification due to these data. NGS MRD positivity at day 33 was a stronger predictor of relapse with 5-year relapse-free survival (RFS) (90% vs. 53%, $p = 0.0003$) compared to RQ-PCR positivity (84% vs. 63%, $p = 0.04$). NGS also allowed for assessment of clonal heterogeneity of the IGH repertoire. Interestingly, patients with lower clonal diversity, or fewer number of distinct clones, at day 78 had a worse 5-year RFS (clones/reads >0.18 5-year RFS of 88 ± 5% vs clones/read <0.18 5-year RFS 50 ± 12%, $p = 0.0005$) [32].

The standard for MRD detection in *BCR::ABL*-positive (Ph+) B-ALL is not as well defined as *BCR::ABL*-negative ALL. MRD assessment by RQ-PCR (IG/TCR) and RQ(RT)–PCR for *BCR::ABL1* fusion proteins are the most accepted methods and are concordant with MRD assessment by MFC, but are more sensitive [33]. It is recommended that more than one method be used to track disease regression, as persistence of the *BCR::ABL* fusion transcript in the absence of MRD by RQ-PCR (IG/TCR) or MFC may indicate chronic myeloid leukemia (CML)-like disease and the need for alternative therapy such as allogeneic stem cell transplant [34].

The predictive value of RQ-PCR was assessed on the EsPhALL study, where the tyrosine kinase inhibitor (TKI) imatinib was integrated into treatment following induction. Patients who were MRD– (10^{-4}) after TP2 (following phase Ib at 10–12 weeks) had a very low CIR (14.3%) compared to patients who attained MRD- status at later timepoints. The level of concordance between RQ-PCR (IG/TCR) and *BCR::ABL1* RQ(RT) PCR was 69%, with RQ(RT)-PCR for *BCR::ABL1* yielding higher values [35]. More recent trials have integrated TKIs earlier in therapy and have utilized MRD to aid treatment decisions.

In two successive international protocols for childhood *BCR::ABL1* positive B-ALL (COG CA180-372/AALL1122 and EsPhALL2017/AALL1631), MRD at week 10–12 (TP3) was used to stratify patients into standard risk ($<5 \times 10^{-4}$, 82% of patients) and high risk ($>5 \times 10^{-4}$, 18% of patients). On EsPhALL, MRD was assessed by RQ-PCR (IGH/TCR). For patients with uninformative IG/TCR results at baseline, MRD assessment for allogeneic hematopoietic cell transplant (allo-HCT) eligibility was substituted by RQ(RT)-PCR (*BCR::ABL1*) or MFC. The concordance between assays was highest for IG/TCR and flow cytometry (98%) and lowest between *BCR-ABL1* transcripts and MFC (82%) [36]. In COG AALL1631, NGS and RQ-PCR were highly concordant, though NGS MRD yielded measurable results 100% of the time, whereas RQ-PCR was less (89.6%) [37].

Monitoring MRD in Relapse/Refractory Setting

MRD is also a prognostic tool for patients with relapsed leukemia in addition to known biomarkers such as time to relapse, site of relapse, and immunophenotype. At relapse, molecular evaluation of IG/TCR markers used for MRD monitoring usually confirms the presence of the same clone as the original diagnosis, but additional clones with unique antigen receptor rearrangements may emerge, and NGS MRD can detect this clonal evolution. Commercial NGS-MRD assays such as Clonoseq are used in the setting of relapse, but initial sequencing of diagnostic leukemic samples is required to identify the original, dominant clone. This is leading many centers to send bank diagnostic samples [38].

The COG AALL01P2 study evaluated the prognostic value of MFC-MRD in the relapsed setting, which included B and T ALL patients [39]. Seventy-five percent of early relapse patients, defined as medullary relapse within 36 months of diagnosis, had detectable EOI MRD at 0.01% compared to 51% of late relapse patients. The 12-month EFS rate for all patients in morphological remission at the end of block one was 80% vs. 58% for MRD− vs. MRD+ patients. In addition, the kinetics of the MRD response at three timepoints identified groups with 12-month EFS of 86% (negative at all three timepoints), 73% (positive after block one but negative at subsequent timepoints and 19% (increasing MRD). This study and subsequent reports serve as a foundation to assess the value of more sensitive molecular MRD methods.

RQ-PCR MRD was evaluated in both the ALLR3 and the ALL-REZ BFM 2002 protocols that included both B and T ALL patients with high-risk (HR) relapse, defined as B ALL relapse within 18 months of diagnosis or isolated medullary relapse within six of stopping therapy [40]. HR T ALL relapse was defined as isolated or medullary relapse at any time. EOI MRD $< 10^{-3}$ was highly prognostic in both protocols (ALLR3 10-year DFS 45.8% vs 32.2%, $P = 0.0018$; ALL-REZ BFM 2002 DFS 58.6% vs. 27.0%, $P = 0.0037$). EOI MRD $< 10^{-4}$ was also prognostic in the ALLR3 protocol (55.9% vs 14.9%, $P = 0.0011$).

There is limited data on the use of NGS-MRD in the relapse setting. A small study of 19 pediatric patients demonstrated that using NGS allowed for a more sensitive MRD detection for patients treated with blinatumomab in the relapsed setting. Particularly, all 19 patients were MRD negative by MFC, but only 13 were MRD negative by NGS. Three NGS-MRD negative patients with available NGS-MRD at pre-, mid-, and post-treatment achieved negative MRD rapidly after blinatumomab treatment through day 28. Three of six NGS-MRD positive patients relapsed after blinatumomab, with three being IGH positive and two being IGL positive [41]. This highlights the prognostic value of NGS in detecting lower levels of MRD in ALL patients treated with immunotherapy and its role in the relapsed setting.

Peri Chimeric Antigen Receptor Cell Therapy MRD Application

CD19-targeted chimeric antigen receptor (CAR) T-cell therapy is currently approved for children, adolescents, and adults with B-cell ALL who have refractory disease or relapse. Real-world outcomes aligned with the results of the landmark ELIANA trial, showing a 12-month OS of 72% and EFS of 50% [42, 43]. CAR T-cell persistence, B-cell aplasia, and MRD are being studied as biomarkers to determine treatment efficacy and relapse risk. B-cell aplasia has been widely used as a surrogate marker of CD19 CAR T-cell persistence; however, standardized definitions have historically been lacking. Recent consensus criteria define B-cell recovery as ≥10 CD19-positive B cells/μL in peripheral blood or ≥1% CD19-positive B cells in the bone marrow, confirmed on repeat testing at least 2 weeks later. Selective pressures generating CD19-negative clones is a known mechanism for CD19-negative relapse [44–46]. Therefore, B-cell aplasia alone is an inadequate biomarker to predict relapse [47, 48]. A collective ELIANA/ENSIGN analysis recently reported the first retrospective comparison between different MRD techniques (i.e., MFC and NGS-MRD) in 143 patients with CD19+ relapsed or refractory B-cell ALL who received tisagenlecleucel [49]. Here, the patients who achieved a complete remission but had detectable MFC-MRD at day 28 and/or month 3 after tisagenlecleucel infusion had poor outcomes. Half of these patients relapsed with a median lead time of 52 days and no prior evidence of positive MFC-MRD. Surprisingly, when analyzing MRD by NGS at a level of 10^{-6} vs detectable levels below this threshold (>0–10^{-6}) at day 28, there was no difference in the 2-year EFS and OS between MRD-positive and negative patients ($P = 0.53$ and $P = 0.46$, respectively), and the median lead time from NGS-MRD detection to relapse was 70 days. In contrast, when NGS-MRD was examined at the lowest feasible threshold (e.g., undetectable [0] vs any level of detection [>0]), its ability to predict outcome improved dramatically with a 2-year EFS of 68% for NGS-MRD negative vs 23% at any level of detection ($P = 0.00047$). Moreover, the median time to overt relapse in patients with NGS MRD at any level of detection (>0) was significantly longer (median 168 days, range 47–330 days), providing time for therapeutic interventions (e.g., second infusion, humanized CAR, clinical trial interventions, and/or hematopoietic cell transplantation, among others). Although Day 28 detectable NGS-MRD independently predicted outcomes, 3 months post-infusion was an even more prognostically significant time point for relapse (detectable bone marrow NGS-MRD at Day 28 HR = 4.87 [$P < 0.001$] vs bone marrow NGS-MRD at Day 90 HR = 12.0 [$P < 0.001$]). These data demonstrated the substantial impact of NGS-MRD in risk stratification and ongoing MRD monitoring by refining the threshold of MRD detection. However, further validation in a prospective multicenter setting integrating other biomarkers, such as B-cell aplasia, is needed.

Peri-Hematopoietic Cell Transplant MRD Application

Allogeneic hematopoietic cell transplantation (HCT) is indicated in patients at high risk for relapse. These include patients with high-risk cytogenetics and MRD positivity after consolidation in first complete remission, or any patient in second or later remissions. Several groups have established the prognostic and predictive impact of MRD status prior to and after transplantation [13, 50–54]. In an analysis of a subset of patients ($n = 41$) with B-ALL enrolled on COG and Pediatric Blood and Marrow Transplant Consortium (PBMTC) trial ASCT0431 (NCT00382109), the 2-year relapse rate was 0% for patients who were pre-HCT NGS-MRD-negative vs 53% for NGS positive MRD patients ($P < 0.0001$), leading to a 2-year OS of 96% vs 48% ($P = 0.03$) [13]. Moreover, NGS-MRD negativity predicted relapse and survival more precisely than MFC-MRD negativity (relapse, 0% vs 16%; $P = 0.02$; 2-year OS, 96% vs 77%; $P = 0.003$). In the same analysis, specifically looking at serial post-transplant MRD monitoring ($n = 53$), detectable NGS-MRD was highly predictive of relapse and survival as early as 30 days after HCT with a hazard ratio of 7.7 ($P = 0.05$). This finding was independent of pre-HCT MRD and the presence of any acute graft vs host disease. In the subset of patients with detectable pre-HCT NGS-MRD, grade I-III acute GVHD (aGVHD) prior to day +55 was associated with better outcomes (73% relapse with no aGVHD vs. 17% relapse with aGVHD).

Traditionally, total body irradiation (TBI) has been a major component in the myeloablative conditioning regimens for patients undergoing HCT for ALL. TBI provides an optimal antileukemic effect, including eradication of disease in sanctuary sites and immunosuppression, ensuring adequate engraftment. Despite these advantages, it is associated with short and long-term toxicities (i.e., mucositis, interstitial pneumonia, veno-occlusive disease, growth delay, secondary malignancies, and endocrine problems) [55–57]. In this context, the randomized, phase III, non-inferiority study FORUM (NCT01949129), demonstrated an improved OS and lower relapse risk in pediatric patients with ALL who received a HCT with TBI-based conditioning regimen vs chemotherapy-only conditioning ($n = 417$; 2-year OS 91% vs 75%, $P = 0.0001$; 2-year cumulative incidence of relapse (CIR) 12% vs 33%, $P < 0.0001$; and treatment-related mortality 2% vs 9%, $P = 0.269$) [58]. In this study, MRD was monitored 2 weeks prior to HCT by MFC ($>10^{-3}$) or RQ-PCR ($>10^{-4}$) in a subset of 340 patients. A recent updated analysis showed a better 3-year EFS (79% vs 62%; $P = 0.003$) and a lower CIR (14% vs 30%; $p = 0.003$) for MRD-negative vs MRD-positive patients, with double the risk of relapse for the subset receiving chemotherapy-based conditioning compared to TBI [59].

A retrospective single institution cohort of 57 patients also showed a significantly better outcome after receiving TBI-based conditioning, as opposed to non-TBI conditioning (3-year EFS 52% vs 77%, $P = 0.03$) [60]. Here, patients with undetectable pre-HCT NGS-MRD had equally outstanding outcomes after TBI or non-TBI conditioning (100% vs 83%, $P = 0.27$), whereas patients with NGS-MRD positivity or unknown status had a higher likelihood of relapse if they received a non-TBI-based regimen (57% vs 24%, $P = 0.03$). In this context, EndRAD (NCT03509961), a phase two prospective clinical trial in patients <25 years, seeks to study the elimination of TBI from the conditioning regimen of patients who are NGS MRD negative pre-transplant. A planned interim analysis showed promising results, with an EFS> 90% in patients with undetectable NGS-MRD pre-HCT, independent of the type of conditioning regimen [61].

Ideally, a deep remission with undetectable NGS-MRD pre-transplant is preferred, however this goal should be individualized in each patient with careful consideration of disease risk, prior lines of therapy, donor selection, donor availability, transplant timing, and patient readiness to proceed. Half of the patients with pre-transplant detectable NGS have a durable disease-free survival, post-transplant NGS-MRD has a higher predictive value compared to pre-transplant NGS-MRD, and there are no predictors of graft vs leukemia effect; therefore, even if a negative NGS-MRD status is not achieved, allo-HCT remains a potential curative approach.

Currently, there is no standardized role for post-allo-HCT interventions in ALL outside TKIs in *BCR::ABL1*-positive ALL to reduce the risk of relapse, where the current recommendation is to consider post–allo-HCT TKI maintenance for at least one year with periodic monitoring for MRD [62–66]. In this context, there are ongoing efforts to develop novel approaches that would eradicate post-transplant MRD and lower relapse risk without compromising graft function in patients without *BCR::ABL1*-positive ALL. An example is the pilot study (NCT03104491) that recently established the safety of low-dose inotuzumab starting between day +40 and +100 after allo-HCT [67]. Eighteen patients were enrolled (14 in first complete remission [CR] and 4 in > second CR). One-year transplant-related mortality was 5.6%, 1-year post–allo-HCT PFS 89%. These promising results served as the framework for a subsequent phase two trial (NCT03104491) focusing on PFS and MRD eradication.

In summary, there is no consensus on the optimal timing of MRD surveillance in the context of transplant, nor in the therapeutic interventions on these results, nor on the de-intensification of transplantation based on MRD, nor in the post-allo-HCT interventions to reduce MRD. However, NGS-MRD has shown superiority over PCR-MRD and MFC-MRD, with growing data demonstrating its critical role for early identification of impending relapse. Novel approaches for intervention incorporating MRD are needed.

Clinical Applications of Molecular MRD in T-Cell Acute Lymphoblastic Leukemia

T-ALL differs from B-ALL as it is biologically distinct, with heterogeneous molecular and epigenetic features, immunophenotypic diversity (including pro-T, pre-T, cortical T, and medullary T), and a slower blast kinetics regression. While EOI MRD has been defined as the time point for disease response risk stratification in B-ALL, in the T-ALL setting, EOC MRD or its equivalent is the most significant predictor of outcome [29]. For patients with persistent EOC MRD, treatment is usually escalated, and allo-HCT is strongly considered. Note, it may be possible to serially monitor peripheral blood (PB) since bone marrow (BM) vs PB MRD appears to be concordant in T-ALL in contradistinction to B-ALL [68–71].

Historically, the genetic alterations in T-ALL do not independently predict outcome, hence risk stratification relies on the evaluation of MRD. NGS-based residual disease monitoring has recently been investigated in T-ALL. Wood et al. analyzed 615 patient samples from COG AALL1231 (NCT02112916) and found that a significant subset of patients with T-ALL did not contain *TCRB* or *TCRG* clonal leukemia-associated sequences and cannot be evaluated for MRD using an NGS approach (31.5% for TCRB, 17.6% using both TCRB and TCRG). EOI MRD was detected in 71% (TCRB) and 90% (TCRG) of samples, while EOC MRD was detected in 64% (TCRB) and 69% (TCRG) of samples. However, there was no correlation between MRD status and clinical outcomes, raising concerns about the disease specificity of clonal sequences at very low levels of detection [72].

While MRD has been known to be a large prognostic factor, FRALLE2000T retrospectively analyzed 220 patients with T ALL and their oncogenetic mutation profiles. Day 35, MRD was available in 191 patients using RQ-PCR (IG/TCR). One hundred and fourteen patients (60%) had MRD $<10^{-4}$ with a CIR of 14% and a 5-year DFS of 86%. Seventy-seven patients (40%) had values $\geq 10^{-4}$, and their outcomes were significantly inferior, with a CIR of 38% and DFS of 58% [73].

Simonin et al provided an update on these earlier studies examining the impact of oncogenetic mutations and MRD [4]. They recently proposed an NGS-based risk classification in T-ALL which effectively stratifies an adult (GRAALL2003/2005, $n = 198$) and pediatric cohort (FRALLE2000T, $n = 242$) into low and high-risk groups. The low-risk group corresponds with *NOTCH1*, *FBXW7*, *PHF6*, or *EP300* mutations, excluding *N-K-RAS*, *PI3K* pathway (*PTEN*, *PIK3CA*, and *PIK3R1*), *TP53*, *DNMT3A*, *IDH1/2*, and *IKZF1* alterations, with a 5-year CIR of 21% and a high-risk group (all remaining alterations) with a 5-year CIR estimated at 47%. When coupled with WBC at diagnosis ($\geq 200 \times 10^9$/L) and EOI MRD by RQ-PCR (IG/TCR) ($\geq 10^{-4}$), this approach identified three subgroups: an adverse risk, intermediate risk, and favorable risk with a 5-year CIR of 51%, 21%, and 12%, respectively [10]. Notably, this analysis excluded induction failure patients, and it is unknown how this classifier influenced the outcome in this subset of patients. Although this work needs to be further validated in independent cohorts undergoing contemporary therapy, it underscores the significant role of NGS in refining risk stratification in T-ALL.

Conclusions

MRD detection has revolutionized risk stratification in ALL and remains the most important prognostic biomarker. The evolution of technical methods, including the application of next-generation sequencing, has improved sensitivity and will likely replace earlier approaches. Finally, cell-free sources of tumor DNA through "liquid biopsies" are being analyzed. The detection of cell-free DNA (cfDNA) composed of extracellular short double-stranded DNA is especially attractive for solid tumors, where serial biopsies are impractical and localized biopsies may fail to address tumor heterogeneity that exists in multiple locations. The application of this technology in hematological cancers is now being investigated, and the application of standardized techniques will be needed for broad applicability [74–76].

References

1. Dworzak MN, et al. Prognostic significance and modalities of flow cytometric minimal residual disease detection in childhood acute lymphoblastic leukemia. Blood. 2002;99(6):1952–8.
2. Borowitz MJ, et al. Clinical significance of minimal residual disease in childhood acute lymphoblastic leukemia and its relationship to other prognostic factors: a Children's Oncology Group study. Blood. 2008;111(12):5477–85.
3. Saygin C, Cannova J, Stock W, Muffly L. Measurable residual disease in acute lymphoblastic leukemia: methods and clinical context in adult patients. Haematologica. 2022;107(12):2783–93.
4. Simonin M, et al. NGS-based stratification refines the risk stratification in T-ALL and identifies a very-high-risk subgroup of patients. Blood. 2024;144(15):1570–80.
5. Theunissen PMJ, et al. Next-generation antigen receptor sequencing of paired diagnosis and relapse samples of B-cell acute lymphoblastic leukemia: clonal evolution and implications for minimal residual disease target selection. Leuk Res. 2019;76:98–104.
6. Bradstock KF, et al. Immunological monitoring of residual disease in treated thymic acute lymphoblastic leukaemia. Leuk Res. 1981;5(4–5):301–9.
7. Li W. Measurable residual disease testing in acute leukemia: technology and clinical significance. In: Li W, editor. Leukemia. Brisbane. 2022.
8. Flores-Montero J, et al. Next Generation Flow for highly sensitive and standardized detection of minimal residual disease in multiple myeloma. Leukemia. 2017;31(10):2094–103.
9. Theunissen P, et al. Standardized flow cytometry for highly sensitive MRD measurements in B-cell acute lymphoblastic leukemia. Blood. 2017;129(3):347–57.
10. Beishuizen A, Verhoeven MA, Mol EJ, van Dongen JJ. Detection of immunoglobulin kappa light-chain gene rearrangement patterns by Southern blot analysis. Leukemia. 1994;8(12):2228–36; discussion 2237-9.
11. Beishuizen A, et al. Analysis of Ig and T-cell receptor genes in 40 childhood acute lymphoblastic leukemias at diagnosis and subsequent relapse: implications for the detection of minimal residual disease by polymerase chain reaction analysis. Blood. 1994;83(8):2238–47.
12. Gaipa G, et al. Time point-dependent concordance of flow cytometry and real-time quantitative polymerase chain reaction for minimal residual disease detection in childhood acute lymphoblastic leukemia. Haematologica. 2012;97(10):1582–93.
13. Pulsipher MA, et al. IgH-V(D)J NGS-MRD measurement pre- and early post-allotransplant defines very low- and very high-risk ALL patients. Blood. 2015;125(22):3501–8.
14. van der Velden VH, et al. Analysis of minimal residual disease by Ig/TCR gene rearrangements: guidelines for interpretation of real-time quantitative PCR data. Leukemia. 2007;21(4):604–11.
15. van der Velden VHJ, et al. Analysis of measurable residual disease by IG/TR gene rearrangements: quality assurance and updated EuroMRD guidelines. Leukemia. 2024;38(6):1315–22.
16. Contreras Yametti GP, et al. Minimal residual disease in acute lymphoblastic leukemia: current practice and future directions. Cancers (Basel). 2021:13(8).
17. Chen X, Wood BL. How do we measure MRD in ALL and how should measurements affect decisions. Re: treatment and prognosis? Best Pract Res Clin Haematol. 2017;30(3):237–48.
18. Coccaro N, et al. Digital PCR: a reliable tool for analyzing and monitoring hematologic malignancies. Int J Mol Sci. 2020:21(9).
19. Della Starza I, Nunes V, Lovisa F, Silvestri D, Cavalli M, Garofalo A, Campeggio M, De Novi LA, Oggioni C, Biondi A, Guarini A, Valsecchi MG, Conter V, Basso G, Foà R, Cazzaniga

G. Digital-droplet PCR, an accurate method for IG/TR PCR-MRD stratification in childhood acute lymphoblastic leukemia. Blood. 2018;132:1544.
20. Ching T, et al. Analytical evaluation of the clonoSEQ Assay for establishing measurable (minimal) residual disease in acute lymphoblastic leukemia, chronic lymphocytic leukemia, and multiple myeloma. BMC Cancer. 2020;20(1):612.
21. Borowitz MJ, et al. Prognostic significance of minimal residual disease in high risk B-ALL: a report from Children's Oncology Group study AALL0232. Blood. 2015;126(8):964–71.
22. Choi JK, Mead PE. Laboratory aspects of minimal/measurable residual disease testing in B-lymphoblastic leukemia. Clin Lab Med. 2021;41(3):485–95.
23. Vora A, et al. Treatment reduction for children and young adults with low-risk acute lymphoblastic leukaemia defined by minimal residual disease (UKALL 2003): a randomised controlled trial. Lancet Oncol. 2013;14(3):199–209.
24. Conter V, et al. Molecular response to treatment redefines all prognostic factors in children and adolescents with B-cell precursor acute lymphoblastic leukemia: results in 3184 patients of the AIEOP-BFM ALL 2000 study. Blood. 2010;115(16):3206–14.
25. Stow P, et al. Clinical significance of low levels of minimal residual disease at the end of remission induction therapy in childhood acute lymphoblastic leukemia. Blood. 2010;115(23):4657–63.
26. Berry DA, et al. Association of minimal residual disease with clinical outcome in pediatric and adult acute lymphoblastic leukemia: a meta-analysis. JAMA Oncol. 2017;3(7):e170580.
27. Wood B, et al. Measurable residual disease detection by high-throughput sequencing improves risk stratification for pediatric B-ALL. Blood. 2018;131(12):1350–9.
28. Pui CH, et al. Clinical impact of minimal residual disease in children with different subtypes of acute lymphoblastic leukemia treated with Response-Adapted therapy. Leukemia. 2017;31(2):333–9.
29. Schrappe M, et al. Late MRD response determines relapse risk overall and in subsets of childhood T-cell ALL: results of the AIEOP-BFM-ALL 2000 study. Blood. 2011;118(8):2077–84.
30. Stutterheim J, et al. Are measurable residual disease results after consolidation therapy useful in children with acute lymphoblastic leukemia? Leukemia. 2024;38(11):2376–81.
31. Wu D, et al. Detection of minimal residual disease in B lymphoblastic leukemia by high-throughput sequencing of. Clin Cancer Res. 2014;20(17):4540–8.
32. Kotrova M, et al. The predictive strength of next-generation sequencing MRD detection for relapse compared with current methods in childhood ALL. Blood. 2015;126(8):1045–7.
33. Tran V, et al. MRD in Philadelphia chromosome-positive ALL: methodologies and clinical implications. Curr Hematol Malig Rep. 2024;19(4):186–96.
34. Zuna J, et al. Minimal residual disease in BCR::ABL1-positive acute lymphoblastic leukemia: different significance in typical ALL and in CML-like disease. Leukemia. 2022;36(12):2793–801.
35. Cazzaniga G, et al. Predictive value of minimal residual disease in Philadelphia-chromosome-positive acute lymphoblastic leukemia treated with imatinib in the European intergroup study of post-induction treatment of Philadelphia-chromosome-positive acute lymphoblastic leukemia, based on immunoglobulin/T-cell receptor and BCR/ABL1 methodologies. Haematologica. 2018;103(1):107–15.
36. Hunger SP, et al. Dasatinib with intensive chemotherapy in de novo paediatric Philadelphia chromosome-positive acute lymphoblastic leukaemia (CA180-372/COG AALL1122): a single-arm, multicentre, phase 2 trial. Lancet Haematol. 2023;10(7):e510–20.
37. Tran TH, et al. Minimal residual disease comparison between Ig/TCR PCR versus NGS assays in children with Philadelphia chromosome-positive acute lymphoblastic leukemia: a report from the COG AALL1631 study. J Clin Oncol. 2022;40(16_suppl):10023.
38. Muffly L, Liang EC, Dolan JG, Pulsipher MA. How I use next-generation sequencing-MRD to plan approach and prevent relapse after HCT for children and adults with ALL. Blood. 2024;144(3):253–61.
39. Raetz EA, et al. Reinduction platform for children with first marrow relapse of acute lymphoblastic Leukemia: a Children's Oncology Group Study [corrected]. J Clin Oncol. 2008;26(24):3971–8.

40. Eckert C, et al. Risk factors and outcomes in children with high-risk B-cell precursor and T-cell relapsed acute lymphoblastic leukaemia: combined analysis of ALLR3 and ALL-REZ BFM 2002 clinical trials. Eur J Cancer. 2021;151:175–89.
41. Gu M, et al. The effectiveness of blinatumomab in clearing measurable residual disease in pediatric B-cell acute lymphoblastic leukemia patients detected by next-generation sequencing. Cancer Med. 2023;12(24):21978–84.
42. Schultz LM, et al. Disease burden affects outcomes in pediatric and young adult B-cell lymphoblastic leukemia after commercial tisagenlecleucel: a pediatric real-world chimeric antigen receptor consortium report. J Clin Oncol. 2022;40(9):945–55.
43. Maude SL. Tisagenlecleucel in pediatric patients with acute lymphoblastic leukemia. Clin Adv Hematol Oncol. 2018;16(10):664–6.
44. Xu X, et al. Mechanisms of relapse after CD19 CAR T-cell therapy for acute lymphoblastic leukemia and its prevention and treatment strategies. Front Immunol. 2019;10:2664.
45. Shah NN, Fry TJ. Mechanisms of resistance to CAR T cell therapy. Nat Rev Clin Oncol. 2019;16(6):372–85.
46. Myers RM, Shah NN, Pulsipher MA. How I use risk factors for success or failure of CD19 CAR T cells to guide management of children and AYA with B-cell ALL. Blood. 2023;141(11):1251–64.
47. Lamble A, et al. Harmonization on defining B-cell recovery post CD19-CAR T-cell therapy in B-cell acute lymphoblastic leukemia: An international consensus statement. Hemasphere. 2025;9(11):e70247. https://doi.org/10.1002/hem3.70247. PMID: 41367923; PMCID: PMC12683365.
48. Molinos-Quintana A, et al. Corrigendum: impact of disease burden and late loss of B cell aplasia on the risk of relapse after CD19 chimeric antigen receptor T Cell (Tisagenlecleucel) infusion in pediatric and young adult patients with relapse/refractory acute lymphoblastic leukemia: role of B-cell monitoring. Front Immunol. 2024;15:1373852.
49. Finney OC, et al. CD19 CAR T cell product and disease attributes predict leukemia remission durability. J Clin Invest. 2019;129(5):2123–32.
50. Pulsipher MA, et al. Next-generation sequencing of minimal residual disease for predicting relapse after tisagenlecleucel in children and young adults with acute lymphoblastic leukemia. Blood Cancer Discov. 2022;3(1):66–81.
51. Knechtli CJ, et al. Minimal residual disease status before allogeneic bone marrow transplantation is an important determinant of successful outcome for children and adolescents with acute lymphoblastic leukemia. Blood. 1998;92(11):4072–9.
52. Bader P, et al. Prognostic value of minimal residual disease quantification before allogeneic stem-cell transplantation in relapsed childhood acute lymphoblastic leukemia: the ALL-REZ BFM Study Group. J Clin Oncol. 2009;27(3):377–84.
53. Leung W, et al. Detectable minimal residual disease before hematopoietic cell transplantation is prognostic but does not preclude cure for children with very-high-risk leukemia. Blood. 2012;120(2):468–72.
54. Eckert C, et al. Use of allogeneic hematopoietic stem-cell transplantation based on minimal residual disease response improves outcomes for children with relapsed acute lymphoblastic leukemia in the intermediate-risk group. J Clin Oncol. 2013;31(21):2736–42.
55. Logan AC, et al. Immunoglobulin and T cell receptor gene high-throughput sequencing quantifies minimal residual disease in acute lymphoblastic leukemia and predicts post-transplantation relapse and survival. Biol Blood Marrow Transplant. 2014;20(9):1307–13.
56. Thomas ED, et al. Marrow transplantation for acute nonlymphoblastic leukemic in first remission using fractionated or single-dose irradiation. Int J Radiat Oncol Biol Phys. 1982;8(5):817–21.
57. Cahu X, et al. Impact of conditioning with TBI in adult patients with T-cell ALL who receive a myeloablative allogeneic stem cell transplantation: a report from the acute leukemia working party of EBMT. Bone Marrow Transplant. 2016;51(3):351–7.

58. Gruen A, et al. Total body irradiation as part of conditioning regimens in childhood leukemia-long-term outcome, toxicity, and secondary malignancies. Strahlenther Onkol. 2022;198(1):33–8.
59. Peters C, et al. Total body irradiation or chemotherapy conditioning in childhood ALL: a multinational, randomized, noninferiority phase III study. J Clin Oncol. 2021;39(4):295–307.
60. Balduzzi A. Impact of minimal residual disease at hematopoietic stem cell transplantation for childhood acute lymphoblastic leukemia within the FORUM trial. In: 50th annual meeting of the EBMT, Glasgow. 2024.
61. Friend BD, et al. The impact of total body irradiation-based regimens on outcomes in children and young adults with acute lymphoblastic leukemia undergoing allogeneic hematopoietic stem cell transplantation. Pediatr Blood Cancer. 2020;67(2):e28079.
62. Abdel-Azim H, et al. Excellent relapse-free and overall survival in pre-HCT next-generation sequencing (NGS-MRD) negative B-ALL patients with or without TBI-based conditioning: outcome of the observational arm of the pediatric transplantation and cellular therapy consortium (PTCTC) ONC1701 endrad study. Transpl Cell Ther. 2023.
63. Anderlini P, et al. Re: Imatinib mesylate administration in the first 100 days after stem cell transplantation. Biol Blood Marrow Transplant. 2004;10(12):883–4.
64. Wassmann B, et al. Early molecular response to posttransplantation imatinib determines outcome in MRD+ Philadelphia-positive acute lymphoblastic leukemia (Ph+ ALL). Blood. 2005;106(2):458–63.
65. Carpenter PA, et al. Prophylactic administration of imatinib after hematopoietic cell transplantation for high-risk Philadelphia chromosome-positive leukemia. Blood. 2007;109(7):2791–3.
66. Brown PA, et al. Acute lymphoblastic leukemia, version 2.2021, NCCN clinical practice guidelines in oncology. J Natl Compr Cancer Netw. 2021;19(9):1079–109.
67. Burke MJ, et al. Allo-hematopoietic cell transplantation for Ph chromosome-positive ALL: impact of imatinib on relapse and survival. Bone Marrow Transplant. 2009;43(2):107–13.
68. Metheny LL, et al. A multicenter study of posttransplantation low-dose inotuzumab ozogamicin to prevent relapse of acute lymphoblastic leukemia. Blood Adv. 2024;8(6):1384–91.
69. Bruggemann M, Kotrova M. Minimal residual disease in adult ALL: technical aspects and implications for correct clinical interpretation. Blood Adv. 2017;1(25):2456–66.
70. Coustan-Smith E, et al. Prognostic importance of measuring early clearance of leukemic cells by flow cytometry in childhood acute lymphoblastic leukemia. Blood. 2002;100(1):52–8.
71. van der Velden VHJ, et al. Minimal residual disease levels in bone marrow and peripheral blood are comparable in children with T cell acute lymphoblastic leukemia (ALL), but not in precursor-B-ALL. Leukemia. 2002;16(8):1432–6.
72. Coustan-Smith E, et al. Use of peripheral blood instead of bone marrow to monitor residual disease in children with acute lymphoblastic leukemia. Blood. 2002;100(7):2399–402.
73. Roy N, et al. Next-generation sequencing (NGS) for residual disease (MRD) monitoring in TLymphoblastic leukemia (T-ALL). Blood. 2023:142.
74. Petit A, et al. Oncogenetic mutations combined with MRD improve outcome prediction in pediatric T-cell acute lymphoblastic leukemia. Blood. 2018;131(3):289–300.
75. Furstenau M, et al. Circulating tumor DNA-based MRD assessment in patients with CLL treated with obinutuzumab, acalabrutinib, and venetoclax. Clin Cancer Res. 2022;28(19):4203–11.
76. Yeh P, et al. Circulating tumour DNA reflects treatment response and clonal evolution in chronic lymphocytic leukaemia. Nat Commun. 2017;8:14756.
77. Schroers-Martin JG, Alizadeh AA. Cell-free DNA in hematologic malignancies. JCO Oncol Pract. 2024;20(11):1491–9.

Molecular Measurable Residual Disease Testing in Acute Myeloid Leukemia

10

Luca Guarnera and Tiziana Ottone

Introduction

Acute myeloid leukemia (AML) is a clonal disorder arising from immature hematopoietic cells that can occur in any age group but is more common in older patients (median of onset ≥65 years) [1], characterized by dismal outcome and a heterogeneous and complex molecular profile. Advances in leukemia biology have brought a broader knowledge of the molecular and cytogenetic abnormalities leading to leukemogenesis and, accordingly, the development of therapeutic strategies more and more tailored to the specific genetic hits underpinning the malignancies. Thus, with the development of target treatments and refinement of patient's clinical care and supportive therapy, we witnessed a significant improvement in the outcomes over the past years [1, 2]. However, despite huge success in specific AML phenotypes [e.g., acute promyelocytic leukemia (APL), defined by *PML-RARA* translocation due to t(15::17) and core-binding factor (CBF) AML, characterized by *RUNX1-RUNX1T1* or *CBFB-MYH11* translocations, due to t(8;21) and inversion(16), respectively], the overall AML prognosis remains dismal (survival at 5 years of 20–30%) [1, 2], due to complication of treatments and/or leukemia relapse.

In this perspective, the early detection of disease relapse with techniques [multicolor flow-cytometry (MFC), polymerase chain reaction (PCR), next-generation sequencing (NGS)] able to identify residual disease beyond morphological assessment of blasts (measurable residual disease, MRD) has gradually gained a central role in AML management. Indeed, MRD has a key role in risk-stratification, drives treatment strategy and consistently predict long-term outcome [3]. Accordingly, the criteria of complete remission (CR), canonically defined as bone marrow (BM) blasts percentage <5%, absence of extramedullary leukemia, absolute neutrophils

L. Guarnera (✉) · T. Ottone
Department of Biomedicine and Prevention, University of Rome Tor Vergata, Rome, Italy
e-mail: luca.guarnera@uniroma2.it; tiziana.ottone@uniroma2.it

W. Li (ed.), *Laboratory Assessments of Pediatric Leukemia*,
https://doi.org/10.1007/978-3-032-26557-9_10

count (ANC) > 1000/μL and platelets >100,000/μL [4], has evolved over time to respect the granularity of hematological recover and the depth of the response. Already in 2017, European LeukemiaNet (ELN) guidelines [5] introduced the definition of CR without minimal residual disease (CR_{MRD}^{-}), paving the way for new response assessment criteria.

In this chapter, we will discuss the principles and methods of molecular-based MRD in AML, the repercussions on clinical practice and the possible future applications.

Principles and Methods

Using PCR technology to amplify a fusion gene from a translocation or a specific point mutation, enables the detection of a few malignant cells within a background of thousands or even millions of normal cells. The PCR technique utilizes a thermostable DNA polymerase and synthetic oligonucleotides flanking the segment of interest. This process can be performed on DNA or, alternatively, RNA extracted from the examined cells, in which case the production of complementary DNA (cDNA) using reverse transcriptase is required. The reaction involves repeated cycles, each consisting of three phases (denaturation, annealing, and extension), and relies on automated instruments. The reaction products are typically visualized using gel electrophoresis or capillary electrophoresis systems. Among the technological advancements of PCR, quantitative PCR (qPCR) stands out. This method provides a measurable result and offers the added advantage of more accurately assessing sample quality. The qPCR combines PCR amplification and detection in a single step, eliminating the need for gel electrophoresis, and importantly, allowing for true quantification. Like traditional PCR, DNA amplification occurs through three repetitive steps: denaturation, annealing, and elongation. However, in qPCR, fluorescent labels enable continuous monitoring of the reaction as it progresses. The main detection chemistry for qPCR is the probe-based dye method. In this technology, specific probes with unique primers tagged with distinct fluorescent dyes can be utilized within the same reaction mixture. Quantitative thermal cyclers with multiple detection channels are designed for this purpose. One of the most common probe types is the hydrolysis probe, which consists of a reporter and a quencher bound to opposite ends of a sequence-specific probe. When the probe is intact, the quencher prevents fluorescence resonance energy transfer (FRET) from the excited reporter. The probe is cleaved during the primer extension phase, separating the quencher from the reporter, which results in an amplification-dependent increase in fluorescence. The fluorescence signal from the cleaved probes correlates with the number of amplicons generated in each PCR cycle, providing quantitative data in real time. The qPCR offers higher specificity and sensitivity for leukemic cells, reduced contamination risk, improved RNA quality assessment, and the ability to track MRD kinetics longitudinally. Due to its high sensitivity (10^{-4}–10^{-5}), qPCR is the most commonly used molecular technique for MRD monitoring in AML [6]. The assay is lesion-specific (there is a selected number of somatic mutations and fusion rearrangements which can be monitored over time, as it will be further discussed in the specific chapters). Considering the frequency of APL, CBF AML, and *NPM1*-mutated AML (Standardized targets of qPCR-based MRD), roughly 30–50% [7–9]. AML patients can be monitored with this tool.

The advent of digital PCR (dPCR) has significantly advanced molecular monitoring in AML patients, offering a high sensitivity and specificity in detecting and quantifying genetic abnormalities. The dPCR method utilizes controlled emulsion technology to partition the PCR reaction into approximately 20,000 independent droplets. The setup for dPCR consists of a reaction buffer formulated with DNA molecules, dNTPs, primers, DNA polymerase, and fluorescent probes (e.g., TaqMan hydrolysis probes) to facilitate the detection of amplification products. Once the sample processing begins, the droplets are aligned and pass through fluorescence detectors, which measure their fluorescence intensity. Due to its high specificity and sensitivity, dPCR is particularly valuable for improving the detection of genetic abnormalities, especially point mutations and fusion genes. After identifying a patient's molecular markers, this technique can be used to monitor these markers during therapeutic follow-up, enabling the assessment of MRD [10, 11].

Further advancements have been made in the field of MRD monitoring with the development of new technologies that offer even higher sensitivity, such as NGS. NGS allows for in-depth analysis of DNA or RNA, allowing the identification of even the smallest traces of residual molecular markers from malignant cells. This is possible due to its ability to sequence millions of DNA fragments in parallel, offering sensitivity down to 0.01% [12, 13]. NGS technology enables the parallel and multiplex reading of individual DNA fragments, allowing millions of base pairs to be analyzed simultaneously in a few hours. With the advent of NGS, the capacity and speed of DNA sequencing have substantially increased, leading to a significant reduction in costs. Today, commercially available NGS platforms vary in terms of fragment length, sequencing speed, and error rate, but they all share a common technological feature: the massive parallel sequencing of clonally amplified DNA molecules or individual DNA molecules spatially separated in a flow cell. This approach marks a dramatic shift compared to the Sanger sequencing method, which relies on the electrophoretic separation of fragments of varying lengths obtained from individual sequencing reactions. The development of targeted-NGS (t-NGS) panels has become increasingly common in clinical practice. These panels have transformed the role of NGS in onco-hematology, evolving from a promising research tool to an essential and highly reliable diagnostic instrument. Following the initial diagnosis, t-NGS panels can be used to identify patient-specific molecular features, which are critical for accurately assessing prognostic scores and determining molecular targets for personalized therapy. The use of smaller panels, consisting of a limited number of genes, has notably reduced the costs associated with the technique, while also decreasing response times and simplifying data analysis. Although various sequencing platforms are available today, targeted-NGS-based DNA sequencing generally follows four main steps: library preparation, amplification, sequencing, and data analysis. In the library preparation step, DNA is fragmented into smaller segments. After fragmentation, adaptors are attached to the

Table 10.1 Comparison between qPCR, dPCR, and NGS

qPCR	dPCR	NGS
Absolute measurement	Absolute measurement	Relative measurement
Greater sensitivity	Greater sensitivity	Lower sensitivity
Easy to operate	Easy to operate	Complex operation
Lower costs	Higher costs	Higher costs
Rapid turnaround time	Rapid turnaround time	Slower turnaround time
Selected targets	Selected targets	Broad panel coverage

dPCR digital PCR, *NGS* next generation sequencing, *qPCR* quantitative PCR

DNA fragments via a DNA ligase enzyme. These adaptors facilitate the binding of the fragments to a complementary counterpart. Multiplexing allows the simultaneous sequencing of multiple libraries in a single sequencing run. To achieve this, unique index sequences are incorporated into each DNA fragment during library preparation, enabling each read to be identified and sorted before final data analysis. For all sequencing methods, except Whole Genome Sequencing (WGS), a capture-enrichment step is required to isolate the specific genomic regions of interest [12]. This technology has significantly advanced the field of molecular genetics, providing powerful tools for detailed DNA and RNA analysis. NGS-based MRD is theoretically feasible for every gene mutation and is based on the evaluation of persistence of gene variants identified at diagnosis (and thus it could be used for almost all AML patients [9]. However, it is still not standardized and only preliminary studies [14–16] are available.

Table 10.1 schematizes the pros and cons of the techniques above described.

History of MRD and Clinical Significance

The introduction of qPCR [17–19], in the 1990s, allowed the detection of minimal levels of pathologic transcripts, and, in a 30-year span, MRD monitoring, from experimental practice, became a common tool in clinical practice and a cornerstone in AML management (Fig. 10.1).

APL

The first proof of concept of the efficacy of MRD monitoring was provided by Miller and colleagues who, thanks to the previous identification of APL breakpoints within the RAR-alpha second intron by Italian researchers [20], were able to detect residual disease in APL [21]. In 1992, Lo Coco and colleagues measured PCR-MRD in 35 patients in CR. 11 of 13 patients who tested positive relapsed 1–4 months later. All 22 patients who tested negative were disease-free after 3 months to 5 years of follow-up [22]. These results were confirmed in 1998 by Diverio and colleagues who analyzed MRD in 163 APL enrolled in the multicenter Gruppo Italiano Malattie Ematologiche Maligne dell' Adulto (GIMEMA) trial AIDA (All-trans retinoic acid

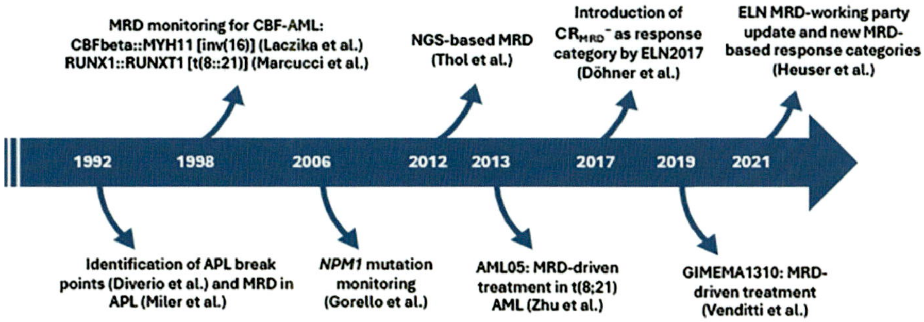

Fig. 10.1 Milestones of PCR-based MRD monitoring. *APL* acute promyelocytic leukemia, *CR* complete remission, *ELN* European LeukemiaNet, *MRD* measurable residual disease, *NGS* next-generation sequencing

plus Idarubicin). All patients achieved CR but, out of 21 who converted to PCR-positive thereafter, 20 underwent hematologic relapse at a median time of 3 months, whereas, of 142 who tested persistently PCR-negative in ≥2 tests after consolidation, 8 had hematologic relapse and 134 remained in CR after a median follow-up of 18 months [23]. Grimwade and colleagues used MRD monitoring to predict relapse of APL and to direct pre-emptive arsenic trioxide therapy in 406 patients. In 30 patients the disease persisted or relapsed and MRD monitoring was able to predict 11 of the 20 relapses. Arsenic trioxide was delivered in 14 of 30 patients and was able to prevent progression to full-blown relapse in 10 patients at a median follow-up of 14.5 months [24].

These findings led to consider PCR-MRD in APL as endpoint in the subsequent seminal trials (e.g. APL0406 [25], which brought to the approval of arsenic-trioxide and all-trans retinoic acid for standard-risk patients, AML17 [26], APOLLO trial [PMID:40825164]), as well as clinical practice [27].

CBF-AML

In a pilot study published in 1998, Laczika and colleagues showed the feasibility of MRD monitoring of *CBFbeta::MYH11* in AML bearing inversion(16) during post-remission chemotherapy, as well as after allogenic hematopoietic stem cell transplantation (allo-HSCT) [28]; these results were confirmed, through real-time PCR, by Marcucci et al. and Buonamici et al. [29, 30] In a similar fashion, in 1998, Marcucci and colleagues and, later, Krauter et al. and Sugimoto et al. were able to monitor AML1/ETO (*RUNX1::RUNXT1*) fusion transcript in t(8;21)-positive AML [31–33].

The identification of the proper timepoints and correct cut-off to assess MRD was at the center of several studies; Tobal et al. serially monitored 25 AML patients bearing t(8;21) and established that a transcript reduction of 2–3 log after induction chemotherapy, followed by a further 2–3 log after consolidation/intensification chemotherapy, was compatible with stable remission [34]. An analysis conducted within the German-Austrian AML Study Group, including 53 patients expressing the *CBFB-MYH11* transcript, defined (i) achievement of PCR negativity in at least one BM sample during consolidation therapy, (ii) achievement of PCR negativity in at least two BM or peripheral blood (PB) samples during consolidation therapy and early follow-up, and (iii) conversion from PCR negativity to PCR positivity with copy ratios of more than 10 after consolidation therapy as clinically relevant checkpoints predicting relapse [35]. A prospective MRD monitoring of a large population of CBF-AML patients (163 with t(8;21) and 115 with inv(16)) within United Kingdom MRC AML-15 trial highlighted a > 3 log reduction in *RUNX1::RUNX1T1* transcripts in BM in t(8;21) patients and a > 10 *CBFB::MYH11* copy number in PB in inv(16) patients after course 1 induction chemotherapy as the most useful prognostic variables for relapse in a multivariable model [36]. The prospective analysis performed within the French CBF-2006 trial showed that, in t(8;21) AML, MRD monitoring on PB every 3 months allowed for the prediction of hematological relapse [37]. Qin et al. investigated the optimal timepoints of MRD assessment after allo-HSCT in in patients with t(8;21) AML and found that *RUNX1::RUNX1T1* transcripts with a <3-log reduction from diagnosis within 12 months and/or a <4-log reduction at ≥12 months after allo-HSCT could accurately predict relapse [38]. A large analysis of 155 intensively treated patients with *RUNX1::RUNX1T1* AML, by AML-Study group, showed that achievement of >2.5 log transcript reduction after treatment cycle 1 and achievement of 3 log reduction after treatment cycle 2 were significantly associated with a reduced risk of relapse; after completion of therapy, achievement of MRD negativity in both BM and PB was an independent, favorable prognostic factor for overall survival (OS) [39]. Of note, a study performed at MD Anderson Cancer Centre showed that the adverse prognostic impact of MRD positivity in CBF-AML could be overcome by allo-HSCT [40].

NPM1-Mutated AML

In 2006, for the first time, an AML-related somatic mutation, *NPM1,* was successfully quantified and monitored, proving its reliability and feasibility in the prediction of hematologic relapse [41]. In 2007, Chou and colleagues analyzed serial samples from 38 *NPM1*-mutated patients showing a high rate of relapses in patients with high mutant copy number following CR achievement. Furthermore, patients with rise of $NPM1^{mut}$ copies during serial follow-up had 3.2-fold increase of relapse risk compared to those with persistently low or undetectable signals and failure to achieve 2 logs of reduction after consolidation predicted shorter OS and relapse free survival (RFS) [42]. A study from the German-Austrian AML Study Group found that higher $NPM1^{mut}$ transcript levels after double induction and after completion of consolidation therapy were an independent predictor of relapse and dismal outcome [43]. An analysis of 174 *NPM1*-mutated AML patients, 155 of whom enrolled in two clinical trials of the Study Alliance Leukemia (SAL) revealed that an increase of more than 1% $NPM1^{mut}$ transcript detection was a prognostic factor for relapse after chemotherapy, whereas an increase of more than 10% was prognostic for relapse after allogeneic transplantation. Univariate and multivariate analysis of RFS and OS showed a significantly worse outcome in patients with >1% *NPM1*^{mut} and >10% *NPM1*^{mut}, respectively [44]. An analysis of patients enrolled in AMLCG trials identified a *NPM1* mutation ratio cut-off of 0.01 after induction therapy as a predictor of relapse [45]. *NPM1* MRD monitoring in patients enrolled in NCRI AML-17 trial showed that the persistence of *NPM1*-mutated transcripts after the second chemotherapy cycle was associated with a greater risk of relapse and a lower rate of survival. Of note, the presence of MRD was the only independent prognostic factor for death in multivariate analysis [46].

Several studies focused on the prognostic impact of *NPM1* MRD assessment in relation to allo-HSCT. Kayser et al. evaluated 67 *NPM1*^{mut} AML patients, of whom 51 in CR. The authors found a significantly inferior prognosis after allo-HSCT in pre-transplant MRD-positive patients. In multivariable analysis pre-transplant NPM1 MRD levels >1% was an independent prognostic factor for poor survival after allo-HSCT. Of note, the outcome of patients with pre-transplant *NPM1* MRD positivity >1% was as poor as that of patients transplanted with resistant disease [47]. In the same line, the French group found a higher incidence of relapse and shorter OS in patients not achieving a 4-log reduction in *NPM1*^{mut} in PB and undergoing allo-HSCT. These findings were confirmed in multivariable analysis [48]. Bill and colleagues confirmed these results, showing inferior outcomes in MRD+ patients undergoing allo-HSCT using dPCR [49]. Finally, a recent analysis of a large population found that the persistence of *FLT3* internal tandem duplication (*FLT3-ITD*) and/or *NPM1* DNA variants before allo-HSCT were associated with increased rates of relapse and worse survival compared with those without these markers [50].

Advances in MRD monitoring led to correlations of this endpoint with specific treatments. The AMLSG 09-09 trial showed significantly lower levels of NPM1 transcript in patients treated with Gemtuzumab Ozogamicin, resulting in a lower incidence of relapse [51]. Othman et al. confirmed the valuable prognostic role of *NPM1* MRD monitoring also in patients treated with less intensive treatment, such as Venetoclax in combination with Azacitidine or low-dose Cytarabine [52]. A subanalysis of AML17 and AML19 trials (NCRI group) found, in a population of patients undergoing allo-HSCT, an OS advantage for MRD+ patients but no benefit for MRD− ones. Restricting the analysis to patients with coexisting *FLT3-ITD*, the advantage in the first subset of patients was confirmed [53]. The Leipzig group retrospectively analyzed their monocentric case series of 81 *NPM1*-mutated AML patients who received an allogeneic HSCT in order to assess the best MRD (measured with dPCR) cut-off to predict relapse. Receiver operator characteristic (ROC) curves identified 0.01% *NPM1/ABL1* as the cut-off with the highest discriminative power for relapse after HSCT. Remarkably, the authors observed a negative correlation between *NPM1/ABL1* MRD levels before HSCT and time to relapse; the higher the *NPM1* MRD burden at HSCT corresponding to an earlier relapse occurrence. This correlation was strongest in patients with *FLT3*-ITD present at diagnosis [54].

FLT3-Mutated AML

The heterogeneity of *FLT3*-ITD mutations, in terms of length and insertion sites, hampered the PCR-based *FLT3* MRD monitoring. However, recent reports showed how NGS is capable of filling this gap: in 2022, a collaboration between UK and Australian groups addressed this issue investigating the impact of pretransplant NGS-based MRD in 104 *FLT3*-mutated AML patients. Of these, 37% had NGS-based *FLT3*-ITD MRD. Of note, only 7 out of 36 MRD+ cases (19%) were positive by capillary electrophoresis. Outcome analysis showed a precise stratification of patients according to MRD status: 2-year RFS was 78%, 32%, 40%, and 0% for *FLT3*-ITD MRD levels <0.001 (negative), ≥0.001 to <0.1%, ≥0.1 to <1%, and ≥1%, respectively. Furthermore, in a multivariate model, pre-HSCT *FLT3*-ITD MRD status, alongside with transplant in CR2 vs CR1, and T-cell depletion were the most important determinants of post-HSCT relapse risk and survival [55]. In 2023, Dillon and colleagues, analyzing a large population of 88w AML patients with *NPM1* and/or *FLT3*-ITD mutation, confirmed these results: pre-HSCT MRD >0.01% correlated with increased relapse and worse survival compared with those without these variants [50]. The same group also performed a specific analysis on the impact of pre-HSCT *FLT3*-ITD MRD status, showing that the detection of residual mutation is associated with dismal outcomes in a dose-dependent manner [56]. Grob and colleagues also explored the *FLT3*-ITD NGS-based MRD in other settings: they performed NGS analysis at diagnosis and in CR after intensive remission induction treatment in 161 patients with de novo *FLT3*-ITD AML. MRD+ was detected in 29% of patients at the second time point and it was associated with increased risk of relapse and inferior OS. At the multivariable analysis, the *FLT3*-ITD MRD status confirmed its independent role in the outcome and, remarkably, outperformed, as a prognostic variable MRD assessment by NGS-based mutant *NPM1* detection and multiparameter flow cytometry [57].

In a similar fashion, in 2024, the German group tested NGS-based *FLT3*-ITD MRD in a population of 157 *FLT3*-ITD AML patients treated with intensive chemotherapy in combination with *FLT3-ITD* inhibitor Midostaurin. The authors confirmed the strong, independent role of MRD+ as a predictor of dismal outcome [14].

MRD-Driven Therapy

The growing body of evidence on residual disease monitoring led to a new role of MRD beyond outcome prognostication, such as efficacy endpoint as well as reliable marker for decision-making in AML management.

In this perspective, in 2013, the AML05 trial prospectively investigated, in a cohort of t(8:21) AML patients, a treatment schedule including allo-HSCT in patients in first CR with MRD positivity (high-risk patients) and chemotherapy/autologous (auto-) HSCT in patients in first CR with MRD negativity (low-risk patients). Patients who could not comply with the risk-directed treatment schedule due to patient bias (low-risk patients undergoing allo-HSCT and high-risk patients undergoing chemotherapy/auto-HSCT) were considered non–risk-directed therapy group. The authors found that allo-HSCT could reduce relapse and improve OS compared with chemotherapy/auto-HSCT for high-risk patients, whereas chemotherapy/auto-HSCT achieved a low relapse rate and high RFS for low-risk patients. In multivariate analysis, MRD status and treatment choice were demonstrated as independent prognostic factors for relapse, RFS, and OS, proving the efficacy and feasibility of an MRD-based, risk-directed AML management [58]. In the same line, recently, a risk-directed treatment according to *KIT/ASXL1* mutations (indicators of poor prognosis) and MRD levels was able to decrease relapse and improve OS of t(8;21) AML patients [59].

In 2019 the results of GIMEMA AML1310 trial, which included all AML types but APL and MRD monitoring through both PCR (*NPM1*-mutated and CBF-AML) and flow-cytometry (all the other types), were published [60]. In this study, the patients were stratified according to the National Comprehensive Cancer Network (NCCN) recommendations and MRD status, identifying 5 categories: favorable-risk (NCCN-FR, undergoing auto-HSCT after induction therapy), poor-risk (NCCN-PR, undergoing allo-HSCT), intermediate-MRD negative (NCCN-IR-Neg, receiving auto-HSCT), intermediate-MRD positive (NCCN-IR-Pos, receiving allo-HSCT) and a fifth group of patients belonging to the IR category, in whom it was not possible to identify any leukemia-associated immunophenotype (LAIP) and thus MRD monitoring was not possible (NCCN-IR-no-LAIP category). The patients of fifth group were allocated to the auto-HSCT post-consolidation option. Overall 2-year OS and RFS were 56% and 54%, respectively. Two-year OS and DFS were 74% and 61% in the FR category, 42% and 45% in the PR category, 79% and 61% in the IR MRD-negative category, and 70% and 67% in the IR MRD-positive category. These results proved the beneficial effect of allo-HSCT in an intermediate risk MRD-positive setting, which conferred outcomes similar to FR category [60].

In pediatric AML, the role of molecular MRD as driver for therapeutic decision is more ill-defined. Despite MFC-based MRD has showed great utility for risk classification and to select patients eligible for HSCT, as showed by AML02 trial [61], there is no solid evidence of molecular-based MRD as tool for decision making. Indeed, when compared to MFC, the monitoring of CBF transcripts proved to be uninformative, while molecular MRD targeting *KMT2A* rearrangements (accounting for 10–15% of adult AML and 80% of pediatric AML [62]) seemed to be more reliable [63]. In this line, two recently published paper explored *KMT2Ar* MRD in adult population: Loo et al. found, a significant correlation between preHSCT MRD+ (≥0.0001%) and 2-year RFS (17% vs 59% in MRD−, $p = 0.001$) and 2-year cumulative incidence of relapse (CIR, 75% vs 25% in MRD−; $p = 0.0004$) [64]. Similarly, Wang et al., analyzing a population of 125 *KMT2Ar* AML patient, found a correlation between MRD+ and 3-year OS (51% vs 82% in MRD−; $p < 0.001$), RFS (42% vs 81% in MRD−; $p < 0.001$), CIR (33% vs 12% in MRD−; $p < 0.001$) and non-relapse mortality (11% vs 5% in MRD−; $p = 0.12$). Of note is that in a multivariable model molecular MRD status held an independent role in predicting OS, RFS and CIR [65].

Current Indications and Future Directions

The growing body of evidence showing the feasibility and reliability of MRD, led to the publication, in 2018, of the first consensus from the ELN MRD working party [66]. In 2021, an updated report from the same working party defined new criteria to assess response based on MRD [13].

The deepest level of response, CR with negative MRD (CR_{MRD}^-) is defined as hematologic CR and MRD negative in all the technologies used; for PCR, specifically, a cycling threshold <40 in ≥2 of 3 replicates. In case of CR and positive MRD, the level of detection defines CR with molecular MRD detection at low level (CR-MRD-LL; in case of PCR < 2% or NGS-MRD < 0.1%) or CR with positive MRD (CR_{MRD}^+; PCR > 2% or NGS-MRD > 0.1%). Finally, MRD relapse is defined by the conversion from MRD negativity to MRD positivity or increase in MRD copy numbers ≥1 log10 between any 2 positive samples in patients with CR-MRD-LL (Table 10.2).

The ELN MRD working party proposed also an MRD assessment algorithm based on different subtypes of AML (Fig. 10.2) [13]. PCR-based MRD (qPCR or dPCR) was recommended for *NPM1*-mutated, CBF AML and APL. Other genetic markers are less specific and not reliable and thus are not recommended for PCR-based MRD assessment [66]. Instead, MFC-based MRD assessment is

Table 10.2 MRD-based assessment of response, adapted from the report by ELN MRD Working party

MRD-based response categories		
Response	Abbreviation	Criteria
CR with negative MRD	CR_{MRD}^-	1. Complete morphologic remission, and 2. MRD− in all MRD technologies that were used: a. FCMRD⁻ in BM (If MFC-MRD was used). b. qPCR-MRD⁻ in BM (or in PB after cycle 2 for *NPM1*- and CBF-MRD) (if qPCR-MRD was used). c. NGS-MRD⁻ in BM (If NGS-MRD was used).
CR with positive MRD	CR_{MRD}^+	1. Complete morphologic remission, and 2. MFC-MRD⁺ in PB and/or BM, or 3. NGS-MRD⁺ in PB and/or BM, or 4. qPCR-MRD⁺ in PB and/or BM.

(continued)

Table 10.2 (continued)

MRD-based response categories		
Response	Abbreviation	Criteria
CR with molecular MRD detection at low level	CR-MRD-LL	1. Morphologic CR, and 2. Molecular MRD detectable at low level in PB and/or BM (i.e., qPCR for NPM1 <2% or NGS-MRD <0.1%, but above the detection limit of the assay).
MRD relapse	–	1. Conversion of MRD negativity to MRD positivity independent of the MRD technique, or 2. Increase in MRD copy numbers $\geq 1 \log_{10}$ between any 2 positive samples in patients with CR-MRD-LL who are monitored by qPCR. 3. The result of (1) or (2) should be rapidly confirmed in a second consecutive sample, preferably from the BM.

BM bone marrow, *CR* complete remission, *dPCR* digital PCR, *LL* low level, *MFC* multicolor flow cytometry, *MRD* measurable residual disease, *NGS* next generation sequencing, *PB* peripheral blood, *qPCR* quantitative PCR

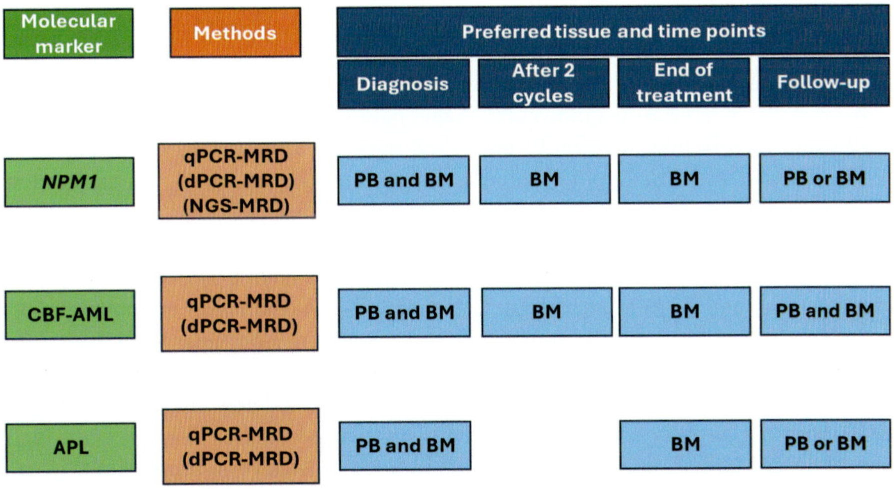

Fig. 10.2 PCR-based MRD assessment algorithm, adapted from the report by ELN MRD Working party. *AML* Acute myeloid leukemia, *APL* Acute promyelocytic leukemia, *BM* Bone marrow, *CBF* Core binding factor, *dPCR* digital PCR, *MRD* measurable residual disease, *NGS* next-generation sequencing, *PB* peripheral blood, *qPCR* real time PCR

recommended, while, due to scarcity of data currently available, NGS is not recommended as a MRD assessment tool, but only to refine prognosis at diagnosis.

In *NPM1*-mutated AML and CBF AML, MRD should be assessed in PB after 2 cycles of therapy (either 2 induction cycles or 1 induction and 1 consolidation cycle), and in BM at the end of consolidation. After the end of consolidation, MRD assessment in *NPM1*-mutated AML should be performed in BM every 3 months or alternatively, from PB every 4–6 weeks, for 24 months; in CBF-AML, it should be assessed in PB every 4–6 weeks for 24 months. MRD follow-up after 24 months should be based on individual prognostic features. In APL the main endpoint is MRD at the end of consolidation, which coincides with the end of treatment in low-risk patients (white blood cell at presentation <10,000/μL), according to current guidelines [27]. On the other hand, high-risk patients require maintenance therapy, and they should be monitored for 24 months, from the end of treatment, from BM every 3 months or, alternatively, from PB every 4–6 weeks.

As widely proven in previous reports, MRD positivity in off-therapy patients and pre-transplant setting correlates with dismal outcome and inferior OS [67]. However, not all the relapses derive from MRD positive status and, conversely, MRD positivity does not always result in overt relapse. In fact, the persistence of low levels of detectable transcript in CBF-AML and *NPM1*-mutant AML is not prognostic of relapse and this subgroup of patients, with stable molecular MRD-LL, do not necessarily require a change in treatment, at the end of treatment or during follow-up [13, 68].

On the other hand, the most recent ELN guidelines for AML management recommend the inclusion of MRD assessment in CR as prognostic factor for long-term outcome and decision-driving variable suggesting allogenic HSCT as post remission treatment for high-risk patients (ELN adverse-risk AML or non-adverse-risk disease with MRD persistence) [68].

New advances, such as the validation of NGS as MRD tool and new techniques may have the potential to grant every AML patient a tool to measure the disease over time: in this line, a recently published paper, addressing MRD in pediatric AML, showed the efficacy of Genomic breakpoint-specific MRD, which showed high concordance with MFC-based techniques and outperformed morphological examination [69].

In conclusion, PCR-based MRD monitoring is nowadays a cornerstone of AML management, and its relevance is going to rise in the future, as an endpoint of several clinical trials [3]. Furthermore, the future holds the promise to include new markers (encouraging results have been published on *WT1* [70]), broadening the population of patients who could benefit from this tool, and new techniques, such as NGS, whose reliability has already been proven in a few studies [14–16] and which hopefully is going to line up with PCR as molecular MRD-monitoring tool in the near future.

References

1. Sasaki K, Ravandi F, Kadia TM, DiNardo CD, Short NJ, Borthakur G, et al. De novo acute myeloid leukemia: a population-based study of outcome in the United States based on the Surveillance, Epidemiology, and End Results (SEER) database, 1980 to 2017. Cancer. 2021;127:2049–61.
2. Kantarjian H, Kadia T, DiNardo C, Daver N, Borthakur G, Jabbour E, et al. Acute myeloid leukemia: current progress and future directions. Blood Cancer J. 2021;11:41.
3. Meddi E, Savi A, Moretti F, Mallegni F, Palmieri R, Paterno G, et al. Measurable residual disease (MRD) as a surrogate efficacy-response biomarker in AML. Int J Mol Sci. 2023;24(4):3062. https://doi.org/10.3390/ijms24043062.
4. Cheson BD, Bennett JM, Kopecky KJ, Büchner T, Willman CL, Estey EH, et al. Revised recommendations of the International Working Group for Diagnosis, Standardization of Response Criteria, Treatment Outcomes, and Reporting Standards for Therapeutic Trials in Acute Myeloid Leukemia. J Clin Oncol. 2003;21:4642–9.
5. Döhner H, Estey E, Grimwade D, Amadori S, Appelbaum FR, Büchner T, et al. Diagnosis and management of AML in adults: 2017 ELN recommendations from an international expert panel. Blood. 2017;129:424–47.
6. van Dongen JJ, Macintyre EA, Gabert JA, Delabesse E, Rossi V, Saglio G, et al. Standardized RT-PCR analysis of fusion gene transcripts from chromosome aberrations in acute leukemia for detection of minimal residual disease. Report of the BIOMED-1 Concerted Action: investigation of minimal residual disease in acute leukemia. Leukemia. 1999;13:1901–28.
7. Falini B. NPM1-mutated acute myeloid leukemia: new pathogenetic and therapeutic insights and open questions. Am J Hematol. 2023;98:1452–64.
8. Falini B, Mecucci C, Tiacci E, Alcalay M, Rosati R, Pasqualucci L, et al. Cytoplasmic nucleophosmin in acute myelogenous leukemia with a normal karyotype. N Engl J Med. 2005;352:254–66.
9. Papaemmanuil E, Gerstung M, Bullinger L, Gaidzik VI, Paschka P, Roberts ND, et al. Genomic classification and prognosis in acute myeloid leukemia. N Engl J Med. 2016;374:2209–21.
10. Vossen RHAM, White SJ. Quantitative DNA analysis using droplet digital PCR. Methods Mol Biol. 2017;1492:167–77.
11. Galimberti S, Balducci S, Guerrini F, Del Re M, Cacciola R. Digital droplet PCR in hematologic malignancies: a new useful molecular tool. Diagnostics (Basel). 2022;12(6):1305. https://doi.org/10.3390/diagnostics12061305.
12. Moritz J, Schwab A, Reinisch A, Zebisch A, Sill H, Wölfler A. Measurable residual disease detection in acute myeloid leukemia: current challenges and future directions. Biomedicine. 2024;12(3):599. https://doi.org/10.3390/biomedicines12030599.
13. Heuser M, Freeman SD, Ossenkoppele GJ, Buccisano F, Hourigan CS, Ngai LL, et al. 2021 Update on MRD in acute myeloid leukemia: a consensus document from the European LeukemiaNet MRD Working Party. Blood. 2021;138:2753–67.
14. Rücker FG, Bullinger L, Cocciardi S, Skambraks S, Luck TJ, Weber D, et al. Measurable residual disease monitoring in AML with FLT3-ITD treated with intensive chemotherapy plus midostaurin. Blood Adv. 2024;8(23):bloodadvances.2024013758.
15. Li Y, Solis-Ruiz J, Yang F, Long N, Tong CH, Lacbawan FL, et al. NGS-defined measurable residual disease (MRD) after initial chemotherapy as a prognostic biomarker for acute myeloid leukemia. Blood Cancer J. 2023;13:59.
16. Kim H-J, Kim Y, Kang D, Kim HS, Lee J-M, Kim M, et al. Prognostic value of measurable residual disease monitoring by next-generation sequencing before and after allogeneic hematopoietic cell transplantation in acute myeloid leukemia. Blood Cancer J. 2021;11:109.
17. Gabert J. Detection of recurrent translocations using real time PCR; assessment of the technique for diagnosis and detection of minimal residual disease. Haematologica. 1999;84(Suppl EHA-4):107–9.

18. van der Velden VHJ, Hochhaus A, Cazzaniga G, Szczepanski T, Gabert J, van Dongen JJM. Detection of minimal residual disease in hematologic malignancies by real-time quantitative PCR: principles, approaches, and laboratory aspects. Leukemia. 2003;17:1013–34.
19. Zimmermann K, Mannhalter JW. Technical aspects of quantitative competitive PCR. BioTechniques. 1996;21:268–72, 274–279.
20. Diverio D, Lo Coco F, D'Adamo F, Biondi A, Fagioli M, Grignani F, et al. Identification of DNA rearrangements at the retinoic acid receptor-alpha (RAR-alpha) locus in all patients with acute promyelocytic leukemia (APL) and mapping of APL breakpoints within the RAR-alpha second intron. Italian Cooperative Study Group 'GIMEMA'. Blood. 1992;79:3331–6.
21. Miller WHJ, Kakizuka A, Frankel SR, Warrell RPJ, DeBlasio A, Levine K, et al. Reverse transcription polymerase chain reaction for the rearranged retinoic acid receptor alpha clarifies diagnosis and detects minimal residual disease in acute promyelocytic leukemia. Proc Natl Acad Sci USA. 1992;89:2694–8.
22. Lo Coco F, Diverio D, Pandolfi PP, Biondi A, Rossi V, Avvisati G, et al. Molecular evaluation of residual disease as a predictor of relapse in acute promyelocytic leukaemia. Lancet. 1992;340:1437–8.
23. Diverio D, Rossi V, Avvisati G, De Santis S, Pistilli A, Pane F, et al. Early detection of relapse by prospective reverse transcriptase-polymerase chain reaction analysis of the PML/RARalpha fusion gene in patients with acute promyelocytic leukemia enrolled in the GIMEMA-AIEOP multicenter 'AIDA' trial. GIMEMA-AIEOP Multicenter 'AIDA' Trial. Blood. 1998;92:784–9.
24. Grimwade D, Jovanovic JV, Hills RK, Nugent EA, Patel Y, Flora R, et al. Prospective minimal residual disease monitoring to predict relapse of acute promyelocytic leukemia and to direct pre-emptive arsenic trioxide therapy. J Clin Oncol. 2009;27:3650–8.
25. Lo-Coco F, Avvisati G, Vignetti M, Thiede C, Orlando SM, Iacobelli S, et al. Retinoic acid and arsenic trioxide for acute promyelocytic leukemia. N Engl J Med. 2013;369:111–21.
26. Burnett AK, Russell NH, Hills RK, Bowen D, Kell J, Knapper S, et al. Arsenic trioxide and all-trans retinoic acid treatment for acute promyelocytic leukaemia in all risk groups (AML17): results of a randomised, controlled, phase 3 trial. Lancet Oncol. 2015;16:1295–305.
27. Sanz MA, Fenaux P, Tallman MS, Estey EH, Löwenberg B, Naoe T, et al. Management of acute promyelocytic leukemia: updated recommendations from an expert panel of the European LeukemiaNet. Blood. 2019;133:1630–43.
28. Laczika K, Novak M, Hilgarth B, Mitterbauer M, Mitterbauer G, Scheidel-Petrovic A, et al. Competitive CBFbeta/MYH11 reverse-transcriptase polymerase chain reaction for quantitative assessment of minimal residual disease during postremission therapy in acute myeloid leukemia with inversion(16): a pilot study. J Clin Oncol. 1998;16:1519–25.
29. Marcucci G, Caligiuri MA, Döhner H, Archer KJ, Schlenk RF, Döhner K, et al. Quantification of CBFbeta/MYH11 fusion transcript by real time RT-PCR in patients with INV(16) acute myeloid leukemia. Leukemia. 2001;15:1072–80.
30. Buonamici S, Ottaviani E, Testoni N, Montefusco V, Visani G, Bonifazi F, et al. Real-time quantitation of minimal residual disease in inv(16)-positive acute myeloid leukemia may indicate risk for clinical relapse and may identify patients in a curable state. Blood. 2002;99:443–9.
31. Marcucci G, Livak KJ, Bi W, Strout MP, Bloomfield CD, Caligiuri MA. Detection of minimal residual disease in patients with AML1/ETO-associated acute myeloid leukemia using a novel quantitative reverse transcription polymerase chain reaction assay. Leukemia. 1998;12:1482–9.
32. Sugimoto T, Das H, Imoto S, Murayama T, Gomyo H, Chakraborty S, et al. Quantitation of minimal residual disease in t(8;21)-positive acute myelogenous leukemia patients using real-time quantitative RT-PCR. Am J Hematol. 2000;64:101–6.
33. Krauter J, Wattjes MP, Nagel S, Heidenreich O, Krug U, Kafert S, et al. Real-time RT-PCR for the detection and quantification of AML1/MTG8 fusion transcripts in t(8;21)-positive AML patients. Br J Haematol. 1999;107:80–5.
34. Tobal K, Newton J, Macheta M, Chang J, Morgenstern G, Evans PA, et al. Molecular quantitation of minimal residual disease in acute myeloid leukemia with t(8;21) can identify patients in durable remission and predict clinical relapse. Blood. 2000;95:815–9.

35. Corbacioglu A, Scholl C, Schlenk RF, Eiwen K, Du J, Bullinger L, et al. Prognostic impact of minimal residual disease in CBFB-MYH11-positive acute myeloid leukemia. J Clin Oncol. 2010;28:3724–9.
36. Yin JAL, O'Brien MA, Hills RK, Daly SB, Wheatley K, Burnett AK. Minimal residual disease monitoring by quantitative RT-PCR in core binding factor AML allows risk stratification and predicts relapse: results of the United Kingdom MRC AML-15 trial. Blood. 2012;120:2826–35.
37. Willekens C, Blanchet O, Renneville A, Cornillet-Lefebvre P, Pautas C, Guieze R, et al. Prospective long-term minimal residual disease monitoring using RQ-PCR in RUNX1-RUNX1T1-positive acute myeloid leukemia: results of the French CBF-2006 trial. Haematologica. 2016;101:328–35.
38. Qin Y-Z, Wang Y, Xu L-P, Zhang X-H, Chen H, Han W, et al. The dynamics of RUNX1-RUNX1T1 transcript levels after allogeneic hematopoietic stem cell transplantation predict relapse in patients with t(8;21) acute myeloid leukemia. J Hematol Oncol. 2017;10:44.
39. Rücker FG, Agrawal M, Corbacioglu A, Weber D, Kapp-Schwoerer S, Gaidzik VI, et al. Measurable residual disease monitoring in acute myeloid leukemia with t(8;21)(q22;q22.1): results from the AML Study Group. Blood. 2019;134:1608–18.
40. Yalniz FF, Patel KP, Bashir Q, Marin D, Ahmed S, Alousi AM, et al. Significance of minimal residual disease monitoring by real-time quantitative polymerase chain reaction in core binding factor acute myeloid leukemia for transplantation outcomes. Cancer. 2020;126:2183–92.
41. Gorello P, Cazzaniga G, Alberti F, Dell'Oro MG, Gottardi E, Specchia G, et al. Quantitative assessment of minimal residual disease in acute myeloid leukemia carrying nucleophosmin (NPM1) gene mutations. Leukemia. 2006;20:1103–8.
42. Chou W-C, Tang J-L, Wu S-J, Tsay W, Yao M, Huang S-Y, et al. Clinical implications of minimal residual disease monitoring by quantitative polymerase chain reaction in acute myeloid leukemia patients bearing nucleophosmin (NPM1) mutations. Leukemia. 2007;21:998–1004.
43. Krönke J, Schlenk RF, Jensen K-O, Tschürtz F, Corbacioglu A, Gaidzik VI, et al. Monitoring of minimal residual disease in NPM1-mutated acute myeloid leukemia: a study from the German-Austrian acute myeloid leukemia study group. J Clin Oncol. 2011;29:2709–16.
44. Shayegi N, Kramer M, Bornhäuser M, Schaich M, Schetelig J, Platzbecker U, et al. The level of residual disease based on mutant NPM1 is an independent prognostic factor for relapse and survival in AML. Blood. 2013;122:83–92.
45. Hubmann M, Köhnke T, Hoster E, Schneider S, Dufour A, Zellmeier E, et al. Molecular response assessment by quantitative real-time polymerase chain reaction after induction therapy in NPM1-mutated patients identifies those at high risk of relapse. Haematologica. 2014;99:1317–25.
46. Ivey A, Hills RK, Simpson MA, Jovanovic JV, Gilkes A, Grech A, et al. Assessment of minimal residual disease in standard-risk AML. N Engl J Med. 2016;374:422–33.
47. Kayser S, Benner A, Thiede C, Martens U, Huber J, Stadtherr P, et al. Pretransplant NPM1 MRD levels predict outcome after allogeneic hematopoietic stem cell transplantation in patients with acute myeloid leukemia. Blood Cancer J. 2016;6:e449.
48. Balsat M, Renneville A, Thomas X, de Botton S, Caillot D, Marceau A, et al. Postinduction minimal residual disease predicts outcome and benefit from allogeneic stem cell transplantation in acute myeloid leukemia with NPM1 mutation: a study by the Acute Leukemia French Association Group. J Clin Oncol. 2017;35:185–93.
49. Bill M, Grimm J, Jentzsch M, Kloss L, Goldmann K, Schulz J, et al. Digital droplet PCR-based absolute quantification of pre-transplant NPM1 mutation burden predicts relapse in acute myeloid leukemia patients. Ann Hematol. 2018;97:1757–65.
50. Dillon LW, Gui G, Page KM, Ravindra N, Wong ZC, Andrew G, et al. DNA sequencing to detect residual disease in adults with acute myeloid leukemia prior to hematopoietic cell transplant. JAMA. 2023;329:745–55.
51. Kapp-Schwoerer S, Weber D, Corbacioglu A, Gaidzik VI, Paschka P, Krönke J, et al. Impact of gemtuzumab ozogamicin on MRD and relapse risk in patients with NPM1-mutated AML: results from the AMLSG 09-09 trial. Blood. 2020;136:3041–50.

52. Othman J, Tiong IS, O'Nions J, Dennis M, Mokretar K, Ivey A, et al. Molecular MRD is strongly prognostic in patients with NPM1-mutated AML receiving venetoclax-based nonintensive therapy. Blood. 2024;143:336–41.
53. Othman J, Potter N, Ivey A, Jovanovic J, Runglall M, Freeman SD, et al. Postinduction molecular MRD identifies patients with NPM1 AML who benefit from allogeneic transplant in first remission. Blood. 2024;143:1931–6.
54. Schwind S, Bischof L, Bill M, Grimm J, Ussmann J, Backhaus D, et al. Quantifying NPM1 MRD in AML patients prior to allogeneic stem cell transplantation: where to draw the line? Hemasphere. 2024;8:e55.
55. Loo S, Dillon R, Ivey A, Anstee NS, Othman J, Tiong IS, et al. Pretransplant FLT3-ITD MRD assessed by high-sensitivity PCR-NGS determines posttransplant clinical outcome. Blood. 2022;140:2407–11.
56. Dillon LW, Gui G, Ravindra N, Andrew G, Mukherjee D, Wong ZC, et al. Measurable residual FLT3 internal tandem duplication before allogeneic transplant for acute myeloid leukemia. JAMA Oncol. 2024;10:1104–10.
57. Grob T, Sanders MA, Vonk CM, Kavelaars FG, Rijken M, Hanekamp DW, et al. Prognostic value of FLT3-internal tandem duplication residual disease in acute myeloid leukemia. J Clin Oncol. 2023;41:756–65.
58. Zhu H-H, Zhang X-H, Qin Y-Z, Liu D-H, Jiang H, Chen H, et al. MRD-directed risk stratification treatment may improve outcomes of t(8;21) AML in the first complete remission: results from the AML05 multicenter trial. Blood. 2013;121:4056–62.
59. Xu D, Yang Y, Yin Z, Tu S, Nie D, Li Y, et al. Risk-directed therapy based on genetics and MRD improves the outcomes of AML1-ETO-positive AML patients, a multi-center prospective cohort study. Blood Cancer J. 2023;13:168.
60. Venditti A, Piciocchi A, Candoni A, Melillo L, Calafiore V, Cairoli R, et al. GIMEMA AML1310 trial of risk-adapted, MRD-directed therapy for young adults with newly diagnosed acute myeloid leukemia. Blood. 2019;134:935–45.
61. Rubnitz JE, Inaba H, Dahl G, Ribeiro RC, Bowman WP, Taub J, et al. Minimal residual disease-directed therapy for childhood acute myeloid leukaemia: results of the AML02 multicentre trial. Lancet Oncol. 2010;11:543–52.
62. Guarnera L, D'Addona M, Bravo-Perez C, Visconte V. KMT2A rearrangements in leukemias: molecular aspects and therapeutic perspectives. Int J Mol Sci. 2024;25(16):9023. https://doi.org/10.3390/ijms25169023.
63. Inaba H, Coustan-Smith E, Cao X, Pounds SB, Shurtleff SA, Wang KY, et al. Comparative analysis of different approaches to measure treatment response in acute myeloid leukemia. J Clin Oncol. 2012;30:3625–32.
64. Loo S, Potter N, Ivey A, O'Nions J, Moon R, Jovanovic J, et al. Pretransplant MRD detection of fusion transcripts is strongly prognostic in KMT2A-rearranged acute myeloid leukemia. Blood. 2024;144:2554–7.
65. Wang L, Chen Y, Zang M, Zhou J, Xiao M, Fu H, et al. Molecular measurable residual disease before transplantation independently predicts survival and relapse risk in adult lysine methyltransferase 2a-rearranged acute myeloid leukemia. Cancer. 2025;131:e35717.
66. Schuurhuis GJ, Heuser M, Freeman S, Béné M-C, Buccisano F, Cloos J, et al. Minimal/measurable residual disease in AML: a consensus document from the European LeukemiaNet MRD Working Party. Blood. 2018;131:1275–91.
67. Short NJ, Zhou S, Fu C, Berry DA, Walter RB, Freeman SD, et al. Association of measurable residual disease with survival outcomes in patients with acute myeloid leukemia: a systematic review and meta-analysis. JAMA Oncol. 2020;6:1890–9.
68. Döhner H, Wei AH, Appelbaum FR, Craddock C, DiNardo CD, Dombret H, et al. Diagnosis and management of AML in adults: 2022 recommendations from an international expert panel on behalf of the ELN. Blood. 2022;140:1345–77.

69. Maurer-Granofszky M, Kohrer S, Fischer S, Schumich A, Nebral K, Larghero P, et al. Genomic breakpoint-specific monitoring of measurable residual disease in pediatric non-standard-risk acute myeloid leukemia. Haematologica. 2024;109:740–50.
70. Liu H, Wang X, Zhang H, Wang J, Chen Y, Ma T, et al. Dynamic changes in the level of WT1 as an MRD marker to predict the therapeutic outcome of patients with AML with and without allogeneic stem cell transplantation. Mol Med Rep. 2019;20:2426–32.

Pharmacogenomics in Pediatric Leukemia

11

Vivek M. Shastri and Jatinder K. Lamba

Introduction

Genomic heterogeneity as a result of somatic, acquired, and inherited genomic variations plays an important role in cancer development and response to treatment [1, 2]. Research in last few decades has advanced our understanding of both malignant and constitutive host genomes providing the impetus to choose the most appropriate anticancer agents to personalize treatment. Many of these discoveries are now part of routine clinical practices and U.S. Food and Drug Administration (U.S. FDA) approved biomarker-specific therapeutic products are proliferating. As of May 05, 2026, 675 drug–biomarker pairs are listed on this site, and of these, 325 are for anticancer agents [3]. Such therapeutic advancements are the results of pharmacogenetic/pharmacogenomic studies. Pharmacogenetics or pharmacogenomics is the field of research that focuses on the impact of genetic variation on the interpatient variation in response to drugs [4, 5]. These studies primarily focus on studying the impact of genes involved in pharmacokinetic (ADME: absorption, distribution, metabolism, and excretion) or pharmacodynamic (drug receptors or enzymes) pathways critical for the safety/efficacy of drugs. Within specific patient populations, outcomes can differ significantly based on individuals who are good responders, non-responders, or those who experience drug-related dose-limiting toxicities. This interpatient variability in drug response and/or toxicity could be due to multiple

V. M. Shastri
Department of Pharmacotherapy & Translational Research, College of Pharmacy, University of Florida, Gainesville, FL, USA

J. K. Lamba (✉)
Department of Pharmacotherapy & Translational Research, College of Pharmacy, University of Florida, Gainesville, FL, USA

UF Health Cancer Institute, University of Florida, Gainesville, FL, USA
e-mail: jlamba@cop.ufl.edu; jatinderklamba@ufl.edu

W. Li (ed.), *Laboratory Assessments of Pediatric Leukemia*,
https://doi.org/10.1007/978-3-032-26557-9_11

factors, including but not limited to environmental, disease characteristics, and interaction with other drugs. However, studies have shown pharmacogenomic diversity to be a significant contributor to the observed inter-patient variability [4]. Over the decades there has been significant progress in emergence actionable pharmacogenomics markers, and this resulted in development of resources and tools to make the discoveries and interpretation uniform across the globe. First of all, development of start allele nomenclature. Secondly, building of resources and databases such as ClinPGx a pharmacogenomics knowledge resource that provides consolidated information on gene-drug associations, genotype phenotype relationships, information on clinical guidelines annotations, drug label annotations, FDA drug label annotations and curated drug pathways along with key literature evidence (https://www.clinpgx.org/). PharmVar is a pharmacogene variation consortium and represents a central repository for pharmacogenomic variation with emphasis on haplotype structure and allele variation. Finally, Clinical Pharmacogenomics Implementation Consortium (CPIC) is an international consortium with goal to further facilitate pharmacogenomic testing to improve patient outcome by addressing barriers to clinical implementation as well as by providing guidelines for therapy modifications for improving patient care. This chapter will summarize pharmacogenetic/pharmacogenomic discoveries from studies in children with acute lymphoblastic leukemia (ALL) and acute myeloid leukemia (AML).

Pharmacogenomics of ALL Treatment

While ALL is the most common cancer in children, survival outcomes have improved to >90% from ~10% in the 1960s [6]. This improvement in treatment outcome can be attributed to risk-adapted therapies, advancements in minimal residual disease (MRD) monitoring, and incorporation of pharmacogenomic markers in making treatment decisions [7]. Childhood ALL treatment protocols are usually generalized and uniform with commonly used drugs including thiopurines, vincristine, methotrexate, and asparagine, allowing for pharmacogenomic discoveries predicting potential efficacy and risk of adverse events [8]. The following section will provide an overview of actionable drug-gene pairs of relevance in ALL.

Thiopurine Pharmacogenomics Thiopurines, including 6-thioguanine, 6-mercaptopurine (6-MP), and azathioprine (a prodrug for 6-MP) , are purine antimetabolites and immunomodulators used in treating acute lymphoblastic leukemia (ALL), inflammatory bowel disease, Crohn's disease, organ transplant immunosuppression, and multiple sclerosis. A core component of ALL chemotherapy is 6-MP, which inhibits DNA and RNA synthesis, promoting leukemic cell death. As a prodrug, 6-MP requires intracellular activation into thioguanine nucleotides (TGNs), particularly 6-thioguanine triphosphate, via enzymes like hypoxanthine-guanine phosphoribosyltransferase and inosine-5′-monophosphate dehydrogenase. The enzyme thiopurine methyl transferase (encoded by *TPMT*) inactivates 6-MP by converting it into less potent methyl-MP, as illustrated in Fig. 11.1. *TPMT* activity

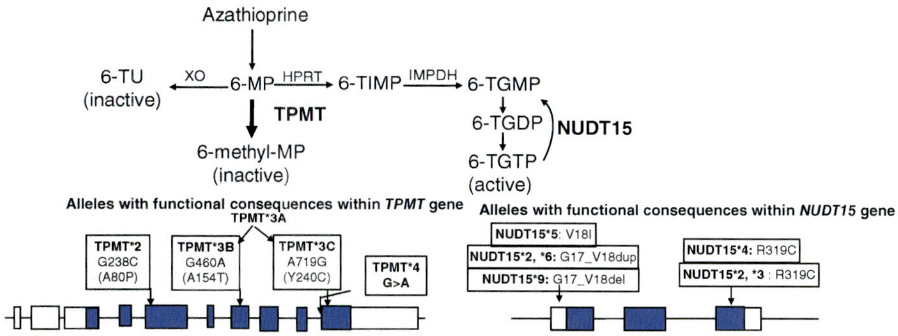

Fig. 11.1 Pathways involved in thiopurine metabolism. While *TPMT* methylates 6-MP to inactivate it, *NUDT15* converts active metabolite 6-TGTP to less toxic 6-TGMP. *TPMT* alleles with major functional consequences. Blue denotes coding region. *NUDT15* alleles with major functional consequences. Blue denotes coding region. *6-MP* 6-mercaptopurine, *6-TGDP* 6-thioguanine diphosphate, *6-TGMP* thioguanine monophosphate, *6-TGTP* 6-thioguanine triphosphate, *6-TIMP* 6-thioinosinic acid, *6-TU* 6-thiouric acid, *HPRT* hypoxanthine phosphoribosyltransferase, *IMPDH* inosine monophosphate dehydrogenase, *TPMT* thiopurine S-methyltransferase, *XO* xanthine oxidase

varies significantly within populations, following a trimodal distribution. Single-nucleotide polymorphisms (SNPs) in *TPMT* contribute to variability in enzymatic activity and thiopurine metabolism. Three deleterious SNPs account for approximately 90% of *TPMT* deficiency, resulting in unstable proteins and increased degradation [9, 10]. Star allele nomenclature has been used to identify and classify the alleles with *1 most commonly referred to as wild-type or reference allele, and *2, *3, *4 referring to functionally altered alleles. Figure 11.1 outlines key *TPMT* variants, including *TPMT*2* (c.238G > C), *TPMT**3A (c.460G > A and c.719A > G in cis), *TPMT*3B (c.460G > A)*, *TPMT**3C (c.719A > G), and *TPMT**4 (intron 9, 626-1A > G), which lead to protein loss-of-function and a reduction in a patient's ability to metabolize 6-MP. Of note, other *TPMT* genotypes have been cataloged by the *TPMT* Nomenclature Committee (Linköping University website: https://liu.se/en/research/*TPMT*-nomenclature-committee). Importantly, patients with two loss-of-function alleles (homozygous or compound heterozygous) are poor metabolizers (*TPMT*-deficient) and face a high risk of severe myelosuppression if given standard doses of thiopurines. Heterozygous individuals, those with one loss of function allele and one wild-type allele, are predicted to have an intermediate activity (~50% enzymatic activity) and termed intermediate metabolizers, also have an elevated risk of myelosuppression with standard doses of thiopurines [11, 12]. Dose reduction in these patients would be recommended.

Nudix hydrolase 15 (encoded by *NUDT15*), another enzyme affecting 6-MP metabolism, converts the active metabolite 6-thioguanine triphosphate into less toxic thioguanine monophosphate. Genome-wide association studies (GWAS) have linked *NUDT15* variants to thiopurine tolerance in ALL and inflammatory bowel disease (IBD) [13–15]. There are over 20 reported variants, cataloged by PharmVar (https://www.pharmvar.org/gene/NUDT15). One variant found in the NUDT15*2 and NUDT15*3 alleles rs116855232 (c.415C > T), which results in the p.R139C amino acid change, leading to enzymatic inactivity. Patients homozygous for this variant tolerate only ~8.3% of the standard 6-MP dose, while heterozygous patients tolerate ~63%, and wild-type patients tolerate ~83.5% [14]. Figure 11.1 illustrates major *NUDT15* alleles. Several studies have shown *NUDT15* variants to be associated with adverse events in ALL, IBD, and ulcerative colitis after treatment with 6-MP [16–23]. Studies have demonstrated that the p.R139C variant is more common among Asian (~6.6% in South Asians) and Latino (~6%) populations compared to groups of Caucasian (non-Finnish 0.38% and Finnish 2.28%) and African (0.1%) ancestry [17]. This led to an increased focus on investigating the p.R139C and other known variants in studies from Guatemala, Singapore, and Japan [17, 24–31]. In the Indian population, 17 studies since 2017 have examined *NUDT15* pharmacogenomics and its toxicity associations in ALL and IBD [9, 20, 29, 32–45]. Overall, variants in *TPMT* are more clinically significant in Caucasians and Africans, whereas *NUDT15* variants have greater relevance in Asians and Hispanics. In certain circumstances, measuring the thiopurine metabolite levels to confirm the metabolizer state for resolving any uncertainty from *TPMT* and *NUDT15* genotypes.

The U.S. FDA has incorporated *TPMT* and *NUDT15* pharmacogenomics into thiopurine drug labels. CPIC provided dosing guidelines for *TPMT* genotypes in 2011 [46], updated in 2013 [47] and 2018, incorporating *NUDT15* [48]. Genotypes for *TPMT* and *NUDT15* are used to define the respective alleles and diplotypes that are associated with enzymatic activity levels or phenotypes for *TPMT* [44]. Patients are categorized as normal, intermediate, possible intermediate, or poor metabolizers based on *TPMT* and *NUDT15* genotypes. Possible intermediate metabolizer are individuals who have one loss of function allele and one allele of uncertain or as yet unknown significance. This classification informs dosing adjustments to minimize thiopurine-related toxicities, such as leukopenia, myelosuppression, and neutropenia. The 2018 CPIC guidelines emphasize combined TPMT and NUDT15 phenotypes in dosing recommendations Summarized in Table 11.1 adapted from the CPIC guidelines [48]. Updates to the current guidelines as well as upcoming new guidelines could be found at https://cpicpgx.org/guidelines/guideline-for-thiopurines-and-tpmt/.

Asparaginase Pharmacogenomics Asparaginase (ASP) , an enzyme that degrades asparagine to aspartic acid and ammonia, has been a key component of ALL chemotherapy in pediatric patients. Leukemic cells are unable to synthesize asparagine due to lack of asparagine synthetase, causing them to rely on extracellular asparagine. The use of ASP thus impacts the proliferation and survival of leukemic cells by depleting extracellular asparagine. Currently available ASP formulations include those from *Escherichia coli*, ASP with polyethylene glycol (PEG-ASP or calaspargase pegol), and that from *Erwinia chrysanthemi* (Erwinia ASP). Despite its efficacy and the known sensitivity of leukemic cells to ASP, one of the biggest clinical challenges associated with the use of ASP is the hypersensitivity reactions in patients, resulting in therapy discontinuation. Efforts to identify pharmacogenomic markers

Table 11.1 Thiopurine methyl transferase (TPMT) and nudix hydrolase 15 (NUDT15)-based dosing guidelines for thiopurines (adapted from CPIC guidelines)

Genotype-based phenotypes	Potential diplotypes	Summary of dosing recommendations*	Implications*	Classification of recommendation
TPMT and *NUDT15* Normal metabolizers	*1/*1 (two normal function alleles)	Start with normal starting dose (e.g., 75 mg/m²/day or 1.5 mg/kg/day for 6-MP, 2–3 mg/kg/day for azathioprine and 40–60 mg/m²/day for thioguanine) and adjust as per standard recommendations*	Normal risk of thiopurine-related toxicity (6-MP, azathioprine, and thioguanine)	Strong for all 3 thiopurines
NUDT15 Normal metabolizer	*1/*1 (two normal function alleles)			
TPMT Intermediate metabolizer	*1/*2, *1/*3A, *1/*3B, *1/*3C, *1/*4 (one normal and one loss of function allele)	Begin with 30–80% of normal dose (e.g., 22.5–60 mg/m²/day or 0.45–1.2 mg/kg/day for 6-MP, 0.6–2.4 mg/kg/day for azathioprine and 20–48 mg/m²/day for thioguanine) and adjust based on myelosuppression and disease-specific guidelines*	Increased risk of thiopurine-related toxicity (6-MP, azathioprine and thioguanine)	Strong for 6-MP and azathioprine and moderate for thioguanine
TPMT Possible intermediate metabolizer	*2/*8, *3A/*7 (one loss of function allele and another with yet unknown functional consequence)			
NUDT15 Intermediate metabolizer	*1/*2, *1/*3 (one normal and one loss of function allele)			
NUDT15 Possible intermediate metabolizer	*2/*5, *3/*5 (one loss of function allele and another with yet unknown functional consequence)			

(continued)

Table 11.1 (continued)

Genotype-based phenotypes	Potential diplotypes	Summary of dosing recommendations*	Implications*	Classification of recommendation
TPMT Poor metabolizer	*3A/*3A, *2/*3A, *2/*3C, *3A/*3C, *3C/*4, *3A/*4 (two loss of function alleles)	In malignant cases, reduce daily dose by 10-fold and frequency to 3 times a week for all 3 thiopurines and further adjust dose based on myelosuppression and disease-specific guidelines*. In nonmalignant cases, consider opting for alternatives	Very high risk of thiopurine-related toxicity (6-MP, azathioprine and thioguanine) due to extremely high thioguanine nucleotide (TGN) levels resulting in fatal toxicity if dose adjustments are not done	Strong for all 3 thiopurines
NUDT15 Poor metabolizer	*2/*2, *3/*3, *2/*3 (two loss of function alleles)			

predicting ASP hyper-sensitivity have identified several variants [49–53]. SNPs associated with ASP hypersensitivity or toxicities include rs4958381 in the glutamate receptor *GRIA1*, rs6021191 in *NFATC2*, as well as variants in *ASNS*, the gene encoding asparagine synthetase enzyme which is critical for asparagine synthesis. Furthermore, variations in the HLA loci, such as HLA-DRB1*07:01, HLA-DQB1*02:02, HLA-DQA1*02:01, and haplotype HLA-DRB1*07:01–HLA-DQA1*02:01–HLA-DQB1*02:02 have been shown to be associated with ASP hypersensitivity in children with ALL [54–62]. Further investigation into the role of these variants in ASP sensitivity is needed. Although several studies have attempted to define factors that predict asparaginase clearance, at present there are no dosing guidelines associated with pharmacogenomics markers for ASP use [63–68].

Methotrexate Pharmacogenomics Methotrexate (MTX) , a folate analog, inhibits dihydrofolate reductase (DHFR) and has been used for treating ALL, non-Hodgkin's lymphoma, osteosarcoma, and rheumatoid arthritis [69]. Inhibition of DHFR blocks the methylene tetrahydrofolate reductase (MTHFR)-mediated conversion of methylene tetrahydrofolate. Methylene tetrahydrofolate, in turn, is an inhibitor of thymidylate synthesis, which is involved in DNA synthesis [69]. Unfortunately, life-threatening myelosuppression and nephrotoxicity are associated with MTX treatment. *SLCO1B1* is a hepatic drug uptake transporter involved in cellular uptake of MTX and several SNPs in this gene have been associated with MTX clearance, including rs4149056 (c.521T > C) and rs2306283 (c.388A > G) [70]. For c.521T > C, MTX clearance was lower when at least one c.521C allele was present compared to the presence of two c.521T alleles. However, the association of c.388A > G with MTX clearance was only apparent with respect to c.521T > C, where the A allele was associated with decreased clearance and the G allele with increased clearance within each c.521T > C genotype [71, 72]. These two SNPs have also been associated with toxicities and survival in a few studies [73–76]. Genetic variants in other key genes in the MTX pathway such as *MTHFR* (rs1801133) and *TYMS* (rs34743033) have mixed evidence showing a role in MTX related toxicities [77], and SNPs in other transcellular transporter genes involved in MTX efflux *ABCB1* (rs1045642), and *ABCG2* (rs12505410, rs1312040, and rs13137622), and *ABCC2* (rs717620) have been shown to impact MTX concentrations [78, 79]. A systematic review of MTX pharmacokinetics in pediatric malignancies from 2021 found results across studies to be inconsistent. However, a recent update showed that *SLCO1B1, ABCB1, ABCC2*, and *MTHFR* genes significantly impact MTX metabolism and clearance [78, 79]. Among all the SNPs reported to be associated with MTX, the strongest evidence exists for *SLCO1B1* to date, though the large intraindividual variability in MTX elimination has precluded clinical implementation of *SLCO1B1*.

Relapse Pharmacogenomics Among the GWASs performed in pediatric ALL, a 2009 study reported an association between rs10821936 in *ARID5B* with susceptibility to ALL and improved treatment response, and rs4132601 in *IKZF1* was linked to higher relapse risk and therapy resistance [80]. Yang et al. in 2012 further confirmed rs4132601 in *IKZF1* and rs10821936 in *ARID5B* to be significantly associated with risk of relapse, while a third SNP rs2239633 (in *CEBPE*) was associated with relapse-free survival [81]. Furthermore, variants in *NR3C1* (rs6189, rs6190) were reported to be linked to glucocorticoid resistance, which is also known to be a significant driver of relapse in patients with ALL [82]. Finally, cis-regulatory SNPs (such as rs6905596) have been associated with disrupted glucocorticoid response, further elucidating the genetic basis of steroid resistance and relapse in childhood ALL [83].

Pharmacogenomics of Acute Myeloid Leukemia Treatment

Acute myeloid leukemia (AML) is the second most common leukemia among children (16% of all leukemias in patients aged 0–19 years), the leading cause of death due to leukemias, and has a 5-year relative survival rate of 70% in pediatric patients compared to a dismal 29% in adults [84–86]. Since 1970s combination of cytarabine and daunorubicin, commonly referred to as a "7 + 3 regimen" has been the front-line induction 1 chemotherapy for the treatment of AML. In pediatric AML, the addition of etoposide to this has been commonly used and is referred to as Ara-C or cytarabine, daunorubicin, and etoposide (ADE). This induction regimen has been shown to induce remission in roughly 85–90% of children [87–90] and 20% of adults [91]. Unfortunately, despite this, among the patients who achieve remission, around 40% of children and 70% of adults experience relapse, with around 90% of patients with resistant or relapsed AML not surviving past 3 years [92–94]. Several new agents have been recently approved by U.S. FDA for the treatment of AML. These include Gemtuzumab Ozogamicin (GO), *FLT3* inhibitors (midostaurin and gilteritinib), the hedgehog pathway inhibitor glasdegib, the *BCL2* inhibitor venetoclax, and CPX-351 (Vyxeos), a dual-drug liposomal encapsulation of Ara-C and daunorubicin in a synergistic 5:1 ratio, and the menin inhibitor Revumenib for relapsed or refractory AML with KMT2A rearrangement [95, 96]. GO is an antibody–drug conjugate that targets CD33, a surface marker that is commonly expressed in AML. Additional molecules that specifically target some somatic mutations recurrently observed in AML are under active investigation. One such example is the efficacy of isocitrate dehydrogenase (IDH) inhibitors (i.e., ivosidenib and enasidenib) for patients with *IDH1* and *IDH2* mutated AML. With the exception of GO and Revumenib, these new agents have been approved for adult AML patients. However, some of these agents are actively being investigated for use in the pediatric population, for example enasidenib (NCT04203316), venetoclax in combination with standard chemotherapy or other agents (NCT05955261, NCT05292664, NCT06177067, NCT06448013), and midostaurin in combination with chemotherapy (NCT03591510). As compared to ALL, pharmacogenomic studies in AML are still not as far ahead in clinical application. Most of the reported work has been focused on cytarabine, the mainstay of AML chemotherapy. Below we will discuss the current state of cytarabine and GO pharmacogenomics in AML.

Cytarabine Pharmacogenomics Cytarabine (also known as "Ara-C") is a cytidine analog and has been the mainstay of AML chemotherapy since the 1970s. Ara-C is a pro-drug requiring activation to Ara-CTP by multiple phosphorylation steps. The antileukemic impact of Ara-C is primarily driven by incorporation of Ara-CTP in place of dCTP blocking DNA and RNA synthesis by triggering chain termination and thus inducing leukemic cell death. Therefore, intracellular abundance of Ara-CTP is critical to its therapeutic impact. Previous in vitro studies have shown that the intracellular concentrations of Ara-CTP are higher in cells that are sensitive to Ara-C as compared to those that are resistant [97]. Furthermore, higher intracellular Ara-CTP levels have been associated with better response in AML patients [98, 99]. Multiple factors can impact the intracellular abundance of Ara-CTP with key genes listed in the metabolic pathway of AML as shown in Fig. 11.2a. Interpatient variability in intracellular levels of Ara-CTP can thus be impacted by variability in expression and/or activity of these genes such as: (a) inefficient cellular uptake due to low expression levels of the uptake transporters (SLC29A1, SLC28A3, and SLC28A1); (b) reduced activation due to alterations in kinases, such as deoxycytidine kinase (DCK), cytidine monophosphate kinases (CMPK1), and nucleoside diphosphate kinases; or (c) increased inactivation rates due to higher levels of cytidine deaminase (CDA), deoxycytidylate deaminase (DCTD), nucleotidase (NT5C2), or deoxynucleoside triphosphate (dNTP) triphosphohydrolase (SAMHD1). In addition, increased cellular dCTP pools, which are regulated ribonucleotide reductases (RRM1 and RRM2), can compete with DNA incorporation of Ara-CTP and impact Ara-CTP mediated chain termination [100].

Studies focused on the pharmacogenomics of Ara-C have shown an association between SNPs within key candidate cytarabine metabolism genes and intracellular Ara-CTP levels as well as clinical response in patients with AML [101–105] and cytarabine in vitro chemosensitvity [106, 107]. Several review articles are available which summarize these findings [108–114].

Given the complexity of multiple genes in the Ara-C activation pathway, a recent approach has been comprehensive evaluation of the whole pathway combined with an assessment of the directionality of gene function in context of the association. Specifically, a polygenic approach using machine learning tools was recently has been used to identify robust cytarabine pharmacogenomic biomarkers [115]. This study defined a polygenic Ara-C Pharmacogenomic Score consists of 10 SNPs in 9 genes (*CDA*, *DCK*, *SLC29A1*, *CMPK*, *CTPS1*, *RRM1*, *RRM2*, *NME1*, *SLC28A3*; referred to as "ACS10") which was predictive of the outcome in pediatric patients with AML (Fig. 11.2b). Patients with low ACS10 scores (score ≤ 0) had worse outcomes (i.e., inferior event-free survival, inferior overall survival, and minimal residual disease after induction 1) as compared with patients within the high-score group (score > 0). Interestingly, the outcomes of patients with low ACS10 scores improved when therapy was augmented with an increased Ara-C dose or by adding another agent, such as gemtuzumab, to the therapy [115]. Furthermore, patients with high ACS10 scores showed desirable outcomes with a standard dose of Ara-C as compared with a high dose of Ara-C, and thus risk of toxicity in the group could be reduced by avoiding therapy intensification.

A follow-up study showed patients with low ACS10 scores also benefitted from an induction regimen with clofarabine and Ara-C combination therapy as compared to standard induction regimen [116, 117]. Additionally, all these studies (which were performed across three different clinical trials, AML02, AML08, and AAML0531) reported a significantly higher frequency of detrimental ACS10 scores in patients with AML who were from African ancestry as compared to those who were from European ancestry. Specifically, approximately 70% of African ancestry patients had have low ACS10 scores in contrast to ~30% of European ancestry patients; this implies that pharmacogenomics may play a role in the historically observed racial disparity in AML outcomes [117–121]. Given that these results

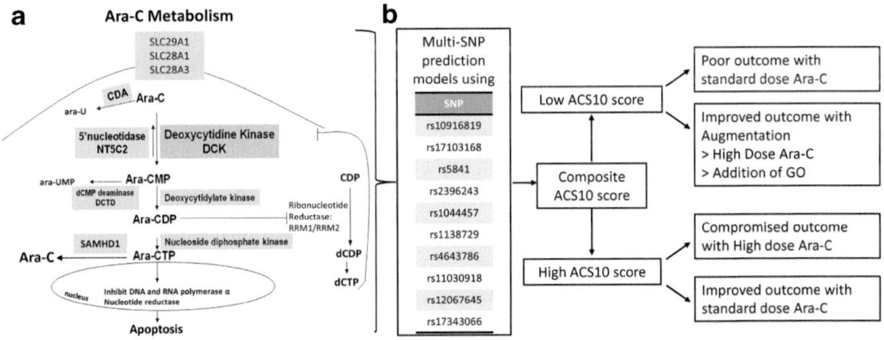

Fig. 11.2 (**a**) Pathways involved in Ara-C formation and metabolism. (**b**) Overview of ACS10 pharmacogenomics score. *Ara-C* cytarabine, *Ara-CDP* cytarabine diphosphate, *Ara-CMP* cytarabine monophosphate, *Ara-CTP* cytarabine triphosphate, *ara-U* uracil arabinoside, *ara-UMP* uracil arabinoside monophosphate

show improved outcomes in the low ACS10 group with an alternative augmented remission induction regimens (e.g., high dose Ara-C or clofarabine+Ara-C or addition of GO to a standard regimen), there is potential to mitigate racial disparity in outcome by using such augmented therapy for the patients with African ancestry with ACS10 low score [116, 117]. These results warrant the need for prospective clinical trials which include AAra-C pharmacogenomics to further establish its clinical utility and eventual incorporation of pharmacogenomics in Ara-C treatment guidelines.

Gemtuzumab Ozogamicin (GO) Pharmacogenomics GO targets *CD33* which belongs to the Siglec family of proteins and is a myeloid marker. ICD33s highly expressed in myeloid leukemia blasts and anti-CD33 antibodies were internalized after binding to the target antigen, which made CD33 a therapeutic target of interest in AML. The most successful CD33-directed agent is an antibody–drug conjugate GO. GO constitutes an anti-CD33 antibody (hP67.6) conjugated to a DNA-damaging cytotoxin, calicheamicin [122]. Figure 11.3 shows the overall GO mechanism; binding of GO to the CD33 antigen on the cell surface triggers its internalization and trafficking to lysosomes. The acidic environment of lysosomes results in further hydrolysis and release of calicheamicin. Calicheamicin is a cytotoxin that when released binds to DNA triggering double and single-strand DNA breaks, thus resulting in leukemic cell apoptosis. GO initially received accelerated approval in 2000 [123], followed by withdrawal in 2010 [124]. However, results from several subsequent follow-up studies demonstrated the benefit of adding GO to adult AML therapeutic regimens, including a well-powered meta-analysis using data from multiple trials (total n = 3325 patients) [125]. In pediatric AML, the Children's Oncology Group initiated trials similarly confirmed the benefit of adding GO in AML treatment [88, 126]. As a result, in September 2017, the U.S. FDA announced the re-approval of GO for the treatment of newly diagnosed and relapsed/refractory pediatric and adult CD33+ AML [127, 128].

CD33 expression varies significantly between patients and is associated with disease characteristics and response to GO [129, 130]. With respect to GO pharmacogenomics studies, SNPs within *CD33* have been studied and found to be associated with CD33 cell surface expression as well as response to GO. So far 6 potentially significant SNPs that hold relevance clinically have been reported, which include a splicing and coding SNP rs12459419C > T (p.A14V, which also occurs in linkage with a promoter SNP) [131]; a CCGG deletion (rs201074739) in exon 4, which results in complete loss of CD33 protein [132]; coding variants rs2455069 (p.R60G), rs35112940 (p.R304G), and rs61736475 (p.S305P); and 3′UTR variant rs1803254 [133, 134]. Of these, all but rs2455069 and rs61736475 have been associated with lower CD33 expression (Fig. 11.3b). Despite the fact that all 6 variants have a significant association with the outcome when compared between standard or GO augmentation and have been used to create a CD33 PGx score [133], the best studied SNP is rs12459419. This SNP results in the substitution of a cytosine to a thymine at c.41 (p.Ala14Val), which leads to an alternatively spliced, shorter isoform of

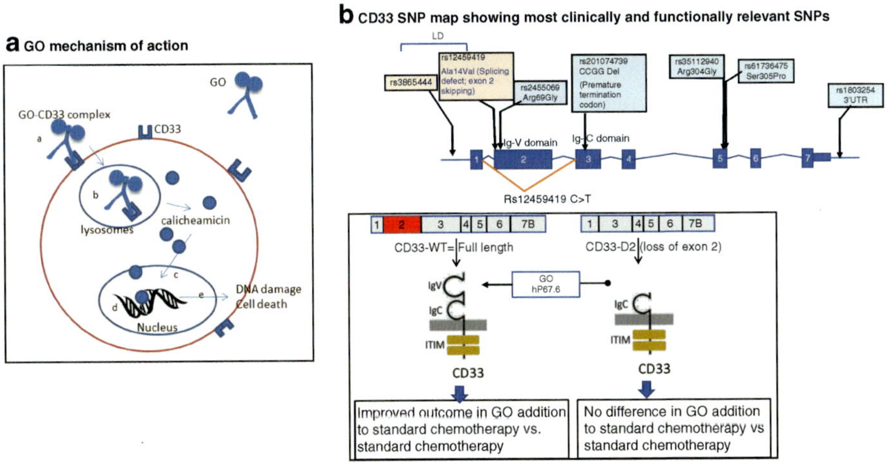

Fig. 11.3 (**A**) GO mechanism of action depicting the steps: (**a**) GO-CD33 complex, (**b**) internalization to lysosomes, (**c**) calicheamicin release, and (**d**, **e**) entry to nucleus triggering DNA damage. (**B**) SNP map showing clinically relevant *CD33* SNPs and the consequence for isoforms from the splicing SNP rs12459419 with respect to GO. *Ig-C domain* C2-set Ig-like domain, *Ig-V domain* V-set Ig-like domain, *ITIM* immunoreceptor tyrosine-based inhibitory motif, *LD* linkage disequilibrium

CD33 that lacks; the most immunogenic domain of CD33–IgV which is targeted by GO. Results from the CD33 pharmacogenomics study in AAML0531, a randomized pediatric AML trial with standard treatment with or without the addition of 2 doses (one in induction and one in consolidation) showed that the benefit from adding GO to standard regimen was observed only in patients who retained the with wild-type (WT) genotype rs12459419 [131]. The presence of the C (WT allele) was associated with higher CD33 cell surface levels, and only patients with the CC genotype experienced a significant reduction in relapse risk and improved disease-free survival when given GO [131]. Patients harboring the T allele (CT or TT genotype) had low CD33 cell surface expression and showed no difference in outcome between standard therapy given with or without the addition of GO [131]. Pediatric KMT2A-rearranged AML patients are a notable exception in that GO is recommended for them regardless of genotype for this splicing SNP [135].

Given the differences in the abundance of the SNPs across different ethnic/racial groups (e.g., rs12459419 (C > T) is more abundant in European ancestry [variant allele frequency = 0.32] and less in African ancestry [variant allele frequency = 0.13], whereas rs1803254 (G > C) and rs61736475 (T > C) are more abundant in African (variant allele frequency = 0.32 and 0.27) versus European ancestry (variant allele frequency = 0.16 and 0.14), a composite *CD33* SNP score based on the 6 SNPs is more global representation of *CD33* genetic variation [133]. Therefore, the *CD33* 6 SNP score holds the potential to predict outcomes across different ethnic groups rather than limiting assessment of GO efficacy to one single SNP. The SNP scoring system is especially promising as patients with scores <0 showed no benefit from adding GO to the standard chemotherapy while patients with scores ≥0 showed significant improvement with the addition of GO to chemotherapy [133]. While not yet a part of official U.S. FDA dosing recommendations, *CD33* splicing SNP or the CD33 6 SNP score in conjunction with other factors are under active investigation and being utilized at selected centers to guide treatment decisions for the use of GO to treat AML.

The antileukemic activity of GO is also dependent upon calicheamicin abundance and calicheamicin-induced DNA damage. ABCB1, also known as PgP or MDR1 has been implicated in cellular efflux of calicheamicin. Interestingly, in patients treated with GO in the AAML0531 trial, the presence of a C > T change at a SNP within *ABCB1* (i.e., rs1045642), the variant T-allele (CT/TT, genotypes) demonstrated was associated with better event free survival and lower risk of relapse as compared to patients with the wild-type CC genotype [136]. In vitro evaluation confirmed the impact of the rs1045642 T allele on calicheamicin-induced DNA damage and cell viability [136]. With respect to the impact of DNA damage response (DDR) pathway genes on the clinical utility of gemtuzumab, one study focused on gene expression levels and a developed a 10-gene expression score referred to as CalDDR-GEx10. High CalDDR-GEx10 score significantly associated with clinical outcome in pediatric AML patients from two pediatric AML trials (AAML03P1 and AAML0531) when they were treated with a GO [137]. In developing the score, the study identified SNPs in DDR pathway genes with significant association with event free survival, risk of relapse, and overall survival in patients treated with ADE+GO but not with the standard ADE group. Further, using a multi-SNP predictive modeling approach, the study created a 7 SNP DDR_PGx7 score, with SNPs associated with worse outcome with negative genotype score and those with better outcome as positive score. Sum of all the 7 SNPs was used to derive DDR_PGx7 score. The results showed that patients with low DDR_PGx7 score (0) experienced significantly worse EFS and higher risk of relapse compared to high DDR_PGx7 score (≥0) when treated with ADE+GO. However, the score was not predictive of outcome in patients treated with standard ADE only. Although the clinical utility of the implementation of these more complex scoring systems requires replication, these results suggest that the underlying pharmacogenomics of multiple SNPs influence the efficacy of GO and could assist in determining which patients are most likely to benefit from its addition within the AML therapeutic regimens [138].

Conclusion

Overall, this chapter provides a summary of recent pharmacogenomic studies and how a patient's genomic landscape impacts response to treatment and outcomes in childhood ALL and AML. Advances in ALL pharmacogenomics have come a long way with clinical implementation of *TPMT* and *NUDT15* actionable genotyping for making treatment decisions, in addition to multiple studies assessing genetic factors that influence response to GO. Additional work is needed to discover and support other pharmacogenomic factors that influence therapeutic response in pediatric leukemia prior to incorporation into clinical decision guidelines.

References

1. Yates LR, Campbell PJ. Evolution of the cancer genome. Nat Rev Genet. 2012;13:795–806. https://doi.org/10.1038/nrg3317.
2. Stratton MR, Campbell PJ, Futreal PA. The cancer genome. Nature. 2009;458:719–24. https://doi.org/10.1038/nature07943.
3. U.S. Food and Drug Administration, 2026. https://www.fda.gov/drugs/science-and-research-drugs/table-pharmacogenomic-biomarkers-drug-labeling. Accessed May 05, 2026.
4. Pirmohamed M. Pharmacogenomics: current status and future perspectives. Nat Rev Genet. 2023;24:350–62. https://doi.org/10.1038/s41576-022-00572-8.
5. Goldstein DB, Tate SK, Sisodiya SM. Pharmacogenetics goes genomic. Nat Rev Genet. 2003;4:937–47. https://doi.org/10.1038/nrg1229.
6. Hunger SP, Mullighan CG. Acute lymphoblastic leukemia in children. N Engl J Med. 2015;373:1541–52. https://doi.org/10.1056/NEJMra1400972.
7. Tran TH, Hunger SP. The genomic landscape of pediatric acute lymphoblastic leukemia and precision medicine opportunities. Semin Cancer Biol. 2022;84:144–52. https://doi.org/10.1016/j.semcancer.2020.10.013.
8. Lee SHR, Yang JJ. Pharmacogenomics in acute lymphoblastic leukemia. Best Pract Res Clin Haematol. 2017;30:229–36. https://doi.org/10.1016/j.beha.2017.07.007.
9. Weinshilboum R. Inheritance and drug response. N Engl J Med. 2003;348:529–37. https://doi.org/10.1056/NEJMra020021.
10. Evans WE. Pharmacogenetics of thiopurine S-methyltransferase and thiopurine therapy. Ther Drug Monit. 2004;26:186–91. https://doi.org/10.1097/00007691-200404000-00018.
11. Schaeffeler E, et al. Comprehensive analysis of thiopurine S-methyltransferase phenotype-genotype correlation in a large population of German-Caucasians and identification of novel TPMT variants. Pharmacogenetics. 2004;14:407–17. https://doi.org/10.1097/01.fpc.0000114745.08559.db.
12. Yates CR, et al. Molecular diagnosis of thiopurine S-methyltransferase deficiency: genetic basis for azathioprine and mercaptopurine intolerance. Ann Intern Med. 1997;126:608–14. https://doi.org/10.7326/0003-4819-126-8-199704150-00003.
13. Walker GJ, et al. Association of genetic variants in NUDT15 with thiopurine-induced myelosuppression in patients with inflammatory bowel disease. JAMA. 2019;321:773–85. https://doi.org/10.1001/jama.2019.0709.
14. Yang JJ, et al. Inherited NUDT15 variant is a genetic determinant of mercaptopurine intolerance in children with acute lymphoblastic leukemia. J Clin Oncol. 2015;33:1235–42. https://doi.org/10.1200/JCO.2014.59.4671.
15. Yang SK, et al. A common missense variant in NUDT15 confers susceptibility to thiopurine-induced leukopenia. Nat Genet. 2014;46:1017–20. https://doi.org/10.1038/ng.3060.
16. Tanaka Y, Saito Y. Importance of NUDT15 polymorphisms in thiopurine treatments. J Pers Med. 2021;11(8):778. https://doi.org/10.3390/jpm11080778.
17. Moyer AM. NUDT15: a bench to bedside success story. Clin Biochem. 2021;92:1–8. https://doi.org/10.1016/j.clinbiochem.2021.02.007.
18. Matsuoka K. NUDT15 gene variants and thiopurine-induced leukopenia in patients with inflammatory bowel disease. Intest Res. 2020;18:275–81. https://doi.org/10.5217/ir.2020.00002.
19. Singh M, Bhatia P, Khera S, Trehan A. Emerging role of NUDT15 polymorphisms in 6-mercaptopurine metabolism and dose related toxicity in acute lymphoblastic leukaemia. Leuk Res. 2017;62:17–22. https://doi.org/10.1016/j.leukres.2017.09.012.
20. Buaboonnam J, et al. Effect of NUDT15 on incidence of neutropenia in children with acute lymphoblastic leukemia. Pediatr Int. 2019;61:754–8. https://doi.org/10.1111/ped.13905.
21. Fei X, et al. NUDT15 R139C variants increase the risk of azathioprine-induced leukopenia in Chinese autoimmune patients. Front Pharmacol. 2018;9:460. https://doi.org/10.3389/fphar.2018.00460.

22. Zhang AL, et al. Association of NUDT15 c.415C>T allele and thiopurine-induced leukocytopenia in Asians: a systematic review and meta-analysis. Ir J Med Sci. 2018;187:145–53. https://doi.org/10.1007/s11845-017-1608-x.
23. Yin D, et al. Impact of NUDT15 polymorphisms on thiopurines-induced myelotoxicity and thiopurines tolerance dose. Oncotarget. 2017;8:13575–85. https://doi.org/10.18632/oncotarget.14594.
24. Khoo XH, et al. Nudix hydroxylase 15 mutations strongly predict thiopurine-induced leukopenia across different Asian ethnicities: implications for screening in a diverse population. Front Med (Lausanne). 2022;9:880937. https://doi.org/10.3389/fmed.2022.880937.
25. Wang CW, et al. Implementation of NUDT15 genotyping to prevent azathioprine-induced leukopenia for patients with autoimmune disorders in Chinese population. Clin Pharmacol Ther. 2022;112(5):1079–87. https://doi.org/10.1002/cpt.2716.
26. Poon KS, Imran IIB, Chew SK, Tan P, Tan KM. A direct sequencing assay for pharmacogenetic testing of thiopurine-intolerant NUDT15 alleles in an Asian population. BMC Res Notes. 2022;15:148. https://doi.org/10.1186/s13104-021-05821-3.
27. Kato M. NUDT15: a major determinant of thiopurine sensitivity in Asians. Pediatr Int. 2021;63:748–9. https://doi.org/10.1111/ped.14558.
28. Jena A, et al. Prevalence of polymorphisms in thiopurine metabolism and association with adverse outcomes: a South Asian region-specific systematic review and meta-analysis. Expert Rev Clin Pharmacol. 2021;14:491–501. https://doi.org/10.1080/17512433.2021.1900729.
29. Bae J, Choe BH, Kang B. Prevention of thiopurine-induced early leukopenia in a Korean pediatric patient with Crohn's disease who turned out to possess homozygous mutations in NUDT15 R139C. Yeungnam Univ J Med. 2020;37:332–6. https://doi.org/10.12701/yujm.2020.00178.
30. Puangpetch A, et al. NUDT15 genetic variants are related to thiopurine-induced neutropenia in Thai children with acute lymphoblastic leukemia. Pharmacogenomics. 2020;21:403–10. https://doi.org/10.2217/pgs-2019-0177.
31. Kakuta Y, et al. NUDT15 codon 139 is the best pharmacogenetic marker for predicting thiopurine-induced severe adverse events in Japanese patients with inflammatory bowel disease: a multicenter study. J Gastroenterol. 2018;53:1065–78. https://doi.org/10.1007/s00535-018-1486-7.
32. Banerjee R, Raghunathan N. Editorial: a paradigm shift in NUDT15 assessment-towards predictive and personalised medicine in Crohn's disease? Aliment Pharmacol Ther. 2022;55:740–1. https://doi.org/10.1111/apt.16798.
33. Bharti N, Banerjee R, Achalere A, Kasibhatla SM, Joshi R. Genetic diversity of 'Very Important Pharmacogenes' in two South-Asian populations. PeerJ. 2021;9:e12294. https://doi.org/10.7717/peerj.12294.
34. Devasia AJ, Illangeswaran RSS, Raj IX, George B, Balasubramanian P. NUDT15 polymorphism explains serious toxicity to azathioprine in Indian patients with chronic immune thrombocytopenia and autoimmune hemolytic anemia: a case series. Drug Metab Pers Ther. 2020;35 https://doi.org/10.1515/dmpt-2020-0128.
35. Grover N, et al. TPMT and NUDT15 polymorphisms in thiopurine induced leucopenia in inflammatory bowel disease: a prospective study from India. BMC Gastroenterol. 2021;21:327. https://doi.org/10.1186/s12876-021-01900-8.
36. Khera S, et al. Prevalence of TPMT, ITPA and NUDT 15 genetic polymorphisms and their relation to 6MP toxicity in north Indian children with acute lymphoblastic leukemia. Cancer Chemother Pharmacol. 2019;83:341–8. https://doi.org/10.1007/s00280-018-3732-3.
37. Kodidela S, et al. Association of NUDT15*3 and FPGS 2572C>T variants with the risk of early hematologic toxicity during 6-MP and low-dose methotrexate-based maintenance therapy in Indian patients with acute lymphoblastic leukemia. Genes (Basel). 2020;11:594. https://doi.org/10.3390/genes11060594.
38. Naushad SM, Janaki Ramaiah M, Kutala VK, Hussain T, Alrokayan SA. Pharmacogenetic determinants of thiopurines in an Indian cohort. Pharmacol Rep. 2021;73:278–87. https://doi.org/10.1007/s43440-020-00158-3.

39. Pai AA, et al. NUDT15 c.415C>T polymorphism predicts 6-MP induced early myelotoxicity in patients with acute lymphoblastic leukemia undergoing maintenance therapy. Pharmgenomics Pers Med. 2021;14:1303–13. https://doi.org/10.2147/PGPM.S325813.
40. Ramalingam R, et al. Pharmacogenetic evaluation of 6-mercaptopurine-mediated toxicity in pediatric acute lymphoblastic leukemia patients from a South Indian population. Pharmacogenomics. 2021;22:401–11. https://doi.org/10.2217/pgs-2020-0193.
41. Shah SAV, Paradkar MU, Desai DC, Ashavaid TF. Preemptive NUDT15 genotyping: redefining the management of patients with thiopurine-induced toxicity. Drug Metab Pers Ther. 2018;33:57–60. https://doi.org/10.1515/dmpt-2017-0038.
42. Shingare A, Dhope N, Bahadur MM. Novel risk factor for valganciclovir toxicity-NUDT15 genetic variant. Transpl Infect Dis. 2022;24:e13799. https://doi.org/10.1111/tid.13799.
43. Suiter CC, et al. Massively parallel variant characterization identifies NUDT15 alleles associated with thiopurine toxicity. Proc Natl Acad Sci USA. 2020;117:5394–401. https://doi.org/10.1073/pnas.1915680117.
44. Yadav A, et al. Fatal thiopurine toxicity: pre-emptive testing of NUDT15 415C>T polymorphism may be life saving in South Asian population. Drug Metab Pers Ther. 2021;36:351–2. https://doi.org/10.1515/dmpt-2021-0120.
45. Shah SA, Paradkar M, Desai D, Ashavaid TF. Nucleoside diphosphate-linked moiety X-type motif 15 C415T variant as a predictor for thiopurine-induced toxicity in Indian patients. J Gastroenterol Hepatol. 2017;32:620–4. https://doi.org/10.1111/jgh.13494.
46. Relling MV, et al. Clinical Pharmacogenetics Implementation Consortium guidelines for thiopurine methyltransferase genotype and thiopurine dosing. Clin Pharmacol Ther. 2011;89:387–91. https://doi.org/10.1038/clpt.2010.320.
47. Relling MV, et al. Clinical Pharmacogenetics Implementation Consortium guidelines for thiopurine methyltransferase genotype and thiopurine dosing: 2013 update. Clin Pharmacol Ther. 2013;93:324–5. https://doi.org/10.1038/clpt.2013.4.
48. Relling MV, et al. Clinical Pharmacogenetics Implementation Consortium guideline for thiopurine dosing based on TPMT and NUDT15 genotypes: 2018 update. Clin Pharmacol Ther. 2019;105:1095–105. https://doi.org/10.1002/cpt.1304.
49. Abaji R, Krajinovic M. Pharmacogenetics of asparaginase in acute lymphoblastic leukemia. Cancer Drug Resist. 2019;2:242–55. https://doi.org/10.20517/cdr.2018.24.
50. Douer D, Gokbuget N, Stock W, Boissel N. Optimizing use of L-asparaginase-based treatment of adults with acute lymphoblastic leukemia. Blood Rev. 2022;53:100908. https://doi.org/10.1016/j.blre.2021.100908.
51. Lopez-Santillan M, Iparraguirre L, Martin-Guerrero I, Gutierrez-Camino A, Garcia-Orad A. Review of pharmacogenetics studies of L-asparaginase hypersensitivity in acute lymphoblastic leukemia points to variants in the GRIA1 gene. Drug Metab Pers Ther. 2017;32:1–9. https://doi.org/10.1515/dmpt-2016-0033.
52. Mei L, et al. Pharmacogenetics predictive of response and toxicity in acute lymphoblastic leukemia therapy. Blood Rev. 2015;29:243–9. https://doi.org/10.1016/j.blre.2015.01.001.
53. Bargal SA, et al. Genome-wide association analysis identifies SNPs predictive of. Oncotarget. 2018;9:34859–75. https://doi.org/10.18632/oncotarget.26163.
54. Liu Y, et al. Class II human leukocyte antigen variants associate with risk of pegaspargase hypersensitivity. Clin Pharmacol Ther. 2021;110:794–802. https://doi.org/10.1002/cpt.2241.
55. Fernandez CA, et al. HLA-DRB1*07:01 is associated with a higher risk of asparaginase allergies. Blood. 2014;124:1266–76. https://doi.org/10.1182/blood-2014-03-563742.
56. Hojfeldt SG, et al. Genetic predisposition to PEG-asparaginase hypersensitivity in children treated according to NOPHO ALL2008. Br J Haematol. 2019;184:405–17. https://doi.org/10.1111/bjh.15660.
57. Chen SH, et al. Genetic variations in GRIA1 on chromosome 5q33 related to asparaginase hypersensitivity. Clin Pharmacol Ther. 2010;88:191–6. https://doi.org/10.1038/clpt.2010.94.
58. Gagne V, et al. HLA alleles associated with asparaginase hypersensitivity in childhood ALL: a report from the DFCI Consortium. Pharmacogenomics. 2020;21:541–7. https://doi.org/10.2217/pgs-2019-0195.

59. Kutszegi N, et al. Two tagging single-nucleotide polymorphisms to capture HLA-DRB1*07:01-DQA1*02:01-DQB1*02:02 haplotype associated with asparaginase hypersensitivity. Br J Clin Pharmacol. 2021;87:2542–8. https://doi.org/10.1111/bcp.14664.
60. Kutszegi N, et al. HLA-DRB1*07:01-HLA-DQA1*02:01-HLA-DQB1*02:02 haplotype is associated with a high risk of asparaginase hypersensitivity in acute lymphoblastic leukemia. Haematologica. 2017;102:1578–86. https://doi.org/10.3324/haematol.2017.168211.
61. Abraham IE, et al. Impact of race on outcomes in intermediate-risk acute myeloid leukemia. Cancer Causes Control. 2021;32:705–12. https://doi.org/10.1007/s10552-021-01422-4.
62. Pastorczak A, et al. Asparagine synthetase (ASNS) gene polymorphism is associated with the outcome of childhood acute lymphoblastic leukemia by affecting early response to treatment. Leuk Res. 2014;38:180–3. https://doi.org/10.1016/j.leukres.2013.10.027.
63. Kloos RQH, Mathot R, Pieters R, van der Sluis IM. Individualized dosing guidelines for PEGasparaginase and factors influencing the clearance: a population pharmacokinetic model. Haematologica. 2021;106:1254–61. https://doi.org/10.3324/haematol.2019.242289.
64. Maese L, et al. Recombinant Erwinia asparaginase (JZP458) in ALL/LBL: complete follow-up of the Children's Oncology Group AALL1931 study. Blood Adv. 2025;9:66–77. https://doi.org/10.1182/bloodadvances.2024013346.
65. McCarty K, et al. Higher rates of hypersensitivity reactions to calaspargase compared with pegaspargase: a single center retrospective review. Pediatr Blood Cancer. 2025;72:e31640. https://doi.org/10.1002/pbc.31640.
66. Brigitha LJ, et al. Pharmacokinetics of PEGasparaginase in infants with acute lymphoblastic leukemia. Pharm Res. 2024;41:711–20. https://doi.org/10.1007/s11095-024-03693-3.
67. Dam M, et al. Increase in peg-asparaginase clearance as a predictor for inactivation in patients with acute lymphoblastic leukemia. Leukemia. 2024;38:712–9. https://doi.org/10.1038/s41375-024-02153-6.
68. Shimonodan H, et al. Silent inactivation of asparaginase in Japan: results of the prospective ALL-ASP19 trial. Int J Hematol. 2024;120:725–34. https://doi.org/10.1007/s12185-024-03856-3.
69. Zarou MM, Vazquez A, Vignir Helgason G. Folate metabolism: a re-emerging therapeutic target in haematological cancers. Leukemia. 2021;35:1539–51. https://doi.org/10.1038/s41375-021-01189-2.
70. Schulte RR, et al. Effect of SLCO1B1 polymorphisms on high-dose methotrexate clearance in children and young adults with leukemia and lymphoblastic lymphoma. Clin Transl Sci. 2021;14:343–53. https://doi.org/10.1111/cts.12879.
71. Ramsey LB, et al. Genome-wide study of methotrexate clearance replicates SLCO1B1. Blood. 2013;121:898–904. https://doi.org/10.1182/blood-2012-08-452839.
72. Ramsey LB, et al. Rare versus common variants in pharmacogenetics: SLCO1B1 variation and methotrexate disposition. Genome Res. 2012;22:1–8. https://doi.org/10.1101/gr.129668.111.
73. Shahrure ZM, et al. SLCO1B1 gene polymorphisms (rs2306283 and rs4149056) and statin-induced myopathy in Jordanian diabetics. Curr Rev Clin Exp Pharmacol. 2021;16:281–8. https://doi.org/10.2174/1574884715666200827105612.
74. Liu SG, et al. Polymorphisms in methotrexate transporters and their relationship to plasma methotrexate levels, toxicity of high-dose methotrexate, and outcome of pediatric acute lymphoblastic leukemia. Oncotarget. 2017;8:37761–72. https://doi.org/10.18632/oncotarget.17781.
75. Goricar K, et al. Influence of the folate pathway and transporter polymorphisms on methotrexate treatment outcome in osteosarcoma. Pharmacogenet Genomics. 2014;24:514–21. https://doi.org/10.1097/FPC.0000000000000083.
76. Han JM, et al. Association between SLCO1B1 genetic polymorphisms and bleeding risk in patients treated with edoxaban. Sci Rep. 2023;13:15967. https://doi.org/10.1038/s41598-023-43179-7.

77. Maagdenberg H, et al. Genetic variants associated with methotrexate-induced mucositis in cancer treatment: a systematic review and meta-analysis. Crit Rev Oncol Hematol. 2021;161:103312. https://doi.org/10.1016/j.critrevonc.2021.103312.
78. Taylor ZL, et al. Systematic review of pharmacogenetic factors that influence high-dose methotrexate pharmacokinetics in pediatric malignancies. Cancers (Basel). 2021;13:2837. https://doi.org/10.3390/cancers13112837.
79. Rahmayanti SU, Amalia R, Rusdiana T. Systematic review: genetic polymorphisms in the pharmacokinetics of high-dose methotrexate in pediatric acute lymphoblastic leukemia patients. Cancer Chemother Pharmacol. 2024;94:141–55. https://doi.org/10.1007/s00280-024-04694-0.
80. Yang JJ, et al. Genome-wide interrogation of germline genetic variation associated with treatment response in childhood acute lymphoblastic leukemia. JAMA. 2009;301:393–403. https://doi.org/10.1001/jama.2009.7.
81. Yang JJ, et al. Genome-wide association study identifies germline polymorphisms associated with relapse of childhood acute lymphoblastic leukemia. Blood. 2012;120:4197–204. https://doi.org/10.1182/blood-2012-07-440107.
82. Autry RJ, et al. Integrative genomic analyses reveal mechanisms of glucocorticoid resistance in acute lymphoblastic leukemia. Nat Can. 2020;1:329–44. https://doi.org/10.1038/s43018-020-0037-3.
83. Bergeron BP, et al. Epigenomic profiling of glucocorticoid responses identifies cis-regulatory disruptions impacting steroid resistance in childhood acute lymphoblastic leukemia. Leukemia. 2022;36:2374–83. https://doi.org/10.1038/s41375-022-01685-z.
84. Cancer Facts & Figures 2024. 2024.
85. Key Statistics for Acute Myeloid Leukemia (AML). 2024. https://www.cancer.org/cancer/types/acute-myeloid-leukemia/about/key-statistics.html
86. SEER Cancer Stat Facts: Acute Myeloid Leukemia (AML). 2024. https://seer.cancer.gov/statfacts/html/amyl.html
87. Tierens A, et al. Residual disease detected by flow cytometry is an independent predictor of survival in childhood acute myeloid leukaemia; results of the NOPHO-AML 2004 study. Br J Haematol. 2016;174:600–9. https://doi.org/10.1111/bjh.14093.
88. Gamis AS, et al. Gemtuzumab ozogamicin in children and adolescents with de novo acute myeloid leukemia improves event-free survival by reducing relapse risk: results from the randomized phase III Children's Oncology Group trial AAML0531. J Clin Oncol. 2014;32:3021–32. https://doi.org/10.1200/JCO.2014.55.3628.
89. Rubnitz JE, et al. Minimal residual disease-directed therapy for childhood acute myeloid leukaemia: results of the AML02 multicentre trial. Lancet Oncol. 2010;11:543–52. https://doi.org/10.1016/S1470-2045(10)70090-5.
90. Wells RJ, et al. Mitoxantrone and cytarabine induction, high-dose cytarabine, and etoposide intensification for pediatric patients with relapsed or refractory acute myeloid leukemia: Children's Cancer Group Study 2951. J Clin Oncol. 2003;21:2940–7. https://doi.org/10.1200/JCO.2003.06.128.
91. Dombret H, Gardin C. An update of current treatments for adult acute myeloid leukemia. Blood. 2016;127:53–61. https://doi.org/10.1182/blood-2015-08-604520.
92. Bose P, Vachhani P, Cortes JE. Treatment of relapsed/refractory acute myeloid leukemia. Curr Treat Options in Oncol. 2017;18:17. https://doi.org/10.1007/s11864-017-0456-2.
93. Dohner H, Weisdorf DJ, Bloomfield CD. Acute myeloid leukemia. N Engl J Med. 2015;373:1136–52. https://doi.org/10.1056/NEJMra1406184.
94. Rowe JM, Tallman MS. How I treat acute myeloid leukemia. Blood. 2010;116:3147–56. https://doi.org/10.1182/blood-2010-05-260117.
95. Forsberg M, Konopleva M. AML treatment: conventional chemotherapy and emerging novel agents. Trends Pharmacol Sci. 2024;45:430–48. https://doi.org/10.1016/j.tips.2024.03.005.
96. Issa GC, et al. Menin inhibition with revumenib for KMT2A-rearranged relapsed or refractory acute leukemia (AUGMENT-101). J Clin Oncol. 2025;43:75–84. https://doi.org/10.1200/JCO.24.00826.

97. Kufe DW, Munroe D, Herrick D, Egan E, Spriggs D. Effects of 1-beta-D-arabinofuranosylcytosine incorporation on eukaryotic DNA template function. Mol Pharmacol. 1984;26:128–34.
98. Anderson E, et al. Intracellular cytarabine triphosphate in circulating blasts post-treatment predicts remission status in patients with acute myeloid leukemia. Exp Hematol. 2019;74:13–18 e13. https://doi.org/10.1016/j.exphem.2019.04.005.
99. Plunkett W, et al. Pharmacologically directed ara-C therapy for refractory leukemia. Semin Oncol. 1985;12:20–30.
100. Verschuur AC, et al. Cyclopentenyl cytosine induces apoptosis and increases cytarabine-induced apoptosis in a T-lymphoblastic leukemic cell-line. Leuk Res. 2001;25:891–900. https://doi.org/10.1016/s0145-2126(01)00047-9.
101. Amaki J, et al. Single nucleotide polymorphisms of cytarabine metabolic genes influence clinical outcome in acute myeloid leukemia patients receiving high-dose cytarabine therapy. Int J Hematol. 2015;101:543–53. https://doi.org/10.1007/s12185-015-1766-4.
102. Pounds S, et al. PROMISE: a tool to identify genomic features with a specific biologically interesting pattern of associations with multiple endpoint variables. Bioinformatics. 2009;25:2013–9. https://doi.org/10.1093/bioinformatics/btp357.
103. Kim KI, et al. Combined interaction of multi-locus genetic polymorphisms in cytarabine arabinoside metabolic pathway on clinical outcomes in adult acute myeloid leukaemia (AML) patients. Eur J Cancer. 2013;49:403–10. https://doi.org/10.1016/j.ejca.2012.07.022.
104. Lamba JK, et al. Pharmacogenetics of deoxycytidine kinase: identification and characterization of novel genetic variants. J Pharmacol Exp Ther. 2007;323:935–45. https://doi.org/10.1124/jpet.107.128595.
105. Mitra AK, et al. Genetic variants in cytosolic 5′-nucleotidase II are associated with its expression and cytarabine sensitivity in HapMap cell lines and in patients with acute myeloid leukemia. J Pharmacol Exp Ther. 2011;339:9–23. https://doi.org/10.1124/jpet.111.182873.
106. Lamba JK. Genetic factors influencing cytarabine therapy. Pharmacogenomics. 2009;10:1657–74. https://doi.org/10.2217/pgs.09.118.
107. Lamba JK. Pharmacogenomics of cytarabine in childhood leukemia. Pharmacogenomics. 2011;12:1629–32. https://doi.org/10.2217/pgs.11.148.
108. Di Francia R, et al. Response and toxicity to cytarabine therapy in leukemia and lymphoma: from dose puzzle to pharmacogenomic biomarkers. Cancers (Basel). 2021;13:966. https://doi.org/10.3390/cancers13050966.
109. Emadi A, Karp JE. The clinically relevant pharmacogenomic changes in acute myelogenous leukemia. Pharmacogenomics. 2012;13:1257–69. https://doi.org/10.2217/pgs.12.102.
110. Maring JG, Groen HJ, Wachters FM, Uges DR, de Vries EG. Genetic factors influencing pyrimidine-antagonist chemotherapy. Pharmacogenomics J. 2005;5:226–43. https://doi.org/10.1038/sj.tpj.6500320.
111. Megias-Vericat JE, Martinez-Cuadron D, Solana-Altabella A, Poveda JL, Montesinos P. Systematic review of pharmacogenetics of ABC and SLC transporter genes in acute myeloid leukemia. Pharmaceutics. 2022;14(4):878. https://doi.org/10.3390/pharmaceutics14040878.
112. Megias-Vericat JE, et al. A systematic review and meta-analysis of the impact of WT1 polymorphism rs16754 in the effectiveness of standard chemotherapy in patients with acute myeloid leukemia. Pharmacogenomics J. 2016;16:30–40. https://doi.org/10.1038/tpj.2015.80.
113. Pinto-Merino A, et al. Role of pharmacogenetics in the treatment of acute myeloid leukemia: systematic review and future perspectives. Pharmaceutics. 2022;14:559. https://doi.org/10.3390/pharmaceutics14030559.
114. Serdjebi C, Milano G, Ciccolini J. Role of cytidine deaminase in toxicity and efficacy of nucleosidic analogs. Expert Opin Drug Metab Toxicol. 2015;11:665–72. https://doi.org/10.1517/17425255.2015.985648.
115. Elsayed AH, et al. Polygenic Ara-C response score identifies pediatric patients with acute myeloid leukemia in need of chemotherapy augmentation. J Clin Oncol. 2022;40(7):Jco2101422. https://doi.org/10.1200/jco.21.01422.

116. Marrero RJ, et al. Pharmacogenomic score effectively personalizes treatment of acute myeloid leukemia. Clin Cancer Res. 2024;30:4388–96. https://doi.org/10.1158/1078-0432.CCR-24-0863.
117. Lamba JK, et al. Pharmacogenomics, race, and treatment outcome in pediatric acute myeloid leukemia. JAMA Netw Open. 2024;7:e2411726. https://doi.org/10.1001/jamanetworkopen.2024.11726.
118. Sekeres MA, et al. Differences in prognostic factors and outcomes in African Americans and whites with acute myeloid leukemia. Blood. 2004;103:4036–42. https://doi.org/10.1182/blood-2003-09-3118.
119. Patel MI, Ma Y, Mitchell B, Rhoads KF. How do differences in treatment impact racial and ethnic disparities in acute myeloid leukemia? Cancer Epidemiol Biomarkers Prev. 2015;24:344–9. https://doi.org/10.1158/1055-9965.EPI-14-0963.
120. Brunner AM, et al. Population-based disparities in survival among patients with core-binding factor acute myeloid leukemia: a SEER database analysis. Leuk Res. 2014;38:773–80. https://doi.org/10.1016/j.leukres.2014.04.001.
121. Larkin KT, et al. High early death rates, treatment resistance, and short survival of Black adolescents and young adults with AML. Blood Adv. 2022;6:5570–81. https://doi.org/10.1182/bloodadvances.2022007544.
122. Bernstein ID, et al. Treatment of acute myeloid leukemia cells in vitro with a monoclonal antibody recognizing a myeloid differentiation antigen allows normal progenitor cells to be expressed. J Clin Invest. 1987;79:1153–9. https://doi.org/10.1172/JCI112932.
123. Bross PF, et al. Approval summary: gemtuzumab ozogamicin in relapsed acute myeloid leukemia. Clin Cancer Res. 2001;7:1490–6.
124. Petersdorf SH, et al. A phase 3 study of gemtuzumab ozogamicin during induction and postconsolidation therapy in younger patients with acute myeloid leukemia. Blood. 2013;121:4854–60. https://doi.org/10.1182/blood-2013-01-466706.
125. Hills RK, et al. Addition of gemtuzumab ozogamicin to induction chemotherapy in adult patients with acute myeloid leukaemia: a meta-analysis of individual patient data from randomised controlled trials. Lancet Oncol. 2014;15:986–96. https://doi.org/10.1016/S1470-2045(14)70281-5.
126. Cooper TM, et al. AAML03P1, a pilot study of the safety of gemtuzumab ozogamicin in combination with chemotherapy for newly diagnosed childhood acute myeloid leukemia: a report from the Children's Oncology Group. Cancer. 2012;118:761–9. https://doi.org/10.1002/cncr.26190.
127. Jen EY, et al. FDA approval: gemtuzumab ozogamicin for the treatment of adults with newly diagnosed CD33-positive acute myeloid leukemia. Clin Cancer Res. 2018;24:3242–6. https://doi.org/10.1158/1078-0432.CCR-17-3179.
128. Norsworthy KJ, et al. FDA approval summary: Mylotarg for treatment of patients with relapsed or refractory CD33-positive acute myeloid leukemia. Oncologist. 2018;23(9):1103–8. https://doi.org/10.1634/theoncologist.2017-0604.
129. Pollard JA, et al. CD33 expression and its association with gemtuzumab ozogamicin response: results from the randomized phase III Children's Oncology Group trial AAML0531. J Clin Oncol. 2016;34:747–55. https://doi.org/10.1200/JCO.2015.62.6846.
130. Pollard JA, et al. Correlation of CD33 expression level with disease characteristics and response to gemtuzumab ozogamicin containing chemotherapy in childhood AML. Blood. 2012;119:3705–11. https://doi.org/10.1182/blood-2011-12-398370.
131. Lamba JK, et al. CD33 splicing polymorphism determines gemtuzumab ozogamicin response in de novo acute myeloid leukemia: report from randomized phase III Children's Oncology Group trial AAML0531. J Clin Oncol. 2017;35:2674–82. https://doi.org/10.1200/JCO.2016.71.2513.
132. Papageorgiou I, et al. CCGG deletion (rs201074739) in CD33 results in premature termination codon and complete loss of CD33 expression: another key variant with potential impact on response to CD33-directed agents. Leuk Lymphoma. 2019;60:2287–90. https://doi.org/10.1080/10428194.2019.1569232.

133. Chauhan L, et al. CD33_PGx6_Score predicts gemtuzumab ozogamicin response in childhood acute myeloid leukemia: a report from the Children's Oncology Group. JCO Precis Oncol. 2019;3:PO.18.00387. https://doi.org/10.1200/PO.18.00387.
134. Mortland L, et al. Clinical significance of CD33 nonsynonymous single-nucleotide polymorphisms in pediatric patients with acute myeloid leukemia treated with gemtuzumab-ozogamicin-containing chemotherapy. Clin Cancer Res. 2013;19:1620–7. https://doi.org/10.1158/1078-0432.CCR-12-3115.
135. Pollard JA, et al. Gemtuzumab ozogamicin improves event-free survival and reduces relapse in pediatric KMT2A-rearranged AML: results from the phase III Children's Oncology Group trial AAML0531. J Clin Oncol. 2021;39:3149–60. https://doi.org/10.1200/JCO.20.03048.
136. Rafiee R, et al. ABCB1 SNP predicts outcome in patients with acute myeloid leukemia treated with gemtuzumab ozogamicin: a report from Children's Oncology Group AAML0531 Trial. Blood Cancer J. 2019;9:51. https://doi.org/10.1038/s41408-019-0211-y.
137. Gbadamosi MO, et al. A ten-gene DNA-damage response pathway gene expression signature predicts gemtuzumab ozogamicin response in pediatric AML patients treated on COGAAML0531 and AAML03P1 trials. Leukemia. 2022;36:2022–31. https://doi.org/10.1038/s41375-022-01622-0.
138. Shastri VM, et al. Genetic variation in DNA damage response pathway and response to gemtuzumab ozogamicin in pediatric AML: a report from the Children's Oncology Group. Clin Cancer Res. 2024;31(5):890–8. https://doi.org/10.1158/1078-0432.CCR-23-2073.

Laboratory Screening of Pediatric Leukemia

12

Geling Li

Introduction

Leukemia is the most common cancer in children and one of the leading causes of death in pediatric age. In the United States, approximately 4000 new cases are diagnosed each year. For practical purposes, one in three children with cancer has leukemia [1].

Clinical suspicion plays a pivotal role as a prognostic indicator for the early detection of pediatric leukemia. Including a complete blood count (CBC) in the diagnostic workup for children presenting with symptoms such as anemia, purpura, splenomegaly, non-growth-related bone pain, and prolonged fever unresponsive to standard treatments is highly recommended [2]. Promptly ordering a CBC for children with cytopenia-related symptoms is imperative and should be viewed as a medical urgency. When interpreting CBC values in pediatric patients, it's important to consider age and sex-based variations for an accurate diagnosis [3].

A CBC is a crucial laboratory test that a pediatrician or primary care physician orders to check for leukemia. Blood samples are processed through automated hematology analyzers to generate CBC results, including white blood cell (WBC) differential count if indicated. An automated CBC, also known as a hemogram, usually includes nine essential parameters: WBC count, red blood cell (RBC) count, hemoglobin (Hb), hematocrit (Hct), mean corpuscular volume (MCV), mean corpuscular hemoglobin (MCH), mean corpuscular Hb concentration (MCHC), red cell distribution width (RDW), and platelet count. WBC differential provides additional WBC differential technology and a reagent system to enumerate nucleated

G. Li (✉)
Department of Pathology and Laboratory Medicine, Children's of Alabama, Birmingham, AL, USA

Department of Pathology, University of Alabama at Birmingham, Birmingham, AL, USA
e-mail: geling.li@childrensal.org

W. Li (ed.), *Laboratory Assessments of Pediatric Leukemia*,
https://doi.org/10.1007/978-3-032-26557-9_12

RBCs (nRBCs). CBC technology has advanced from manual count to modern technologies for an accurate automated CBC with WBC differential in a short turnaround time.

In scenarios where blasts are abundant in the peripheral blood, the identification of these blasts in a well-established clinical laboratory is rarely a problem, and the blood sample is usually diagnostic. However, the diagnostic process becomes more complex for patients with scarce or absent blasts in the peripheral blood. This chapter highlights the vital importance of laboratory testing in the early detection of pediatric leukemia, emphasizing the key role of hematology analyzers as an essential initial diagnostic tool.

Hematology Analyzers

Manufacturers produced different models of hematology analyzers for various clinical laboratory needs. Small hematology analyzers are found in small clinics and physician offices and used as backups in hospital and commercial laboratories. They offer a limited test menu, including CBC with WBC and RBC count, Hb level, MCV, and platelet count, and some provide an up to five-part automated WBC differential. They are known for reliability, high-quality results, simple operation, speed (especially in point-of-care testing), low operating expense, and small sample requirements. Throughput, however, usually does not exceed 30 tests per hour. In patients with leukemia or lymphoma, they could provide a "flag" in the presence of abnormal WBCs, blasts, or atypical lymphocytes, which should prompt operators to examine the blood film morphology and treat the results cautiously if suspicious cells are present or refer the sample to a specialized regional center for further evaluation. Midsize hematology systems are used in large clinics and hospitals, offering similar tests with an up to 6-part WBC differential and higher throughput ranging from approximately 50–100 tests per hour. Modern midsize hematology analyzers demonstrate a strong correlation coefficient in the CBC parameters and outstanding comparative flagging performance when evaluated against larger hematology analyzers [4]. Large hematology analyzers are designed for high-volume laboratories with high throughput (>100 tests per hour) and automate every aspect of hematology testing. They interface with a laboratory information system and network with one another, performing complex tasks such as reflex testing and rerun samples, and are capable of rule-based analysis. Some hematology analyzers, including large analyzers, are equipped with microsample capability, which may be especially useful for pediatric patients [5]. Additionally, some hematology analyzers have a low WBC count mode to provide a more precise extended count and an accurate differential when the WBC count is below 500/μL [6], which may be very useful for leukemic patients receiving chemotherapy. Instrument flags generated by the automated hematology analyzers prompt further microscopic morphological review. Over the past two decades, digital imaging coupled with artificial intelligence (AI) has introduced new tools for performing WBC differential.

Technology Evolution of Hematology Analyzers

The CBC count and WBC differential rely on two basic principles: electrical resistance or impedance and optical analysis. The impedance principle, first developed by Coulter in 1949, allows cytometers to count and measure the volume of cells [7]. In 1968, the Coulter Model-S revolutionized hematological laboratories by introducing features sampling valve and automatic correction for coincidence [8, 9]. TOA medical electronics, now operating as Sysmex in Kobe, Japan, utilized a comparable methodology rooted in capacitance measurements instead of resistance to launch their first commercial analyzers. The contemporary use of both low and high frequency currents allows for the examination of the size, composition, and internal structure of different cells. These bi-parametric measurements were first commercially applied by Coulter and Sysmex in the 1980s (Fig. 12.1) [10–14].

The optical method was developed earlier than the impedance by Moldavan back in 1934 [15]. In 1953, the use of dark field analysis and the introduction of sheath flow by Crosland-Taylor significantly advanced relatively accurate cell count [16]. The amplitude of scattered light was collected at a narrow (forward scatter) and greater angles (side scatter) to inform the cell volume and cellular structural complexity, respectively. In the early 1960s, Kamentsky et al. built the first flow cytometer "Rapid Cell Spectrophotometer," that was capable of evaluating cell volume based on scattering and absorbance [17]. In 1974, Technicon (now Siemens, Erlangen, Germany) commercialized these two methods and developed Hemalog D analyzer, which allows for a WBC differential [18].

Adding the capability of detecting a fluorescence signal that captures the lights emitted from internal cellular components that are stained with a fluorescence dye or bound to monoclonal antibodies further enhanced the potential of optical technology. Fluorescence flow cytometry is used by some manufacturers to obtain reticulocyte count, as well as WBC differential or platelet count [19–22]. The ongoing evolution of technology facilitates the accurate and consistent classification of WBCs into seven distinct subpopulations of nucleated cells. These subpopulations encompass neutrophils, lymphocytes, monocytes, eosinophils, basophils, immature granulocytes (which include metamyelocytes, myelocytes, and promyelocytes), as well as nRBCs. Moreover, this technological advancement significantly improves the sensitivity and accuracy in the morphological identification of blasts and

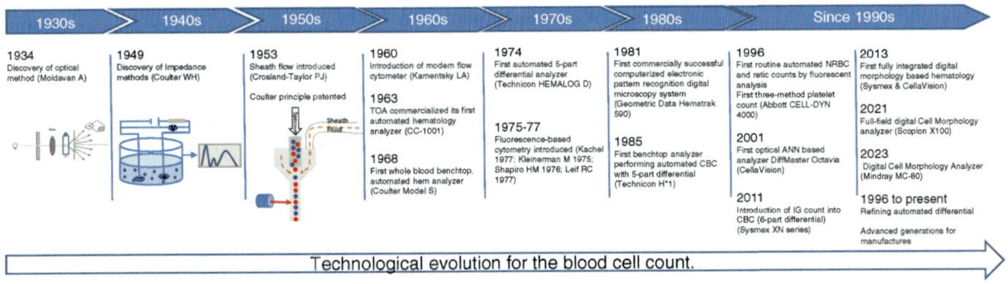

Fig. 12.1 Technology evolution of hematology analyzers

atypical lymphocytes, enhancing diagnostic capabilities. Additionally, it enhances the sensitivity and accuracy of morphological flagging for blasts and atypical lymphocytes.

Being the gold standard for morphological examination of blood smears, conventional manual light microscopy has its limitations, particularly regarding labor intensity and interobserver variability. The introduction of flow-based analyzers in the 1980s significantly advanced the diagnosis of blood samples by enabling the subclassification of WBCs and the detection of abnormalities in WBCs, RBCs, and platelets through instrument flags. Despite these advancements, a morphological review of blood smears remained a necessary step in the diagnostic process. Automated systems like Cellscan, Hematrack, and Cydac were introduced in the 1960s, but they were slow and had limited automation [23–25]. In the 1980s and 1990s, advancements in AI led to the development of artificial neural networks (ANNs) and modern digital cell analyzers [26]. AI enables machines to perform human-like tasks such as problem solving, language comprehension, and image recognition [27]. Machine learning, as a subset of AI, uses statistical methods to enable computers to learn from data [28]. Deep learning is a specialization within machine learning that utilizes algorithms to identify data patterns through multiple layers of processing, establishing ANNs capable of tasks like image and pattern recognition and medical diagnosis [29]. In the early 2000s, CellaVision developed the first optical ANN-based automated digital cell analyzer, DiffMaster Octavia, which located and imaged cells and provided classification[30]. Today, digital cell analyzers, like those from CellaVision, accept continuously loaded, automatically stained slides, locate cells in a blood smear, capture images, and classify them using image analysis software. In a clinical trial (clinicalTrials.gov identifier: NCT04466059), an AI model demonstrated a 95% agreement rate with hematologists' annotations in classifying single-cell images of peripheral blood smears from patients with suspected hematologic neoplasms. Given the dynamic nature of leukemia and the atypical features of various cells, an AI-powered digital cell analyzer offers a more rapid, accurate, and efficient examination of blood cell morphology. This technology would reduce turnaround time for patient diagnosis, minimize interpersonal variation, support remote consultations and quality assurance access, and enhance healthcare delivery [31].

Principle of Operation

Hb Measurement

Hb is a standard diagnostic parameter in blood tests. The International Committee for Standardization in Hematology (ICSH) recommends the cyan-methemoglobin method. Other methods, like Sysmex, use cyanide-free sodium lauryl sulfate (SLS) as a reagent. This reagent breaks down red and white blood cells in the sample and forms a stable, colored complex (SLS-Hb), which is analyzed using a photometric method. A light emitting diode emits monochromatic light, which passes through the mixture. The SLS-Hb complexes absorb the light, and a photosensor measures the absorbance, which is proportional to the Hb concentration of the sample [32].

Auto CBC (Hemogram) Measurement

The impedance procedure is commonly used to determine RBC, WBC, and platelet counts. This method forces cells suspended in an isotonic saline solution through an aperture in a single file. Each cell causes a momentary decrease in electrical current, creating a pulse proportional to the size of the responsible cell. Using flow cytometry with a semiconductor laser, modern hematology analyzers measure WBC count in multiple channels for increased accuracy and automatically correct WBC count in the presence of RBCs. Flow cytometry is also employed in some analyzers to measure platelet count using a specific fluorescence marker that labels platelet organelles, reducing interference from fragmented WBCs and RBCs or microcytic RBCs [33].

WBC Differential Measurement

The current hematology analyzers use technologies such as laser, impedance, radio frequency (RF), direct current (DC), optimized temperatures, volumes, and staining to automate the WBC differential. For instance, Beckman Coulter analyzers in Miami, FL perform impedance-based CBC analysis and use a differential based on volume, conductivity, and scatter (VCS) technology (Fig. 12.2). VCS is the only single-channel analysis that utilizes three independent energy sources (DC, RF, and scatter) to probe approximately 8192 cells simultaneously in their near native state, in an environment as close to the human body as possible and without stains. The latest analyzer, DxH900, employs five angles of laser-light scatter to establish WBC differential count and nRBC enumeration using a flow cell. Modern DataFusion technology incorporates information from multiple modules per run to overcome sample-specific challenges in real time and avoid reruns [34, 35]. Abbott Diagnostics' hematology analyzers use laser optical and multi-angle polarized scattered

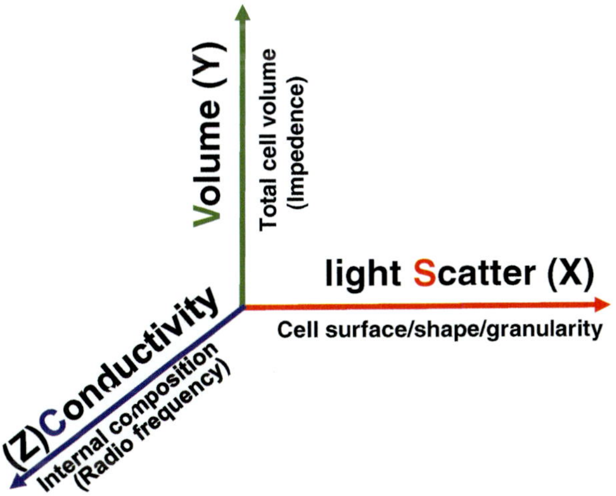

Fig. 12.2 VCS technology utilized by Beckman Coulter analyzers for WBC differential. Three probes = impedance, RF and light scatter-simultaneously analyze each cell, generating X, Y, and Z 3D coordinates (V, C, S) for precise leukocyte differentiation

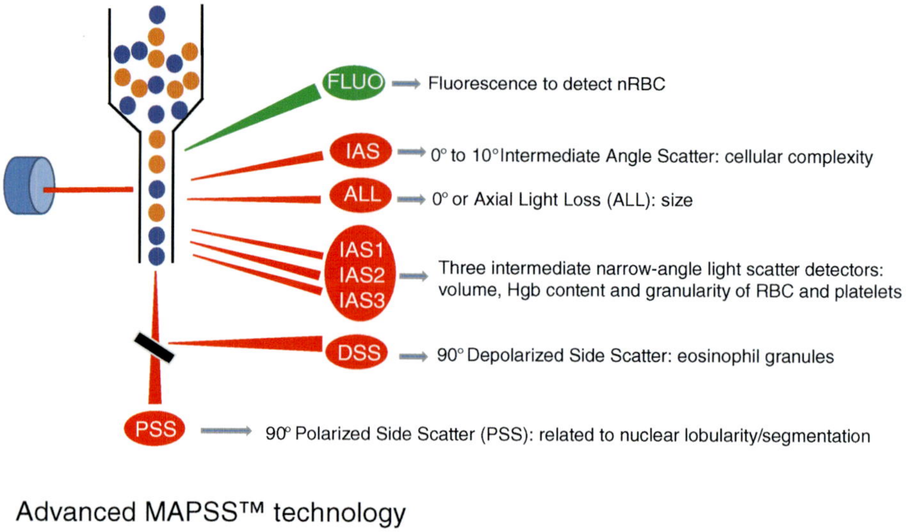

Fig. 12.3 MAPSS™ technology used by Abbott Diagnostics analyzers for WBC differential

separation (MAPSS™) technology for classify WBC subpopulations and provide morphological flagging. The latest Alinity h-series analyzer uses advanced MAPSS™ technology by introducing three additional narrow-angle light scattered detectors and one fluorescent detector to create a unique signal signature of each cell. This allows for the counting of nRBCs and simultaneous analysis of six-part WBC differential including immature granulocytes (Fig. 12.3). Sysmex hematology analyzers use RF/DC to count and classify cell types. Another channel detects immature WBCs by lysing the cytoplasm of normal WBCs while leaving immature WBCs intact to be counted. It performs the WBC differential count by combining three kinds of optical information with the pre-established impedance/IMI methods [36].

The Sysmex analyzers utilize fluorescence flow cytometry with chemical modification of cell membranes to gather combined information on internal complexity (side scatter, SSC), nucleic acid content (fluorescence, SFL), and cell size (forward scatter, FSC) for WBC differential count (Fig. 12.4a). Lysis reagents perforate cell

Fig. 12.4 Technology by Sysmex hematology analyzer. (**a**) Sysmex analyzers use fluorescence intensity of the cells and cell complexity after chemical modification of the cell membrane for optimal WBC differential. The intensity of forward scatter (FSC) indicates the cell volume, while the side scatter (SSC) provides information about the internal cell structure and its content, such as the nucleus and granules. Side fluorescence (SFL) indicates the amount of nucleic acids. Cells with similar physical and chemical properties form a cluster in a graph known as a scattergram, which is depicted in two-axis or, alternatively 3D format (shown here, image courtesy of Sysmex). (**b**) Sysmex integrates CellaVision's ANN technology and digital imaging into its automated hematology workflows to pre-classify WBCs, which are shown in a gallery view of selected cell type's images. (**c**) WPC application differentiates samples initially flagged as "Blasts/Abn Lympho?" by the WBC differential (WDF) channel to two specific flags: "blasts" or "Abn lympho" or removes the flags if no blasts or abnormal lymphocytes were present

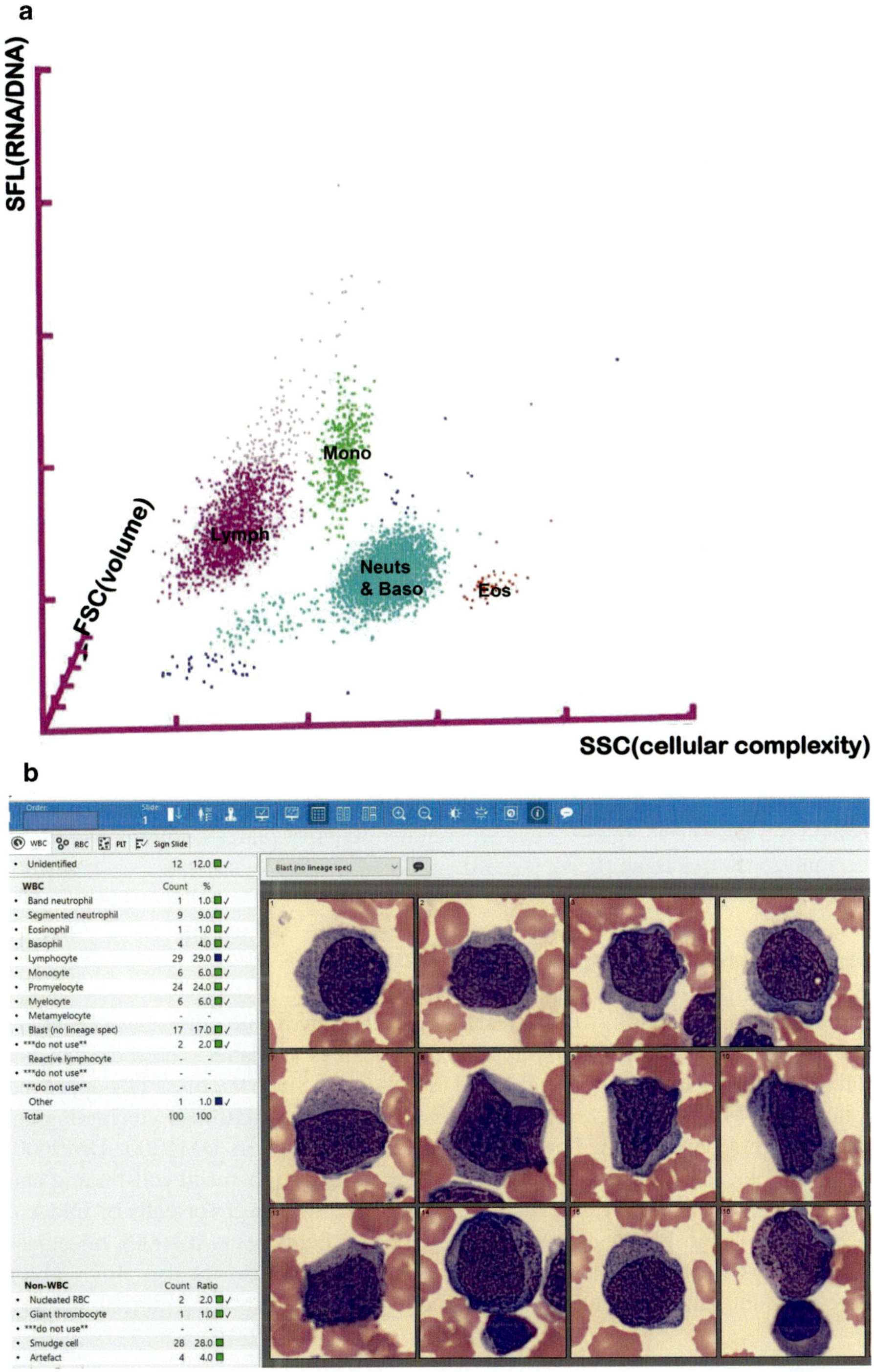
a
SFL(RNA/DNA)
FSC(volume)
SSC(cellular complexity)
Mono
Lymph
Neuts
& Baso
Eos
b
Order:
Slide:
1
WBC
RBC
PLT
Sign Slide
Blast (no lineage spec)
Unidentified 12 12.0
WBC Count %
Band neutrophil 1 1.0
Segmented neutrophil 9 9.0
Eosinophil 1 1.0
Basophil 4 4.0
Lymphocyte 29 29.0
Monocyte 6 6.0
Promyelocyte 24 24.0
Myelocyte 6 6.0
Metamyelocyte - -
Blast (no lineage spec) 17 17.0
***do not use** 2 2.0
Reactive lymphocyte - -
***do not use** - -
***do not use** - -
Other 1 1.0
Total 100 100
Non-WBC Count Ratio
Nucleated RBC 2 2.0
Giant thrombocyte 1 1.0
***do not use** - -
Smudge cell 28 28.0
Artefact 4 4.0

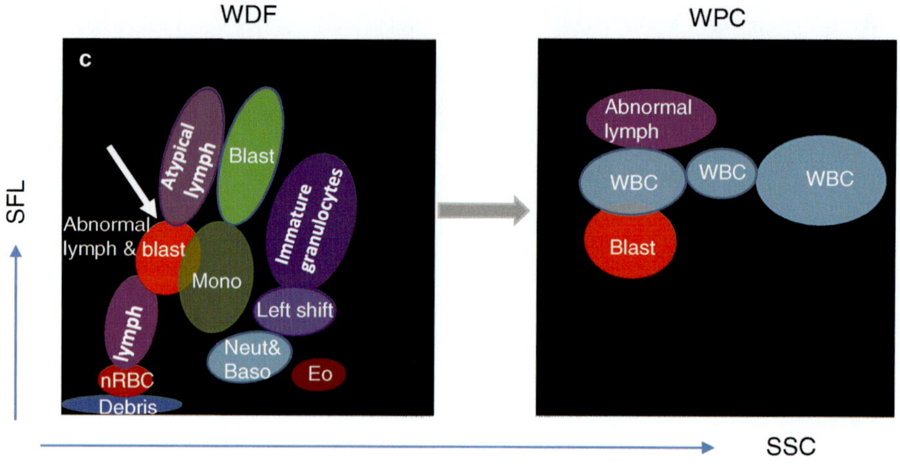

Fig. 12.4 (continued)

membranes at different degree, followed by fluorescent markers labeling the nucleic acids (DNA, RNA) inside the cells. By using lysing reagents with different potency, adjusting incubation time, and applying fluorescence reagents with a higher polymethine concentration for DNA labeling, modern Sysmex analyzers refine WBC differential and flagging capability. In the Platelet-F channel, a fluorescent marker labels the RNA in the platelets, which helps avoid confusion from other cells or debris. This method enhances platelet results, especially in samples with counts below 3000/μL, and minimizes falsely low counts caused by giant platelets or fragmented RBCs. The Platelet-F channel can also identify platelet clumps and alerts the analyzer to this issue [6, 31, 37, 38].

AI-Guided Morphological Examination

The use of AI in hematology in clinical labs is still limited, with only a few U.S. Food and Drug Administration (FDA)-approved AI devices available. These devices are mainly used to examine peripheral blood morphology. Since the first FDA-approved optical ANN-based analyzer by CellaVision in 2001, significant technological advancements have resulted in newer models (CellaVision DM1200, DM9600, DC-1) that incorporate robotics and AI for automating high-speed cell-finding and image acquisition [31]. The device scans slides at low power for cells of interest, then acquires high-power images of representative fields using a 1000x oil objective. An "overview image" corresponding to eight 1000x fields is also provided for platelet count estimation and RBC morphology. After capturing digital images, specialized image analysis software processes and analyzes the data. The software can enhance image quality and perform quantitative measurements. The ANN allows the device to recognize patterns and quickly and efficiently, preclassify WBCs and RBCs into 18 and 22 categories, respectively. The pre-classified cells are typically shown in a gallery view of each cell type's images, including blasts, artifacts, and unclassified cells (Fig. 12.4b). Human operators review the cells on a computer screen, reclassify cells if necessary, and release the results, wherein the software calculates the differential count. The device links multiple analyzers in multiple locations and allows remote review of digital slides.

In 2013, CellaVision and Sysmex codeveloped a product DI-60, the first fully integrated digital cell morphology-based hematology analyzer on the market (Fig. 12.1). DI-60 consists of two Sysmex XN hematology analyzers, the Sysmex slide-making/staining device SP-10, and a CellaVision Digital Cell Analyzer. The DI-60 system utilizes identical software and modified hardware (camera lens system) to the CellaVision DM1200 analyzer. Thus, a single sample placed on this automated device can provide a CBC result, perform a blood smear preparation, and determine cell location and identification. Whole blood samples are mixed and aspirated, and a wedge-type blood smear is prepared using Hct information from the host computer (if available) to determine optimum smearing criteria. Prepared and labeled smears are shuttled to the stain area, where they will then be transferred through the various sections to be stained, rinsed, and dried. The laboratory defines the intervals within each section of the staining process. Completed smears from the staining process are placed into slide magazines for review. The analyzer has a manual mode for processing samples that do not meet rack operation requirements. Some system also allows for pre-made smears to be routed to the staining process. For the first time, digital cell morphology has been successfully integrated with a cell counter and slide preparation device, eliminating the need to manually load the slide for analysis, thus further streamlining the hematology workflow [39, 40].

The Scopio Labs X100 is a recently developed image analyzer that uses innovative technology to capture and analyze the entire field of a blood smear (Fig. 12.1). This is a significant improvement over previous digital cell analyzer, as it allows for the capture of platelet clumps and rare but clinically relevant cells that may be distributed throughout the slide. The X100 utilizes advanced image processing, storage, and deep convolutional learning to classify cells, providing a larger full-field of view corresponding to 1000 high-power fields on a blood smear, from the monolayer to the feathered edge. It can perform a complete smear with a differential in around 8 min. By scanning peripheral blood smear samples at 100× resolution, users can digitally pan or zoom to seamlessly go from the full context of a slide down to individual cells. The larger image obtained by the Scopio system allows users to see where cells of interest are located within the peripheral blood smear. However, it is still a decision support system and human input is required to classify the cells [40, 41].

Point-of-Care (POC) CBC Measurement

The rising need for POC CBC testing has driven the creation of smaller, more advanced analyzers with enhanced capabilities. The Sight OLO analyzer offers a new approach to POC and automated analysis of peripheral blood [42]. Unlike conventional techniques that rely on flow cytometry or stained slides reviewed by a human technologist, this innovative device only requires a small blood sample (27 μL) to be added to a self-sufficient cartridge. Inside the cartridge, blood cells are diluted onto a suspension matrix, settling into a monolayer at the focal plane of an optical receiver. The optical data is then processed through machine learning classification algorithms to produce a five-part WBC differential, providing results in under 10 min [43]. It also generates flags for WBC distributional and morphological abnormalities, including blasts, atypical lymphocytes, nRBCs, and immature granulocytes, and demonstrated 86.5% agreement compared to light microscopy [42]. Clinical studies have shown the clinical usefulness of this device in monitoring WBCs and absolute neutrophil count in outpatient chemotherapy settings and for routine monitoring of patients on clozapine therapy [43]. Implementing the Sight OLO analyzer in an outpatient oncology clinic reduced overall turnaround time and test utilization, including manual smear reviews, without compromising patient safety [44].

The HemoScreen represents a novel advancement in hematology analysis, functioning as a POC device. It employs a unique viscoelastic focusing technique to achieve single-file cell flow using reduced fluid volumes compared to traditional hydrodynamic focusing. This compact tabletop unit is capable of measuring 20 CBC parameters, including a five-part WBC differential and platelet count, with the assistance of AI-powered machine vision [45]. Comparative analyses with centralized hematology analyzers have demonstrated generally acceptable agreement and decreased turnaround time [46]. Its ability to provide laboratory-quality results within 5 min using a small quantity of venous or capillary blood positions it as a viable alternative to centralized hematology analyzers in a post-chemotherapy environment [47]. However, limitations exist, such as potential challenges in identifying abnormal samples with increased blasts, likely stemming from increased sample viscosity that may interfere with the innovative viscoelastic focusing technology during extreme cases of leukocytosis [48].

Table 12.1 summarizes representative hematology analyzers from different vendors [34, 36, 48–56]. Individual manufacturers' websites provide detailed information.

Table 12.1 A summary of representative hematology analyzers from different manufacturers

Manufacturers	Model First launch in USA/ Outside USA	WBC differential	Differential method(s)	Blast sensitivity & specificity	Max. CBC and diff per hour	Minimal sample volume/ Microsample capability
Abbott Diagnostics	Alinity h-series 2023/2017	6-part diff	advanced MAPSS with 7 light scatter and 1 fluorescent detectors	≥1% blast: 38% & 96% ≥5% blasts: 71% & 96% Combined with other WBC diff flags: ≥1% blast: 75% & 96% ≥5% blasts: 100% & 96% [36]	119	≤100 μL/no
Beckman Coulter	DxH 900 2018/2018	5-part diff plus sepsis indicator: MDW	5 angles of light scatter for size and refractive capabilities, direct volume Coulter principle	>1% blast: 47% & 99% >5% blasts: 88% & 99% [49]	300	165 μL/yes
Beckman Coulter	DxH 560 AL 2020/2021	5-part diff	flow cytometry with proprietary dynamic gating		55–60	16.7 μL(ideal for infants and difficult draws)/yes

(continued)

Table 12.1 (continued)

Manufacturers	Model First launch in USA/ Outside USA	WBC differential	Differential method(s)	Blast sensitivity & specificity	Max. CBC and diff per hour	Minimal sample volume/ Microsample capability
Beckman Coulter	DxH slide maker/stainer II 2018/2018(designed to connect with Scopio X100HT digital cell platform)	–	–	No difference in identification and enumeration of blasts, variant lymphocytes compared to manually prepared blood films [50]	140 slides	90 μL/yes
Beckman Coulter	DxH Connected Workcell 2014/2014	5-part diff plus sepsis indicator: MDW	Biophysical characterization with 5 angles of light scatter for size and refractive capabilities, direct volume, conductivity for intracellular and nuclear complexity	–	300	165 μL/yes
CellaVision	CellaVision DC-1 2021/2019	18 WBC Preclassif, 6 RBC morphology and platelet estimate	Automated brightfield microscopy, image analysis, AI	High precision and specificity (>99%) in 12 WBC cell classes, high NPV(>98%), but zero PPV in 7 cell classes (metamyelocytes, myelocytes, promyelocytes, blasts, plasma cells, nRBC, and unidentified cells)[51]	10	–/–

CellaVision	CellaVision DM9600/ DM1200 2004/2003	18 WBC Pre-classif, 22 RBC morphology and platelet estimate	Light microscopy, image analysis, ANN	Misidentify blasts as monocytes in one of 100 leukemic patients Blasts counts lower in preclassif (38.8 ± 25.2%) and similar in classif (49.6 ± 29.1%) compared to manual (46.6 ± 27.4%) [52]	35	–/–
PixCell Medical	HemoScreen 2018/2016	5-part diff (POC)	digital microscopy and computer-vision algorithms	All samples with blasts displaying either flagging or measurement failure [48]	10	40 μL,results in 5 min/yes
Scopio Labs	X100/X100HT with Full-Field Peripheral Blood Smear Application	14 WBC preclassi, 22 RBC morph, platelet estimate	computational photography, image analysis, artificial intelligence	–	15/40	–/–
Siemens Healthineers	Advia 560/560AL Hematology System 2015/2015	5-part diff	Laser-based optical measurement		60	100 μL/yes

(continued)

Table 12.1 (continued)

Manufacturers	Model First launch in USA/ Outside USA	WBC differential	Differential method(s)	Blast sensitivity & specificity	Max. CBC and diff per hour	Minimal sample volume/ Microsample capability
Sight Diagnostics	Sight OLO 2019/2018	5-part diff	Digital microscopy and computer-vision algorithms	93.0% sens and 80.6% spec for WBC abnormalities (blasts, immature granulocytes, nRBC, and atypical lymphocytes) [53]	5	2 drops of blood (27 μL) from finger prick or venous sample for patients 3 months or older; results in <10 min/ yes
Sysmex America	XN-9100 Series 2017/2017	6-part diff	Fluorescent flow cytometry with side fluorescent light, forward-scattered and side-scattered light	>1% blast: 88% & 86% >5% blasts: 100% & 85% [49]	>100	88 μL/yes

Automatic Blast/Abnormal Cell Identification and Reflex to Blood Smear Review

The contemporary hematology analyzer utilizes advanced technology to flag samples requiring morphology review. Some hematology analyzers, such as Sysmex XN and Abbott Affinity h-series, offer the immature granulocyte count, which reduces the number of smears due to immature granulocyte flags [37]. In the Sysmex XN-20 configuration, a new WBC precursor channel (WPC) has been introduced to enhance the detection and separation of blasts and abnormal lymphocytes with greater sensitivity and specificity [36–38, 54, 57].

The WPC application further differentiates samples initially flagged as "Blasts/Abn Lympho?" by the WBC differential (WDF) channel to two specific flags: "blasts" or "Abn lympho" (Fig. 12.4c) or removes the flags if no blasts or abnormal lymphocytes were present. Compared to WDF which employs a lysing regent to perforate cell membrane and utilizes a fluorescent dye to label mostly RNA in the cytoplasm, the WPC channel leverages a chemical reagent that has a greater effect on the membrane lipid and a fluorescent dye targeting DNA in the nucleus, allowing for improved differentiation between blasts and abnormal lymphocytes [58]. Compared to resting mature and immature cells, malignant and activated mature cells have a higher concentration of lipid rafts in their cell membranes and are more susceptible to lysis by reagents. As a result, blasts are less permeable to lysis reagents, which leads to relatively low fluorescence signals and high forward scatter light signals since they mostly remain intact. On the other hand, neoplastic lymphocytes are more easily permeated and possess a higher DNA content due to their rapid proliferation, resulting in increased fluorescence signals. WPC may reduce smear review in a busy lab. A recent study found that WPC reduced false positive flags for blasts and abnormal lymphocytes on neonatal samples by 50% and removed a false positive flag from WDF channel on 46% of samples [59]. Another study showed that WPC channel removed 13% of false positive flags in the WDF channel in adult samples. It also removed 8% of false positive "blasts/Abn lymphocytes" flag from pediatric samples. Besides, WPC reflex testing was highly sensitivity (99%) in detecting blasts and abnormal lymphocytes in adult and pediatric samples [54].

A study comparing Sysmex XN-3000 and Beckman Coulter DxH 800 analyzers found good correlations between both analyzers for specific blood components including neutrophils and lymphocytes ($r > 0.80$). However, there was a limited correlation between basophils and monocytes. The Sysmex XN-3000 showed higher sensitivity in detecting blasts (72.2% in Sysmex vs. 55.5% in DxH800) and atypical lymphocytes (50% vs. 28.5%). However, the specificity of the Sysmex XN-3000 in detecting blasts (67.8% vs. 89.2%) and atypical lymphocytes (64.7% vs. 93.3%) appeared to be lower. The two analyzers were comparable in nRBC detection and when compared to manual microscopy. The Sysmex WPC channel, which allows optimized detection of blast cells, was speculated to be the reason for the higher flagging sensitivity [55]. Another study compared the Sysmex XN20 and the new generation of DxH900, showing a more negligible difference in blast flag sensitivity, although the sample size was smaller. The XN20 equipped with WPC, compared to DxH900 appeared to have better blast flag sensitivity (88.2% in XN20 vs. 47% in DxH900) when the blast cut-off was set at >1%. However, when the blast cut-off was set higher at >5%, both analyzers showed similar flagging sensitivity (100% vs. 87.5%); this was the case with >20% blasts (100% vs. 85.7%) (Table 12.1). As for abnormal lymphocyte detection, flagging sensitivity was 75.8% for Sysmex XN20 and 62.5% for DxH900. When comparing the two analyzers, Sysmex has greater sensitivity but lower specificity [49]. DxH900 analyzer integrates cell morphology parameters (CMP) and cell population data (CPD), which are raw measurement signals that reflect the morphological and functional characteristics of WBC subpopulations in pathological conditions. This integration allows the introduction of a new parameter known as monocyte distribution width (MDW) [49]. MDW measures the standard deviation of the volume of the circulating monocyte population, and it can be reported as part of the routine CBC on the DxH900 analyzer. The MDW value has been proven a reliable biomarker for the early detection of patients at risk of sepsis in the emergency department [60, 61].

Hematology analyzers from other manufactures, such as Abbott Alinity hq, also demonstrated a remarkable sensitivity and specificity in detecting blasts. Specifically, they reported a sensitivity of 75% and a specificity of 96% at a 1% threshold, while achieving 100% of sensitivity when using a 5% blast threshold (Table 12.1) [36]. These findings show that modern hematology analyzers are accurate and efficient systems for screening leukemia in the pediatric population. They are highly sensitive in detecting abnormal cells and feature extensive flagging capabilities, which provides high-volume clinical laboratories with increased confidence. This leads to improved workflow, fewer slide reviews, and faster turnaround times.

In addition to clinical applications, researchers worldwide have been using raw measurement signals, such as CMP and CPD from hematology analyzers, to gain a deeper understanding of cellular morphological changes in various disease states. This approach has also been applied to enhance the sensitivity and specificity of detecting blast and abnormal lymphocyte. Through the development and customization of CPD rules to prompt smear review, studies have demonstrated that a combination of flags and CPD rules and tailored CPD rules outperforms WBC-related flags in detecting low levels of blasts [62]. The implementation of customized CPD rules has showed significant value in aiding the differential diagnosis of macrocytic anemia and myelodysplastic syndrome in various research studies [63]. The research has the potential to facilitate the integration of these technologies within clinical laboratory settings.

Improvement in Morphological Review Using AI-Powered Digital Cell Analyzer

In modern clinics, FDA-approved digital cell analyzers automate most peripheral smear reviews. Analyzer-generated instrument flags prompt a morphology review by an Imaging analyzer, which locates cells in a blood smear, captures images, reclassifies cells using image analysis software, and displays the images on a computer screen. Cell type recognition is based on an ANN. Skilled lab technologists review and reclassify the pre-classified cell population if necessary [64]. CellaVision was an early provider of digital cell analyzers in laboratory hematology for at least 20 years. Current literature has mainly focused on evaluating the specific features, abilities, and limitations of CellaVision.

Data indicates CellaVision accelerates the review process, particularly in samples with fewer abnormal cells. CellaVision saves approximately 10–25% of times than a manual differential, even after manual reclassification [64]. However, CellaVision significantly increases the time needed to count cells in samples with low WBC counts, particularly in cases of severe leukopenia. Although it reduces risks during the analytical phase, laboratories must evaluate their own circumstances regarding turnaround time and sample type. Each lab can establish its own threshold for leukopenia that necessitates a manual review under a microscope [65].

The accuracy of pre-classifying WBCs using CellaVision was found to be particularly high for segmented neutrophils (92.5% accuracy), lymphocytes (96.4%), and monocytes (81.4%) [41, 66]. The reproducibility for basophils was also considered similar, but the accuracy for immature granulocytes, plasma cells, and eosinophils was notably lower. Technologists agreed with the analyzer's classifications between 82% and 89.2% of the time [66, 67]. In a large multi-center academic hospital study, CellaVision demonstrated an accuracy of 93% in adult cancer center, 87.3% in adult general hospital, and 95.4% in children's hospital. Cell types that comprise a lower frequency of the total events, such as blasts, showed lower accuracy at some site. However, blast identification in the pediatric population had excellent positive predictive value and sensitivity with rates of 94.7% and 90.5%, respectively [68].

The CellaVision Advanced RBC Application accurately classified all examined red cell conditions into 22 categories and diagnosed RBC pathology faithfully [69, 70]. It also provides comparable platelet count to automated hematology analyzers and manual platelet count. It saves technologists time, and by scanning the same area of the slide, the result could be more consistent across different samples in clinical practice.

As a newly developed AI-assistant digital cell analyzer, Scopio's Full Field PBS allows for comprehensive screening of the peripheral blood smear with high accuracy for WBCs, RBCs, and platelet count estimation [41]. Blast count and RBC morphology were compatible to manual microscopic review. Platelet clumps were reliably detected in all the samples tested. However, more data and studies are needed for evaluation of its efficiency in identifying blasts and abnormal lymphocytes. The benefits of digital cell analyzer over manual microscopy are summarized in Table 12.2.

Table 12.2 Benefits of digital cell analyzers over manual review

Reduction in turnaround time on WBC differential, platelet count and RBC morphology classification
Reduction in eye fatigue
Reduction in labor costs
Standardization of blood cell differential and morphology
Remote review and sign out, peer review of questionable cells
Digital archiving, easy retrieval of blood film imaging
Education and training, creating cell library, and quality assurance
Locate and label cells on the smear (for certain digital cell analyzer)

Limitation of AI-Assistant Digital Cell Analysis

The pre-classification feature of CellaVision can confirm if there are no blasts in flagged samples. If it detects blasts, an experienced technologist must verify or reclassify the results. However, CellaVision DM96 may produce false negatives, both in pre-classification and after reclassification. Eilertsen et al. compared the results of pre- and reclassifications and inter-smear and technologist variability in blast count. They found a significant difference in blast count between preclassification and reclassification ($P = 0.009$) [71].

The CellaVision system encountered challenges in accurately pre-classifying blasts, particularly in newborns and infants. Although the system demonstrated good sensitivity (94%) in recognizing fewer than 3% of blasts in pediatric samples, it tended to underestimate blast count, with statistical significance found for acute lymphoblastic leukemia (ALL) at $p = 0.03$ and for acute myeloid leukemia (AML) at $p = 0.06$, even after reclassification by the user. The preclassification agreement for ALL was relatively low at 74%, with a significant number of cells misclassified as lymphocytes by the CellaVision system. After user reclassification, the blast count remained close to, but still lower than, the results obtained from manual microscopy. In pediatric samples, newborns exhibited the lowest rates of overall accuracy and classification agreement. The authors suggest that the high misclassification rate may stem from increased cell fragility in young children, as elevated Hct levels can lead to a higher number of damaged cells [69]. Additionally, there are significant differences in the appearance of slides that are manually prepared and stained compared to those made with automated machines [72]. While automated methods provide consistent smears and stains, the operators may not fully appreciate the details of cell shapes and color differences [64, 73]. In pediatric samples with abnormal cells, variations in size, thickness, and color can lead to mistakes in identifying cells. The quality of the digital image may further complicate the appreciation of chromatin structure on screen, which may result in counting too many or too few blast cells [69]. The blasts cells confined to the slide margins will not be scanned [64], which may also explain the underestimation of blast count [71, 73].

Platelet aggregates are frequently observed in the pediatric population. CellaVision cannot be used to exclude analyzer generated "platelet aggregates" flag unless they are in large numbers in the smear or if the user identifies them in the

RBC digitized field. The vast majority of platelet aggregates and fibrin are not recognized by the CellaVision system [69].

Practical Consideration of AI-Assistant Digital Cell Analysis

Automated cell analyzers have largely replaced traditional manual assessments for initial screening and detection of hematological abnormalities. However, the peripheral blood smear remains the most important method for identifying abnormalities that analyzers cannot detect. Most analyzers provide "flags," for conditions, including one for blasts. However, other conditions, such as reactive lymphocytes, atypical lymphocytes, monocytosis, and degenerated cells, can also trigger a blast flag. Additionally, there are instances where analyzers may fail to flag abnormal cells, potentially missing the rare blasts.

In practice, the absence of "blasts" or "abnormal lymphocytes" flags in the CBC analysis by automatic hematology analyzer does not preclude a diagnosis of leukemia. For example, a CBC analysis of a 16-year-old patient who presented to the clinic with fatigue showed pancytopenia with a single flag "neutropenia" by hematology analyzer (Fig. 12.5a). According to our lab-established criteria, samples with "neutropenia" flag will be examined by CellaVision. CellaVision preclassified the WBCs and identified a single atypical lymphocyte (Fig. 12.5b). However, the digital image of the single atypical lymphocyte on CellaVision was equivocal for further classification. A manual smear was made; 4% of blasts were identified under light microscope (Fig. 12.5C). A subsequent bone marrow biopsy confirmed the diagnosis of AML (not shown). In AML with monocytic differentiation, hematology analyzer may generate a "monocytosis" without a "blast" flag (Fig. 12.6a). A reflexed CellaVision review identified monoblasts (Fig. 12.6b, c). In ALL patients, the blasts are often flagged as atypical lymphocytes (reactive lymphocytes) rather than blasts or abnormal lymphocytes (neoplastic lymphocytes) (Fig. 12.7). Therefore, samples with no blast/abnormal lymphocytes flags, but with other flags defined by the laboratory established criteria would be reviewed by morphological analysis.

In the presence of a high percentage of blasts, leukemia is usually diagnosed or highly suspected. However, rare or low levels of blasts can also be found in a variety of conditions aside from leukemia. These include patients with sepsis who present with a leukemoid reaction and those receiving growth factors [74, 75]. A single blast may be seen in a peripheral blood in a healthy individuals or patients with benign hematological disorder and non-neoplastic neoplasms/disorders [76]. Atypical lymphocytes (Type II Downey cells) and, occasionally, abnormal monocytes may be mistaken for blasts [77, 78]. It is important to identify blasts, even when they are present in low numbers. When only a few blasts are detected, a thorough clinical history and assessment of symptoms (such as fever, bone pain, bleeding, and weight loss) should be conducted. A blood count, physical examination (to check for lymphadenopathy or hepatosplenomegaly), and blood chemistry tests (including blood urea, uric acid, lactic dehydrogenase (LDH), liver function, coagulation profiles and immunoglobulin levels) may also be considered. A follow-up CBC with a

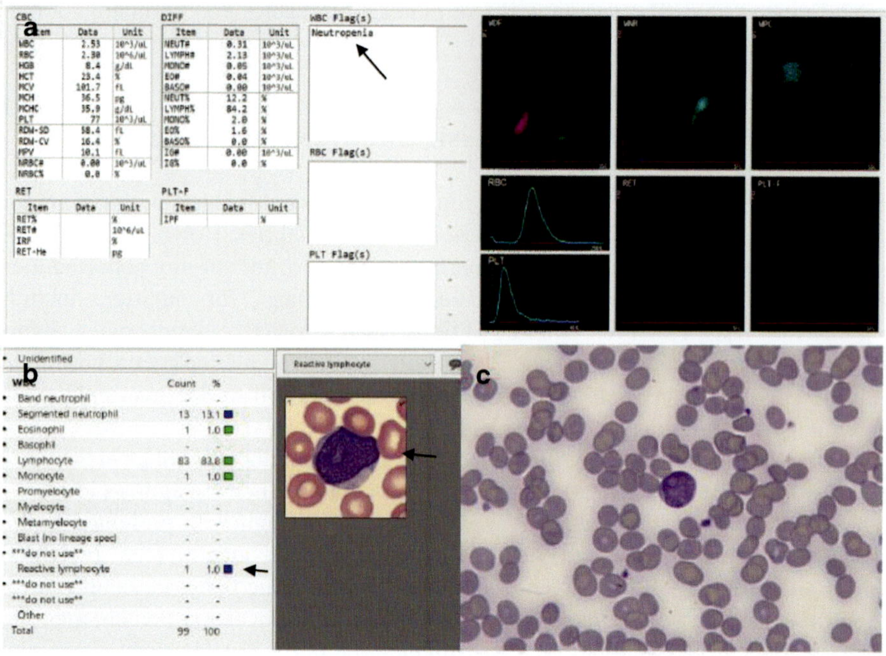

Fig. 12.5 A 16-year-old patient presented with pancytopenia. "Neutropenia" was the only flags prompted by analyzer (**a**). A reflex CellaVision identified a single atypical lymphocyte with a morphology suspicious of a blast by technologists (**b**). According to lab-established criteria, a reflex manual smear was made and a microscopic review showed 4% blasts. A representative blast was shown in the field (**c**)

smear review can provide additional insights. In suspicious cases, flow cytometry might be considered for further evaluation.

Manual Review in the Context of Modern Hematology Analyzer Integrated with Digital Cell Analyzer

Due to limitations of digital cell analyzer, traditional microscopy remains necessary. It is estimated that about 10–20% of all slides require manual microscopic review [64]. Samples from newborns and pediatric patients suspected of having leukemia may particularly necessitate manual microscopy, especially when the number of blasts identified by digital image is low. The same applies to suspected abnormal cells. However, the morphology of pathological cells, such as dysplastic cells, can be assessed using images produced by digital microscopy systems. They typically acquire images of a limited number of cells, commonly set at 100 cells for peripheral blood smears. Therefore, a microscopic review of the slides may be essential to examine a greater number of abnormal cells.

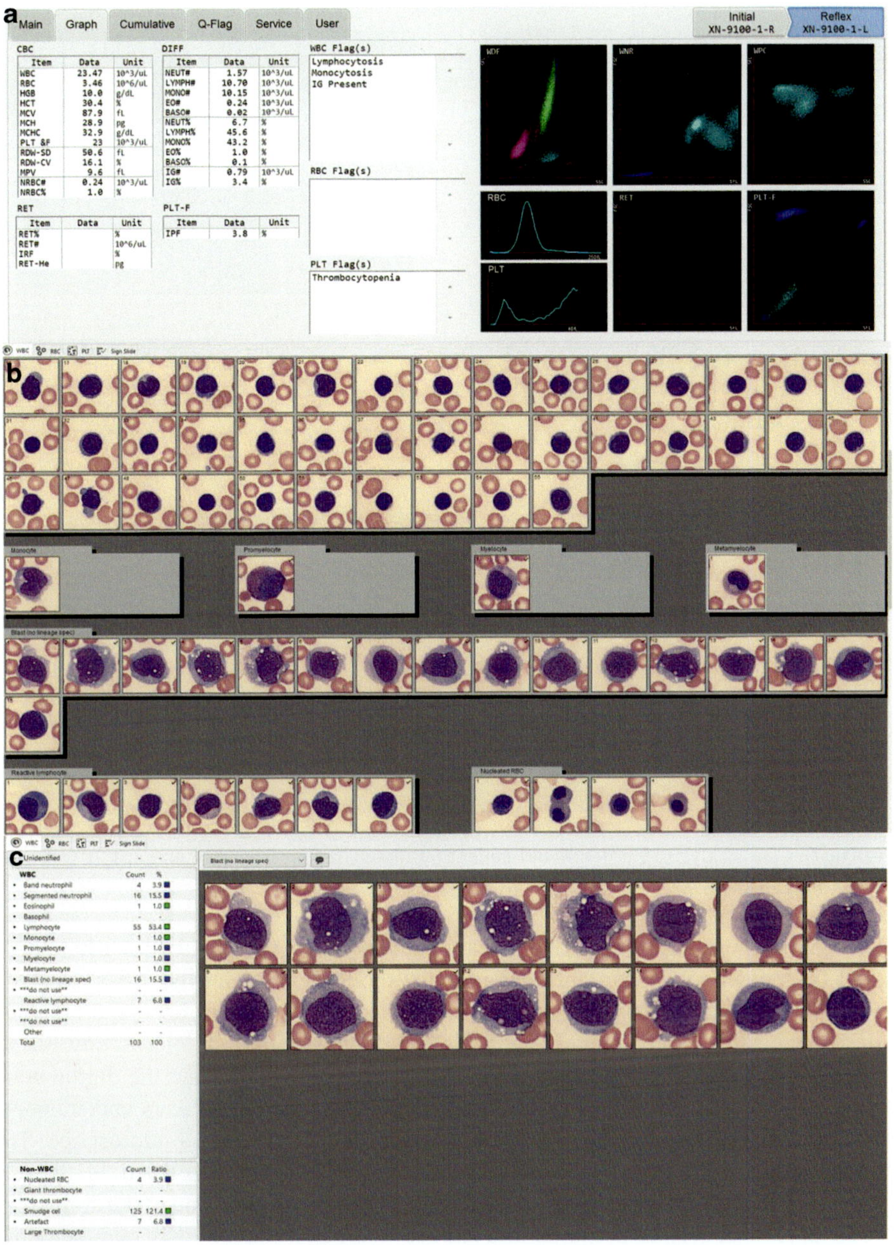

Fig. 12.6 A 2-year-old patient with history of ear infection. CBC analysis triggered "lymphocytosis, monocytosis, immature granulocytes, and thrombocytopenia" flags (**a**). Reflex CellaVision analysis identified monoblasts and left shift myeloid maturation. Monoblasts are shown in full screen view with other WBC subsets (**b**) and are shown in one WBC gallery view (**c**)

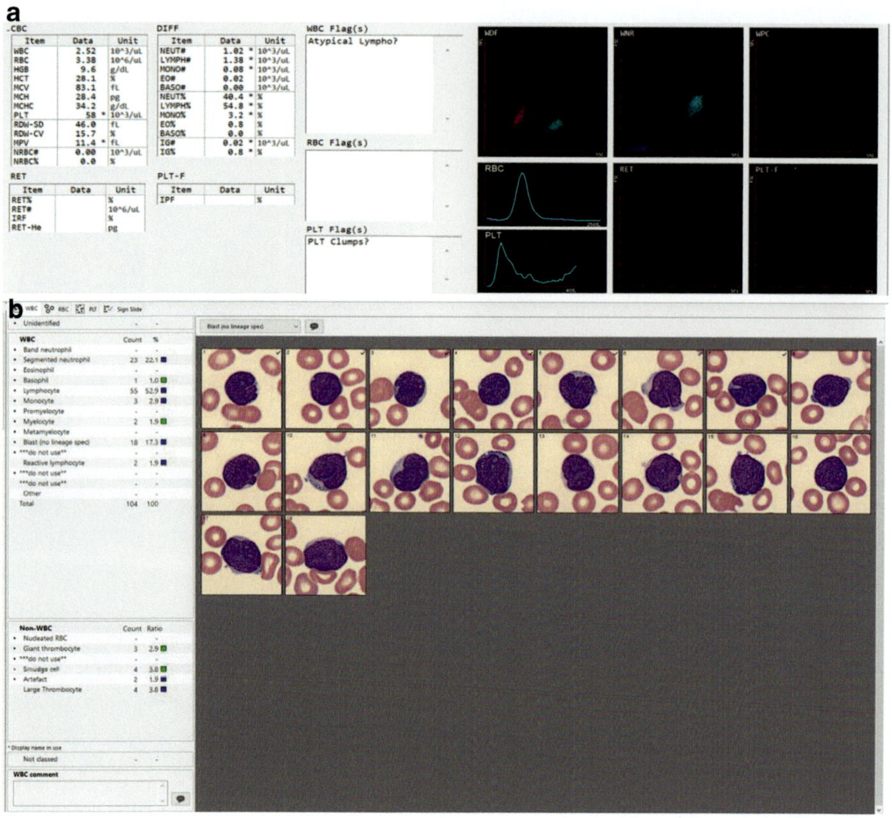

Fig. 12.7 CBC analysis of a 9-year-old patient prompted "atypical lymph" flag (**a**). A reflexed CellaVision morphological review confirmed the blasts (17.3%) (**b**)

In cases where image quality is questionable, such as when examining lymphoblasts from newborns and infants, technologist should re-examine the slides scanned by digital cell analyzer using traditional microscopy. If concerns persist, a manual microscopic slide can be prepared and evaluated again with light microscopy.

If a significant disparity exists between the automated CBC and the digital cell differential, review of slides that are made by automated slide makers and stainers and scanned by digital cell analyzer should be conducted under a microscope. To compare the cell morphology and differentials with those displayed in digital images is imperative. If deemed necessary, technologists may undertake a microscopic review of a slide prepared and stained manually. Pathologists may be consulted if pathology review criteria are met. Specific situations where digital cell analyzer has limitations and a manual microscopic review may be necessary are summarized in Table 12.3, while a pathology review that may be necessary is summarized in Table 12.4. These recommendations are primarily based on scientific studies highlighting the benefits of CellaVision and other automatic digital cell

Table 12.3 A manual microscopic review may be considered

Samples from patients with newly identified blasts, especially blast count by CellaVision being low
Severe cytopenia when no enough cells captured by the digital cell analyzer
Suspected dysplastic cells or other pathological cells such as Pelger-Huet anomaly
Blasts concentrated on feature edge or relatively thick smear area (blast count may be underestimated in the image analyzer) resulting in significant underestimate of blast count
Rare blasts with unclear image
Unclassified cells
RBC agglutinates
Platelet clumps (due to location in feather and lateral edges)

Table 12.4 Pathology review may be considered

CellaVision image with greater than 10% reactive lymph
Any number of newly identified blasts in patients with no prior history of leukemia or history of leukemia in remission
Greater than 1% promyelocytes
Cells classified as "OTHERS"
Microorganisms
If requested by a physician for abnormal morphology

analyzers, along with ICSH guidelines. There measurement have demonstrated improved accuracy in screening leukemia in both adult and pediatric population [64, 79, 80].

Conclusion

Clinical hematology laboratories promptly analyze a high volume of samples while ensuring high accuracy and minimizing false-negative results. Therefore, workflow optimization and increased efficiency are essential indicators of each laboratory's operations [81, 82]. Modern hematology analyzers have improved CBC analysis, mainly by refining WBC subclassification and enhancing flagging efficiency for blasts and abnormal lymphocytes.

Integrating AI-assisted digital cell analyzers has standardized and accelerated the morphology review process. Nevertheless, the expertise of skilled morphologists remains indispensable for the classification of digital images and for the triaging of cases that necessitate manual examination under a light microscope.

Pediatric hematology laboratories encounter unique challenges, primarily due to the analysis of a significant volume of complex and abnormal samples, with an increased percentage of pediatric samples requiring morphology review—especially those originating from newborns and infants. To achieve reliable and efficient leukemia diagnoses, laboratories need to establish flagging criteria tailored to the specific patient population and reviewed regularly. Factors influencing this process include the type of analyzers employed, digital cell or manual microscopic review, the proficiency of laboratory technicians, manufacturer recommendations, and insights drawn from contemporary literature review [79, 82, 83]. This approach aims to balance detecting blasts with reducing the necessity for manual reviews. The ongoing development and enhancement of automated and digital cell analyzers, which offer improved accuracy in cell recognition and leukemia screening, continue to be a pivotal topic of interest in the field.

Disclosures The author has no conflicts of interest or funding to disclose.

References

1. Hutter JJ. Childhood leukemia. Pediatr Rev. 2010;31(6):234–41.
2. Liano OG. The complete blood count in the early diagnosis of acute leukemia in children. Med Univ. 2016;18(73):216–8.
3. Jones PM, Dietzen DJ, Haymond S, Bennett MJ. Pediatric laboratory medicine. New York: McGraw-Hill Education; 2017.
4. Ashley Ortiz JD. Performance comparision of Sysmex Hematology Analyzers XN-550 and XN-10. Sysmex J Int. 2020;30(1):9–15.
5. Chapman D. Hematology analyzers offer new technology and user-friendliness. Lab Med. 2000;31(3):146–50.
6. Seo JY, Lee ST, Kim SH. Performance evaluation of the new hematology analyzer Sysmex XN-series. Int J Lab Hematol. 2015;37(2):155–64.
7. Coulter W. Inventor means for counting particles suspended in a fluid patent 2656508. 1949.
8. Van Dilla MA, Fulwyler MJ, Boone IU. Volume distribution and separation of normal human leucocytes. Proc Soc Exp Biol Med. 1967;125(2):367–70.
9. Gauthier J, Harel P. Human leukocytes: their size distribution and mean corpuscular volume. Can Med Assoc J. 1967;97(13):793–6.
10. Okada T. Development and problem of automated hematology analyzers. Sysmex J Int. 1999;9:52–7.
11. Coulter WH. Inventor signal modulated apparatus for generating and detecting resistive and reactive changes in a modulated current path for particle classification on analysis. 1966.
12. Hoffman RA, Britt WB. Flow-system measurement of cell impedance properties. J Histochem Cytochem. 1979;27(1):234–40.
13. Leif RC, Thomas RA. Electronic cell-volume analysis by use of the AMAC 1 Transducer. Clin Chem. 1973;19(8):853–70.
14. Thomas RA, Yopp TA, Watson BD, Hindman DH, Cameron BF, Leif SB, et al. Combined optical and electronic analysis of cells with the AMAC transducers. J Histochem Cytochem. 1977;25(7):827–35.
15. Moldavan A. Photo-electric technique for the counting of microscopical cells. Science. 1934;80(2069):188–9.
16. Crosland-Taylor PJ. A device for counting small particles suspended in a fluid through a tube. Nature. 1953;171(4340):37–8.
17. Kamentsky LA, Melamed MR, Derman H. Spectrophotometer: new instrument for ultrarapid cell analysis. Science. 1965;150(3696):630–1.
18. Mansberg HP, Saunders AM, Groner W. The Hemalog D white cell differential system. J Histochem Cytochem. 1974;22(7):711–24.
19. Kleinerman M. Inventor differential counting of leukocytes and other cells. 1975.
20. Kachel V, Glossner E, Kordwig E, Ruhenstroth-Bauer G. Fluvo-metricell, a combined cell volume and cell fluorescence analyzer. J Histochem Cytochem. 1977;25(7):804–12.

21. Shapiro HM, Schildkraut ER, Curbelo R, Laird CW, Turner B, Hirschfeld T. Combined blood cell counting and classification with fluorochrome stains and flow instrumentation. J Histochem Cytochem. 1976;24(1):396–401.
22. Leif RC, Thomas RA, Yopp TA, Watson BD, Guarino VR, Hindman DH, et al. Development of instrumentation and fluorochromes for automated multiparameter analysis of cells. Clin Chem. 1977;23(8):1492–8.
23. Preston K. High-resolution leukocyte analyzers: retrospective and prospective. Appl Opt. 1987;26(16):3258–65.
24. Rock WA Jr, Miale JB, Johnson WD. Detection of abnormal cells in white cell differentials: comparison of the HEMATRAK automated system with manual methods. Am J Clin Pathol. 1984;81(2):233–6.
25. Prewitt JM, Mendelsohn ML. The analysis of cell images. Ann N Y Acad Sci. 1966;128(3):1035–53.
26. Lewis JE, Pozdnyakova O. Digital assessment of peripheral blood and bone marrow aspirate smears. Int J Lab Hematol. 2023;45(Suppl 2):50–8.
27. Shouval R, Fein JA, Savani B, Mohty M, Nagler A. Machine learning and artificial intelligence in haematology. Br J Haematol. 2021;192(2):239–50.
28. Wong ANN, He Z, Leung KL, To CCK, Wong CY, Wong SCC, et al. Current developments of artificial intelligence in digital pathology and its future clinical applications in gastrointestinal cancers. Cancers (Basel). 2022;14(15).
29. Allegra A, Tonacci A, Sciaccotta R, Genovese S, Musolino C, Pioggia G, et al. Machine learning and deep learning applications in multiple myeloma diagnosis, prognosis, and treatment selection. Cancers (Basel). 2022;14(3).
30. Cellavision. The history of CellaVision. 21 September 2024. Available from: https://www.cellavision.com/about/history-cellavision.
31. Bowers KA, Nakashima MO. Digital Imaging and AI Pre-classification in Hematology. Clin Lab Med. 2024;44(3):397–408.
32. Brown BA. Hematology: principles and procedures. subsequent ed. Lea & Febiger; 1993.
33. Chabot-Richards DS, George TI. White blood cell counts: reference methodology. Clin Lab Med. 2015;35(1):11–24.
34. Martinez-Iribarren A, Tejedor X, Sala Sanjaume A, Leis A, Dolade Botias M, Morales-Indiano C. Performance evaluation of the new hematology analyzer UniCel DxH 900. Int J Lab Hematol. 2021;43(4):623–31.
35. Coulter B. Instructions for use. UniCel DxH900 Coulter Cellular analysis system and UniCell DxH slidemaker stainer II coulter cellular analysis system. Nyon: Beckman Coulter Eurocenter SA; 2017.
36. Van der Beken Y, Van Dalem A, Van Moer G, Segers E, Damiaens S, Hoffmann J, et al. Performance evaluation of the prototype Abbott Alinity hq hematology analyzer. Int J Lab Hematol. 2019;41(4):448–55.
37. Kim H, Hur M, Choi SG, Oh KM, Moon HW, Yun YM. Comparison of white blood cell counts by WNR, WDF, and WPC channels in Sysmex XN hematology analyzer. Int J Lab Hematol. 2015;37(6):869–75.
38. Schoorl M, Schoorl M, Chevallier M, Elout J, van Pelt J. Flagging performance of the Sysmex XN2000 haematology analyser. Int J Lab Hematol. 2016;38(2):160–6.
39. Kim HN, Hur M, Kim H, Kim SW, Moon HW, Yun YM. Performance of automated digital cell imaging analyzer Sysmex DI-60. Clin Chem Lab Med. 2017;56(1):94–102.
40. Lapic I, Milos M, Dorotic M, Drenski V, Coen Herak D, Rogic D. Analytical validation of white blood cell differential and platelet assessment on the Sysmex DI-60 digital morphology analyzer. Int J Lab Hematol. 2023;45(5):668–77.
41. Katz BZ, Feldman MD, Tessema M, Benisty D, Toles GS, Andre A, et al. Evaluation of Scopio Labs X100 Full Field PBS: the first high-resolution full field viewing of peripheral blood specimens combined with artificial intelligence-based morphological analysis. Int J Lab Hematol. 2021;43(6):1408–16.

42. Bachar N, Benbassat D, Brailovsky D, Eshel Y, Gluck D, Levner D, et al. An artificial intelligence-assisted diagnostic platform for rapid near-patient hematology. Am J Hematol. 2021;96(10):1264–74.
43. Atkins M, McGuire P, Balgobin B, Desouza N, Taylor D. Haematological point of care testing for clozapine monitoring. J Psychiatr Res. 2023;157:66–71.
44. Jatoi A, Jaromin R, Jennings L, Nguyen PL. Using the absolute neutrophil count as a stand-alone test in a hematology/oncology clinic: an abbreviated test can be preferable. Clin Lab Manage Rev. 1998;12(4):256–60.
45. Bransky A, Larsson A, Aardal E, Ben-Yosef Y, Christenson RH. A novel approach to hematology testing at the point of care. J Appl Lab Med. 2021;6(2):532–42.
46. Larsson A, Carlsson L, Karlsson B, Lipcsey M. Rapid testing of red blood cell parameters in primary care patients using HemoScreen point of care instrument. BMC Fam Pract. 2019;20(1):77.
47. Kristian Kur D, Thogersen D, Kjeldsen L, Friis-Hansen L. The HemoScreen hematology point-of-care device is suitable for rapid evaluation of acute leukemia patients. Int J Lab Hematol. 2021;43(1):52–60.
48. Linko-Parvinen AM, Keranen K, Kurvinen K, Tienhaara A. HemoScreen hematology analyzer compared to Sysmex XN for complete blood count, white blood cell differential, and detection of leukocyte abnormalities. EJHaem. 2022;3(4):1126–34.
49. Serrando Querol M, Nieto-Moragas J, Marull Arnall A, Figueras MD, Jimenez-Romero O. Evaluation of the new beckmann coulter analyzer DxH 900 compared to Sysmex XN20: analytical performance and flagging efficiency. Diagnostics (Basel). 2021;11(10).
50. Brown W, Keeney M, Hedley BD. Initial performance evaluation of the UniCel(R) DxH slide maker/stainer Coulter(R) cellular analysis system. Int J Lab Hematol. 2014;36(2):172–83.
51. Lee GH, Yoon S, Nam M, Kim H, Hur M. Performance of digital morphology analyzer CellaVision DC-1. Clin Chem Lab Med. 2023;61(1):133–41.
52. Merino A, Laguna J, Rodriguez-Garcia M, Julian J, Casanova A, Molina A. Performance of the new MC-80 automated digital cell morphology analyser in detection of normal and abnormal blood cells: comparison with the CellaVision DM9600. Int J Lab Hematol. 2024;46(1):72–82.
53. Leite R, Woodcock S, Brady S, Bigsby C, Webber K, Daniel Y. Performance analysis of the compact haematology analyser Sight OLO. Int J Lab Hematol. 2022;44(6):1078–87.
54. Blomme S, Boeckx N, Brusselmans C, Claerhout H, Van Laer C. The integration of Sysmex XN-9100' WPC channel reflex testing in the detection of reactive versus malignant blood samples. Int J Lab Hematol. 2021;43(2):191–8.
55. Genc S, Dervisoglu E, Erdem S, Arslan O, Aktan M, Omer B. Comparison of performance and abnormal cell flagging of two automated hematology analyzers: Sysmex XN 3000 and Beckman Coulter DxH 800. Int J Lab Hematol. 2017;39(6):633–40.
56. Slim CL, Wevers BA, Demmers M, Lakos G, Hoffmann J, Adriaansen HJ, et al. Multicenter performance evaluation of the Abbott Alinity hq hematology analyzer. Clin Chem Lab Med. 2019;57(12):1988–98.
57. today C. Hematology analyzer. CAP today. 2023.
58. Hotton J, Broothaers J, Swaelens C, Cantinieaux B. Performance and abnormal cell flagging comparisons of three automated blood cell counters: cell-Dyn Sapphire, DxH-800, and XN-2000. Am J Clin Pathol. 2013;140(6):845–52.
59. Jones AS, Tailor H, Liesner R, Machin SJ, Briggs CJ. The value of the white precursor cell channel (WPC) on the Sysmex XN-1000 analyser in a specialist paediatric hospital. J Clin Pathol. 2015;68(2):161–5.
60. Crouser ED, Parrillo JE, Seymour C, Angus DC, Bicking K, Tejidor L, et al. Improved early detection of sepsis in the ED with a novel monocyte distribution width biomarker. Chest. 2017;152(3):518–26.
61. Crouser ED, Parrillo JE, Seymour CW, Angus DC, Bicking K, Esguerra VG, et al. Monocyte distribution width: a novel indicator of sepsis-2 and sepsis-3 in high-risk emergency department patients. Crit Care Med. 2019;47(8):1018–25.

62. Kim H, Hur M, Yi JH, Lee GH, Lee S, Moon HW, et al. Detection of blasts using flags and cell population data rules on Beckman Coulter DxH 900 hematology analyzer in patients with hematologic diseases. Clin Chem Lab Med. 2024;62(5):958–66.
63. Di Luise D, Giannotta JA, Ammirabile M, De Zordi V, Torricelli S, Bottalico S, et al. Cell Population Data NE-WX, NE-FSC, LY-Y of Sysmex XN-9000 can provide additional information to differentiate macrocytic anaemia from myelodysplastic syndrome: a preliminary study. Int J Lab Hematol. 2022;44(1):e40–3.
64. Kratz A, Lee SH, Zini G, Riedl JA, Hur M, Machin S, et al. Digital morphology analyzers in hematology: ICSH review and recommendations. Int J Lab Hematol. 2019;41(4):437–47.
65. Nam M, Yoon S, Hur M, Lee GH, Kim H, Park M, et al. Digital morphology analyzer Sysmex DI-60 vs. Manual counting for white blood cell differentials in leukopenic samples: a comparative assessment of risk and turnaround time. Ann Lab Med. 2022;42(4):398–405.
66. Kratz A, Bengtsson HI, Casey JE, Keefe JM, Beatrice GH, Grzybek DY, et al. Performance evaluation of the CellaVision DM96 system: WBC differentials by automated digital image analysis supported by an artificial neural network. Am J Clin Pathol. 2005;124(5):770–81.
67. Briggs C, Longair I, Slavik M, Thwaite K, Mills R, Thavaraja V, et al. Can automated blood film analysis replace the manual differential? An evaluation of the CellaVision DM96 automated image analysis system. Int J Lab Hematol. 2009;31(1):48–60.
68. Rollins-Raval MA, Raval JS, Contis L. Experience with CellaVision DM96 for peripheral blood differentials in a large multi-center academic hospital system. J Pathol Inform. 2012;3:29.
69. Billard M, Lainey E, Armoogum P, Alberti C, Fenneteau O, Da Costa L. Evaluation of the CellaVision DM automated microscope in pediatrics. Int J Lab Hematol. 2010;32(5):530–8.
70. Egele A, Stouten K, van der Heul-Nieuwenhuijsen L, de Bruin L, Teuns R, van Gelder W, et al. Classification of several morphological red blood cell abnormalities by DM96 digital imaging. Int J Lab Hematol. 2016;38(5):e98–e101.
71. Eilertsen H, Henriksson CE, Hagve TA. The use of CellaVision DM96 in the verification of the presence of blasts in samples flagged by the Sysmex XE-5000. Int J Lab Hematol. 2017;39(4):423–8.
72. Kim HN, Hur M, Kim H, Park M, Kim SW, Moon HW, et al. Comparison of three staining methods in the automated digital cell imaging analyzer Sysmex DI-60. Clin Chem Lab Med. 2018;56(12):e280–3.
73. Simson E, Gascon-Lema MG, Brown DL. Performance of automated slidemakers and stainers in a working laboratory environment—routine operation and quality control. Int J Lab Hematol. 2010;32(1 Pt 1):e64–76.
74. Meyerson HJ, Farhi DC, Rosenthal NS. Transient increase in blasts mimicking acute leukemia and progressing myelodysplasia in patients receiving growth factor. Am J Clin Pathol. 1998;109(6):675–81.
75. Sakka V, Tsiodras S, Giamarellos-Bourboulis EJ, Giamarellou H. An update on the etiology and diagnostic evaluation of a leukemoid reaction. Eur J Intern Med. 2006;17(6):394–8.
76. Shuaeb Bhat SS, Hussain S. Single circulating blast in the peripheral blood film in normal individuals and patients of non-neoplastic haematological disorders and non-hematological neoplasms/disorders- a study at a tertiary care centre. Int J Contemp Med Res. 2019;6(1):A1–4.
77. Brigden ML, Au S, Thompson S, Brigden S, Doyle P, Tsaparas Y. Infectious mononucleosis in an outpatient population: diagnostic utility of 2 automated hematology analyzers and the sensitivity and specificity of Hoagland's criteria in heterophile-positive patients. Arch Pathol Lab Med. 1999;123(10):875–81.
78. McKenna RW. Infectious mononucleosis: Part 1. Morphologic aspects. Lab Med. 1979;10:135–9.
79. Pratumvinit B, Wongkrajang P, Reesukumal K, Klinbua C, Niamjoy P. Validation and optimization of criteria for manual smear review following automated blood cell analysis in a large university hospital. Arch Pathol Lab Med. 2013;137(3):408–14.
80. Guo LF, Gao XF, Chen Y, Ma L, Liu Y, Zhang J, et al. Establishment and verification of review criteria for blood cell analysis in children. Int J Lab Hematol. 2023;45(3):e75–8.

81. Loo E, Rodrigues Simoes NJ, Browne LJ, Mindiola Romero AE, Kaur P. Hematology lab waste reduction through implementation of peripheral smear review criteria. Int J Lab Hematol. 2023;45(5):813–5.
82. Hur M, Cho JH, Kim H, Hong MH, Moon HW, Yun YM, et al. Optimization of laboratory workflow in clinical hematology laboratory with reduced manual slide review: comparison between Sysmex XE-2100 and ABX Pentra DX120. Int J Lab Hematol. 2011;33(4):434–40.
83. Buoro S, Mecca T, Seghezzi M, Manenti B, Azzara G, Ottomano C, et al. Validation rules for blood smear revision after automated hematological testing using Mindray CAL-8000. J Clin Lab Anal. 2017;31(4).

Prognostic and Predictive Biomarkers in B-Lymphoblastic Leukemia

13

Lei Zhang, Sahibu Sultan M. Habeebu, John Herriges, and Weijie Li

Introduction

B-cell acute lymphoblastic leukemia (B-ALL) is a hematologic malignancy resulting from clonal proliferation of abnormal B-cell precursors (B-lymphoblasts) in bone marrow (BM). Most B-ALL cases are diagnosed in young children, although it can occur at any age. The estimated number of new B-ALL cases in the USA is close to 5000 each year [1]. In recent years, due to the progression of molecular biology and the development of new technologies, significant advances have been made in understanding the pathophysiology of B-ALL, identifying prognostic and predictive biomarkers, risk stratification, and risk-adjusted therapy as well as targeted therapy based on genetic abnormalities. Currently, 80–90% of B-ALL patients are cured with a long-term survival rate close to 90% [2]. However, a significant number of patients develop treatment resistance and relapse, which results in a poor prognosis [3]. Relapse and chemotherapy-related morbidity and mortality remain the big challenges to oncologists, and B-ALL continues to be the leading cause of cancer-related death in children and young adults. Therefore, a thorough understanding of the spectrum of genetic lesions in B-ALL is needed to identify new biomarkers that may be open to potential therapeutic targeting, better risk stratification, and personalized adjustment of primary therapy for better disease management over time, thus improving patient survival and reducing adverse outcomes [4]. Additionally, identification of specific biomarkers, such as genetic changes, may lead to better monitoring of the course of the disease.

Risk stratification of B-ALL is currently based on age, white blood cell count (WBC), early therapeutic response, cytogenetic abnormalities such as ploidy, and

L. Zhang (✉) · S. S. M. Habeebu · J. Herriges · W. Li
Department of Pathology and Laboratory Medicine, Children's Mercy Kansas City, University of Missouri-Kansas City School of Medicine, Kansas City, MO, USA
e-mail: lzhang@cmh.edu

W. Li (ed.), *Laboratory Assessments of Pediatric Leukemia*,
https://doi.org/10.1007/978-3-032-26557-9_13

translocations. There are many types of prognostic/predictive biomarkers for B-ALL, which include genetic, morphologic, radiographic, physiological, or immunophenotypic categories. The genetic biomarker category alone can have many types, including characteristic chromosome numerical or structural alterations, DNA sequence variants including indels, altered RNA, and altered/aberrant or new proteins. Molecular biomarkers play an increasingly important role in risk-stratification and risk-adapted therapy of B-ALL. The application of advanced molecular diagnostic techniques has led to the discovery of many new genetic biomarkers, which show promise for a more accurate risk stratification, improved individualized therapeutic strategy, and the design of molecularly targeted therapies. Immunophenotypic markers can predict the therapeutic responses to certain immunotherapies, and some of them are correlated with certain cytogenetic/molecular subtypes. In this chapter, we will review the genetic biomarkers, immunophenotypic biomarkers, as well as other prognostic and/or predictive biomarkers.

Common Approaches for Investigating Molecular Biomarkers

The diagnostic testing run on B-ALL samples can be at different levels with corresponding techniques:

- Proteins: Flow cytometry (FCM), immunohistochemistry, and cytochemistry.
- Traditional cytogenetic techniques: Karyotyping, fluorescence in-situ hybridization (FISH).
- Molecular techniques:
  - DNA: polymerase chain reaction (PCR), Sanger sequencing, microarray, Optical Genome Mapping (OGM), Multiplex Ligation-dependent Probe Amplification (MLPA), and next-generation sequencing (NGS, single gene, targeted panel, whole exome, and whole genome).
  - RNA: RNASeq, gene expression profiling, reverse transcription-PCR (RT-PCR).

Standard-of-care techniques for clinical study of B-ALL include cytogenetic analysis, FISH, RT-PCR, MLPA, and Single Nucleotide Polymorphism (SNP) arrays. Almost 70% of children affected by B-ALL are characterized by well-known cytogenetic abnormalities. However, the integration of results from genomics, transcriptomics, proteomics, and metabolomics has enabled a deeper definition of the molecular scenario of B-ALL and the identification of new genetic alterations [5]. Therefore, whole exome, whole genome, transcriptome sequencing, OGM, as well as long-read sequencing are starting to be employed for clinical testing.

Genetic Biomarkers

Cytogenetic abnormalities serve as the basis for B-ALL subtype classification in the 5th edition of the WHO [6]. In the past few years, the integration of genomic analysis, especially whole genome sequencing (WGS) and whole transcriptome sequencing (WTS), into the clinical workup has revealed multiple new subtypes not evident on cytogenetic analysis due to cryptic rearrangements or sequence level mutations. So far, more than 20 distinct genetic subtypes of B-ALL have been described [7], and the subtype list is still expanding. The recognized genetic biomarkers help stratify B-ALL patients into standard, intermediate, and high-risk groups; and not only aid in diagnosis and prognostication, but many also offer opportunities for targeted treatment. Significant abnormalities are described below and summarized in Fig. 13.1, and Tables 13.1 and 13.2.

ETV6::RUNX1 Fusion

The cytogenetically cryptic t(12;21)(p13.2;q22.1) results in the fusion of the *ETS* variant 6 (*ETV6*) and Runt-related transcription factor 1 (*RUNX1*) genes, historically known as *TEL-AML1* fusion [8]. It affects approximately 25% of children (age 3–10 years old) and is considered the most common genetic alteration among children with B-ALL, but only affects <3% in adult B-ALL [9]. Early studies showed that the *ETV6:: RUNX1* chimeric product converts *RUNX1* from an activator to a repressor; however, recent data points to a more complex mechanism [10]. Despite the prevalence of *ETV6::RUNX1* fusion in childhood B-ALL, the consensus now is that this fusion alone is unlikely to be responsible for causing overt leukemia, as up to 5% of newborns were found to have this alteration at birth, with most cases not developing overt leukemia [11]. In addition, *ETV6::RUNX1* fusion has been found in cord blood, consistent with the rearrangement originating prenatally. Due to the

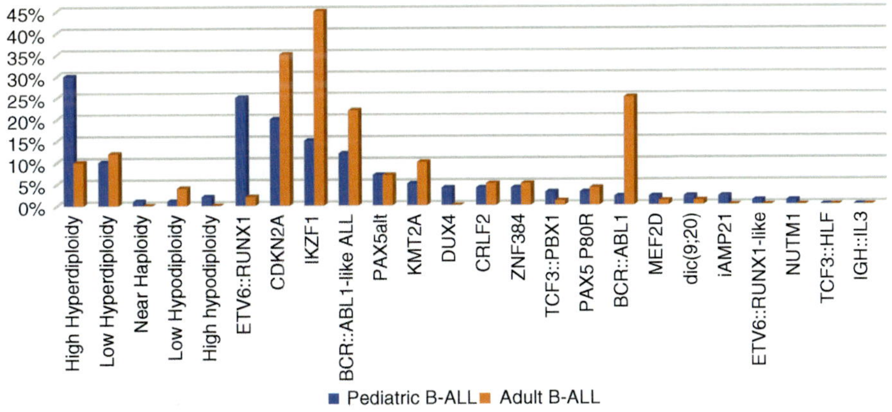

Fig. 13.1 Frequencies of the common genetic abnormalities in B-ALL

Table 13.1 Established genetic biomarkers in B-ALL

Biomarker	Alterations	Function	Prognosis	Predictive	Comment
High hyperdiploidy	51–65 chromosomes	N/A	Excellent	N/A	Associated with mutations in genes encoding histone modifiers (e.g., *CREBBP*) and RTK-RAS pathway (e.g., *FLT3*)
Low hyperdiploidy	47–50 chromosomes	N/A	Poor	N/A	–
Near haploidy	24–29 chromosomes	N/A	Very poor	BCL2 inhibitors	May be associated with alterations in *NF1, NRAS, KRAS, FLT3*, etc.
Low hypodiploidy	30–39 chromosomes	N/A	Very poor	BCL2 inhibitors	Associated with *TP53* mutations (>90%)
High hypodiploidy	40–44 chromosomes	N/A	Poor	N/A	–
BCR::ABL1	t(9;22)(22q11;9q34.12)	The fusion can constitutively activate tyrosine kinase that can activate many pathways	Poor, improved by TKIs	Positive; responds to ABL1 TKIs	High-risk ALL, 80% with *IKZF1* deletion
BCR::ABL1-like	Gene fusions (Tables 13.3 and 13.4)	Majority has constitutively active kinase or cytokine receptor signaling	Poor	N/A	High-risk ALL
CRLF2	t(X;14)(p22.3;q32)-*IGH::CRLF2* PAR1 deletion-*P2RY8::CRLF2*	B cell development through activation of the JAK-STAT pathway	Poor	Negative; trial of JAK TKIs	Standard and high-risk ALL
ETV6::RUNX1	t(12;21)(p13;q22)	Transcriptional regulation	Excellent	N/A	–
ETV6::RUNX1-like	N/A	N/A	Poor	N/A	>80% occur in children; *ETV6* and *IKZF1* alterations
iAMP21	Amplification within 21q	N/A	Poor	N/A	High-risk ALL, Associated with RAS signaling pathway gene mutations

Biomarker	Alterations	Function	Prognosis	Predictive	Comment
KMT2A	11q23, translocation/ inversion/deletion	Transcription factor; regulates gene expression during hematopoiesis	Very poor	Resistance to glucocorticoids	High-risk ALL. CD10 negative, CD15, CD33 and CD68 positive
TCF3::HLF	t(17;19)(q22;p13.3)	*TCF3*: Lymphopoiesis; required for B and T cell development; *HLF*: Transcriptional activator	Very poor	N/A	High-risk ALL. *PAX5* deletion and RAS pathway gene mutations
TCF3::PBX1	t(1;19)(q23.3;p13.3)	*TCF3*: See above. *PBX1* regulates many embryonic processes including hematopoiesis	Intermediate to excellent prognosis	N/A	Intermediate risk ALL due to modern therapy. High-risk of CNS leukemia and relapse. Expresses cytoplasmic immunoglobulin μ heavy chain
IGH::IL3	t(5;14)(q31.1;q32)	*IL3*: cytokine controlling the production and differentiation of hematopoietic progenitor cells	Poor	N/A	Present with reactive hypereosinophilia and lack of peripheral blasts

Table 13.2 New genetic biomarker in B-ALL

Biomarker	Location	Function	Alteration	Prognostic	Predictive	Comment
DUX4	4q35.2	*DUX4*: Transcriptional activator	Gene fusions	Good	N/A	Most frequent partner is *IGH*. CD2 and CD371 positive.
ERG	21q22.2	*ERG*: Transcriptional regulator of hematopoiesis	Deletion	Good	N/A	Occurs exclusively in the DUX4-r subgroup.
IKZF1	7p12.2	B-cell development regulation	Deletion/point mutation/gene fusion	Poor	Resistance to ABL1 TKIs	High-risk ALL;. Older age at diagnosis;. Emerging subtype IKZF1^{plus} with very poor prognosis.
IKZF1 N159Y	7p12.2	B-cell development regulation	Point mutation	Intermediate	Good response to treatment	Gain of chromosome 21 common
IKZF1^{plus}	7p12.2	B-cell development regulation	Co-deletion with CDKN2A/B/PAX5/PAR1 without *ERG* deletion	Very poor	Resistance to ABL1 TKIs	*VPREB1* deletion frequent
MEF2D	1q22	Control of cell growth, survival and apoptosis	Gene fusions	Poor	Responds to HDAC9 inhibitors	CD10 negative, CD38 bright;. *IKZF1* and *CDKN2A/B* deletion
NUTM1	15q14	Role in regulating cell proliferation.	Gene fusions	Excellent	Responds to HDAC inhibitors	Rare; occurs mainly in infants
PAX5 P80R	9p13	Transcription factor; regulates B-lineage specific genes	Hotspot mutation (PAX5 p.Pro80Arg mutation)	Intermediate to poor	N/A	Accompanied by inactivation of the second *PAX5* allele in all cases.
PAX5alt	9p13	Transcription factor; regulates early stages of B cell development	Gene fusions/ mutations/focal amplification	Intermediate to poor	N/A	High-risk ALL;. More than 20 fusion partners including *ETV6*

ZNF384	12p12	Transcription factor	Gene fusions	Intermediate, prognosis varies with different partners	*FLT3* inhibitors	CD13 and CD33 positive, negative or weak CD10.
UBTF	17q21.31	Plays a crucial role in the transcription of ribosomal RNA (rRNA) genes	Gene fusions	Poor	Reduced chemosensitivity	CDX2 overexpression, CD10 negative, immunoglobulin M positive
ZEB2 H1038R	2q22.3	Transcription factor	Point mutation	Poor	N/A	Expression profile close to *IGH::CREBP*

long latency and low concordance (~10%) in monozygotic twins, it has been proposed that a postnatal second-hit is required for completion of B-ALL leukemic transformation [11]. Numerous secondary abnormalities have been reported in the *ETV6::RUNX1* group with deletion of the non-translocated *ETV6* allele being the most common one (16–69%), followed by deletion of *VPREB1* (55%), 6q (13–37%), 9p (*CDKN2A/B, PAX5, JAK2*) (7–29%), *CDKN1B* (15%), *BTG1* (15%), and gain of chromosome 21 or der(21)t(12;21) *(RUNX1)* (10–25%) [12–15]. Rarer findings include deletions of *RB1* (8%), *IKZF1* (5%) and *EBF1* (4%), along with recurrent mutations in *KRAS* (10%) and *NRAS* (6%) genes [12, 14, 15].

ETV6::RUNX1 fusion in B-ALL is associated with excellent prognosis, with overall survival (OS) estimated at 94% at 5 years and 88% at 10 years [16]. Larger studies have shown that the good prognosis associated with *ETV6::RUNX1* fusion remains even in the presence of additional genetic abnormalities [13, 17]. However, approximately 5% of *ETV6::RUNX1* patients experience relapse, accounting for nearly 20% of all B-ALL relapses [18]. Measurable residual disease (MRD) level have been the only identified biomarker that predicts treatment failure in *ETV6::RUNX1* leukemia [19]. However, just recently focal deletion on 15q containing *INO80* locus has been shown to be associated with treatment resistance [20]. Subsequently, the finding of 15q deletion portending a poorer prognosis has been validated in a statistically significant manner in an independent, retrospectively analyzed cohort of 1580 *ETV6::RUNX1* positive national cancer institute (NCI) standard-risk (SR) patients enrolled in AALL0932, a legacy children's oncology group (COG) NCI SR trial [21, 22]. In addition, studies did show that treatment fast responders frequently exhibited the *APOBEC* mutational signature and the gene expression signature of high cell cycle activity, while slow responders frequently harbor rearrangements of *IGK* genes [23]. Focal deletions on chromosome 3 (centered on *TBL1XR1*), 9p (*PAX5*), as well as gain of 12p may also associate with treatment resistance [14, 20, 23].

ETV6::RUNX1 Fusion-Like

A new subtype, *ETV6::RUNX1*-Like ALL, was recently identified using integrated genomic analysis [24]. This type of ALL shares a similar gene expression profile and immunophenotype (CD27 positive, CD44 low to negative) with *ETV6::RUNX1* ALL, although there is an absence of *ETV6::RUNX1* fusion. More than 80% of *ETV6::RUNX1*-like cases occur in children, accounting for 2–3% of pediatric B-ALL. When compared to other types of B-ALL, it was found through WGS that cases of *ETV6::RUNX1*-like, on average, have a higher mutational load than other B-ALL subtypes [25]. Enriched genetic abnormalities in this subtype include *ETV6* deletion or rearrangement with *IKZF1* or *ELMO1*; deletions of *IKZF1, ATP10A,* and *ARPP21*; deletions of the histone gene cluster on 6p22.2, *BTG1* aberrations, as well as other chromosome rearrangements such as *TCF3::FLI1* and *FUS::ERG* fusions [7, 25–27]. The prognosis of this subtype is considered to be intermediate-to-poor with reported 5-year event-free survival (EFS) and OS rates at ~66.7% and

87.5%, respectively [28]. Both favorable [7, 27] and poor outcomes [4, 29] have been reported in comparison to the *ETV6::RUNX1* subtype. Higher-intensity therapy may be considered for this subtype [4].

Aneuploidy

Hyperdiploidy (>46 chromosomes) represents the largest cytogenetic subgroup in childhood B-ALL. It can be subdivided into two groups: high hyperdiploidy (51–65 chromosomes or DNA index (DI) ≥ 1.16) and low hyperdiploidy (47–50 chromosomes or DI 1.0–1.16) [30] with different prognosis in each group.

High hyperdiploidy (HHyper) is a favorable prognostic factor, presenting in up to 30% of children and 10% of adults with B-ALL [31]. Typically, children with HHyper B-ALL achieve negative MRD after induction treatment and have excellent cure rates, with 5-year EFS and OS rates of ~75% and ~90%, respectively [30]. The most commonly gained chromosomes are 4, 6, 8, 10, 14, 17, 18, 21, and X with the presence of either double trisomy (+4, +10) or triple trisomy (+4, +10, +17) associated with a very low risk of relapse by children's cancer group (CCG), pediatric oncology group (POG), or children's oncology group (COG) [32]. Trisomy 18 has also been associated with a favorable prognosis, while gain of extra copies of chromosomes 5 and 20 has been associated with a relatively poor prognosis. A retrospective study for pediatric B-ALL found that the good risk profile included karyotypes with +17 and +18 or +17 or +18 in the absence of +5 and +20, and its prognostic effect was independent of MRD [33]. Another recent study showed that gain of chromosome 6 with disomy of chromosomes 10 and 17 was associated with relapse [20].

Although HHyper is generally associated with a favorable prognosis, there are still approximately 20% of pediatric HHyper B-ALL cases that experience relapse [34]. A recent study showed a high degree of clonal heterogeneity and a hierarchical order of chromosome gains in diagnostic samples of HHyper B-ALL with the rates of specific chromosome gains and clonal heterogeneity different between HHyper B-ALL patients with favorable or unfavorable clinical outcomes. This study found that low levels of trisomies 10 and 18 and low levels of clonal heterogeneity are robust relapse risk factors in MRD-negative childhood HHyper B-ALL patients [35]. In addition, several co-existent or secondary genetic abnormalities have been suggested to impact HHyper prognosis. Mutations targeting genes encoding histone modifiers (*CREBBP, WHSC1, SUV420H1, SETD2*, and *EZH2*) and the RTK-RAS pathway (*FLT3, NRAS, KRAS, and PTPN11*) are common (~50% and 25%, respectively) in patients with HHyper B-ALL [20, 36–38]. Mutations in these genes as well as *IKZF1* deletion are believed to occur after chromosome gain [37, 38] and have been detected at a higher incidence in relapsed versus diagnostic B-ALL samples [36]. The recurrent translocations, t(9;22)(q34;q11)-*BCR::ABL1*, t(12;21)(p13;q22)-*ETV6::RUNX1*, t(1;19)(q23;p13)-*TCF3::PBX1*, and t(4;11)(q21;q23)-*KMT2A::AFF1*, have also been reported in 1–4% of HHyper B-ALL [39]. In such cases, the prognostic impact of the translocation is believed to override the beneficial effect of HHyper [30]. Of note, the most commonly gained chromosomes in the t(9;22) group are chromosomes 9, 11, 14, 16, 17, and 22, different from those in classic HHyper without t(9;22) [39]. It has been considered that t(9;22) was the primary event with hyperdiploidy being the secondary event in this group. Previous data showed that patients with both t(9;22) and hyperdiploidy have a better outcome compared to t(9;22) in a diploid background [39].

The structural abnormality of i(17q) has been correlated with poorer outcome in some [40], although not all studies [34] on HHyper B-ALL. Gain of 1q through duplication or unbalanced translocation is the most common structural abnormality in HHyper B-ALL, being reported in approximately 20% of HHyper B-ALL [39, 41], and is significantly associated with trisomy 5 [41]. The prognostic significance of 1q gain has been controversial [39, 42], with more recent studies showing evidence that duplication 1q is an independent adverse parameter on disease-free survival (DFS) of HHyper patients [39, 43].

Low hyperdiploidy (LHyper) is present in 10–11% of children and 10–15% of adults with increasing incidence with age [16]. Almost any chromosome can be gained, but generally chromosomes X, 8, 10, 21, and 14 are involved. The most common variant in this group seems to be patients with 47 chromosomes [44]. Patients with low hyperdiploid have worse OS and relapse-free survival (RFS), a significantly shorter median time to first relapse, and less frequently achieve second complete remission than patients with normal karyotype and miscellaneous abnormalities [44]. The relapse in patients with LHyper accounts for 10% of B-ALL relapses [16, 44].

Hypodiploidy can be defined as the loss of one or more chromosomes and constitutes ~5% of B-ALL cases across all age groups [45]. Hypodiploidy B-ALL can be further divided into three groups: (i) high-hypodiploid (40–44 chromosomes), (ii) low-hypodiploid (30–39 chromosomes), and (iii) near-haploid (24–29 chromosomes) [45]. Near-haploid and low-hypodiploid pediatric B-ALL display significantly poorer clinical outcomes in comparison with high-hypodiploid [16, 46].

Near-haploidB-ALL presents in approximately 0.5% of pediatric B-ALL and has not been reported in adult ALL. Disomies for chromosomes 8, 10, 14, 18, 21, and sex chromosomes are usually retained in this subtype [45]. Up to 70.6% of patients with this subtype may harbor mutations in receptor tyrosine kinase (RTK) and RAS pathway genes including *NF1* (≥44%), *NRAS* (15%), *KRAS* (3%), *FLT3* (9%), and *PTPN1* (1.5%) [47]. In addition, deletions of *IKZF3* (13.2%) and histone cluster at chromosome band 6p22 (19.1%) are frequently observed [47]. Other frequently detected abnormalities in this subtype include alterations in *CREBBP* and *PAG1*, deletions involving *CDKN2A/B*, *RB1*, and *PAX5*, and point mutations in *EP300* and *EZH2* [47]. Near-haploid B-ALL is not well characterized in association with any known hereditary predisposition syndrome, but Noonan syndrome patients with germline mutations in *PTPN11* and *NRAS* have been reported [47].

Low Hypodiploid B-ALL (LHypo) presents in 0.5% of children and approximately 4% of adult patients [48]. In the pediatric population, older children are more likely to present with low hypodiploidy than those with near-haploidy, with a median age at diagnosis of 12.9 years [46]. The retained chromosomes generally include 1, 5, 6, 8, 10, 11, 14, 18, 19, 21, 22, X and Y, with the most frequently retained disomies being chromosomes 1, 6, 11, and 18, and the most typical lost chromosomes being 3, 7, 9, 15, 16, and 17 [49]. The characteristic molecular abnormality in LHypo B-ALL is *TP53* mutation which can be detected in >90% of both pediatric and adult patients with this subtype [47, 50]. Most *TP53* variants are missense mutations involving exons 5–8, affecting the DNA binding domain and the nuclear localization sequence [47, 50]. Moreover, due to the frequent loss of chromosome 17, *TP53* mutations are found to be homozygous in virtually all LHypo B-ALL. In approximately 50% of pediatric LHypo B-ALL, *TP53* mutations are germline in origin, which should prompt consideration of Li-Fraumeni syndrome, and genetic counselling should be recommended [47]. In contrast to pediatric cases, *TP53* mutations in adult LHypo B-ALL are somatic [47, 50].

In addition to *TP53* mutations, other cryptic cytogenetic or molecular genetic abnormalities frequently found in LHypo B-ALL include *IKZF2/Helios* loss at 2q34 (53% in children and 36% in adults), *RB1* alterations (41% in children and 19% in adults), *CDKN2A/B* alterations (22% in both children and adults), and *CREBBP* mutations (60%) [47, 50]. It has been reported that *CDKN2A/B* mutations are often mutually exclusive with *RB1* mutations in the background of *TP53* mutated LHypo B-ALL [51]. *IKZF2* deletion is the most recurrent alteration among genes associated with B-cell differentiation in LHypo B-ALL in comparison with focal deletions involving other lymphocyte developing genes, such as *IKZF1*, *EBF1* and *LEF1*, and is more frequently observed in LHypo B-ALL than any other subtypes including near-haploid B-ALL [47]. *IKZF2* is highly expressed in common lymphoid progenitors and in pre-pro-B progenitor cells, which supports the hypothesis that low-hypodiploidy targets a more immature lymphoid progenitor (pro-B stage or earlier) than other B-ALL subtypes with a pre-B immunophenotype [47].

Both near-haploid and low hypodiploid genomes can undergo endoreduplication, resulting in doubling of the hypodiploid chromosome complement, which occurs in 60–65% of hypodiploid B-ALL and is commonly observed as a mosaic with both hypodiploid and hyperdiploid (doubled) clones visible by standard cytogenetics [45]. A doubled clone has a modal chromosome number of 50–78, so-called "masked hypodiploidy," which may not be differentiated from a high-hyperdiploid or triploid clone cytogenetically if it is the only clone detected at diagnosis [45]. As hyperdiploidy with more than 50 chromosomes and hypodiploidy are associated with different prognosis, it is crucial to distinguish between true hyperdiploidy and masked hypodiploid B-ALL. Cytogenetically, doubled clones commonly show tetrasomy for chromosomes 14, 18, 21, and the sex chromosome, as well as doubled structural abnormalities from specific chromosomes. A method to screen for genome wide loss of heterozygosity (LOH) (e.g., a SNP microarray) should be performed to detect loss of heterozygosity (LOH), which is a very characteristic feature for masked hypodiploidy [48].

High hypodiploidy (HHypo) presents in approximately 4% of diagnosed cases with hypodiploid B-ALL in both children and adults [45, 49]. Based on the limited number of studies on HHypo patients, this group of B-ALL seems to have a better prognosis than that of the group with <40 chromosomes [46]. High incidence of complex chromosomal abnormalities has been observed, with a high prevalence of abnormalities involving chromosomes 7, 9, and 12 [45].

BCR::ABL1 (Ph+) B-ALL

BCR::ABL1 fusion is present in 1–3% of children and approximately 25% of adult B-ALL [52] and is a poor prognostic factor [53]. The majority of *BCR::ABL1* fusion results from t(9;22)(q34.1;q11.2) [Philadelphia chromosome positive (Ph+)] and gives rise to a constitutively active tyrosine kinase that can activate many pathways including RAS, RAC, PI3K/AKT/mTOR, NF-κB, and JAK/STAT [54]. The t(9;22) leads to the fusion of the 5′ region of the *BCR* gene with the sequences upstream of the second exon of the *ABL1* gene (almost the entire gene coding for this tyrosine kinase). *BCR::ABL1* chimeric proteins may differ in molecular weight depending on the site of *BCR* gene disruption. Fusion of exon 1 of *BCR* (minor breakpoint) with exon 2 of *ABL1* (e1a2 transcript) gives rise to the p190 fusion protein found in approximately 85% of Ph+ pediatric ALL and 50–70% of Ph+ adult B-ALL. Fusion of exon 13 or 14 of *BCR* (major breakpoint) with exon 2 of *ABL1* (e13a2 or e14a2 transcripts) gives rise to the p210 fusion protein found in 15% of Ph+ pediatric ALL and 30–50% of Ph+ adult ALL [54]. Of note, *BCR::ABL1* fusion is also the main driver of chronic myelogenous leukemia (CML), with p210 protein being seen in >95% of CML cases [55].

Other genetic abnormalities frequently associated with Ph+ B-ALL include deletions of *IKZF1* (80%), *PAX5* (50%), *CDKN2A/B* (50%), and *EBF1* (14%) [56]. *IKZF1* deletion is associated with shorter DFS and shorter cumulative incidence of relapse in Ph+ B-ALL [57]. One study has shown that *CDKN2A/B* deletion was also associated with worse outcomes compared to patients without this deletion [58].

The introduction of tyrosine kinase inhibitors (TKIs) has led to a dramatic improvement in outcomes for Ph+ B-ALL. Different TKIs as well as different treatment regimens, such as combined TKI and chemotherapy, have been developed [59]. However, despite recent therapeutic advances, Ph+ ALL is still an adverse subtype [60].

BCR::ABL1-Like(Ph-Like) B-ALL

This type of B-ALL was initially discovered because it had a gene expression profile similar to Ph+ B-ALL despite lacking *BCR::ABL1* fusion. Ph-like B-ALL presents in 10–15% of pediatric and approximately 20–24% of adult cases, peaking in adolescents and adults [6, 61, 62], and is associated with inferior outcomes compared with other B-ALL subtypes [62]. A wide spectrum of genetic alterations has been described in Ph-like B-ALL cases, including translocations, cryptic gene rearrangements, sequence mutations, and copy number changes. The majority of these alterations lead to constitutively active kinase or cytokine receptor signaling, and many of them have been shown to be targetable with a variety of TKIs [63, 64]. These alterations may be grouped into four groups: (i) JAK/STAT alterations. This group has been reported in 24.1% of children, 32% of adolescents (16–21 years), 14.6% of young adults (21–39 years), and 11.2% of adults (40–86 years) [65]. The genetic alterations include mutations activating cytokine receptors (e.g., *CRLF2* and *IL7R*); gene fusions hijacking cytokine receptor expression (e.g., *IGH::CRLF2* and *P2RY8::CRLF2*); gene fusions and/or mutations activating kinases (e.g., *JAK1, JAK2, JAK3, TYK2*); and rearrangements hijacking and truncating cytokine receptor expression (e.g., cryptic *EPOR* rearrangements) [62, 65, 66] (Table 13.3). (ii) ABL class gene rearrangements. This group has been reported in 16.7% of children, 9% of adolescents (16–21 years), 10.4% of young adults (21–39 years), and 9.2% of adults (40–86 years) [65]. The fusions involve ABL-class genes including *ABL1, ABL2, CSF1R, LYN, PDGFRA, PDGFRB,* etc. [66, 67] (Table 13.4); (iii) Mutations activating Ras signaling (*NRAS, KRAS, PTPN11*). This group has been reported in 4% of B-ALL [65, 66]; (iv) Less common fusions involving *FLT3, FGFR1, NTRK3, PTK2B,* etc., with a growing number due to the application of sequencing techniques. This group has been reported in 2.8% of children, 3% of adolescents (16–21 years), 5.2% of young adults (21–39 years), and 3.1% of adults (40–86 years) [62, 64–67].

In addition to the alterations in kinase or cytokine receptor signaling, deletions involving B-cell developmental genes are also common genetic abnormalities in Ph-like B-ALL. Similar to Ph+ ALL, *IKZF1* alterations are a hallmark of Ph-like ALL, presenting in 70–80% Ph-like B-ALL [66] and confer a poor prognostic outcome. *IKZF1* deletions are significantly more common in patients carrying *CRLF2* rearrangement, especially in Hispanic/Latino (H/L) children with B-ALL (29% in H/L compared to 15% of non-Hispanic Whites) [66], demonstrating that both *IGH::CRLF2* translocation and *IKZF1* deletion could be contributing factors to the higher death rate of B-ALL in H/L patients [68]. *PAX5* is another gene frequently altered, presenting in approximately 30% of Ph-like B-ALL cases. *IKZF1* and *PAX5* alterations often occur together [69].

CRLF2 Deregulation

CRLF2 rearrangements occur in approximately 5% of B-ALL patients with a higher frequency in *BCR-ABL1*-like and B-ALL NOS subgroups (>30%) as well as patients with Down syndrome (50%) [63, 70]. *CRLF2* rearrangements are associated with unfavorable prognosis in the *BCR-ABL1*-like subgroup due to poor response to current chemotherapy, high rate of positive MRD, and high incidence of relapse [71]. For other B-ALL subtypes in which *CRLF2* rearrangement is a secondary abnormality and often presents only within low level subclones, its presence may not be relevant to prognosis in the context of other risk factors [72].

CRLF2 overexpression can result from interstitial deletions within the pseudoautosomal region (PAR1) located at Xp22.3 or Yp11.3, which bring *CRLF2* to the *P2RY8* promoter [73] (Fig. 13.2). Overexpression of *CRLF2* can also arise from an *IGH* translocation and, more rarely, an activating mutation [74]. In comparison with *CRLF2::P2RY8* fusion, *IGH::CRLF2* is more common in adults and may have a worse prognosis [75]. *CRLF2* rearrangements have been associated with *IKZF1* deletion and activation of the JAK-STAT, ERK and mTOR/PI3K pathways, with

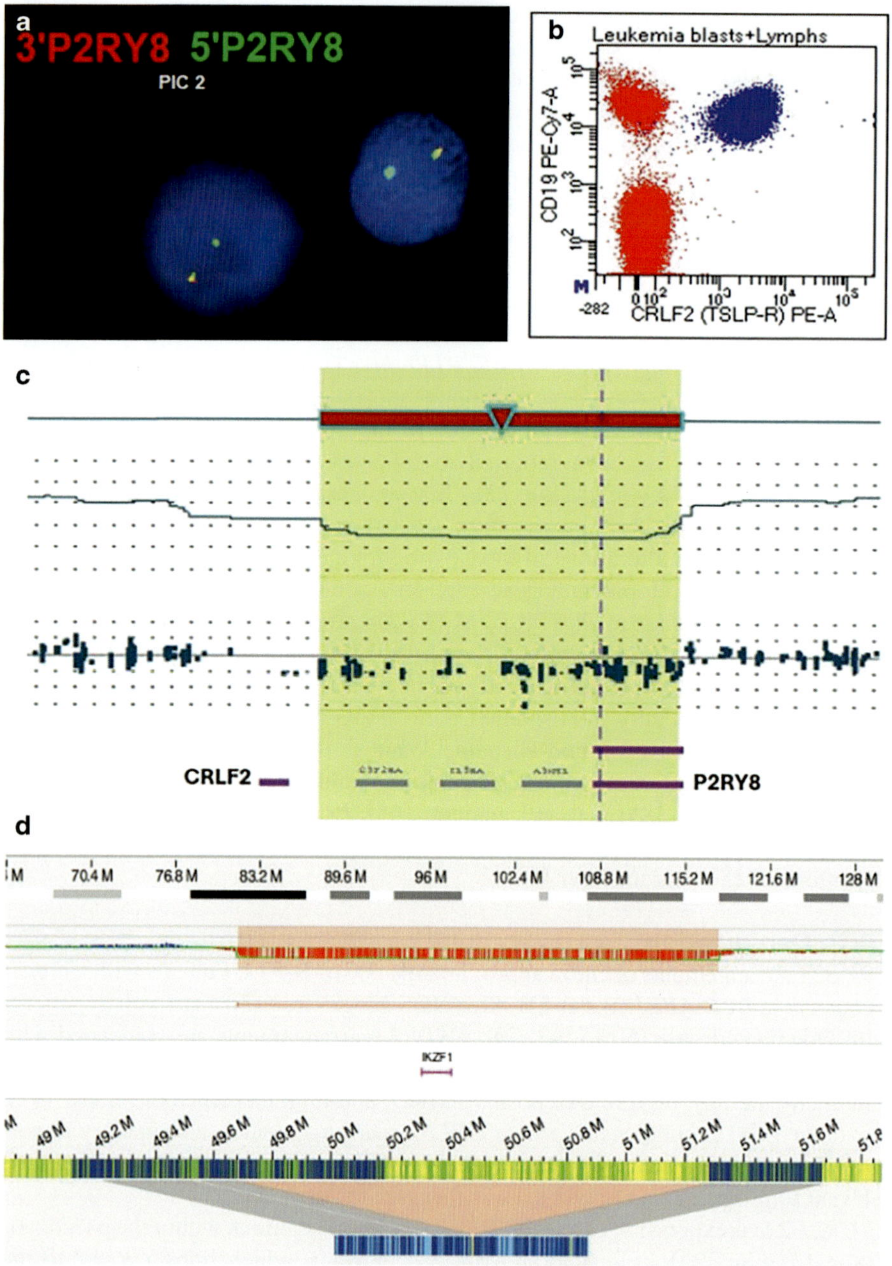

Fig. 13.2 Ph-like B-ALL with *P2RY8::CRLF2* fusion and *IKZF1*^{plus} biomarkers. (**a**) FISH analysis shows 3′*P2RY8* deletion suggesting *P2RY8::CRLF2* fusion. (**b**) Flow cytometry study shows the expression of thymic stromal lymphopoietin receptor (TSLPR), the protein encoded by the *CRLF2* gene, in leukemia cells (blue) but not in normal lymphocytes (red). (**c**) Microarray identifies a deletion within Xp22.3 resulting in *P2RY8::CRLF2* fusion. (**d**) OGM identifies *IKZF1* deletion. (**e**) Chromosome analysis identifies an isochromosome 9q (arrow) resulting in loss of *CDKN2A/CDKN2B and PAX5* on 9p, which, together with *IKZF1* deletion and absence of *ERG* deletion, forms *IKZF1*^{plus} subtype

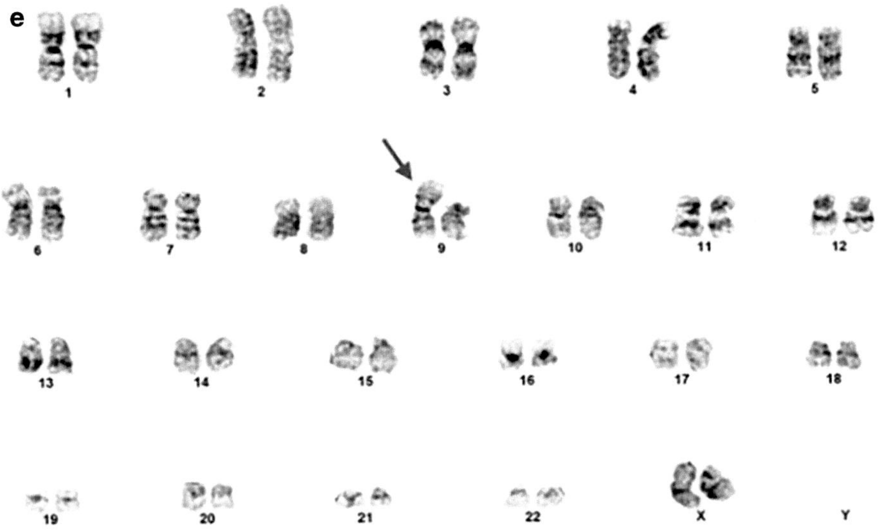

Fig. 13.2 (continued)

50% of cases harboring mutations in *JAK* family genes [76]. The concomitance of *CRLF2* overexpression and *JAK2* mutations is associated with inferior outcomes [76].

Although the rearrangements of *CRLF2* are the most common alteration in *BCR::ABL1*-like ALL, approximately 5–10% of *CRLF2*-rearranged ALL cases are not *BCR::ABL1*-like ALL [77]. *P2RY8::CRLF2* fusion is often a secondary lesion in leukemias with iAMP21, hyperdiploidy, or dic(9;20) [78]. Although rare, at least one study has reported that *P2RY8::CRLF2* fusion has been observed in all subtypes of B-ALL except the *KMT2A* rearranged group, including *ETV6::RUNX1*, *TCF3::PBX1* and *BCR::ABL1* fusions [79].

KMT2A Rearrangements

KMT2A rearrangement is present in 70–80% of infants (frequently being acquired in utero), 5% of children, and 10% of adults with B-ALL [80]. It is a poor prognostic factor, characterized by hyperleukocytosis, aggressive behavior with early relapse, and relatively high incidence of central nervous system (CNS) involvement in infants [81]. The immunophenotype associated with *KMT2A*-rearranged (*KMT2A*-r) B-ALL includes expression of CD19, lack of CD10, and also co-expression of myeloid markers such as CD15, CD33, and CD68 [82]. More than 90 fusion partners of *KMT2A* have been documented in acute leukemia [83]. In B-ALL, the most common partner is *AFF1* (formerly named *AF4*) at 4q21. The *KMT2A::AFF1* fusion [t(4;11)(q21;q23)] is estimated to be present in 50% of infants with *KMT2A*-r

B-ALL with an especially poor prognosis [81, 83]. The second most common fusion is *KMT2A::MLLT3* (*AF9*) resulting from t(9;11)(p22;q23) followed by *KMT2A::MLLT1 (ENL)* originated from t(11;19)(q23;p13.3) [83]. Fusions with *KMT2A* breakpoint in intron 11 were reported to have a poorer outcome [84]. Other major partner genes in infant ALL patients include *MLLT10 (AF10*), *MLLT6* (*AF17*), and *MLLT4* (*AF6*) [83].

Although *KMT2A*-r infant B-ALL may have the lowest somatic mutations in sequenced cancers [85], activating mutations in tyrosine kinase-PI3K-RAS signaling pathway components can be detected in 47% of cases including recurrent ones in *KRAS* and *NRAS*, and also non-recurrent mutations in *FLT3, NF1, PTPN11*, and *PIK3R1* [85], thus may serve as possible treatment target in the subgroup of *KMT2A*-r B-ALL with somatic mutations [86].

TCF3 Rearrangement

Although not as numerous as *KMT2A, TCF3* (*E2A*) rearrangements can involve many different partner genes in B-ALL. The most common fusion partner is *PBX1*, resulting from t(1;19)(q23;p13.3), occurring in both adults and children with B-ALL at an overall frequency of 5–6% [9]. Originally considered to be a poor prognosis mainly due to higher CNS involvement and relapse, it is now associated with a favorable or intermediate outcome with contemporary treatment [9]. The translocation t(1;19) can be in balanced form or more often in unbalanced form with the derivative chromosome 19—der (19)t(1.19). B-ALL patients with *TCF3::PBX1* fusion usually have a pre-B immunophenotype that expresses cytoplasmic μ [87].

Another fusion partner is *HLF*, resulting from t(17;19)(q22;p13.3), occurring in less than 1% of childhood B-ALL and rarely in adults with extremely poor prognosis [61]. There are two types of *TCF3::HLF* fusion with the same intron 3 breakpoint in the *HLF* gene, but different breakpoints in *TCF3*. Type I rearrangement has a breakpoint in intron 13 of *TCF3* associated with disseminated intravascular coagulation (DIC), while type II has a breakpoint in intron 12 of *TCF3* associated with hypercalcemia [88]. Other genetic abnormalities, frequently associated with *TCF3::HLF* fusion, include *PAX5* and *VPREB1* deletions and aberrations in the RAS pathway genes [3]. A number of other gene partners have been reported, including *ZNF384, NOL1* and *TFPT* [89, 90].

IGH::IL3 Fusion—t(5;14)

IgH::IL3 fusion is seen in less than 1% of B-ALL and represents an aggressive subtype with poor outcomes [91]. It results from t(5;14)(q31.1; q32.3), leading to overexpression of *IL3* as a result of its juxtaposition to the potent *IGH* enhancer. These cases are rare and poorly characterized, but are observed predominantly in males and the adolescent/young adult (AYA) age group. Patients with this translocation clinically present with reactive hypereosinophilia and lack of peripheral blasts [92].

Intrachromosomal Amplification of Chromosome 21 (iAMP21)

B-ALL with iAMP21 is present in approximately 2% of pediatric patients and is associated with worse prognosis when treated with a low-intensity National Cancer Institute (NCI) standard-risk regimen [93]. It is extremely rare in adult B-ALL, and its prognostic effect in adult cases is unclear [53]. Patients with iAMP21 are usually older children or adolescents (median 9.4 years) with a common pre-B immunophenotype and generally have a low WBC [94]. Individuals carrying balanced constitutional Robertsonian translocation rob(15;21)(q10;q10)c and trisomy 21 have a 2700-fold and 10–12-fold, respectively, increased risk of developing B-ALL with iAMP21 compared to children without these genetic anomalies [95].

The iAMP21 chromosome is a single abnormal chromosome 21 occurring through Breakage–Fusion–Bridge (BFB) cycles followed by chromothripsis, thus containing multiple regions of gain, amplification, inversion, and deletion [96]. The iAMP21-ALL has been defined as the presence of three or more extra copies of *RUNX1* on a single abnormal chromosome 21 (a total of five or more *RUNX1* signals per cell) by FISH [93]. However, a recent study has shown that approximately 9% of iAMP21 B-ALL failed to meet the FISH definition, but amplifications were confirmed by microarray, indicating the unbalanced result from iAMP21 may not contain *RUNX1* [97]. Common secondary abnormalities in B-ALL with iAMP21 include gain of chromosomes X, 10, or 14; monosomy 7/deletion of 7q; deletions of 11q including the *ATM* and *KMT2A* genes; as well as abnormalities affecting *IKZF1, CDKN2A, PAX5, ETV6*, and *RB1* [94]. More than 60% of iAMP21-ALL patients had a mutation of genes related to the RAS signaling pathway, and 20% of patients had a *P2RY8::CRLF2* gene fusion [98].

dic(9;20)

The dic(9;20) is a rare aberration seen in 2% of children and 1% of adults with B-ALL [99]. Both favorable and poor prognosis associated with dic(9;20) have been reported [99]. Relapses in these patients are fairly common; however, post relapse treatment is often successful [100]. Additional studies are needed to accurately define the prognostic value of dic(9;20). The dic(9;20) arises from the fusion of two centromeres of chromosomes 9 and 20, resulting in the loss of 9p and 20q material, which masquerades as monosomy 20. The breakpoints on 9p target *PAX5*, and the breakpoints on 20q target *ASXL1*. However, the breakpoints are heterogeneous at the molecular level, suggesting that loss of genetic material rather than gene fusion is the functional consequence of this aberration [101].

DUX4 Rearrangement

DUX4 rearrangement (*DUX4*-r) is present in 4–7% of pediatric B-ALL cases with a slightly higher incidence in AYA patients and rarely seen in adult B-ALL [90, 102]. *DUX4*-r B-ALL has a unique immunophenotype (CD2 and CD371 positive) with CD371 expression being pathognomonic of this leukemia [103]. *DUX4* is a transcription factor located within repetitive subtelomeric arrays on chromosomes 4q35 and 10q26, where it is nested within each 3.3 kb repeat unit of a macrosatellite array [104]. The most frequent translocation partner is the immunoglobulin heavy chain locus (*IgH*). The rearrangement involves insertion of a partial repeat copy, or one complete and one partial copy of *DUX4* (out-of-frame) from the D4Z4 or 10q26 loci into the *IGH* locus in either strand orientation [105], resulting in truncation of the highly conserved C terminus of *DUX4* and expression of this truncated protein [102]. This truncated form binds to an intragenic region of the ETS-family transcription factor *ERG* (ETS-related gene) and commonly results in the expression of a C-terminal ERG protein fragment that is a dominant-negative inhibitor of wild-type ERG function contributing to leukemogenesis [103]. Other partners, such as *ERG* and *ZNF384*, have also been reported [105, 106].

A critical secondary event in *DUX4*-r B-ALL is intragenic *ERG* deletions (ERGdel) which occur almost exclusively in this subtype [107] with multiple studies showing that >95% of B-ALL cases with ERGdel harbor a *DUX4* rearrangement [108]. *ERG* deletions are focal, most commonly involving exons 3–7 or 3–9 [108]. In addition to *ERG* focal deletion (~50% of *DUX4*-r cases), other intragenic structural alterations have also been frequently reported including deletions involving *CDKN2A/B* (~31%), *IKZF1* (~19%), and *PAX5* (~13%) [109], although incidence of other chromosomal alterations is characteristically low compared to other B-ALL subtypes [110]. Mutation analysis of *DUX4*-r cases showed that 44.7% of cases carry mutations affecting genes involved in the RAS/MAPK pathway, while 32.3% carry mutations in epigenetic pathway genes, and 21.3% of cases carry mutations affecting transcription factor genes [111].

DUX4-r is associated with excellent prognosis, with an 8-year EFS and 8-year OS of 86.4% and 95.6%, respectively [112]. Although the patients often present with poor initial treatment responses, they typically achieve excellent long-term survival rates with intensive chemotherapy regimens [106]. *ERG* deletion is reported to be associated with a good outcome which is not attenuated by the presence of poor-risk features, such as *IKZF1* deletion and intermediate MRD levels [108].

Due to the cryptic nature of *DUX4* rearrangements, they cannot be detected by traditional cytogenetic technologies (karyotyping and FISH). Recent advancements in RNA-seq and long-read sequencing provide the potential to both markedly improve and simplify the detection of this notoriously cryptic subtype. Deletion of *ERG* is considered a surrogate marker for *DUX4*-r in B-ALL cases, and thus the deletion detection through microarray, MLPA, or optical genome mapping (OGM) can be used as an indirect detection method for *DUX4*-r. In addition, Immunophenotyping, in particular, flow cytometry of CD371 has demonstrated great reliability to detect *DUX4*-r cases [106].

***ZNF384* Rearrangement and *ZNF384*-r-Like**

ZNF384-r is present in 3–5% of childhood and 3–8% of adult patients with B-ALL [89, 113]. Overall, its prognostic impact is intermediate but varies with different partner genes [89, 114]. The fusion genes include almost all of the coding sequence of the *ZNF384* gene translocated to a range of 5′ partner genes [115]. *ZNF384* rearrangements cause perturbed DNA binding and drive transcriptional deregulation [116]. More than 19 different *ZNF384* fusion partners have been identified, with *EP300, TCF3, TAF15*, and *CREBBP* being the most common ones. Others include *ARIDIB, BMP2K, CLTC, EWSR1, NIPBL, SMARCA2*, and *SYNRG* [117]. The *EP300::ZNF384* fusion outcome was reported to be better than the *TCF3::ZNF384* fusion [114]. Patients with *ZNF384* fusions share a characteristic immunophenotype of negative or weak CD10 expression and aberrant expression of myeloid antigens CD13/33 [113].

In 60% of the patients with *ZNF384* fusions, alterations in *NRAS, KRAS, NF1, PTPN11,* and *FLT3* were observed [43]. In addition, mutations in genes associated with epigenetic regulation (*KMT2D, CREBBP, and EZH2*) were common [43]. Deletions in lymphoid regulator genes, including *LEF1, EBF1, CDKN2A, FBXW7,* and *ETV6,* have also been detected in *ZNF384*-r B-ALL [117].

ZNF384-r-Like is present in 0.5% of patients with B-ALL [118]. This subtype shares the same expression profile with *ZNF384*-r B-ALLs without canonical *ZNF384* fusions [5, 115, 119, 120]. *ZNF362* rearrangement has been identified in this group [120]; however, in some ZNF384-r-like cases, no established primary aberration has been found.

***MEF2D* Rearrangement**

MEF2D-r is present in 1–4% of pediatric B-ALL (usually older children and adolescents) and 1% of adult patients [121]. It is associated with high white cell count and classified as an intermediate to high-risk factor [29, 121]. The leukemic blasts with the *MEF2D* fusion gene have an immunophenotype of low or no CD10 expression, common expression of immunoglobulin μ chain and CD5, and high CD38 expression [121, 122]. *MEF2D*-r is characterized by the fusion of an N-terminal region of *MEF2D* to the C-terminal region of multiple, different partner genes [122]. The most associated fusion partners are *BCL9* and *HNRNPUL1*, while *DAZAP1, CSF1R, SS18, TAT6, HNRNPH1, PYGO2, BCL9L*, and *FOXJ2* have also been reported [120, 122, 123]. One recent study showed that the most common secondary abnormality was *CDKN2A/B* deletion, occurring in ~71% of *MEF2D*-r cases with *PAX5* co-deleted in 25% of *CDKN2A/B*-deleted cases, while *IKZF1* deletions and *NRAS/KRAS* mutations were rare, occurring in ≤10% cases [122].

***NUTM1* Rearrangement**

NUTM1-r is a rare subtype observed in 5–7% of all infants with B-ALL (21.7% of *KMT2A*-wild type infant B-ALL) and 1% in children, with no report in adults [7, 120, 124]. The current limited data suggests *NUTM1* rearrangement is a favorable prognostic factor in B-ALL. Reported partner genes include *ACIN1, CUX1, BRD9,* and *ZNF618* [124]. Chromosome analysis may show 15q abnormalities or a normal karyotype (cryptic) [125]; thus, unbiased technologies, for example, RNA sequencing, OGM or long-read sequencing, may be better suited to detect this finding. Co-occurrence of *NUTM1::BRD9* fusion (resulting from t(5;15)) and *P2RY8::CFLF2* has been reported in one infant B-ALL [126] (Fig. 13.3).

UBTF Rearrangement

UBTF-r is present in 1–2% of B-ALL patients and has been more common in females [118, 127]. This subtype is characterized by an *UBTF::ATXN7L3* fusion which results from a ~10 kb deletion within 17q21.31 leading to in-frame readthrough between *UBTF* exon 15 (or later exons) and a 5′UTR splice site of *ATXN7L3*. It is associated with *CDX2* overexpression and an immunophenotype of CD10 negativity and immunoglobulin M positivity. This subtype is high-risk, associated with failure to achieve remission after induction therapy and high post-induction MRD levels [127].

IGH Rearrangement

Although individually rare, *IGH* rearrangements are overall present in approximately 5% of B-ALL cases, and form part of the B-ALL NOS subgroup. *IGH* rearrangements can be detected in all age groups with the peak incidence in adolescents and young adults. Collectively, they have been associated with an adverse outcome in adults, although they did not represent an independent prognostic factor in children and adolescents [123]. In addition to previously mentioned *IL3, CRLF2,* and *DUX4*, other reported partners include *MYC* at 8q24 [128], *ID4* at 6p14 [129], *EPOR* at 19p13 [130], and 5 members of the CEBP gene family: *CEBPA* (19q13), *CEBPB* (20q13), *CEBPD* (8q11), *CEBPE* (14q11), and *CEBPG* (19q13) [131]. The important molecular consequence of all *IGH* translocations is high levels of overexpression of the partner genes as a result of juxtaposition of the gene to *IGH*. With few exceptions, the karyotypes are relatively simple and near-diploid, with many showing cooperating deletions of *CDKN2A* and/or *PAX5* [132].

MYC, BCL2, BCL6 Rearrangement

Rearrangements involving these genes are known to be associated with B-cell non-Hodgkin's lymphoma. In B-ALL, translocations of *MYC, BCL2,* and/or *BCL6* with immunoglobulin genes (*IGH/ IGL/IGK*) form a rare subgroup, which is predominantly in adult patients and is associated with a poor prognosis [133].

ZEB2 H1038R Mutation

Recurrent *ZEB2* mutations, H1038R and Q1072, have been reported in <1% of B-ALL overall and 2.7–3.8% of B-ALL NOS [120, 134]. Although *ZEB2* mutations have been observed in association with other subtype-defining lesions (*DUX4*-r, *TCF3::PBX1*, and *ZNF384*-r) and at low mutant allele frequencies, pointing to cooperating activity rather than initiating, the majority of *ZEB2* mutations do not belong to any established subtype, and some have an expression profile close to

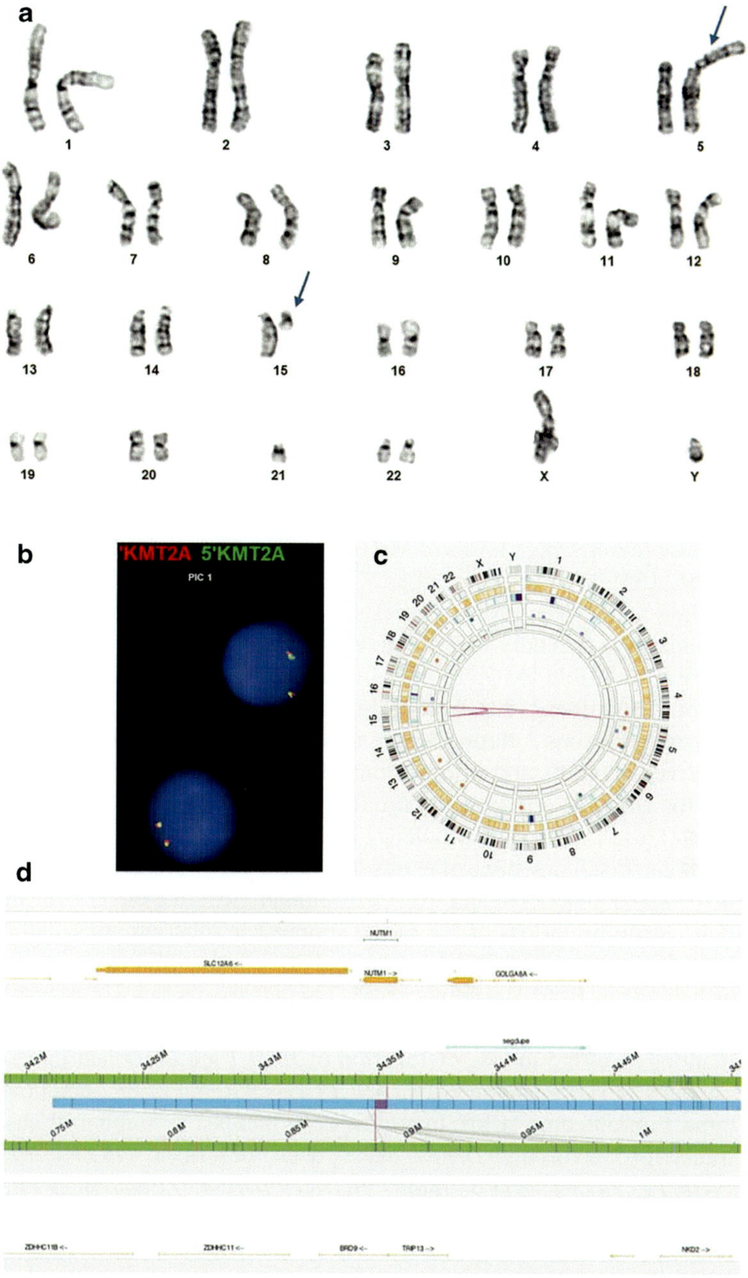

Fig. 13.3 Infant B-ALL with *NUTM1* rearrangement. (**a**) Chromosome analysis shows an apparent t(5;15)(p15.3;q11.2). (**b**) FISH is negative for *KMT2A* rearrangement. (**c**) OGM Circos Plot view suggests insertion of 15q material into 5p. (**d**) *BRD9::NUTM1* fusion is shown on the genome browser analysis

IGH::CREBP [134]. The few *ZEB2* mutation studies showed that Ras pathway-activating mutations (mutations in *NRAS, PTPN11* and *FLT3*) tended to be more frequent in cases with the H1038 mutation, and *ZEB2* mutations seemed to be enriched in relapsed B-ALL cases [120, 134].

IKZF1

IKZF1 alterations occur in approximately 15% of pediatric and 40–50% of adult patients with B-ALL and are highly prevalent in *BCR::ABL1*-positive ALL (~85%) and *BCR::ABL1*-like ALL (~70%) subtypes [70]. It is also overrepresented in Down syndrome-ALL and in patients with other features of high-risk disease, but rarely detected in *TCF3*-rearrangements (3%) and *ETV6::RUNX1*-positive B-ALL (3%), and ranges from 15% to 20% among other subtypes such as hyperdiploid and B-ALL NOS [135]. Patients with *IKZF1* deletion usually have advanced age and high white blood cell count [136]. Various studies have found *IKZF1* aberrations to have a negative prognostic impact, driving resistance to cytarabine or tyrosine kinase inhibitor therapy, high levels of MRD, poor survival, and increased frequency of relapse [56, 135].

IKZF1 plays a key role in hematopoiesis, differentiation, and proliferation of all lymphoid lineages, especially in the activation and development of B cells [137]. Deletions are responsible for up to 90% of cases with *IKZF1* alterations, with the rest being point mutations [138]. Among patients with *IKZF1* deletions, whole gene deletions involving exons 1 through 8 are observed in 25–40%, deletions of exons 4–7 are observed in ~25%, and other partial deletions comprise the remainder [139]. Deletion of the entire *IKZF1* gene or partial deletions that affect at least the starting codon (exon 2) result in haploinsufficiency and constitute up to 55% of B-ALL with *IKZF1* deletions. Focal deletions of exons 4–7 of the DNA binding domain account for ~33% of *IKZF1* deletions, and exert a dominant–negative effect over the unaffected allele, resulting in loss of the tumor suppressor function attributed to wild-type *IKZF1* [140]. Exons 4–7 deletions lead to a more severe phenotype than haploinsufficiency in B-ALL patients [141]. The adverse prognosis normally associated with *IKZF1* deletion is abrogated in the presence of *ERG* deletions [109]. Point mutations resulting in loss-of-function of *IKZF1* are described in up to 10% of *BCR::ABL1*+ and ~1% of non-*BCR::ABL1* cases without *IKZF1* deletion, with a similar impact on outcome [136]. In addition, an increasing number of cases with fusion transcripts involving *IKZF1* have been described (*IKZF1::PRDM16, IKZF1::NUMT1, IKZF1::ETV6, IKZF1::CDK2, IKZF1::ZEB2, IKZF1::SETD5, IKZF1::STIM2*) [120].

Two emerging B-ALL subtypes are related to *IKZF1* alterations, *IKZF1* N159Y and *IKZF1*^{plus}. The *IKZF1* N159Y comprises less than 1% of cases and is associated with intermediate prognosis [7, 120]. The *IKZF1* N159Y mutation is heterozygous, located in exon 5, and is also recurrently associated with the partial tandem duplication of the mutated exon 5 [139, 142]. This mutation affects the DNA banding domain, resulting in abnormal nuclear localization and enhanced cell-cell adhesion

[7, 142]. *IKZF1* N159Y is associated with a subtype-defining, characteristic gene expression pattern with overexpression of *YAP1, SALL1, and ARHGEF28;* and downregulation of JAK-STAT and B cell receptor signaling [119]. Abnormal karyotype can be found in 90% of *IKZF1* N159Y cases, with somatic gain of chromosome 21 being the most common chromosome abnormality (83%). Notably, additional mutations are uncommon, with the most frequent mutations (15%) involving in the RAS signaling pathway (*KRAS* and *FLT3*) [143]. *IKZF1*^{plus} is characterized by the co-existence of *IKZF1* deletions with deletions of *CDKN2A, CDKN2B,* and/or *PAX5* or the PAR1 region in the absence of *ERG* deletion [144] (Fig. 13.2), and presents in ~12.8% of overall B-ALL patients with strong association with Hispanic/Latino (H/L) ethnicity (19.6% in H/L vs. 4.8% in non-H/L). It is a poor prognostic factor and confers the most unfavorable outcome in MRD-positive patients with childhood B-ALL [145]. The *IKZF1*^{plus} subtype has a high frequency of *VPREB1* deletions and additional mutually exclusive deletions in the *CD200* and *BTLA* genes. Concomitant *IKZF1*^{plus} and *VPREB1* deletion has been reported to have significantly worse outcomes compared to patients with *IKZF1*^{plus} and non-*VPREB1* deletion [144, 146]. *IKZF1*^{plus} had also been associated with markedly up and down of *KCNA5* and *GREB1* [144].

PAX5

PAX5 is the B-lymphoid transcription factor that is essential for early stages of B cell development [147]. PAX5 alterations have been observed in approximately 30% of B-ALL cases, with copy number changes being the most common, followed by point mutations and rearrangements [148, 149]. Deletion and mutations have been considered as secondary events because they are present in many subtypes of B-ALL [148], except those co-deleted with *IKZF1* and *CDKN2A/B* to define the *IKZF1*^{plus} subtype with poorer outcome [145]. *PAX5* deletions have been noted to be associated with a complex karyotype [150]. However, two categories of distinct alterations in the *PAX5* gene have been identified as the driver: the *PAX5* p.Pro80Arg (PAX5 P80R) point mutation and the *PAX5*-altered (PAX5alt), which have different gene expression profiles and are now considered as distinct genetic subtypes [7].

PAX5 **P80R** subtype has an occurrence of 3–4% of children and 4% of adults with B-ALL. It confers a poor prognosis in children but is suggested to have a relatively good prognosis in adults [151]. The *PAX5* P80R mutation has been accompanied by inactivation of the second *PAX5* allele (biallelic events) through deletion or a second mutation (homozygous or compound heterozygous) or loss of heterozygosity in all reported cases. This mutation also frequently co-occurs with biallelic *CDKN2A/B* deletion and mutations in the RAS or JAK-STAT pathways as well as *FLT3, BRAF* and *PIK3CA* [7].

*PAX5***alt** subtype represents ~7.4% of B-ALL and confers an intermediate prognosis in children treated with intensive chemotherapy, but a poor prognosis in adults

[7]. This subtype contains diverse *PAX5* alterations, including rearrangements, sequence mutations and focal/intragenic amplifications [149]. More than 20 fusion partners have been reported for *PAX5* rearrangements, with *ETV6, NOL4L, AUTS2, ZCCHC7,* and *CBFA2T3* being the most involved. Others, such as *HIPK1, POM121, JAK2, DACH1, BRD1, ELN, FOXP1, ZNF521, PML,* and *C20orf112,* have also been reported [16, 152]. *PAX5* fusions are commonly observed in a relatively normal karyotype, suggesting that they are founder lesions [150, 152]. The *PAX5* intragenic amplification (*PAX5*^{amp}) in this *PAX5*alt subtype usually involves exons 2–5, exon 5 only, or exon 2 only, encoding the DNA-binding and octapeptide domains. It is present in ~1% of B-ALL and 3% of the B-ALL NOS. *PAX5*^{AMP} is frequently accompanied by trisomy 5, *CDKN2A/B* loss, and deletion of *IKZF1* and PAR1 region [26, 153] (Fig. 13.4). Cases with *PAX5*^{AMP} lack stratifying genetic markers and are mutually exclusive from other risk-stratifying alterations [153]. Transcriptome sequencing (RNA-seq) has revealed that *PAX5*^{AMP} can be grouped into the PAX5alt subtype [7].

CDKN2A

CDKN2A encodes p16, a cyclin-dependent kinase inhibitor participating in cell cycle regulation. The most common changes in the *CDKN2A* gene are deletions, found in 15–35% of children and 30–45% of adults with B-ALL, commonly involving both *CDKN2A* and *CDKN2B* as well as *PAX5* deletions due to their co-location on chromosome 9p. The deletions may be homozygous or heterozygous and appear to occur at approximately the same frequency [154]. The deletions are more frequently found in *BCR::ABL1*+ and *BCR::ABL1*-like ALL than in *ETV6::RUNX1* and Hyperdiploid ALL [79]. *CDKN2A/B* losses have been reported to be associated with an inferior outcome in adults, but do not appear to affect the outcome in pediatric B-ALL in the United Kingdom ALL (UKALL) study as well as other risk-stratification studies [154, 155]. However, recent studies have reported that deletion of *CDKN2A/B* is associated with poor prognosis [156]. *CDKN2A* promoter hypermethylation is also described, but it is less common than gene deletions. Very few studies have analyzed the effect of methylation status in the *CDKN2A/B* promoters, most of which have not shown a significant effect on B-ALL progression [154].

RB1, BTG1, EBF1, and Other Genes

Genes involved in cell cycle control, lymphoid development, signaling, or tumor suppressor genes are frequently altered in B-ALL. *RB1* gene deletions are present in 2–4% children with B-ALL. It is frequently deleted (39%) in children with iAMP21 and low hypodiploidy [157]. *BTG1* gene deletions are seen in up to 10% children with B-ALL and are known to be clustered with *ETV6::RUNX1* (15%) translocations [158]. *EBF1* deletions occur in 6% of B-ALL and are enriched in *BCR-ABL1*-like cases (15%), but absent in *KMT2A*-rearranged and *TCF3-PBX1*

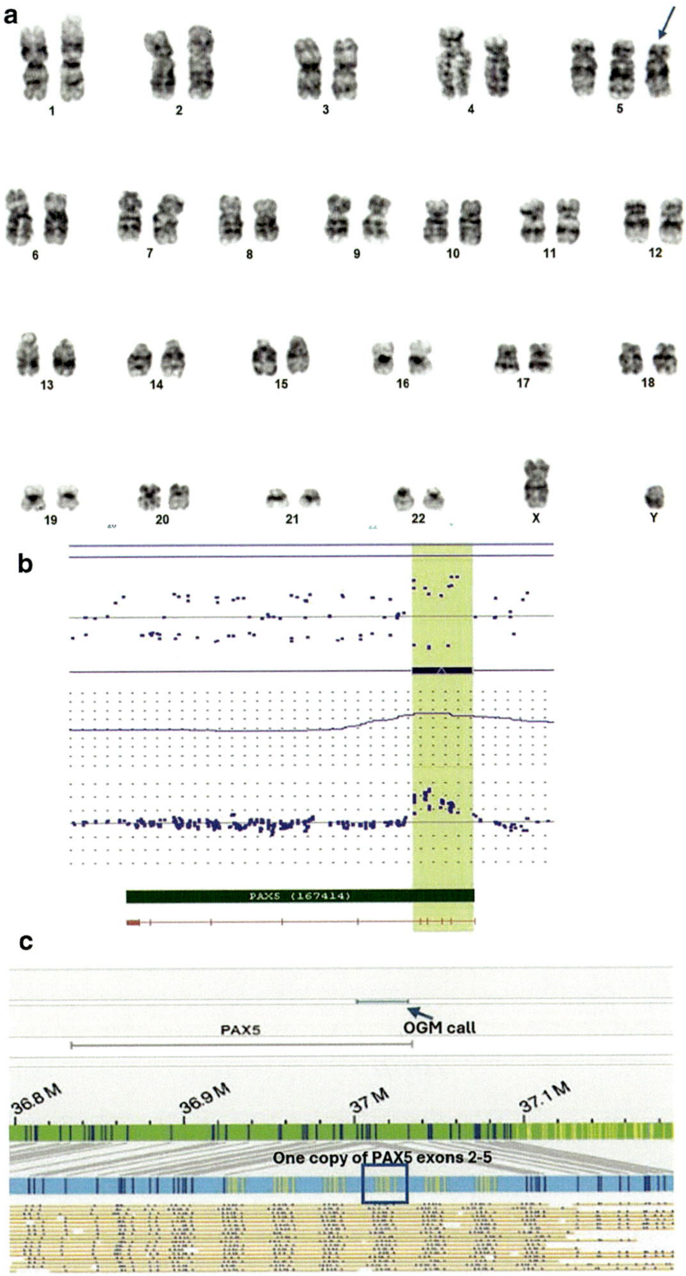

Fig. 13.4 B-ALL with *PAX5* exons 2–5 amplification. (**a**) Chromosome analysis shows the gain of chromosome 5, a common secondary abnormality in this subtype. (**b**) Microarray shows gain of *PAX5* exons 2–5. (**c**) OGM detects molecules containing intragenic tandem amplification (at least 7 copies of *PAX5* exons 2–5 amplicon)

Table 13.3 JAK-STAT alterations

Alteration classification	Fusion partner genes	Targeted therapy
CRLF2	*IGH, P2RY8*	JAK inhibitors PI3K/mTOR inhibitors
JAK2	*ATF7IP, BCR, EBF1, ETV6, GOLGA5, HMBOX1, OFD1, PAX5, PCM1, PFIBP1, RFX3, SMU1, SNX29, SSBP2, STRN3, TERF2, TPR, USP25, ZNF274, ZBTB46*	JAK inhibitors PI3K/mTOR inhibitors
EPOR	*IGH, IGK, LAIR1, THADA*	JAK inhibitors
IL2RB	*MYH9*	JAK inhibitors
TYK2	*MYB, SMARCA4, ZNF340*	TYK2 inhibitors
JAK1, JAK3, IL7R, SH2B3	N/A, can be mutations	JAK inhibitors

Table 13.4 *ABL* class rearrangements, Ras activating, and other rare fusions

Alteration groups		Fusion partner genes	Targeted therapy
ABL	*ABL1*	*CENPC, ETV6, FOXP1, LSM14, NUP214, NUP153, RCSD1, NBP2, SNX2, SFPQ, SPTAN1, ZMIZ1*	Dasatinib
	ABL2	*PAG1, RCSD1, ZC3HAV1*	Dasatinib
	CSF1R	*MEF2D, SSBP2, TBL1XR1*	Dasatinib
	LYN	NCOR1, GATAD2A	Dasatinib
	PDGFRA	FIP1L1	Dasatinib
	PDGFRB	ATF7IP, EBF1, ETV6, SSBP2, NIP1, ZEB2, ZMYND8	Dasatinib
Ras pathway	*KRAS, NRAS, PTNP11, CBL1, NF1, BRAF*	N/A	MEK inhibitors
Rare fusions	*NTRK3*	*ETV6*	TKI
	FLT3	*ZMYM2*	FLT3 inhibitors
	FGFR1	*BCR*	FGFR inhibitors
	BLNK	*DNIT*	Unknown
	PT2KB	*KDM6A, STAG2, TMEM2*	FAK inhibitors

cases. Patients carrying *EBF1* deletion tend to have higher MRD levels compared with those without *EBF1* deletion [159]. Other genes, which have been reported to be deleted in B-ALL, include *ABL1, CASP8AP2, CD200/BTLA, MLLT3, IKZF2, NF1, PHF6, PTEN, PTPN2, TBL1XR1, TP53*, and *VPREB1*. Deletions in *VPREB1, RB1, IKZF2,* and *TBL1XR1* can be biallelic [155].

Immunophenotypic Biomarkers

As mentioned above, genetic and molecular biomarkers play a critically important role in prognostic prediction and risk stratification in B-ALL. The prognostic value provided by immunophenotyping is likely attributed to its ability to predict certain cytogenetic/molecular subtypes. Innovative therapies targeting leukemia surface antigens, such as monoclonal antibodies, bispecific T cell engagers, antibody-drug conjugates, and chimeric antigen receptor T cells (CAR-Ts), have shown significant effectiveness in treating relapsed/refractory B-ALL (R/R B-ALL) [160]. The targeted surface antigens in leukemic cells are important predictors of the responses to these treatments. A small number of antigens might work as an independent prognostic biomarker, and their presence or absence is associated with a better or worse prognosis.

Immunophenotypic Biomarkers Associated with Genetic Subtypes

B-ALL can be subclassified as pro-B-ALL (CD10–), common ALL (CD10+), and pre-B-ALL (cytoplasmic IgM+) based on the developmental stage demonstrated by immunophenotyping [161]. Pro-B-ALL is commonly seen in B-ALL with *KMT2A* rearrangement, a prognostically unfavorable subtype that is commonly positive for CD15 or other myeloid markers. Pre-B-ALL is commonly seen in B-ALL cases with *TCF3::PBX1* or *MEF2D* fusions. CD5, a T-cell marker, can be expressed in B-ALL with *MEF2D* rearrangement, and its presence is associated with a worse prognosis [162]. CD25 is commonly associated with *BCR::ABL1*+ B-ALL, a subtype with poor prognosis [163]. Expression of the *CRLF2* gene product (TSLPR) assessed by FCM (Fig. 13.2b) is associated with *CRLF2* gene alteration that is commonly seen in *BCR::ABL1*-like ALL, a subtype associated with inferior prognosis [164]. Surface CD371 expression is specifically associated with B-ALL with *DUX4* rearrangement, a subtype with a good prognosis, which also commonly expresses CD2, a T/NK cell marker [103, 165]. CD2 is also commonly seen in *PAX5*-P80R B-ALL [165]. Surface CD36 expression is a characteristic feature of B-ALL with ABL/JAK-class kinase fusions [166].

Antigens Targeted by Immunotherapy

The most common targeted surface antigens for B-ALL treatment are CD19 and CD22. The expression of these antigens in leukemic cells is a prerequisite for the success of these treatments, and loss of the antigen is associated with antigen-negative relapse [167–169]. Moreover, the expression level or intensity of these antigens may also affect the therapeutic efficacy.

CD19 is a transmembrane glycoprotein present in over 90% of B-ALL cases. Blinatumomab is a bispecific T cell engager (BiTE) monoclonal antibody directed against CD19 and CD3. By binding to CD19+ leukemic cells and CD3+ T cells simultaneously, it induces antibody-dependent cellular cytotoxicity against the leukemic cells, thereby eliminating the CD19+ blasts. The efficacy of blinatumomab in R/R B-ALL is well established and superior to high-dose chemotherapy in children and young adults [170, 171]. The cases with dim CD19 expression on leukemia cells tend to have lower response rates to blinatumomab compared to those with bright CD19 expression [172]. Tisagenlecleucel (Kymriah), an anti-CD19 CAR-T treatment, is the first U.S. Food and Drug Administration (FDA)-approved and most commonly used CAR-T therapy for B-ALL, which has shown a remarkable efficacy for R/R B-ALL [173]. The study conducted by Majzner et al. demonstrated the association of CD19 density with the activity of CAR-Ts, that is, reduced killing capacity, proliferation, and cytokine production in response to cell lines with decreased CD19 expression [174]. This study also found that different costimulatory domains in CAR constructs influenced the CAR-T response to low antigen density threshold, that is, axicabtagene ciloleucel (CD19-CD28ζ) outperforming tisagenlecleucel (CD19-4-1BBζ) against antigen-low tumor cells [174]. The association of pre-treatment low surface CD19 density with poor response was also demonstrated in another study on adult patients with large B-cell lymphoma or B-ALL [175]. However, in a large cohort study on pediatric or young adult patients treated with Tisagenlecleucel [176], no association between pre-treatment CD19 intensity and CAR-T therapeutic response was found. The presence of dimly CD19+ or rare CD19- blasts by FCM did not predict nonresponse or recurrence after CAR-T therapy. Therefore, the presence of dimly CD19+ and rare CD19- blasts should not exclude patients from anti-CD19 CAR-T therapy. Prior blinatumomab treatment is associated with the emergence of CD19-dim or negative leukemia cells and inferior therapeutic response to anti-CD19 CAR-T therapy [172, 176].

CD22 is an inhibitory B-cell co-receptor, which is positive in more than 90% of B-ALL cases. Inotuzumab ozogamicin (InO) is a monoclonal anti-CD22 antibody attached to calicheamicin. Clinical trials involving both pediatric and adult patients have shown that InO produced better therapeutic outcomes compared to standard chemotherapy in R/R B-ALL [177, 178]. CD22 surface expression varies in leukemia cells, not only between patients but also within the same patient. The impact of varying CD22 levels on the response to InO has been investigated in several clinical trials. The results indicated that the favorable benefic-risk profile in InO treatment was not significantly influenced by CD22 expression based on the percentage of CD22 positivity [177, 179]. Even in patients with <90% CD22 positivity, the therapeutic responses with InO were still more effective than those with conventional chemotherapy. In CD22 fluorescence intensity quartile analysis, the quartile with the lowest CD22 had a trend of having the least benefit from InO treatment compared to chemotherapy, indicating the response to InO could be limited by low CD22 expression [179]. However, dim CD22 expression may not predict non-response or poor response to InO [180], and thus it cannot be used as a criterion to exclude patients for this therapy. CD22 CAR-T therapy and dual CD19/CD22 CAR-T therapy are also at different stages of clinical development [175]. One study showed that low CD22 expression reduced CD22 CAR-T functionality in vitro and in vivo and impeded in vivo CART persistence [181]. This study also showed that increased CD22 on leukemia and lymphoma cell lines by Bryostatin1 improved CAR-T functionality and in vivo persistence.

Other Immunophenotypic Biomarkers

CD20 is a B-lymphocyte-specific membrane protein expressed in late-stage B-cell precursors and mature B cells. Approximately 40–50% of B-ALL cases show CD20 expression, which is often dim and variable. The prognostic impact of CD20 on pediatric B-ALL is contradictory among different studies [182, 183], which questions the role of CD20 as a prognostic biomarker in pediatric B-ALL. In contrast, the studies in adult B-ALL patients consistently demonstrated that CD20 positivity was generally associated with an inferior outcome [184, 185]. As a commonly used target by immunotherapy for B-cell non-Hodgkin lymphomas, the expression of CD20 in B-ALL provides a therapeutic option for adding Rituximab (anti-CD20 monoclonal antibody) into the treatment regimen of B-ALL. A randomized clinical study has demonstrated that the addition of Rituximab to the B-ALL chemotherapy protocol can improve the outcome for younger adults with CD20+ Ph-negative B-ALL [186]. The study in pediatric patients with newly diagnosed B-ALL didn't show any benefits of adding Rituximab into the treatment regimen [187].

CD45, also known as leukocyte common antigen, is a receptor-type protein tyrosine phosphatase expressed in all leukocytes and most hematopoietic precursors. Most B-ALL cases express low-level CD45. There have been a few studies demonstrating the adverse prognostic impact of high CD45 expression on pediatric ALL [183, 188, 189]. The early POG study on 1231 pediatric B-ALL cases showed that high CD45 intensity (>75th percentile) was associated with a worse EFS, and the association was not related to other known poor prognostic factors such as NCI risk group, ploidy, and unfavorable translocations [183]. A Japanese study conducted several years later confirmed the negative impact of high CD45 intensity on EFS only in the NCI HR pediatric B-ALL patients [188]. Later, a German team also found a shorter EFS in the high-CD45 group due to a higher cumulative incidence of relapse (CIR). And they also found that high CD45 expression was associated with NCI HR, presence of unfavorable genetic biomarkers, and poor prednisone response [189].

CD36 is a membrane glycoprotein present on monocytes/ macrophages, platelets, erythroblasts, adipocytes, and some epithelia. It is a scavenger receptor involved in many physiologic functions. A one-center retrospective study has shown the negative impact of CD36 expression on the outcome of pediatric B-ALL cases. In this study, 5-year EFS and OS of the NCI-SR patients were significantly worse in the CD36+ group compared with the CD36- group [190]. The prognostic value of CD36 may be attributed to its association with Ph-like kinase fusions [166].

CD34 is a transmembrane glycoprotein expressed on lymphohematopoietic progenitor cells. A large proportion of B-ALL cases demonstrate CD34 expression, which is commonly partial or variable. The study by Modvig et al. demonstrated high CD34 expression as a predictor of poor induction therapy response. The CD34+ cases were approximately 6.5 times more likely to have a positive MRD result at the end of induction compared with CD34− cases [191]. The lack of CD34 was found to be associated with a favorable prognosis [192]. Further studies with an increased number of patients are needed to confirm these results.

Other Prognostic and/or Predictive Biomarkers

Initial WBC, a measure of extramedullary leukemia burden, has been one of the historical strongest risk factors. It has been used for NCI risk stratification [193] in pediatric B-ALL. The two groups of patients with NCI-SR (WBC <50,00/μL and age 1–9 years) or NCI-HR (all others) had significantly different 4-year EFS (80% vs. 60%) [193]. NCI risk stratification is currently still in use to guide risk-adapted treatment for pediatric B-ALL. A study involving 2666 ALL patients from five Nordic countries showed that WBC was not associated with risk of event for B-ALL or T-ALL in patients with day 29 MRD (MRDd29) <0.1%. In contrast, for patients with MRDd29 ≥ 0.1% and <5%, the 5-year EFS for patients with WBC ≥ 100,000/μL was significantly shorter than that of patients with WBC < 100,000/μL [194]. Other blood cell counts, such as platelet and neutrophil counts, may also have some prognostic value in certain patient groups; however, their independent prognostic values are in question and should be further studied.

Initial cerebrospinal fluid (CSF) findings (CNS involvement) have also been found to have an impact on the outcome of pediatric B-ALL patients. A COG study published in 2017 demonstrated significantly lower 5-year EFS and OS rates in the CNS2 group (76% and 86.8%) and CNS3 group (76% and 82.1%) than those in the CNS1 (no blasts) group (85% and 92.7%), regardless of NCI risks [195]. These findings indicate that the presence of blasts in CSF, regardless of CSF cell count, is an independent predictor of adverse outcome in pediatric B-ALL patients.

Conclusion

Many prognostic and predictive biomarkers have been identified in B-ALL. These biomarkers enable categorizing B-ALL cases into risk groups, allowing for a customized treatment approach for each case. This risk-adapted treatment strategy has led to the very high cure rates in newly diagnosed pediatric ALL cases. However, a significant portion of B-ALL cases will experience relapse, and the prognosis of these relapsed cases is often poor. Additionally, therapy-related mortality and morbidity continue to pose risks for B-ALL patients. Recent advances in sequencing technology and integrated analyses of large-scale data have facilitated the discovery of many new genetic biomarkers, which have the potential to enhance the accuracy of risk stratification, identify new genetic/molecular defects that may serve as potential therapeutic targets, and eventually improve the overall clinical outcomes.

References

1. Malard F, Mohty M. Acute lymphoblastic leukaemia. Lancet. 2020;395(10230):1146–62.
2. American Cancer Society Cancer Facts & Figures 2020. Available online: https://www.cancer.org/research/cancer-factsstatistics/all-cancer-facts-figures/cancer-facts-figures-2020.html. Accessed on 6 Jan 2022.
3. Inaba H, Pui CH. Advances in the diagnosis and treatment of pediatric acute lymphoblastic leukemia. J Clin Med. 2021;10(9):1926.
4. Lee SHR, Li Z, Tai ST, Oh BLZ, Yeoh AEJ. Genetic alterations in childhood acute lymphoblastic leukemia: interactions with clinical features and treatment response. Cancers (Basel). 2021;13(16):4068.
5. Vllahu M, Savarese M, Cantiello I, Munno C, Sarcina R, Stellato P, et al. Application of omics analyses in pediatric B-cell acute lymphoblastic leukemia. Biomedicine. 2025;13(2):424.
6. Alaggio R, Amador C, Anagnostopoulos I, Attygalle AD, Araujo IBO, Berti E, et al. The 5th edition of the World Health Organization classification of haematolymphoid tumours: lymphoid neoplasms. Leukemia. 2022;36(7):1720–48.
7. Gu Z, Churchman ML, Roberts KG, Moore I, Zhou X, Nakitandwe J, et al. PAX5-driven subtypes of B-progenitor acute lymphoblastic leukemia. Nat Genet. 2019;51(2):296–307.
8. Pui CH, Relling MV, Downing JR. Acute lymphoblastic leukemia. N Engl J Med. 2004;350(15):1535–48.
9. Burmeister T, Gokbuget N, Schwartz S, Fischer L, Hubert D, Sindram A, et al. Clinical features and prognostic implications of TCF3-PBX1 and ETV6-RUNX1 in adult acute lymphoblastic leukemia. Haematologica. 2010;95(2):241–6.
10. Sundaresh A, Williams O. Mechanism of ETV6-RUNX1 leukemia. Adv Exp Med Biol. 2017;962:201–16.
11. Schafer D, Olsen M, Lahnemann D, Stanulla M, Slany R, Schmiegelow K, et al. Five percent of healthy newborns have an ETV6-RUNX1 fusion as revealed by DNA-based GIPFEL screening. Blood. 2018;131(7):821–6.
12. Sun C, Chang L, Zhu X. Pathogenesis of ETV6/RUNX1-positive childhood acute lymphoblastic leukemia and mechanisms underlying its relapse. Oncotarget. 2017;8(21):35445–59.
13. Enshaei A, Schwab CJ, Konn ZJ, Mitchell CD, Kinsey SE, Wade R, et al. Long-term follow-up of ETV6-RUNX1 ALL reveals that NCI risk, rather than secondary genetic abnormalities, is the key risk factor. Leukemia. 2013;27(11):2256–9.

14. Li Z, Zhao H, Yang W, Maillard M, Yoshimura S, Hsiao YC, et al. Molecular and pharmacological heterogeneity of ETV6::RUNX1 acute lymphoblastic leukemia. Nat Commun. 2025;16(1):1153.
15. Lilljebjorn H, Soneson C, Andersson A, Heldrup J, Behrendtz M, Kawamata N, et al. The correlation pattern of acquired copy number changes in 164 ETV6/RUNX1-positive childhood acute lymphoblastic leukemias. Hum Mol Genet. 2010;19(16):3150–8.
16. Lejman M, Chalupnik A, Chilimoniuk Z, Dobosz M. Genetic biomarkers and their clinical implications in B-cell acute lymphoblastic leukemia in children. Int J Mol Sci. 2022;23(5):2755.
17. Barbany G, Andersen MK, Autio K, Borgstrom G, Franco LC, Golovleva I, et al. Additional aberrations of the ETV6 and RUNX1 genes have no prognostic impact in 229 t(12;21)(p13;q22)-positive B-cell precursor acute lymphoblastic leukaemias treated according to the NOPHO-ALL-2000 protocol. Leuk Res. 2012;36(7):936–8.
18. Kuster L, Grausenburger R, Fuka G, Kaindl U, Krapf G, Inthal A, et al. ETV6/RUNX1-positive relapses evolve from an ancestral clone and frequently acquire deletions of genes implicated in glucocorticoid signaling. Blood. 2011;117(9):2658–67.
19. O'Connor D, Enshaei A, Bartram J, Hancock J, Harrison CJ, Hough R, et al. Genotype-specific minimal residual disease interpretation improves stratification in pediatric acute lymphoblastic leukemia. J Clin Oncol. 2018;36(1):34–43.
20. Chang TC, Chen W, Qu C, Cheng Z, Hedges D, Elsayed A, et al. Genomic determinants of outcome in acute lymphoblastic leukemia. J Clin Oncol. 2024;42(29):3491–503.
21. Wang'ondu RW, Kairalla JA, Shago M, Angiolillo A, Breidenbach HM, et al. Chromosome 15q deletions confer inferior outcomes among children with ETV6::RUNX1 B-cell acute lymphoblastic leukemia. Blood Adv. 2026:bloodadvances.2026019599. https://doi.org/10.1182/bloodadvances.2026019599. Online ahead of print
22. Wang'ondu RW, Loh ML. Revisiting novel genomic classifiers in the era of immunotherapy for pediatric B-ALL. Hematology Am Soc Hematol Educ Prog. 2025;5(1):252–61.
23. Oksa L, Moisio S, Maqbool K, Kramer R, Nikkila A, Jayasingha B, et al. Genomic determinants of therapy response in ETV6::RUNX1 leukemia. Leukemia. 2025;39(9):2125–39.
24. Zaliova M, Kotrova M, Bresolin S, Stuchly J, Stary J, Hrusak O, et al. ETV6/RUNX1-like acute lymphoblastic leukemia: a novel B-cell precursor leukemia subtype associated with the CD27/CD44 immunophenotype. Genes Chromosomes Cancer. 2017;56(8):608–16.
25. Kaczmarska A, Derebas J, Pinkosz M, Niedzwiecki M, Lejman M. The landscape of secondary genetic rearrangements in pediatric patients with B-cell acute lymphoblastic leukemia with t(12;21). Cells. 2023;12(3):357.
26. Zaliova M, Stuchly J, Winkowska L, Musilova A, Fiser K, Slamova M, et al. Genomic landscape of pediatric B-other acute lymphoblastic leukemia in a consecutive European cohort. Haematologica. 2019;104(7):1396–406.
27. Lilljebjorn H, Fioretos T. New oncogenic subtypes in pediatric B-cell precursor acute lymphoblastic leukemia. Blood. 2017;130(12):1395–401.
28. Murthy A, Lee B, Zavala A, Tirado CA. ETV6::RUNX1-like acute lymphoblastic leukemia. J Assoc Genet Technol. 2024;50(2):61–3.
29. Jeha S, Choi J, Roberts KG, Pei D, Coustan-Smith E, Inaba H, et al. Clinical significance of novel subtypes of acute lymphoblastic leukemia in the context of minimal residual disease-directed therapy. Blood Cancer Discov. 2021;2(4):326–37.
30. Paulsson K, Johansson B. High hyperdiploid childhood acute lymphoblastic leukemia. Genes Chromosomes Cancer. 2009;48(8):637–60.
31. Inaba H, Mullighan CG. Pediatric acute lymphoblastic leukemia. Haematologica. 2020;105(11):2524–39.
32. Sutcliffe MJ, Shuster JJ, Sather HN, Camitta BM, Pullen J, Schultz KR, et al. High concordance from independent studies by the Children's Cancer Group (CCG) and Pediatric Oncology Group (POG) associating favorable prognosis with combined trisomies 4, 10, and 17 in children with NCI Standard-Risk B-precursor Acute Lymphoblastic Leukemia: a Children's Oncology Group (COG) initiative. Leukemia. 2005;19(5):734–40.

33. Enshaei A, Vora A, Harrison CJ, Moppett J, Moorman AV. Defining low-risk high hyperdiploidy in patients with paediatric acute lymphoblastic leukaemia: a retrospective analysis of data from the UKALL97/99 and UKALL2003 clinical trials. Lancet Haematol. 2021;8(11):e828–e39.
34. Moorman AV, Richards SM, Martineau M, Cheung KL, Robinson HM, Jalali GR, et al. Outcome heterogeneity in childhood high-hyperdiploid acute lymphoblastic leukemia. Blood. 2003;102(8):2756–62.
35. Ramos-Muntada M, Trincado JL, Blanco J, Bueno C, Rodriguez-Cortez VC, Bataller A, et al. Clonal heterogeneity and rates of specific chromosome gains are risk predictors in childhood high-hyperdiploid B-cell acute lymphoblastic leukemia. Mol Oncol. 2022;16(16):2899–919.
36. Chen C, Bartenhagen C, Gombert M, Okpanyi V, Binder V, Rottgers S, et al. Next-generation-sequencing of recurrent childhood high hyperdiploid acute lymphoblastic leukemia reveals mutations typically associated with high risk patients. Leuk Res. 2015;39(9):990–1001.
37. Paulsson K, Lilljebjorn H, Biloglav A, Olsson L, Rissler M, Castor A, et al. The genomic landscape of high hyperdiploid childhood acute lymphoblastic leukemia. Nat Genet. 2015;47(6):672–6.
38. Studd JB, Cornish AJ, Hoang PH, Law P, Kinnersley B, Houlston R. Cancer drivers and clonal dynamics in acute lymphoblastic leukaemia subtypes. Blood Cancer J. 2021;11(11):177.
39. El Ashry MS, Elsayed GM, Madney Y, Arafah O, Allam RM, Rasekh EO. Duplication 1q is highly correlated with poor prognosis in high hyperdiploid pediatric B-acute lymphoblastic leukemia. Int J Lab Hematol. 2021;43(2):235–43.
40. Pui CH, Raimondi SC, Williams DL. Isochromosome 17q in childhood acute lymphoblastic leukemia: an adverse cytogenetic feature in association with hyperdiploidy? Leukemia. 1988;2(4):222–5.
41. Paulsson K, Forestier E, Lilljebjorn H, Heldrup J, Behrendtz M, Young BD, et al. Genetic landscape of high hyperdiploid childhood acute lymphoblastic leukemia. Proc Natl Acad Sci USA. 2010;107(50):21719–24.
42. Paulsson K, Forestier E, Andersen MK, Autio K, Barbany G, Borgstrom G, et al. High modal number and triple trisomies are highly correlated favorable factors in childhood B-cell precursor high hyperdiploid acute lymphoblastic leukemia treated according to the NOPHO ALL 1992/2000 protocols. Haematologica. 2013;98(9):1424–32.
43. Yasuda T, Sanada M, Kawazu M, Kojima S, Tsuzuki S, Ueno H, et al. Two novel high-risk adult B-cell acute lymphoblastic leukemia subtypes with high expression of CDX2 and IDH1/2 mutations. Blood. 2022;139(12):1850–62.
44. Groeneveld-Krentz S, Schroeder MP, Reiter M, Pogodzinski MJ, Pimentel-Gutierrez HJ, Vagkopoulou R, et al. Aneuploidy in children with relapsed B-cell precursor acute lymphoblastic leukaemia: clinical importance of detecting a hypodiploid origin of relapse. Br J Haematol. 2019;185(2):266–83.
45. Harrison CJ, Moorman AV, Broadfield ZJ, Cheung KL, Harris RL, Reza Jalali G, et al. Three distinct subgroups of hypodiploidy in acute lymphoblastic leukaemia. Br J Haematol. 2004;125(5):552–9.
46. Pui CH, Rebora P, Schrappe M, Attarbaschi A, Baruchel A, Basso G, et al. Outcome of children with hypodiploid acute lymphoblastic leukemia: a retrospective multinational study. J Clin Oncol. 2019;37(10):770–9.
47. Holmfeldt L, Wei L, Diaz-Flores E, Walsh M, Zhang J, Ding L, et al. The genomic landscape of hypodiploid acute lymphoblastic leukemia. Nat Genet. 2013;45(3):242–52.
48. Creasey T, Enshaei A, Nebral K, Schwab C, Watts K, Cuthbert G, et al. Single nucleotide polymorphism array-based signature of low hypodiploidy in acute lymphoblastic leukemia. Genes Chromosomes Cancer. 2021;60(9):604–15.
49. Moorman AV, Harrison CJ, Buck GA, Richards SM, Secker-Walker LM, Martineau M, et al. Karyotype is an independent prognostic factor in adult acute lymphoblastic leukemia (ALL): analysis of cytogenetic data from patients treated on the Medical Research Council (MRC) UKALLXII/Eastern Cooperative Oncology Group (ECOG) 2993 trial. Blood. 2007;109(8):3189–97.

50. Muhlbacher V, Zenger M, Schnittger S, Weissmann S, Kunze F, Kohlmann A, et al. Acute lymphoblastic leukemia with low hypodiploid/near triploid karyotype is a specific clinical entity and exhibits a very high TP53 mutation frequency of 93%. Genes Chromosomes Cancer. 2014;53(6):524–36.
51. Comeaux EQ, Mullighan CG. TP53 mutations in hypodiploid acute lymphoblastic leukemia. Cold Spring Harb Perspect Med. 2017;7(3):a026286.
52. Kurzrock R, Kantarjian HM, Druker BJ, Talpaz M. Philadelphia chromosome-positive leukemias: from basic mechanisms to molecular therapeutics. Ann Intern Med. 2003;138(10):819–30.
53. Moorman AV. New and emerging prognostic and predictive genetic biomarkers in B-cell precursor acute lymphoblastic leukemia. Haematologica. 2016;101(4):407–16.
54. Pane F, Intrieri M, Quintarelli C, Izzo B, Muccioli GC, Salvatore F. BCR/ABL genes and leukemic phenotype: from molecular mechanisms to clinical correlations. Oncogene. 2002;21(56):8652–67.
55. Deininger MW, Goldman JM, Melo JV. The molecular biology of chronic myeloid leukemia. Blood. 2000;96(10):3343–56.
56. Fedullo AL, Messina M, Elia L, Piciocchi A, Gianfelici V, Lauretti A, et al. Prognostic implications of additional genomic lesions in adult Philadelphia chromosome-positive acute lymphoblastic leukemia. Haematologica. 2019;104(2):312–8.
57. Martinelli G, Iacobucci I, Storlazzi CT, Vignetti M, Paoloni F, Cilloni D, et al. IKZF1 (Ikaros) deletions in BCR-ABL1-positive acute lymphoblastic leukemia are associated with short disease-free survival and high rate of cumulative incidence of relapse: a GIMEMA AL WP report. J Clin Oncol. 2009;27(31):5202–7.
58. Notta F, Mullighan CG, Wang JC, Poeppl A, Doulatov S, Phillips LA, et al. Evolution of human BCR-ABL1 lymphoblastic leukaemia-initiating cells. Nature. 2011;469(7330):362–7.
59. Shen S, Chen X, Cai J, Yu J, Gao J, Hu S, et al. Effect of dasatinib vs imatinib in the treatment of pediatric Philadelphia chromosome-positive acute lymphoblastic leukemia: a randomized clinical trial. JAMA Oncol. 2020;6(3):358–66.
60. Yeung DTO, Osborn MP, White DL. B-cell acute lymphoblastic leukaemia: recent discoveries in molecular pathology, their prognostic significance, and a review of the current classification. Br J Haematol. 2022;197(1):13–27.
61. Arber DA, Orazi A, Hasserjian R, Thiele J, Borowitz MJ, Le Beau MM, et al. The 2016 revision to the World Health Organization classification of myeloid neoplasms and acute leukemia. Blood. 2016;127(20):2391–405.
62. Jain S, Abraham A. BCR-ABL1-like B-acute lymphoblastic leukemia/lymphoma: a comprehensive review. Arch Pathol Lab Med. 2020;144(2):150–5.
63. Plotka A, Lewandowski K. BCR/ABL1-like acute lymphoblastic leukemia: from diagnostic approaches to molecularly targeted therapy. Acta Haematol. 2022;145(2):122–31.
64. Chuang S, Chu A, Hurtado R, Tirado CA. Integrative insights into Philadelphia-like B-cell acute lymphoblastic leukemia: a genetic and molecular landscape. Diagnostics (Basel). 2025;15(3):385.
65. Yadav V, Ganesan P, Veeramani R, Kumar VD. Philadelphia-like acute lymphoblastic leukemia: a systematic review. Clin Lymphoma Myeloma Leuk. 2021;21(1):e57–65.
66. Roberts KG, Li Y, Payne-Turner D, Harvey RC, Yang YL, Pei D, et al. Targetable kinase-activating lesions in Ph-like acute lymphoblastic leukemia. N Engl J Med. 2014;371(11):1005–15.
67. Reshmi SC, Harvey RC, Roberts KG, Stonerock E, Smith A, Jenkins H, et al. Targetable kinase gene fusions in high-risk B-ALL: a study from the Children's Oncology Group. Blood. 2017;129(25):3352–61.
68. Raca G, Abdel-Azim H, Yue F, Broach J, Payne JL, Reeves ME, et al. Increased incidence of IKZF1 deletions and IGH-CRLF2 translocations in B-ALL of Hispanic/Latino children-a novel health disparity. Leukemia. 2021;35(8):2399–402.
69. Ou Z, Sherer M, Casey J, Bakos HA, Vitullo K, Hu J, et al. The genomic landscape of PAX5, IKZF1, and CDKN2A/B alterations in B-cell precursor acute lymphoblastic leukemia. Cytogenet Genome Res. 2016;150(3–4):242–52.

70. Mullighan CG, Su X, Zhang J, Radtke I, Phillips LA, Miller CB, et al. Deletion of IKZF1 and prognosis in acute lymphoblastic leukemia. N Engl J Med. 2009;360(5):470–80.
71. Meyer LK, Delgado-Martin C, Maude SL, Shannon KM, Teachey DT, Hermiston ML. CRLF2 rearrangement in Ph-like acute lymphoblastic leukemia predicts relative glucocorticoid resistance that is overcome with MEK or Akt inhibition. PLoS One. 2019;14(7):e0220026.
72. Morak M, Attarbaschi A, Fischer S, Nassimbeni C, Grausenburger R, Bastelberger S, et al. Small sizes and indolent evolutionary dynamics challenge the potential role of P2RY8-CRLF2-harboring clones as main relapse-driving force in childhood ALL. Blood. 2012;120(26):5134–42.
73. Russell LJ, Capasso M, Vater I, Akasaka T, Bernard OA, Calasanz MJ, et al. Deregulated expression of cytokine receptor gene, CRLF2, is involved in lymphoid transformation in B-cell precursor acute lymphoblastic leukemia. Blood. 2009;114(13):2688–98.
74. Yano M, Imamura T, Asai D, Moriya-Saito A, Suenobu S, Hasegawa D, et al. An overall characterization of pediatric acute lymphoblastic leukemia with CRLF2 overexpression. Genes Chromosomes Cancer. 2014;53(10):815–23.
75. Frisch A, Ofran Y. How I diagnose and manage Philadelphia chromosome-like acute lymphoblastic leukemia. Haematologica. 2019;104(11):2135–43.
76. Russell LJ, Jones L, Enshaei A, Tonin S, Ryan SL, Eswaran J, et al. Characterisation of the genomic landscape of CRLF2-rearranged acute lymphoblastic leukemia. Genes Chromosomes Cancer. 2017;56(5):363–72.
77. Harvey RC, Tasian SK. Clinical diagnostics and treatment strategies for Philadelphia chromosome-like acute lymphoblastic leukemia. Blood Adv. 2020;4(1):218–28.
78. Panzer-Grumayer R, Kohrer S, Haas OA. The enigmatic role(s) of P2RY8-CRLF2. Oncotarget. 2017;8(57):96466–7.
79. Schwab CJ, Chilton L, Morrison H, Jones L, Al-Shehhi H, Erhorn A, et al. Genes commonly deleted in childhood B-cell precursor acute lymphoblastic leukemia: association with cytogenetics and clinical features. Haematologica. 2013;98(7):1081–8.
80. El Chaer F, Keng M, Ballen KK. MLL-rearranged acute lymphoblastic leukemia. Curr Hematol Malig Rep. 2020;15(2):83–9.
81. Pui CH, Gaynon PS, Boyett JM, Chessells JM, Baruchel A, Kamps W, et al. Outcome of treatment in childhood acute lymphoblastic leukaemia with rearrangements of the 11q23 chromosomal region. Lancet. 2002;359(9321):1909–15.
82. Khalidi HS, Chang KL, Medeiros LJ, Brynes RK, Slovak ML, Murata-Collins JL, et al. Acute lymphoblastic leukemia. Survey of immunophenotype, French-American-British classification, frequency of myeloid antigen expression, and karyotypic abnormalities in 210 pediatric and adult cases. Am J Clin Pathol. 1999;111(4):467–76.
83. Meyer C, Burmeister T, Groger D, Tsaur G, Fechina L, Renneville A, et al. The MLL recombinome of acute leukemias in 2017. Leukemia. 2018;32(2):273–84.
84. Emerenciano M, Meyer C, Mansur MB, Marschalek R, Pombo-de-Oliveira MS. Brazilian Collaborative Study Group of Infant Acute L. The distribution of MLL breakpoints correlates with outcome in infant acute leukaemia. Br J Haematol. 2013;161(2):224–36.
85. Andersson AK, Ma J, Wang J, Chen X, Gedman AL, Dang J, et al. The landscape of somatic mutations in infant MLL-rearranged acute lymphoblastic leukemias. Nat Genet. 2015;47(4):330–7.
86. Salzer WL, Jones TL, Devidas M, Dreyer ZE, Gore L, Winick NJ, et al. Decreased induction morbidity and mortality following modification to induction therapy in infants with acute lymphoblastic leukemia enrolled on AALL0631: a report from the Children's Oncology Group. Pediatr Blood Cancer. 2015;62(3):414–8.
87. Hunger SP. Chromosomal translocations involving the E2A gene in acute lymphoblastic leukemia: clinical features and molecular pathogenesis. Blood. 1996;87(4):1211–24.
88. Hunger SP, Devaraj PE, Foroni L, Secker-Walker LM, Cleary ML. Two types of genomic rearrangements create alternative E2A-HLF fusion proteins in t(17;19)-ALL. Blood. 1994;83(10):2970–7.

89. Sudutan T, Erbilgin Y, Hatirnaz Ng O, Karaman S, Karakas Z, Kucukcankurt F, et al. Zinc finger protein 384 (ZNF384) impact on childhood mixed phenotype acute leukemia and B-cell precursor acute lymphoblastic leukemia. Leuk Lymphoma. 2022;63(12):1–9.
90. Zhong CH, Prima V, Liang X, Frye C, McGavran L, Meltesen L, et al. E2A-ZNF384 and NOL1-E2A fusion created by a cryptic t(12;19)(p13.3; p13.3) in acute leukemia. Leukemia. 2008;22(4):723–9.
91. McClure BJ, Heatley SL, Rehn J, Breen J, Sutton R, Hughes TP, et al. High-risk B-cell acute lymphoblastic leukaemia presenting with hypereosinophilia and acquiring a novel PAX5 fusion on relapse. Br J Haematol. 2020;191(2):301–4.
92. Fournier B, Balducci E, Duployez N, Clappier E, Cuccuini W, Arfeuille C, et al. B-ALL with t(5;14)(q31;q32); IGH-IL3 rearrangement and eosinophilia: a comprehensive analysis of a peculiar IGH-rearranged B-ALL. Front Oncol. 2019;9:1374.
93. Harrison CJ. Blood spotlight on iAMP21 acute lymphoblastic leukemia (ALL), a high-risk pediatric disease. Blood. 2015;125(9):1383–6.
94. Harrison CJ, Moorman AV, Schwab C, Carroll AJ, Raetz EA, Devidas M, et al. An international study of intrachromosomal amplification of chromosome 21 (iAMP21): cytogenetic characterization and outcome. Leukemia. 2014;28(5):1015–21.
95. Harrison CJ, Schwab C. Constitutional abnormalities of chromosome 21 predispose to iAMP21-acute lymphoblastic leukaemia. Eur J Med Genet. 2016;59(3):162–5.
96. Stephens PJ, Greenman CD, Fu B, Yang F, Bignell GR, Mudie LJ, et al. Massive genomic rearrangement acquired in a single catastrophic event during cancer development. Cell. 2011;144(1):27–40.
97. Koleilat A, Smadbeck JB, Zepeda-Mendoza CJ, Williamson CM, Pitel BA, Golden CL, et al. Characterization of unusual iAMP21 B-lymphoblastic leukemia (iAMP21-ALL) from the Mayo Clinic and Children's Oncology Group. Genes Chromosomes Cancer. 2022;61(12):710–9.
98. Ryan SL, Matheson E, Grossmann V, Sinclair P, Bashton M, Schwab C, et al. The role of the RAS pathway in iAMP21-ALL. Leukemia. 2016;30(9):1824–31.
99. Letouzey M, Penther D, Roche-Lestienne C, Nelken B, Devoldere C, Vannier JP, et al. Detection of dicentric chromosome (9;20) in paediatric B-cell acute lymphoblastic leukaemia: prognostic significance. Ann Hematol. 2015;94(2):187–93.
100. Johansson B, Mertens F, Mitelman F. Clinical and biological importance of cytogenetic abnormalities in childhood and adult acute lymphoblastic leukemia. Ann Med. 2004;36(7):492–503.
101. An Q, Wright SL, Moorman AV, Parker H, Griffiths M, Ross FM, et al. Heterogeneous breakpoints in patients with acute lymphoblastic leukemia and the dic(9;20)(p11-13;q11) show recurrent involvement of genes at 20q11.21. Haematologica. 2009;94(8):1164–9.
102. Rehn JA, O'Connor MJ, White DL, Yeung DT. DUX hunting-clinical features and diagnostic challenges associated with DUX4-rearranged leukaemia. Cancers (Basel). 2020;12(10):2815.
103. Schinnerl D, Mejstrikova E, Schumich A, Zaliova M, Fortschegger K, Nebral K, et al. CD371 cell surface expression: a unique feature of DUX4-rearranged acute lymphoblastic leukemia. Haematologica. 2019;104(8):e352–e5.
104. Dixit M, Ansseau E, Tassin A, Winokur S, Shi R, Qian H, et al. DUX4, a candidate gene of facioscapulohumeral muscular dystrophy, encodes a transcriptional activator of PITX1. Proc Natl Acad Sci USA. 2007;104(46):18157–62.
105. Lilljebjorn H, Henningsson R, Hyrenius-Wittsten A, Olsson L, Orsmark-Pietras C, von Palffy S, et al. Identification of ETV6-RUNX1-like and DUX4-rearranged subtypes in paediatric B-cell precursor acute lymphoblastic leukaemia. Nat Commun. 2016;7:11790.
106. Bakewell J, Moorman AV, Ryan SL. DUX4-rearranged B-ALL: deciphering a biological and clinical conundrum. Leukemia. 2025;39:2835–47.
107. Schinnerl D, Riebler M, Schumich A, Haslinger S, Brambock A, Inthal A, et al. Risk factors in DUX4-positive childhood and adolescent B-cell acute lymphoblastic leukemia. Blood Cancer J. 2024;14(1):119.

108. Zaliova M, Zimmermannova O, Dorge P, Eckert C, Moricke A, Zimmermann M, et al. ERG deletion is associated with CD2 and attenuates the negative impact of IKZF1 deletion in childhood acute lymphoblastic leukemia. Leukemia. 2014;28(1):182–5.
109. Zaliova M, Potuckova E, Hovorkova L, Musilova A, Winkowska L, Fiser K, et al. ERG deletions in childhood acute lymphoblastic leukemia with DUX4 rearrangements are mostly polyclonal, prognostically relevant and their detection rate strongly depends on screening method sensitivity. Haematologica. 2019;104(7):1407–16.
110. Vendramini E, Giordan M, Giarin E, Michielotto B, Fazio G, Cazzaniga G, et al. High expression of miR-125b-2 and SNORD116 noncoding RNA clusters characterize ERG-related B cell precursor acute lymphoblastic leukemia. Oncotarget. 2017;8(26):42398–413.
111. Brady SW, Roberts KG, Gu Z, Shi L, Pounds S, Pei D, et al. The genomic landscape of pediatric acute lymphoblastic leukemia. Nat Genet. 2022;54(9):1376–89.
112. Aberuyi N, Rahgozar S, Ghodousi ES, Ghaedi K. Drug resistance biomarkers and their clinical applications in childhood acute lymphoblastic leukemia. Front Oncol. 2019;9:1496.
113. Hirabayashi S, Ohki K, Nakabayashi K, Ichikawa H, Momozawa Y, Okamura K, et al. ZNF384-related fusion genes define a subgroup of childhood B-cell precursor acute lymphoblastic leukemia with a characteristic immunotype. Haematologica. 2017;102(1):118–29.
114. Hirabayashi S, Butler ER, Ohki K, Kiyokawa N, Bergmann AK, Moricke A, et al. Clinical characteristics and outcomes of B-ALL with ZNF384 rearrangements: a retrospective analysis by the Ponte di Legno Childhood ALL Working Group. Leukemia. 2021;35(11):3272–7.
115. Zaliova M, Winkowska L, Stuchly J, Fiser K, Triska P, Zwyrtkova M, et al. A novel class of ZNF384 aberrations in acute leukemia. Blood Adv. 2021;5(21):4393–7.
116. Qian M, Zhang H, Kham SK, Liu S, Jiang C, Zhao X, et al. Whole-transcriptome sequencing identifies a distinct subtype of acute lymphoblastic leukemia with predominant genomic abnormalities of EP300 and CREBBP. Genome Res. 2017;27(2):185–95.
117. Shago M, Abla O, Hitzler J, Weitzman S, Abdelhaleem M. Frequency and outcome of pediatric acute lymphoblastic leukemia with ZNF384 gene rearrangements including a novel translocation resulting in an ARID1B/ZNF384 gene fusion. Pediatr Blood Cancer. 2016;63(11):1915–21.
118. Benjamin M, Singh J, Pandey AK, Thukral N, Kumari S, Palanichamy JK, et al. Integrative genetic and transcriptomic subtyping improves prognosis prediction in B-lineage acute lymphoblastic leukemia. Lab Investig. 2025;105(9):104201.
119. Davis K, Sheikh T, Aggarwal N. Emerging molecular subtypes and therapies in acute lymphoblastic leukemia. Semin Diagn Pathol. 2023;40(3):202–15.
120. Li JF, Dai YT, Lilljebjorn H, Shen SH, Cui BW, Bai L, et al. Transcriptional landscape of B cell precursor acute lymphoblastic leukemia based on an international study of 1,223 cases. Proc Natl Acad Sci USA. 2018;115(50):E11711–E20.
121. Gu Z, Churchman M, Roberts K, Li Y, Liu Y, Harvey RC, et al. Genomic analyses identify recurrent MEF2D fusions in acute lymphoblastic leukaemia. Nat Commun. 2016;7:13331.
122. Ohki K, Butler ER, Kiyokawa N, Hirabayashi S, Bergmann AK, Moricke A, et al. Clinical characteristics and outcomes of B-cell precursor ALL with MEF2D rearrangements: a retrospective study by the Ponte di Legno Childhood ALL Working Group. Leukemia. 2023;37(1):212–6.
123. Schwab C, Harrison CJ. Advances in B-cell precursor acute lymphoblastic leukemia genomics. Hema. 2018;2(4):e53.
124. Boer JM, Valsecchi MG, Hormann FM, Antic Z, Zaliova M, Schwab C, et al. Favorable outcome of NUTM1-rearranged infant and pediatric B cell precursor acute lymphoblastic leukemia in a collaborative international study. Leukemia. 2021;35(10):2978–82.
125. Pincez T, Landry JR, Roussy M, Jouan L, Bilodeau M, Laramee L, et al. Cryptic recurrent ACIN1-NUTM1 fusions in non-KMT2A-rearranged infant acute lymphoblastic leukemia. Genes Chromosomes Cancer. 2020;59(2):125–30.
126. McClure BJ, Pal M, Heatley SL, Rehn J, Schutz C, Breen J, et al. Two novel cases of NUTM1-rearranged B-cell acute lymphoblastic leukaemia presenting with high-risk features. Br J Haematol. 2022;196(6):1407–11.

127. Passet M, Kim R, Gachet S, Sigaux F, Chaumeil J, Galland A, et al. Concurrent CDX2 cis-deregulation and UBTF::ATXN7L3 fusion define a novel high-risk subtype of B-cell ALL. Blood. 2022;139(24):3505–18.
128. Bomken S, Enshaei A, Schwalbe EC, Mikulasova A, Dai Y, Zaka M, et al. Molecular characterisation and clinical outcome of B-cell precursor acute lymphoblastic leukaemia with IG-MYC rearrangement. Haematologica. 2022;108(3):717–31.
129. Russell LJ, Akasaka T, Majid A, Sugimoto KJ, Loraine Karran E, Nagel I, et al. t(6;14)(p22;q32): a new recurrent IGH@ translocation involving ID4 in B-cell precursor acute lymphoblastic leukemia (BCP-ALL). Blood. 2008;111(1):387–91.
130. Russell LJ, De Castro DG, Griffiths M, Telford N, Bernard O, Panzer-Grumayer R, et al. A novel translocation, t(14;19)(q32;p13), involving IGH@ and the cytokine receptor for erythropoietin. Leukemia. 2009;23(3):614–7.
131. Akasaka T, Balasas T, Russell LJ, Sugimoto KJ, Majid A, Walewska R, et al. Five members of the CEBP transcription factor family are targeted by recurrent IGH translocations in B-cell precursor acute lymphoblastic leukemia (BCP-ALL). Blood. 2007;109(8):3451–61.
132. Harrison CJ. Cytogenetics of paediatric and adolescent acute lymphoblastic leukaemia. Br J Haematol. 2009;144(2):147–56.
133. Stratmann JA, von Rose AB, Koschade S, Wendelin K, Kohler F, Heinsch M, et al. Clinical and genetic characterization of de novo double-hit B cell precursor leukemia/lymphoma. Ann Hematol. 2019;98(3):647–56.
134. Zaliova M, Potuckova E, Lukes J, Winkowska L, Starkova J, Janotova I, et al. Frequency and prognostic impact of ZEB2 H1038 and Q1072 mutations in childhood B-other acute lymphoblastic leukemia. Haematologica. 2021;106(3):886–90.
135. Marke R, van Leeuwen FN, Scheijen B. The many faces of IKZF1 in B-cell precursor acute lymphoblastic leukemia. Haematologica. 2018;103(4):565–74.
136. Stanulla M, Cave H, Moorman AV. IKZF1 deletions in pediatric acute lymphoblastic leukemia: still a poor prognostic marker? Blood. 2020;135(4):252–60.
137. Heizmann B, Kastner P, Chan S. The Ikaros family in lymphocyte development. Curr Opin Immunol. 2018;51:14–23.
138. Mullighan CG. The molecular genetic makeup of acute lymphoblastic leukemia. Hematology Am Soc Hematol Educ Program. 2012;2012:389–96.
139. Paolino J, Tsai HK, Harris MH, Pikman Y. IKZF1 alterations and therapeutic targeting in B-cell acute lymphoblastic leukemia. Biomedicine. 2024;12(1):89.
140. Agarwal M, Seth R, Chatterjee T. Recent advances in molecular diagnosis and prognosis of childhood B cell lineage acute lymphoblastic leukemia (B-ALL). Indian J Hematol Blood Transfus. 2021;37(1):10–20.
141. Kastner P, Dupuis A, Gaub MP, Herbrecht R, Lutz P, Chan S. Function of Ikaros as a tumor suppressor in B cell acute lymphoblastic leukemia. Am J Blood Res. 2013;3(1):1–13.
142. Churchman ML, Low J, Qu C, Paietta EM, Kasper LH, Chang Y, et al. Efficacy of retinoids in IKZF1-mutated BCR-ABL1 acute lymphoblastic leukemia. Cancer Cell. 2015;28(3):343–56.
143. Alvey EN, Yap KL, Rathbun P, Fitzpatrick C, Gong S, Richardson AI. B-cell lymphoblastic leukemia/lymphoma with mutated IKZF1 N159Y: clinical and genetic features of an emerging entity. Haematologica. 2025;110(12):3078–82.
144. Blunck CB, Poubel CP, Lopes BA, Barbosa TC, Maciel ALT, da Costa ES, et al. Characterisation of cells markers associated with IKZF1(plus) in BCP-ALL. Transl Oncol. 2024;50:102127.
145. Stanulla M, Dagdan E, Zaliova M, Moricke A, Palmi C, Cazzaniga G, et al. IKZF1(plus) defines a new minimal residual disease-dependent very-poor prognostic profile in pediatric B-cell precursor acute lymphoblastic leukemia. J Clin Oncol. 2018;36(12):1240–9.
146. Mangum DS, Meyer JA, Mason CC, Shams S, Maese LD, Gardiner JD, et al. Association of combined focal 22q11.22 deletion and IKZF1 alterations with outcomes in childhood acute lymphoblastic leukemia. JAMA Oncol. 2021;7(10):1521–8.
147. Cobaleda C, Schebesta A, Delogu A, Busslinger M. Pax5: the guardian of B cell identity and function. Nat Immunol. 2007;8(5):463–70.

148. Mullighan CG, Goorha S, Radtke I, Miller CB, Coustan-Smith E, Dalton JD, et al. Genome-wide analysis of genetic alterations in acute lymphoblastic leukaemia. Nature. 2007;446(7137):758–64.
149. Crepinsek K, Klobucar N, Tesovnik T, Sket R, Jenko Bizjan B, Kovac J, et al. PAX5 alterations in a consecutive childhood B-cell acute lymphoblastic leukemia cohort treated using the ALL IC-BFM 2009 protocol. Cancers (Basel). 2024;16(6):1164.
150. Jia Z, Gu Z. PAX5 alterations in B-cell acute lymphoblastic leukemia. Front Oncol. 2022;12:1023606.
151. Passet M, Boissel N, Sigaux F, Saillard C, Bargetzi M, Ba I, et al. PAX5 P80R mutation identifies a novel subtype of B-cell precursor acute lymphoblastic leukemia with favorable outcome. Blood. 2019;133(3):280–4.
152. Coyaud E, Struski S, Prade N, Familiades J, Eichner R, Quelen C, et al. Wide diversity of PAX5 alterations in B-ALL: a Groupe Francophone de Cytogenetique Hematologique study. Blood. 2010;115(15):3089–97.
153. Schwab C, Nebral K, Chilton L, Leschi C, Waanders E, Boer JM, et al. Intragenic amplification of PAX5: a novel subgroup in B-cell precursor acute lymphoblastic leukemia? Blood Adv. 2017;1(19):1473–7.
154. Gonzalez-Gil C, Ribera J, Ribera JM, Genesca E. The Yin and Yang-like clinical implications of the CDKN2A/ARF/CDKN2B gene cluster in acute lymphoblastic leukemia. Genes (Basel). 2021;12(1):79.
155. Kiss R, Gango A, Benard-Slagter A, Egyed B, Haltrich I, Hegyi L, et al. Comprehensive profiling of disease-relevant copy number aberrations for advanced clinical diagnostics of pediatric acute lymphoblastic leukemia. Mod Pathol. 2020;33(5):812–24.
156. Ampatzidou M, Papadhimitriou SI, Paisiou A, Paterakis G, Tzanoudaki M, Papadakis V, et al. The prognostic effect of CDKN2A/2B gene deletions in pediatric acute lymphoblastic leukemia (ALL): independent prognostic significance in BFM-based protocols. Diagnostics (Basel). 2023;13(9):1589.
157. Studniak E, Maloney E, Ociepa T, Urasinski T, Skonieczka K, Haus O, et al. Allelic loss of selected tumor suppressor genes in acute lymphoblastic leukemia in children. Pol J Pathol. 2013;64(2):121–8.
158. Waanders E, Scheijen B, van der Meer LT, van Reijmersdal SV, van Emst L, Kroeze Y, et al. The origin and nature of tightly clustered BTG1 deletions in precursor B-cell acute lymphoblastic leukemia support a model of multiclonal evolution. PLoS Genet. 2012;8(2):e1002533.
159. Steeghs EMP, Boer JM, Hoogkamer AQ, Boeree A, de Haas V, de Groot-Kruseman HA, et al. Copy number alterations in B-cell development genes, drug resistance, and clinical outcome in pediatric B-cell precursor acute lymphoblastic leukemia. Sci Rep. 2019;9(1):4634.
160. Salvaris R, Fedele PL. Targeted therapy in acute lymphoblastic leukaemia. J Pers Med. 2021;11(8):715.
161. Bene MC, Castoldi G, Knapp W, Ludwig WD, Matutes E, Orfao A, et al. Proposals for the immunological classification of acute leukemias. European Group for the Immunological Characterization of Leukemias (EGIL). Leukemia. 1995;9(10):1783–6.
162. Ohki K, Takahashi H, Fukushima T, Nanmoku T, Kusano S, Mori M, et al. Impact of immunophenotypic characteristics on genetic subgrouping in childhood acute lymphoblastic leukemia: Tokyo Children's Cancer Study Group (TCCSG) study L04-16. Genes Chromosomes Cancer. 2020;59(10):551–61.
163. Gaikwad AS, Donohue RE, Elghetany MT, Sheehan AM, Lu XY, Gramatges MM, et al. Expression of CD25 is a specific and relatively sensitive marker for the Philadelphia chromosome (BCR-ABL1) translocation in pediatric B acute lymphoblastic leukemia. Int J Clin Exp Pathol. 2014;7(9):6225–30.
164. Konoplev S, Lu X, Konopleva M, Jain N, Ouyang J, Goswami M, et al. CRLF2-positive B-cell acute lymphoblastic leukemia in adult patients: a single-institution experience. Am J Clin Pathol. 2017;147(4):357–63.

165. Novakova M, Zaliova M, Fiser K, Vakrmanova B, Slamova L, Musilova A, et al. DUX4r, ZNF384r and PAX5-P80R mutated B-cell precursor acute lymphoblastic leukemia frequently undergo monocytic switch. Haematologica. 2021;106(8):2066–75.
166. Strullu M, Caye-Eude A, Robert E, Renard JM, Chaye A, Galimand J, et al. CD36 cell surface expression as a surrogate marker to identify ABL/JAK-class kinase fusions in pediatric BCP-ALL. Leukemia. 2025;39(1):64–74.
167. Sotillo E, Barrett DM, Black KL, Bagashev A, Oldridge D, Wu G, et al. Convergence of acquired mutations and alternative splicing of CD19 enables resistance to CART-19 immunotherapy. Cancer Discov. 2015;5(12):1282–95.
168. Reinert J, Beitzen-Heineke A, Wethmar K, Stelljes M, Fiedler W, Schwartz S. Loss of CD22 expression and expansion of a CD22(dim) subpopulation in adults with relapsed/refractory B-lymphoblastic leukaemia after treatment with Inotuzumab-Ozogamicin. Ann Hematol. 2021;100(11):2727–32.
169. Aparicio-Perez C, Carmona M, Benabdellah K, Herrera C. Failure of ALL recognition by CAR T cells: a review of CD 19-negative relapses after anti-CD 19 CAR-T treatment in B-ALL. Front Immunol. 2023;14:1165870.
170. Locatelli F, Zugmaier G, Rizzari C, Morris JD, Gruhn B, Klingebiel T, et al. Effect of blinatumomab vs chemotherapy on event-free survival among children with high-risk first-relapse B-cell acute lymphoblastic leukemia: a randomized clinical trial. JAMA. 2021;325(9):843–54.
171. Kantarjian H, Stein A, Gokbuget N, Fielding AK, Schuh AC, Ribera JM, et al. Blinatumomab versus chemotherapy for advanced acute lymphoblastic leukemia. N Engl J Med. 2017;376(9):836–47.
172. Myers RM, Taraseviciute A, Steinberg SM, Lamble AJ, Sheppard J, Yates B, et al. Blinatumomab nonresponse and high-disease burden are associated with inferior outcomes after CD19-CAR for B-ALL. J Clin Oncol. 2022;40(9):932–44.
173. Myers RM, Dolan J, Teachey DT. Chimeric antigen receptor T cell therapy for pediatric and young adult B cell acute lymphoblastic leukemia. Expert Rev Clin Immunol. 2020;16(10):1029–42.
174. Majzner RG, Rietberg SP, Sotillo E, Dong R, Vachharajani VT, Labanieh L, et al. Tuning the antigen density requirement for CAR T-cell activity. Cancer Discov. 2020;10(5):702–23.
175. Spiegel JY, Patel S, Muffly L, Hossain NM, Oak J, Baird JH, et al. CAR T cells with dual targeting of CD19 and CD22 in adult patients with recurrent or refractory B cell malignancies: a phase 1 trial. Nat Med. 2021;27(8):1419–31.
176. Pillai V, Muralidharan K, Meng W, Bagashev A, Oldridge DA, Rosenthal J, et al. CAR T-cell therapy is effective for CD19-dim B-lymphoblastic leukemia but is impacted by prior blinatumomab therapy. Blood Adv. 2019;3(22):3539–49.
177. Kantarjian HM, Stock W, Cassaday RD, DeAngelo DJ, Jabbour E, O'Brien SM, et al. Inotuzumab ozogamicin for relapsed/refractory acute lymphoblastic leukemia in the INO-VATE trial: CD22 pharmacodynamics, efficacy, and safety by baseline CD22. Clin Cancer Res. 2021;27(10):2742–54.
178. Rubinstein JD, O'Brien MM. Inotuzumab ozogamicin in B-cell precursor acute lymphoblastic leukemia: efficacy, toxicity, and practical considerations. Front Immunol. 2023;14:1237738.
179. Sartor C, Arpinati M, Chirumbolo G, Dozza L, Cristiano G, Nanni J, et al. Baseline cluster of differentiation 22 fluorescent intensity correlates with patient outcome after inotuzumab ozogamicin treatment. Hematol Oncol. 2022;40(4):734–42.
180. Fingrut W, Davis W, McGinnis E, Dallas K, Ramadan K, Merkeley H, et al. Reevaluating patient eligibility for inotuzumab ozogamicin based on CD22 expression: is dim expression sufficient? Curr Oncol. 2020;28(1):252–9.
181. Ramakrishna S, Highfill SL, Walsh Z, Nguyen SM, Lei H, Shern JF, et al. Modulation of target antigen density improves CAR T-cell functionality and persistence. Clin Cancer Res. 2019;25(17):5329–41.
182. Jeha S, Behm F, Pei D, Sandlund JT, Ribeiro RC, Razzouk BI, et al. Prognostic significance of CD20 expression in childhood B-cell precursor acute lymphoblastic leukemia. Blood. 2006;108(10):3302–4.

183. Borowitz MJ, Shuster J, Carroll AJ, Nash M, Look AT, Camitta B, et al. Prognostic significance of fluorescence intensity of surface marker expression in childhood B-precursor acute lymphoblastic leukemia. A Pediatric Oncology Group Study. Blood. 1997;89(11):3960–6.
184. Thomas DA, O'Brien S, Jorgensen JL, Cortes J, Faderl S, Garcia-Manero G, et al. Prognostic significance of CD20 expression in adults with de novo precursor B-lineage acute lymphoblastic leukemia. Blood. 2009;113(25):6330–7.
185. Maury S, Huguet F, Leguay T, Lacombe F, Maynadie M, Girard S, et al. Adverse prognostic significance of CD20 expression in adults with Philadelphia chromosome-negative B-cell precursor acute lymphoblastic leukemia. Haematologica. 2010;95(2):324–8.
186. Maury S, Chevret S, Thomas X, Heim D, Leguay T, Huguet F, et al. Rituximab in B-lineage adult acute lymphoblastic leukemia. N Engl J Med. 2016;375(11):1044–53.
187. Hoshitsuki K, Zhou Y, Miller AM, Choi JK, Swanson HD, Bhakta NH, et al. Rituximab administration in pediatric patients with newly diagnosed acute lymphoblastic leukemia. Leukemia. 2023;37(9):1782–91.
188. Nakamura A, Tsurusawa M, Kato A, Taga T, Hatae Y, Miyake M, et al. Prognostic impact of CD45 antigen expression in high-risk, childhood B-cell precursor acute lymphoblastic leukemia. Leuk Lymphoma. 2001;42(3):393–8.
189. Cario G, Rhein P, Mitlohner R, Zimmermann M, Bandapalli OR, Romey R, et al. High CD45 surface expression determines relapse risk in children with precursor B-cell and T-cell acute lymphoblastic leukemia treated according to the ALL-BFM 2000 protocol. Haematologica. 2014;99(1):103–10.
190. Newton JG, Horan JT, Newman S, Rossi MR, Ketterling RP, Park SI. CD36-positive B-lymphoblasts predict poor outcome in children with B-lymphoblastic leukemia. Pediatr Dev Pathol. 2017;20(3):224–31.
191. Modvig S, Wernersson R, Obro NF, Olsen LR, Christensen C, Rosthoj S, et al. High CD34 surface expression in BCP-ALL predicts poor induction therapy response and is associated with altered expression of genes related to cell migration and adhesion. Mol Oncol. 2022;16(10):2015–30.
192. Jiang Z, Wu D, Lin S, Li P. CD34 and CD38 are prognostic biomarkers for acute B lymphoblastic leukemia. Biomark Res. 2016;4:23.
193. Smith M, Arthur D, Camitta B, Carroll AJ, Crist W, Gaynon P, et al. Uniform approach to risk classification and treatment assignment for children with acute lymphoblastic leukemia. J Clin Oncol. 1996;14(1):18–24.
194. Vaitkeviciene G, Forestier E, Hellebostad M, Heyman M, Jonsson OG, Lahteenmaki PM, et al. High white blood cell count at diagnosis of childhood acute lymphoblastic leukaemia: biological background and prognostic impact. Results from the NOPHO ALL-92 and ALL-2000 studies. Eur J Haematol. 2011;86(1):38–46.
195. Winick N, Devidas M, Chen S, Maloney K, Larsen E, Mattano L, et al. Impact of initial CSF findings on outcome among patients with National Cancer Institute standard- and high-risk B-cell acute lymphoblastic leukemia: a report from the Children's Oncology Group. J Clin Oncol. 2017;35(22):2527–34.

Prognostic and Predictive Biomarkers in T-Lymphoblastic Leukemia

14

Elena A. Repnikova, Dmitry A. Lyalin, and Madina Sukhanova

Introduction

T-cell acute lymphoblastic leukemia (T-ALL) is an aggressive hematologic malignancy characterized by the diffuse infiltration of the bone marrow by malignant hematopoietic cells expressing immature T-cell markers [1]. It is a relatively uncommon and aggressive form of cancer, representing approximately 15% of newly diagnosed pediatric acute lymphoblastic leukemia (ALL) cases. The disease has been studied extensively and based on gene expression signatures, it has been previously shown that the genes involved in T-cell development appear to be dysregulated in T-ALL [2, 3]. T-ALL is characterized by distinctive clinical and biological features, with numerous oncogenes and tumor suppressors implicated in its onset and progression. Over the past few years, multiple efforts have been undertaken to classify T-ALL based on distinct genetic findings, several of which will be discussed in this chapter. However, despite significant progress in the genomic characterization of T-ALL, due to the complexity of its underlying oncogenic drivers, clinical classification still relies primarily on immunophenotypic findings.

E. A. Repnikova (✉)
Department of Pathology and Laboratory Medicine, Children's Mercy Kansas City, University of Missouri-Kansas City School of Medicine, Kansas City, MO, USA
e-mail: erepnikova@cmh.edu

D. A. Lyalin
Department of Pathology, Virginia Commonwealth University Health System, Richmond, VA, USA
e-mail: dmitry.lyalin@vcuhealth.org

M. Sukhanova
Department of Pathology, Division of Molecular Pathology, Feinberg School of Medicine, Northwestern University, Chicago, IL, USA
e-mail: madina.sukhanova@nm.org

W. Li (ed.), *Laboratory Assessments of Pediatric Leukemia*,
https://doi.org/10.1007/978-3-032-26557-9_14

Treatment protocols for pediatric T-ALL are similar to those used for B-cell acute lymphoblastic leukemia (B-ALL). However, many clinical studies have reported that outcomes for T-ALL patients tend to be less favorable [4–6]. As in B-ALL, T-ALL prognosis is also influenced by genetic abnormalities. Relapse rate is higher among T-ALL patients, with relapses occurring earlier during therapy. Therefore, it is essential to improve our understanding of this heterogeneous disease to identify prognostic markers that can predict treatment response or resistance, develop targeted therapies based on unique molecular markers, and detect markers indicative of relapse. Several factors may serve as prognostic indicators in T-ALL, including age at diagnosis, clinicopathologic features, central nervous system involvement, tumor molecular profile, and response to therapy assessed by minimal residual disease (MRD).

Demographic Characteristics of Patients with T-ALL

The differences in survival rates between B-ALL and T-ALL can, in part, be attributed to age of onset: B-ALL typically occurs between the ages of 2 and 5 years, whereas T-ALL diagnoses in pediatric patients range broadly from several months to 15 years of age, with higher prevalence observed in older children and adolescents. In addition to age, the patient's sex may also influence prognosis in T-ALL, as a significant male predominance (approximately 70%) has been observed among T-ALL patients [7–9]. Additionally, male patients exhibit lower survival rates and a higher risk of relapse [10]. Conversely, no evident racial disparities in survival outcomes have been identified for T-ALL [11, 12]. However, the incidence of T-ALL varies among racial groups, with a higher prevalence observed in Black pediatric patients compared to those of Caucasian or Hispanic/Latino descent [11, 12].

Clinicopathologic Subclassification of T-ALL

Clinical Prognostic Markers

T-ALL is characterized by the malignant proliferation of immature T-cells in the bone marrow, peripheral blood, and other tissues. Prior to the development of MRD monitoring based on molecular markers and flow cytometry, clinical risk assessment relied on markers such as elevated white blood cell counts (WBC), the presence of mediastinal masses and/or splenomegaly, and central nervous system (CNS) involvement [13, 14]. Although, initial WBC is still considered one of the strongest independent predictors of induction failure and risk of relapse in pediatric B-ALL, it is significantly less predictive in T-ALL [8, 15]. Additionally, T-ALL patients with either an initially low or high WBC count were found to have a significantly lower survival rate than those with an intermediate count [16]. Currently, T-ALL risk stratification is determined by MRD response, with age and CNS involvement continuing to serve as strongest independent prognostic factors across various treatment regimens [5, 17, 18].

Thus, T-ALL patients can be categorized into three age groups, each corresponding to specific risk categories:

1. *Standard risk: children between 1 and 10 years of age.* This group has a better prognosis compared to two other age groups [19–21].
2. *High risk: adolescent patients older than 10 years of age.* The overall survival rate for patients in this group is lower compared to children aged 1–10 years. Additionally, the outcomes for patients older than 16 years are further reduced in comparison to those aged between 10 and 15 years [9, 22, 23].
3. *Very high risk: infantile patients (<1 year old).* T-ALL is exceedingly rare in infants, and limited data are available. The current consensus indicates that outcomes are generally poorer in this age group, with a 5-year overall survival rate of approximately 21.5%, compared to approximately 35.5% in older pediatric patients. Additionally, infants with T-ALL experience higher rates of early relapses [24–27].

T-ALL Subclassification by CNS Involvement

1. *CNS-1* (absence of blasts in cerebrospinal fluid [CSF] on cytospin preparation, regardless of WBC count).
2. *CNS-2* (blasts present in CSF on cytospin preparation and WBC count was <5/μL).
3. *CNS-3* (blasts present in CSF on cytospin preparation and WBC count ≥5/μL).

Children's Oncology Group (COG) subclassified T-ALL into three groups based on CNS involvement [28, 29] with gradually worse overall survival (OS) with increasing group number and with the CNS-3 group having a significantly worse OS regardless of treatment intensity, whereas the outcome for the CNS-2 group greatly depended on treatment.

T-ALL Subclassification by Immunophenotype

Leukemic blasts in T-ALL are consistently positive for cytoplasmic CD3 (cCD3), usually positive for TdT, CD7, CD38, and CD45. They may also exhibit variable positivity for other pan-T-cell antigens, including surface CD3 (sCD3), CD2, CD4, CD5, CD8, the T-cell receptor, as well as CD10 and other immature markers such as CD1a, CD34, and CD99. In some cases, T-ALL may aberrantly express CD56, CD79a, or myeloid markers such as CD13 or CD33.

Pediatric T-ALL can be classified into several subtypes based on immunophenotypic features. The European Group for Immunological Classification of Leukemia (EGIL) scale is commonly used to classify these subtypes, which reflect different stages of T-cell maturation [30]. With current treatment protocols, these subtypes carry no or very limited prognostic values. The main subtypes are:

1. *Pro-T (EGIL T-I):* Characterized by expression of cCD3 and CD7 but lacking other markers like CD5 or CD2. This resembles an early stage of T-cell development.
2. *Pre-T (EGIL T-II):* Positive markers include cCD3, CD7, CD5, and CD2. This subtype represents a slightly more differentiated stage than pro-T.
3. *Cortical-T (EGIL T-III):* Defined by the presence of cCD3, CD1a, and variable expression of sCD3. This subtype is derived from thymocytes at the cortical stage of T-cell development.
4. *Mature-T (EGIL T-IV):* This subtype is characterized by the expression of mature T-cell markers such as sCD3, and the absence of CD1a. The leukemic cells show an immunophenotype representing a late stage of T-cell development.
5. *T-γ/δ Subtype:* This is a rarer subtype characterized by T-lymphoblasts that express the γ/δ T-cell receptor instead of the α/β receptor, which is more common in T cells. It is seen in about 10–13% of pediatric T-ALL cases, and likely has a poor therapeutic response and decreased overall survival [31].
6. *Early T-Cell Precursor (ETP) ALL:* This recently identified subtype is associated with poorer prognosis and chemoresistance [32]. ETP-ALL is defined immunophenotypically by the absence of both CD1a and CD8 and weak or absent CD5 expression, and the exprcssion of at least one of the myeloid or stem cell markers. It shows a gene expression profile resembling that of early stages of T-cell precursors. In pediatric T-ALL, the ETP-ALL subgroup represents 12–17% cases. In the recently published COG studies, there was no significant difference in the outcomes between EPT-ALL and other T-ALL patients, although ETP-ALL patients showed higher induction failure [33].

Existing Molecular Subclassification of T-ALL

Two major classification systems for T-ALL, the fifth edition of the WHO classification (WHO-HAEM5) and International Consensus Classification (ICC), share some categorization criteria based on morphology, immunophenotype, and degree of leukemic cell maturation. Thus, both systems generally break T-ALL into less differentiated early T-precursor (based on WHO) or early T-cell precursor (based on ICC) lymphoblastic leukemia/lymphoma (ETP) and more differentiated T-ALL. Diagnosis of ETP T-ALL is made based on immunophenotype [34, 35].

In the publication of the WHO-HAEM5, no genetically defined entity was included for T-ALL, as the classification based on genetic features remained complex and exhibited significant variability in reproducibility across different studies [1, 36, 37].

However, the implementation of comprehensive molecular high-throughput methodologies, including whole-transcriptome sequencing (WTS), whole-exome sequencing (WES) and whole-genome sequencing (WGS) in routine clinical settings, enriched the knowledge about genetic alterations in T-ALL and their association with patient's outcome. T-ALL is characterized by genomic alterations leading to activation of transcriptional programs related to T-cell development; therefore, gene rearrangements leading to deregulated expression of the target genes are expected to be common, while cytogenetic abnormalities common in B-ALL (e.g., hypodiploidy or hyperdiploidy) are rare. As a result of the molecular advances, ICC has incorporated several provisional genetically defined entities (Table 14.1 and Fig. 14.1). ICC classification has also included a subtype of ETP T-ALL characterized by activated *BCL11B* [40].

Brief Overview of Major Genetic Subtypes

BCL11B-Activated

BCL11B encodes a C2H2-type transcriptional repressor zinc finger protein involved in T-lineage development. At least two characterized molecular mechanisms can result in the activation of *BCL11B*: interchromosomal rearrangements (80%) with the partner genes such as *ARID1B* (6q25), *CCDC26/MYC* (8q24.2), *CDK6* (7q21), *SATB1* (3p24), *ETV6* (12p13), *ZEB2* (2q22), *RUNX1* (21q22) often referred as enhancer hijacking events and amplification of the enhancer distal to *BCL11B* (20%) [41]. Enhancer hijacking mechanism is a type of rearrangement whereby structural variants (e.g., translocations, deletions, or inversions) result in the "re-wiring" of enhancer-promoter interactions. Patients with this subtype frequently harbor mutations in *FLT3* (*FLT3*-ITD) and *WT1*, but lack mutations in *NOTCH1* and *PHF6,* and *CDKN2A* deletions. Additionally, this subtype demonstrates decreased expression of *RAG1* and *RAG2* and increased expression of *KIT* and *LMO2*. The level of BCL11B expression does not appear to influence pediatric patient clinical outcome [42].

While no single method can detect all types of rearrangements, various techniques—each with its own limitations—can be employed, including fluorescence *in situ* hybridization (FISH), chromosome analysis, RNA sequencing (RNAseq), quantitative reverse transcription polymerase chain reaction (qRT-PCR), and optical genome mapping (OGM).

HOXA-Dysregulated

The *HOXA* locus located in the short arm of chromosome 7 (7p15.3) contains the HOXA gene cluster, a group of homeobox genes essential for embryonic development. HOXA contains at least 11 genes: *HOXA1, HOXA2, HOXA3, HOXA4, HOXA5, HOXA6, HOXA7, HOXA9, HOXA10, HOXA11,* and *HOXA13.* These genes encode transcription factors which contain DNA-binding homeodomain and are involved in the regulation of gene expression, morphogenesis, and differentiation [43]. HOXA dysregulation frequently leads to an immature immunophenotype

Table 14.1 ICC provisional genetic classification of T-ALL

Subtype	Frequency in pediatric population	Prognosis % OS by 5 years	Immunophenotype	Primary genetic abnormalities	Molecular mechanism
BCL11B-altered	1.4% of T-ALL and 94% of ETP-ALL	Intermediate (88%)	Mostly ETP	Juxtaposition of *BCL11B* (14q32) to enhancers of the partner genes *ARID1B* (6q25), *CCDC26/MYC* (8q25), *CDK6* (7q21), *SATB1* (3p24), *ETV6* (12p13), *ZEB2* (2q22), *RUNX1* (21q22), or *BCL11B* enhancer tandem amplification	Overexpression of the transcription factor, *BCL11B*
HOXA dysregulated	Up to 20%	Intermediate (87%)	Immature immunophenotype resembling ETP-ALL	*TCR::HOXA (KMT2A*-rearranged*; PICALM::MLLT10; SET::NUP214)*	Overexpression of *HOXA* genes
TLX1-rerarranged	Up to 10%	Good (92%)	CD4+, CD8+/−, CD1a+, cortical thymocyte	t(7;10)(q34;q24) *TRB::TLX1* t(10;14)(q24;q11.2) *TCRA/D::TLX1*	Ectopic expression of the DNA-binding transcription factor, *TLX1*
TLX3-rerarranged	Up to 14%	Good (91%)	CD4+, CD8+/−, CD1a+, cortical thymocyte, some ETP or near ETP	t(5;14)(q35.1;q11.2) *TRD::TLX3* t(5;14)(q35;q32) *BCL11B::TLX3* t(5;7)(q35.1;q21) *CDK6::TLX3*	Ectopic expression of the DNA-binding transcription factor, *TLX3; BCL11B* overexpression different from ETP group
NKX2-rearranged	Up to 5%	Good (93%)	CD4+, CD8+	t(5;14)(q35.1;q32.2) *BCL11B::NKX2* t(5;14)(q35.1;q11.2) *TRD::NKX2*	Ectopic expression of the DNA-binding transcription factor, *NKX2*
TAL1-rearranged	Up to 30%	Intermediate (~75%)	CD3+, mature late cortical	t(1;7)(p32;q34) *TRB::TAL1* t(1;14)(p32;q11) *TRAD::TAL1* del(1)(p32p32) *STIL::TAL1* Intergenic SNV (generating super enhancer)	Ectopic expression of the DNA-binding transcription factor, *TAL1*
TAL2-rearranged	Up to 3%	Intermediate (75%)	CD3+, mature, late cortical	t(7;9)(q34;q32) *TRB::TAL2*	Ectopic expression of the DNA-binding transcription factor, *TAL2*

LMO1-rearranged	Up to 5%	Intermediate (88%)	Immature but not ETP	t(11;14)(p15;q11) *TRAD::LMO1*	Ectopic extremely high expression of the DNA-binding transcription factor, *LMO1*
LMO2-rearranged	Up to 5%	Intermediate to poor	Immature but not ETP	t(11;14)(p13;q11) *TRAD::LMO2* t(7;11)(q34;p13) *TRB::LMO2* del(11)(p12p13) 11p13/*LMO2*—insertional mutagenesis	Ectopic extremely high expression of the DNA-binding transcription factor, *LMO2*
SPI1-rerarranged	<5%	Very poor (34%)	CD4-, CD8+/−, DR+	t(1;11)(p36;p11) *STMN1::SPI1* *t(5;11)(q31;p11) TCF7::SPI1* *BCL11B::SPI1*	Aberrant expression of the *SPI1* transcription factor
LYL1-rearranged	<2%	Poor (62%)	CD4-, CD8-, CD3-, some cases with aberrant expression of LMO1/LMO2	t(7;19)(q35;p13) *TCB::LYL1*	Extremely high LMO expression LYL1-R shows stem cell-like signature
OLIG2 (BHLHB1)	<2%	Poor (62%)	High LMO expression	*t(14;21)(q11.2;q22.1) TRA::BHLHB1*	Aberrant and overexpression of transcription factor *BHLHB1*

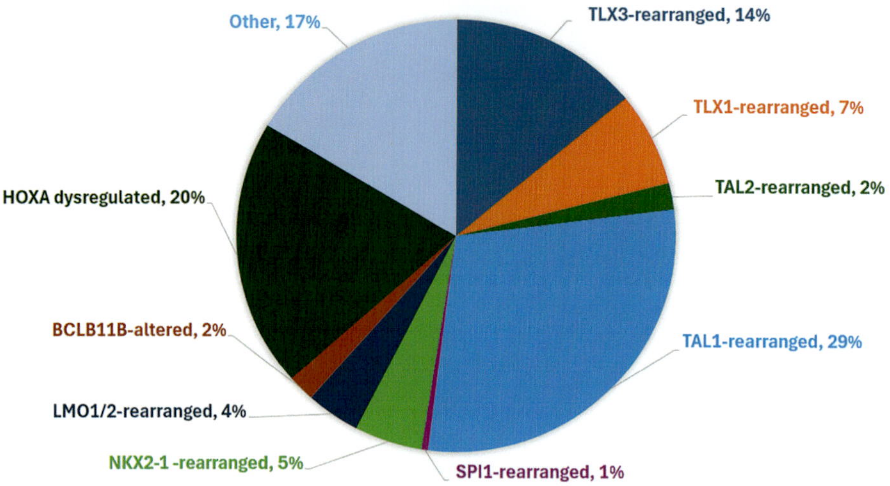

Fig. 14.1 Major T-ALL genomic subtypes with relative frequencies in the pediatric population. Numbers are based on information provided by several publications [29, 38, 39]

resembling ETP-ALL and can either result from *cis* mechanisms (HOXA translocations often involving noncoding regions of the genome, e.g., enhancer hijacking events) or *trans* mechanisms (fusion events involving other oncogenes resulting in HOXA cluster activation) [44].

The patient outcome data available for each HOXA family member is limited, given the rarity of the events. Currently, *HOXA11*-altered T-ALL has been associated with intermediate-risk disease, while *HOXA13*-altered T-ALL has been associated with a high-risk disease exhibiting significantly worse relapse-free survival and MRD [45, 46].

The most common rearrangement involving HOXA includes a cryptic inv(7)(p15q34) and t(7;7)(p15;q34), where the *TRB* locus is juxtaposed to the *HOXA*. These rearrangements lead to transcriptional activation of HOXA genes, including *HOXA10* and *HOXA11,* which can be detected using FISH or OGM and they account for ~2–3% of T-ALL cases [47]. However, HOXA gene expression is increased in approximately 20% of T-ALL cases even in the absence of these chromosomal rearrangements [48]. Elevated HOXA expression has also been observed in T-ALL cases with *KMT2A::MLLT1* and *PICALM::MLLT10* translocations, as well as in cases with *NOTCH1*-activating mutations and deletions of 9p21. These findings suggest that *HOXA* cluster genes play a significant role in T-cell oncogenesis. In a larger study, patients with the *TRB::HOXA* fusion exhibited outcomes similar to those of other T-ALL patients who did not carry the fusion transcript [49].

Chromosome analysis, FISH, OGM, or RNAseq could be utilized to detect translocations involving *HOXA* and *TRB*. Upregulation of HOXA caused by promoter hijacking events can be detected using RNA transcript analysis.

TAL1/2-Rearranged

TAL1/TAL2 encode bHLH transcription factors involved in mediating hematopoietic stem cell fate by regulating gene expression in megakaryocytic/erythroid progenitors [50]. The *TAL1* oncogene is one of the most frequently deregulated in T-ALL. The first description of the genomic alteration involving *TAL1* and resulting in the chimeric fusion *STIL::TAL1* was reported back in 1990 [51]. This fusion is detected in nearly 30% of T-ALL pediatric cases and is a result of an interstitial deletion between the two genes, placing *TAL1* under the regulatory control of the *STIL* promoter (Fig. 14.2) and resulting in aberrant expression of TAL1 [52]. *STIL::TAL1* requires cooperation with other genomic events involving *LMO1* or *LMO2* or activation of the NOTCH pathway. In some cases (<5%), *TAL1* is translocated into either the T-cell receptor B (TRB) locus or, more often, the T-cell receptor δ (TRD) locus and overexpressed by being placed under the control of T-cell receptor cis-regulatory elements [53–55]. Furthermore, TAL1 overexpression may result from super-enhancer formation driven by mutations in the noncoding enhancer region upstream of the *TAL1* transcription start site. These mutations generate novel binding motifs for the MYB transcription factor, leading to robust transcriptional activation and increased expression of TAL1 [56]. Additional alternative alterations leading to TAL1 overexpression may include enhancer gain, enhancer alteration via missense/indel variants, intergenic inversions and noncoding rearrangements [45]. *TAL1* alterations usually exhibit secondary activating mutations in the PI3K-AKT pathway with some of them being clinically targetable [45, 57].

In rare instances of T-ALL (1–2%), alterations of the other member of that transcription factor family, *TAL2*, have also been described [58, 59]. *TAL2* shares a high sequence homology with *TAL1*. Most commonly, *TAL2* is juxtaposed with sequences from the T-cell receptor beta-chain locus on chromosome 7, leading to recurring t(7;9)(q34;q32) which results in overexpression of TAL2. Both *TAL1* and *TAL2* rearrangements confer a poor prognosis [40]. *TAL1*-rearranged T-ALL cells are

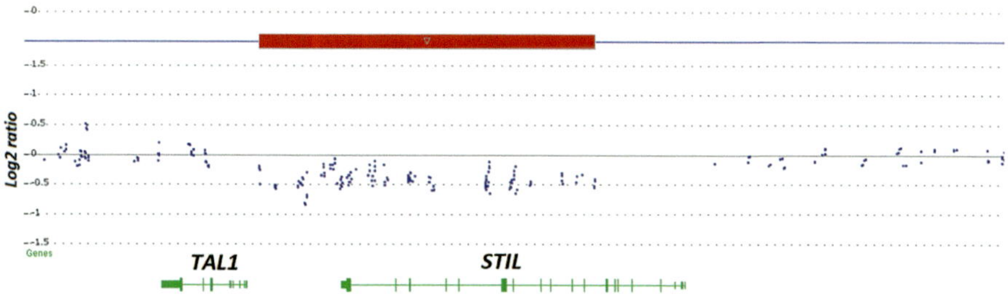

Fig. 14.2 Microarray analysis shows a ~63 kb loss between the 5′ untranslated region (UTR) of the *TAL1* and the *STIL* genes. Disruption of *TAL1* is frequently associated with a submicroscopic interstitial deletion between the 5′ untranslated region (UTR) of the *TAL1* and the *STIL* genes. The *STIL::TAL1* fusion product gives rise to the high expression of TAL1, which, in turn, promotes T-cell leukemogenesis

frequently CD2+ and lack CD10 (CALLA) expression. *TAL1*-rearrangement-positive patients may have a higher frequency of extramedullary relapses.

TLX1-Rearranged

Rearrangements of *TLX1* are recurrent in T-ALL and seen in ~30% of pediatric patients. The immunophenotypic profile demonstrates positivity for CD4, CD8, and CD1a antigens; the associated prognosis is generally favorable [60].

TLX1 (*HOX11L2*) belongs to the TLX family, consisting of a subset of the homeobox family of genes. During embryonic development, it is expressed in various regions including the spleen, spinal cord, and branchial arches.

Aberrant expression of *TLX1* has been reported in up to 20% of pediatric T-ALL cases, most frequently resulting from t(10;14)(q24;q11) and t(7;10)(q35;q24) translocations. The most common rearrangement is t(10;14)(q24;q11), which involves the juxtaposition of *TLX1* on chromosome 10 with the T-cell receptor beta (*TCRB*) or gamma (*TCRG*) loci. However, approximately 30% of *TLX1* rearrangements occur independently of the TCR locus, involving translocations resulting from paracentric inversions and/or cryptic interstitial deletions that juxtapose *TLX1* to nearby regulatory sequences within 10q23 [61].

Immunophenotype of the *TLX1*-rearranged cases demonstrates CD1 expression and differentiation arrest at the cortical stage [62].

The most common secondary genomic alterations in the *TLX1*-rearranged subgroup include co-deletions of *ETV6* and *CDKN1B*, deletions of *CDKN2A/B* (mono- and bi-allelic), and *PTPN2* deletions, resulting in aberrant activation of the PI3K-AKT-mTOR pathway [61]. Additionally, the inactivation of *PHF6* (through mutations or deletions) is frequently reported in T-ALL cases driven by aberrant expression of the *TLX1* and *TLX3* genes [63]. Recent studies suggest that *PHF6* alterations confer sensitivity to 5-azacytidine and venetoclax combination therapy in T-ALL, providing a potentially novel approach for targeted treatment [64].

Overall, *TLX1*-rearranged T-ALL with high levels of TLX1 expression is considered a molecular subgroup with extraordinarily favorable prognosis, achieving a 3-year overall survival rate that exceeds 90%. However, the presence of *NUP214::ABL1* fusion, frequently accompanying *TLX1*-rearrangements in T-ALL cases, may negatively impact event-free survival and overall survival [65].

Detection methods include chromosome analysis, FISH, qRT-PCR, RNAseq, OGM or low-pass WGS [61] (Fig. 14.3).

TLX3-Rearranged

TLX3 rearrangements are about as frequent in pediatric T-ALL, as *TLX1* alterations. It should be noted that, although *BCL11B* is a frequent fusion partner for *TLX3*, the *BCL11B::TLX3* fusion does not result in the activation of *BCL11B* and should not

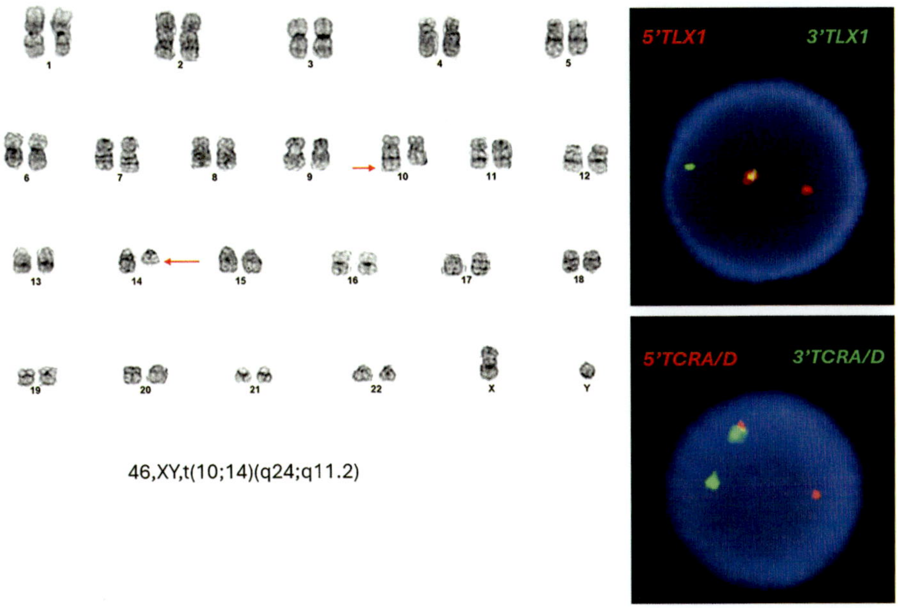

Fig. 14.3 Chromosome analysis shows a balanced translocation between the long arms of chromosome 10 and 14 suggestive of a *TCRA/D::TLX1* rearrangement. FISH analysis using break-apart probes, TLX1 and TCRA/D, shows one fused, one red, and one green patterns consistent with rearrangement of both genes

be interpreted as a criterion for ETP-ALL. The *BCL11B::TLX3* fusion results in deregulated expression of *TLX3* [60].

TLX3 belongs to the TLX family, a subset of homeobox genes that are predominantly expressed in the nervous system and play a crucial role in vertebrate brain development. Under normal physiological conditions, *TLX3* is not expressed during T-cell development. However, approximately 20% of pediatric T- ALL cases exhibit aberrant *TLX3* expression.

In T-ALL patients, *TLX3* activation typically occurs as a result of the cryptic translocation t(5;14)(q35;q32), which predominantly juxtaposes *TLX3* to the *BCL11B* gene—a gene normally expressed during T-cell maturation [66]. Several alternative *TLX3* translocations have been reported, including t(5;14)(q32;q11), which juxtaposes *TLX3* to the *TCRα/δ* locus [67], and t(5;7)(q35;q21), which translocates *TLX3* next to the *CDK6* gene [68].

TLX3-rearranged T-ALL cases frequently harbor additional genomic abnormalities, including *NOTCH1* and *PHF6* mutations, *CDKN2A/B* deletions, and *NUP214::ABL1* fusion and subsequent amplification. The immunophenotype of T-ALL cases with *TLX3* alterations often resembles that of the ETP-ALL subgroup.

TLX3 dysregulation shows a male predominance across all age groups. In childhood T-ALL, *TLX3* expression (TLX3+) was initially associated with poor prognosis when patients were treated with regimens lacking early and/or late re-intensification therapy elements. However, outcomes improved significantly with the implementation of such therapeutic interventions. Notably, the presence of the *NUP214::ABL1* fusion and its subsequent amplification in T-ALL, a late event co-occurring with *TLX3*-rearrangement, was reported in association with increased relapse risk, suggesting that these cases may represent a high-risk *TLX3*+ subgroup that could benefit from targeted tyrosine kinase inhibitor therapy [66, 69]. When treated with Berlin-Frankfurt-Münster (BFM)—based therapy protocols, the *TLX3*-positive group demonstrated no significant difference in disease-free survival rates or 5-year disease-free survival compared to the *TLX3*-negative group [70].

Standard methods for *TLX3* rearrangement detection may include FISH, chromosome analysis, RNAseq, qRT-PCR, or OGM.

NKX2-Rearranged

NKX2-1 is a homeobox-containing transcription factor, also known as TTF-1, which plays a critical role in lung and thyroid gland development and function. In T-ALL, chromosomal rearrangements result in the aberrant expression of *NKX2-1* in T-lymphoblasts, where it is not normally present. Multiple mechanisms drive *NKX2-1* activation in T-ALL, including rearrangements with T-cell receptor delta (TCRD) loci on chromosome 14, recurrent chromosome 14 chromothripsis, intergenic deletions, rare enhancer hijacking events, and enhancer gains [45]. *NKX2-1* rearrangements account for approximately 3–5% of all pediatric T-ALL cases. Notably, *NKX2-1* rearrangements are associated with favorable clinical outcomes, with patients achieving 5-year event-free survival (EFS) rates exceeding 98% when day 29 MRD levels remain below 0.1%.

NKX2-5 is another member of the NKX2 family, which is also found to be involved in pediatric T-ALL. In pediatric T-ALL, the *NKX2-5* subtype is characterized by chromosomal rearrangements involving *NKX2-5* and T-cell receptor beta/delta (TCRβ/δ) loci or *BCL11B* enhancer hijacking events [71]. Additionally, *NKX2-5*-positive T-ALL cases show enrichment for PI3K pathway alterations. Patients with *NKX2-5* rearrangements present distinct clinical characteristics, including younger age at diagnosis and a higher female predominance. In contrast to *NKX2-1*, *NKX2-5* rearrangements are associated with adverse outcomes, with 5-year EFS rates below 60%. The *NKX2* rearrangements frequently co-occur with *MYB* alterations or chromothripsis-like genomic instability events [72].

Interestingly, younger pediatric patients with *NKX2* rearrangements (infants and toddlers), despite presenting with higher rates of hyperleukocytosis and demonstrating slower treatment responses, achieve survival outcomes comparable to older pediatric patients, with a 5-year overall survival rate of 75.4% [72].

Current diagnostic approaches for identifying *NKX2* rearrangements include FISH, RNAseq, RT-PCR or OGM.

LMO1/2-Rearranged

The *LMO1* and *LMO2* genes encode members of a family of nuclear transcription co-regulators that modulate gene expression by binding other proteins rather than directly interacting with DNA [73]. Both genes were initially identified as T-cell oncogenes through their association with specific chromosomal translocations occurring in patients with T-ALL. These oncogenes become upregulated through juxtaposition with T-cell receptor enhancers following chromosomal rearrangement. While *LMO1/LMO2* translocations occur in only 9% of pediatric T-ALL cases, aberrant *LMO2* expression can be detected in up to 45% of T-ALL patients, indicating the presence of additional activation mechanisms beyond chromosomal translocations. One such alternative mechanism involves the cryptic chromosomal deletion del(11)(p12p13) [74], which can lead to *LMO2* dysregulation without translocations detectable by conventional cytogenetics.

LMO1 and *LMO2* alterations are thought to be mutually exclusive [75]. Dysregulation of *LMO2* often co-occurs with *LYL1* overexpression, while dysregulation of *LMO1* is often observed together with deregulation of *TAL1* [42]. Overexpression of *LMO1* or *LMO2* contributes to leukemogenesis by blocking normal T-cell differentiation and promoting continuous thymocyte self-renewal [42, 76]. *TAL1* and/or *LMO2* rearrangements form a single TAL-LMO gene expression cluster, explained by the fact that TAL1 and LMO2 participate in the same transcriptional complex and regulate similar downstream pathways [77].

LMO1/LMO2-rearranged cases are more commonly identified in T-ALL in pediatric compared to adult patients. *LMO2* rearrangements are associated with poor clinical outcomes in pediatric T-ALL patients [74]. However, recent studies suggest that LMO2 overexpression may confer increased sensitivity to PARP inhibitors [78], potentially providing a novel targeted treatment avenue for patients with LMO2-rearranged T-ALL.

Current methods of detection of *LMO1/LMO2* alterations involve FISH or chromosomal microarray analysis (CMA) to identify deletions cryptic to the resolution of standard cytogenetic methods, OGM and RNAseq.

SPI1-Rearranged

SPI1 encodes an ETS-domain transcription factor that is crucial for normal hematopoiesis, particularly in early T-cell development. Translocations involving the *SPI1* locus, located on the short arm of chromosome 11 (11p11.2), are rare (<5%) recurrent rearrangements in pediatric T-ALL. Typical fusion partners include *STMN1* (1p36.11), *TCF7* (5q31.1) or *BCL11B* (14q32.2). The presence of *SPI1* fusions is linked to an immature T-cell phenotype and a higher enrichment for an ETP-ALL signature suggesting a potential role in leukemia development from early thymic progenitors. Immunophenotype shows a double-negative (DN; CD4-CD8-) or CD8+ single-positive (SP) phenotype. Rearrangements of *SPI1* are associated with poor prognosis. Patients with *SPI1*-fusion positive T-ALL showed significantly shorter OS—a reported 2-year OS is ~50% [79].

A recent study reported that the *SPI1* T-ALL subtype frequently develops secondary cancers related to Langerhans cell histiocytosis and myeloid sarcomas, with dismal outcomes [45].

Rearrangements involving *SPI1* can be detected by FISH, OGM or RNAseq methods.

LYL1-Rearranged

The Lymphoid leukemia 1 (*LYL1*) gene encodes a basic helix-loop-helix (bHLH) transcription factor that shares high amino acid homology in the bHLH domain with *TAL1* [80]. *TAL1* and *LYL1* demonstrate overlapping expression patterns during hematopoietic development and can exert identical functions in certain regulatory pathways [81, 82].

The most frequently reported translocation involving *LYL1* is t(7;19)(q34;p13), resulting in the *TRB::LYL1 fusion* juxtaposing the *LYL1* gene with T-cell receptor regulatory sequences and resulting in aberrant *LYL1* expression. *LYL1* overexpression commonly co-occurs with *LMO2* dysregulation, likely reflecting established protein-protein interactions between these transcription factors. Additionally, mutations in genes within the JAK-STAT or Ras signaling pathways (including *FLT3, NRAS,* and *JAK3*) are enriched in the *LMO2/LYL1* subtype as well as HOXA subgroup [42].

Pediatric patients harboring *LYL1* rearrangements demonstrate inferior EFS and persistent MRD, indicating an adverse prognosis [45].

LYL1 rearrangements can be detected using FISH, RT-PCR, OGM, or RNAseq [77].

OLIG2

OLIG2 (originally designated as *BHLHB1*) encodes a basic helix-loop-helix transcription factor located on chromosome 21q22.11. While *OLIG2* expression is normally restricted to neural tissues, overexpression has been observed in patients with T-ALL/ T-cell lymphoblastic lymphoma (T-ALL/LBL). *OLIG2* rearrangements are rare in T-ALL, occurring in less than 2% of cases, typically resulting from the translocation t(14;21)(q11;q22). This genetic alteration demonstrates a strong male predominance, with a male-to-female ratio of 4:1 based on available data, and may be associated with adverse prognosis [83]. The oncogenic mechanism appears to involve *OLIG2* overexpression, functioning as an inhibitor of TCF3-mediated transcription activation, disrupting the normal T-cell differentiation required for proper lymphoid development [84].

The *OLIG2* rearrangement can be suspected in G-banded karyotype based on chromosome morphology, but ultimately needs to be confirmed by FISH, OGM, RT-PCR or RNAseq analysis.

Emerging Molecular Markers of Prognostic Importance for Further T-ALL Classification

The reduced cost of sequencing and the increased availability of WGS, WES, WTS, and methylation sequencing in clinical diagnostics and clinical research have drastically enriched knowledge of T-ALL genomics, adding gene expression or methylation profiles and further improving classification of T-ALL. Interestingly, T-ALL genomic landscape biology is mostly driven by noncoding alterations in comparison to B-ALL. It is noteworthy that chromosomal rearrangements resulting in the formation of chimeric fusion oncoproteins are observed in approximately 50% of B-ALL cases, whereas these events are present in approximately 20% of T-ALL cases. By contrast, enhancer hijacking appears to be a prevalent way for oncogene activation, impacting nearly 50% of T-ALL cases and nearly 61 oncogenes, while appearing to be rare in B-ALL cases.

Thus, the recent international AALL0434 COG Clinical Trial utilized complete sequencing approaches, WGS, WES, WTS of tumors and WGS of matched normal samples, for 1309 T-ALL patients between ages 1 and 30 years [45] and subclassified T-ALL based on clustering by expression profiles into 15 distinct molecular classes: *NKX2* (−1 and −5), *TLX1, TLX3, TAL1* (DP-like and αß-like), *LMO2* γδ-like, *STAG2/LMO2*, TME-enriched, *SPI1*, ETP-like (*KMT2A*-rearranged, *HOXA13*-rearranged, *MLLT10*-rearranged, *NUP214*-rearranged, *NUP98*-rearranged, *ZFP36L2*-rearranged, *ETV6*-altered, and loss of function mutations in *MED12*), *BCL11B, KMT2A, MLLT10, HOXA9* TCR, *NUP98*, and *NUP214*—rearranged (Table 14.2 and Fig. 14.4). Almost all cases with *BCL11B* overexpression revealed ETP immunophenotype, highlighting this group as a distinct entity of T-ALL. At the same time, *TAL1*-rearranged and *TLX3*-rearranged T-ALL subgroups revealed ETP, near-ETP, and even non-ETP immunophenotypes, showing significant overlap between T-ALL subtypes defined by immunophenotype and by genetic markers. In addition, *KMT2A, MLLT10, NUP98* and *NUP214* cases were noted in the ETP-like cluster and in clusters with more differentiated immunophenotype; despite the common genetic driver, the 5-year survival rates and gene expression profiles differed.

In addition to the genetic subtypes proposed by the COG group, which are characterized by key genetic abnormalities and characteristic expression profile, T-ALL cases frequently exhibit secondary aberrations, which include genetic variants in NOTCH1 (*NOTCH1, FBXW7*), JAK-STAT (*JAK1, JAK2, JAK3, STAT5A/B, IL7R, PTPN2*), RAS (*NRAS, KRAS, PTPN11, NF1*), PI3K-AKT-mTOR (*PTEN, PTPN2, PIK3CD, PIK3CA, PIK3R1, AKT1, MTOR*) signaling pathway genes as well as cell cycle and apoptosis regulating genes, *CDKN2A/B* and *CDKN1B*, ribosome *RPL10*, oncogene *MCYN* and tumor suppressor gene *RB1* (Fig. 14.5). Identifying variants in

Table 14.2 Genotypic T-ALL subtypes proposed by Children Oncology Group [45]

Subtype	Oncogene expression pattern	Common genetic aberration	Frequently observed TCR rearrangement status (molecular assay)	Blast percentage proportion	ETP status	Prevalence in age groups/ Genotypic sex
BCL11B	*BCL11B* overexpression	*BCL11B::ARID1B*, *BCL11B* enhancer amplification, *BCL11B*::other partner genes	No TCR-R	Majority of cases: 75–100%	Mostly ETP; small number of non-ETP	Most 7–15 years old (y.o.) and some >15; M > F
ETP-like	*HOXA13*-high; *TAL1/LMO2/ LYL1*-high; *NKX2-5*-high	*NUP98::RAP1GDS1; SET::NUP214; BCL11B::v, ETV6* fusion, *ZFP36L2* fusion, *MED12* mutation; *HOXA13* fusion; *HOXA13-BCL11B* enhancer hijacking; *HOXA13 TCR; NUP98* fusion; *SET::NUP214* fusion	No TCR-R	Majority of cases: 75–100%	ETP, near-ETP, non-ETP	All ages, rare in 0–2 y.o.; M > F
KMT2A	*HOXA9*-high	*KMT2A* fusion	N/A	Majority of cases: 75–100%	Most non-ETP, rare cases with ETP	All ages, common in 7–15 y.o., rare in 0–2 y.o.; M > F
MLLT10	*HOXA9*-high	*MLLT10* fusion	N/A	Majority of cases: 75–100%	Non-ETP and near-ETP	All ages, common in 2–7 y.o. and 7–15 y.o., rare in 0–2 y.o.; M > F
HOXA9 TCR	*HOXA9*-high	*HOXA9::TCR*	TCRß, TCRαß, TCRγδ, TCRγ/δ	Majority of cases: 75–100%	Non-ETP and near-ETP	More common in 7–15 y.o., absent in 0–2 y.o., M = F

TLX3	*TLX3*-high	*TLX3::BCL11B*; *TLX3* fusion; *TLX3* copy number gain; *TLX3* missense alteration	N/A	Majority of cases: 75–100%	ETP, near-ETP, non-ETP	More common in 2–7 y.o., absent in 0–2 y.o., M > F
TLX1	*TLX1*-high	*TLX1::TCR; TLX1* intergenic loss; *TLX1* intergenic inversion	TCRß, TCRαß, TCRγδ, TCRγ/δ	Majority of cases: 75–100%	Non-ETP	More common in 2–7 y.o., rare in 0–2 y.o., M > F
NKX2-1	*NKX2-1*-high	*NKX2-1::TCR*; *NKX2-1* chromothripsis; *NKX2-1*::v; *NKX2-1* copy number gain	TCRß, TCRαß, TCRγδ, TCRγ/δ	Majority of cases: 75–100%	Non-ETP, unknown	In all ages; M > F
TAL1 DP-like	*TAL2*-high, *LMO1*-high (rare *NKX2-1*-high and *NKX2-5*-high)	*STIL::TAL1*; *TAL1* enhancer SNV/indel; *TAL11::TCR*; *TAL1* enhancer gain; *TAL1* fusion	TCRß, TCRαß, TCRγ/δ, no TCR-R	Majority of cases: 75–100%	Non-ETP	All ages, common in 2–7 and 7–15 y.o., M > F
TAL1 αß-like	*TAL2*-high, *LMO1*-high	*STIL::TAL1*; *TAL1* enhancer SNV/indel; *TAL11::TCR*; *TAL1* enhancer gain; *TAL1* fusion	TCRαß	Majority of cases: 75–100%	Near-ETP, non-ETP	All ages, common in 2–7 and 7–15 y.o., M > F
LMO2 γδ-like	*LMO2*-high	*LMO2* TCR; *LMO2* enhancer SNV/indel; *LMO2* enhancer gain; LMO2 fusion; *LMO2* intergenic loss (*RAG2*); *LMO2* intergenic loss (*CAPRIN1*); *LMO2*::v fusions	TCRγδ	Majority of cases: 75–100%	Non-ETP	All ages groups, more common in 2–15 y.o.; M = F

(continued)

Table 14.2 (continued)

Subtype	Oncogene expression pattern	Common genetic aberration	Frequently observed TCR rearrangement status (molecular assay)	Blast percentage proportion	ETP status	Prevalence in age groups/ Genotypic sex
NKX2–5	*NKX2-5* high	*NKX2-5* fusion	TCRδ	Half of cases: 75–100%; a quarter of cases 10–50%	Non-ETP	Common in 0–7 y.o., absent in older children; M = F
SPI-1	*SPI1*-high	*SPI1* fusion	N/A	Majority of cases: 75–100%	Non-ETP	Present in 0–15, absent in >15; M > F
STAG2/LMO2	*LMO2*-high, *STAG2*-low	Dual hit *LMO2* activation and *STAG2* inactivation: *LMO2::STAG2, LMO2::TCR, LMO2 SNV*		Majority of cases: 75–100%; a quarter of cases: 10–50%	Non-ETP	Common in 0–2 y.o., may be seen in 2–7, absent in older children; F > M
Tumor microenvironment (TME)-enriched	*NKX2-5*-high *NKX2-1*-high *TAL2*-high *TAL1/LMO2/ LYL1*-high *TLX3*-high *HOXA13*-high	*SET::NUP214*; *MLLT10* fusion; *HOXA9::TCR*; *TLX3 BCL11B* enhancer; *TLX3* fusion; *TLX1*::v; *NKX2-1* fusion; *TAL1* enhancer SNV/ indel; *LMO2* fusion	TCRαß, TCRß, TCRγ/δ, TCRγδ, no TCR-R	Majority of cases: 10–50%; some cases with 50–100%	ETP, near-ETP, non-ETP, unknown	More common in 2–15 y.o., rare in 0–2 y.o. and > 15 y.o.; M > F

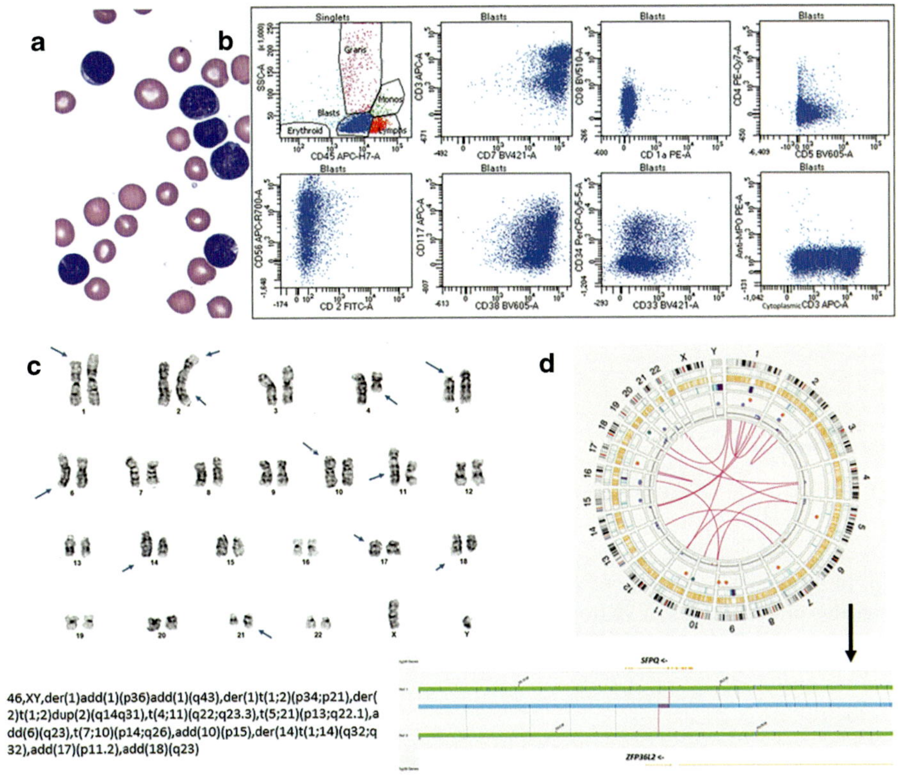

Fig. 14.4 (**a**) The blasts are small to medium in size with round or convoluted nuclei, immature chromatin, inconspicuous nucleoli, and a scant basophilic cytoplasm. Wright-Giemsa stained bone marrow aspirate smear, original magnification ×1000. (**b**) Representative flow cytometry dot plots of the bone marrow specimen. The blasts show low side scatter (SSC), are positive for CD45, CD7, and CD38, mostly and variably positive for surface and cytoplasmic CD3, partially positive for CD56, CD34, CD117, and CD33, negative for CD1a, CD2, CD8, and myeloperoxidase (MPO), and mostly negative for CD4 and CD5. (**c**) G-banded chromosome analysis shows a complex karyotype. (**d**) OGM confirms a complex karyotype and identifies the fusion *SFPQ::ZFP36L2* which resulted from the reciprocal translocation, t(1;2)(p34.3;p21). This fusion is associated with ETP phenotype in T-ALL

these genes is important for developing potential therapies [37, 85, 86]. Additionally, T-ALL cases frequently exhibit biallelic losses of the T-cell receptor alleles. These can be detected by microarray or quantitative PCR analysis (Fig. 14.6). Some studies have found that the absence of biallelic deletion of the TCR-gamma locus was associated with early treatment failure in patients with T-ALL [44, 87].

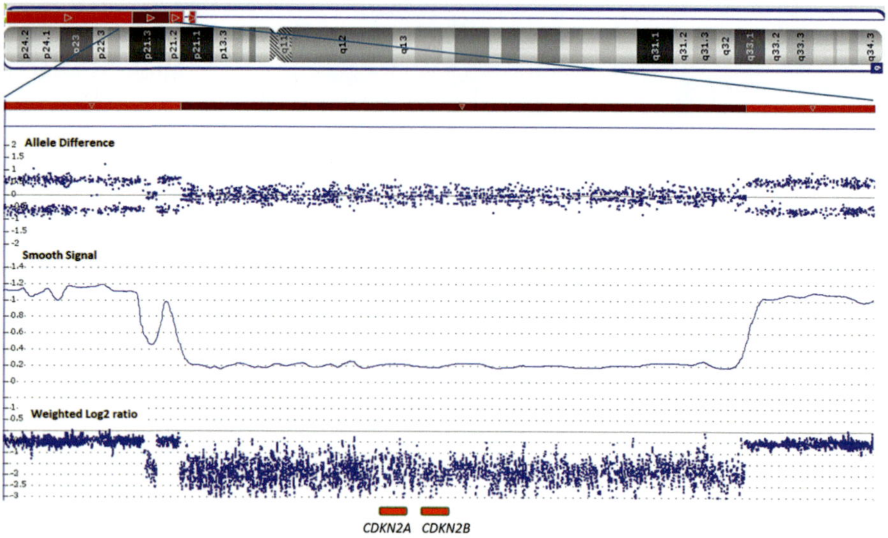

Fig. 14.5 Microarray analysis of a bone marrow specimen from the patient with T-ALL showed a deletion of the majority of 9p from 9pter to 9p21.1 which encompasses an ~6 Mb biallelic loss containing *CDKN2A* and *CDKN2B*, an abnormality observed in about 70% of T-ALL pediatric cases

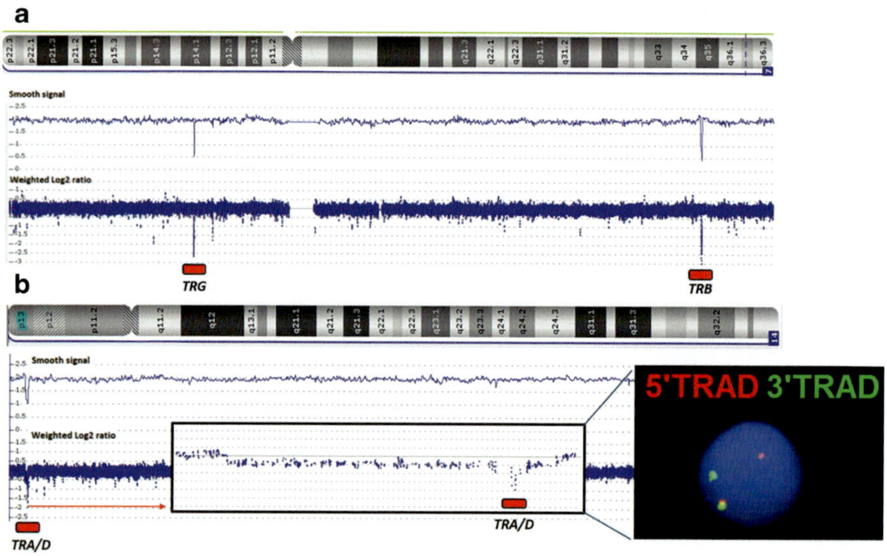

Fig. 14.6 Microarray analysis of a bone marrow specimen from the patient with T-ALL shows biallelic losses involving T-cell receptor loci: *TRG* (7p14.1), *TRB* (7q34) and *TRA/D* (14q11.2). Clonal losses of the T-cell receptor sites are common to T-ALL. Biallelic loss as seen by microarray may indicate their clonal rearrangements. However, confirmation of these rearrangements are required by a separate testing. In B, an example of a biallelic loss of *TRA/D* locus which was confirmed to be rearranged by FISH testing

Concluding Remarks

Recent guidelines integrated multiple molecular markers into the subclassification and risk assessment of T-ALL. In addition to that, an explosive growth of pre-clinical and clinical studies described in this chapter highlights not only the diverse transcriptome and methylome profiles associated with T-ALL but also identifies additional genetic markers. These advancements contribute to more accurate diagnosis and improved prognostic assessment of this highly heterogeneous disease. Although conventional cytogenetics and FISH analyses are still employed as a front-line genetic tests assisting flow cytometry in T-ALL classification, limitations of these conventional methodologies highlight the need of incorporation of molecular high-throughput methods, such as more expensive whole-genome transcriptome or cost-effective targeted RNA sequencing that analyze specific genetic fusions associated with T-ALL. This integrated approach should be complemented by highly sensitive methods for MRD detection, such as multiparameter flow cytometry and/or NGS-based MRD testing.

References

1. Gianni F, Belver L, Ferrando A. The genetics and mechanisms of T-cell acute lymphoblastic leukemia. Cold Spring Harb Perspect Med. 2020;10(3):a035246.
2. Graux C, et al. Cytogenetics and molecular genetics of T-cell acute lymphoblastic leukemia: from thymocyte to lymphoblast. Leukemia. 2006;20(9):1496–510.
3. Ferrando AA, et al. Biallelic transcriptional activation of oncogenic transcription factors in T-cell acute lymphoblastic leukemia. Blood. 2004;103(5):1909–11.
4. Burns MA, et al. Identification of prognostic factors in childhood T-cell acute lymphoblastic leukemia: results from DFCI ALL Consortium Protocols 05-001 and 11-001. Pediatr Blood Cancer. 2021;68(1):e28719.
5. Schrappe M, et al. Late MRD response determines relapse risk overall and in subsets of childhood T-cell ALL: results of the AIEOP-BFM-ALL 2000 study. Blood. 2011;118(8):2077–84.
6. Vora A, et al. Augmented post-remission therapy for a minimal residual disease-defined high-risk subgroup of children and young people with clinical standard-risk and intermediate-risk acute lymphoblastic leukaemia (UKALL 2003): a randomised controlled trial. Lancet Oncol. 2014;15(8):809–18.
7. Jaime-Perez JC, Santos J, Gomez-Almaguer D. Childhood T-cell acute lymphoblastic leukemia in a single Latin American center: impact of improved treatment scheme and support therapy on survival. Hematol Transfus Cell Ther. 2020;42(4):320–5.
8. Lustosa de Sousa DW, et al. Acute lymphoblastic leukemia in children and adolescents: prognostic factors and analysis of survival. Rev Bras Hematol Hemoter. 2015;37(4):223–9.
9. Teachey DT, Pui CH. Comparative features and outcomes between paediatric T-cell and B-cell acute lymphoblastic leukaemia. Lancet Oncol. 2019;20(3):e142–54.
10. Gupta S, et al. Sex-based disparities in outcome in pediatric acute lymphoblastic leukemia: a Children's Oncology Group report. Cancer. 2022;128(9):1863–70.
11. Pui CH, et al. Results of therapy for acute lymphoblastic leukemia in black and white children. JAMA. 2003;290(15):2001–7.
12. Gupta S, et al. Racial and ethnic disparities in childhood and young adult acute lymphocytic leukaemia: secondary analyses of eight Children's Oncology Group cohort trials. Lancet Haematol. 2023;10(2):e129–41.

13. Polonen P, Mullighan CG, Teachey DT. Classification and risk stratification in T-lineage acute lymphoblastic leukemia. Blood. 2025;145(14):1464–74.
14. Vega-Garcia N, et al. Measurable residual disease assessed by flow-cytometry is a stable prognostic factor for pediatric T-cell acute lymphoblastic leukemia in consecutive SEHOP protocols whereas the impact of oncogenetics depends on treatment. Front Pediatr. 2020;8:614521.
15. Pullen J, et al. Significance of commonly used prognostic factors differs for children with T cell acute lymphocytic leukemia (ALL), as compared to those with B-precursor ALL. A Pediatric Oncology Group (POG) study. Leukemia. 1999;13(11):1696–707.
16. Yanada M, et al. Clinical features and outcome of T-lineage acute lymphoblastic leukemia in adults: a low initial white blood cell count, as well as a high count predict decreased survival rates. Leuk Res. 2007;31(7):907–14.
17. Raetz EA, et al. Children's Oncology Group blueprint for research: acute lymphoblastic leukemia. Pediatr Blood Cancer. 2023;70(Suppl 6):e30585.
18. Patrick K, Vora A. Update on biology and treatment of T-cell acute lymphoblastic leukaemia. Curr Opin Pediatr. 2015;27(1):44–9.
19. Bhojwani D, Howard SC, Pui CH. High-risk childhood acute lymphoblastic leukemia. Clin Lymphoma Myeloma. 2009;9(Suppl 3):S222–30.
20. Gupta S, et al. Blinatumomab in standard-risk B-cell acute lymphoblastic leukemia in children. N Engl J Med. 2025;392(9):875–91.
21. Hayashi H, Makimoto A, Yuza Y. Treatment of pediatric acute lymphoblastic leukemia: a historical perspective. Cancers (Basel). 2024;16(4):723.
22. Wang Y, et al. Impact of age on the survival of pediatric leukemia: an analysis of 15083 children in the SEER database. Oncotarget. 2016;7(50):83767–74.
23. O'Connor D, et al. The clinicogenomic landscape of induction failure in childhood and young adult T-cell acute lymphoblastic leukemia. J Clin Oncol. 2023;41(19):3545–56.
24. Baig N, Muhammad S, Shaikh S. Infantile T-cell acute lymphoblastic leukaemia: a case report. J Cancer Allied Spec. 2022;8(1):e459.
25. Doerrenberg M, et al. T-cell acute lymphoblastic leukemia in infants has distinct genetic and epigenetic features compared to childhood cases. Genes Chromosom Cancer. 2017;56(2):159–67.
26. Kotecha RS. Updates in infant acute lymphoblastic leukemia and the potential for targeted therapy. Hematology Am Soc Hematol Educ Program. 2022;2022(1):611–7.
27. Reaman G, et al. Acute lymphoblastic leukemia in infants less than one year of age: a cumulative experience of the Children's Cancer Study Group. J Clin Oncol. 1985;3(11):1513–21.
28. Gossai NP, et al. Central nervous system status is prognostic in T-cell acute lymphoblastic leukemia: a Children's Oncology Group report. Blood. 2023;141(15):1802–11.
29. O'Connor D, et al. Cranial radiotherapy has minimal benefit in children with central nervous system involvement in T-ALL. Blood Adv. 2023;7(23):7231–4.
30. Bene MC, et al. Proposals for the immunological classification of acute leukemias. European Group for the Immunological Characterization of Leukemias (EGIL). Leukemia. 1995;9(10):1783–6.
31. Pui CH, et al. Treatment response and outcome of children with T-cell acute lymphoblastic leukemia expressing the gamma-delta T-cell receptor. Onco Targets Ther. 2019;8(8):1599637.
32. Coustan-Smith E, et al. Early T-cell precursor leukaemia: a subtype of very high-risk acute lymphoblastic leukaemia. Lancet Oncol. 2009;10(2):147–56.
33. Wood BL, et al. Prognostic significance of ETP phenotype and minimal residual disease in T-ALL: a Children's Oncology Group study. Blood. 2023;142(24):2069–78.
34. Alaggio R, et al. The 5th edition of the World Health Organization classification of haematolymphoid tumours: lymphoid neoplasms. Leukemia. 2022;36(7):1720–48.
35. Duffield AS, Mullighan CG, Borowitz MJ. International Consensus Classification of acute lymphoblastic leukemia/lymphoma. Virchows Arch. 2023;482(1):11–26.
36. Iacobucci I, Mullighan CG. Genetic basis of acute lymphoblastic leukemia. J Clin Oncol. 2017;35(9):975–83.
37. Van Vlierberghe P, Ferrando A. The molecular basis of T cell acute lymphoblastic leukemia. J Clin Invest. 2012;122(10):3398–406.

38. Brady SW, et al. The genomic landscape of pediatric acute lymphoblastic leukemia. Nat Genet. 2022;54(9):1376–89.
39. Girardi T, et al. The genetics and molecular biology of T-ALL. Blood. 2017;129(9):1113–23.
40. Arber DA, et al. International Consensus Classification of Myeloid Neoplasms and Acute Leukemias: integrating morphologic, clinical, and genomic data. Blood. 2022;140(11):1200–28.
41. Montefiori LE, et al. Enhancer hijacking drives oncogenic BCL11B expression in lineage-ambiguous stem cell leukemia. Cancer Discov. 2021;11(11):2846–67.
42. Liu Y, et al. The genomic landscape of pediatric and young adult T-lineage acute lymphoblastic leukemia. Nat Genet. 2017;49(8):1211–8.
43. Mark M, Rijli FM, Chambon P. Homeobox genes in embryogenesis and pathogenesis. Pediatr Res. 1997;42(4):421–9.
44. Yang YL, et al. Absence of biallelic TCRgamma deletion predicts induction failure and poorer outcomes in childhood T-cell acute lymphoblastic leukemia. Pediatr Blood Cancer. 2012;58(6):846–51.
45. Polonen P, et al. The genomic basis of childhood T-lineage acute lymphoblastic leukaemia. Nature. 2024;632(8027):1082–91.
46. Yang L, et al. 3D genome alterations associated with dysregulated HOXA13 expression in high-risk T-lineage acute lymphoblastic leukemia. Nat Commun. 2021;12(1):3708.
47. Speleman F, et al. A new recurrent inversion, inv(7)(p15q34), leads to transcriptional activation of HOXA10 and HOXA11 in a subset of T-cell acute lymphoblastic leukemias. Leukemia. 2005;19(3):358–66.
48. Soulier J, et al. HOXA genes are included in genetic and biologic networks defining human acute T-cell leukemia (T-ALL). Blood. 2005;106(1):274–86.
49. Cauwelier B, et al. Clinical, cytogenetic and molecular characteristics of 14 T-ALL patients carrying the TCRbeta-HOXA rearrangement: a study of the Groupe Francophone de Cytogenetique Hematologique. Leukemia. 2007;21(1):121–8.
50. Vagapova ER, et al. The role of TAL1 in hematopoiesis and leukemogenesis. Acta Nat. 2018;10(1):15–23.
51. Brown L, et al. Site-specific recombination of the tal-1 gene is a common occurrence in human T cell leukemia. EMBO J. 1990;9(10):3343–51.
52. Mansur MB, et al. SIL-TAL1 fusion gene negative impact in T-cell acute lymphoblastic leukemia outcome. Leuk Lymphoma. 2009;50(8):1318–25.
53. Bernard O, et al. Two distinct mechanisms for the SCL gene activation in the t(1;14) translocation of T-cell leukemias. Genes Chromosom Cancer. 1990;1(3):194–208.
54. Le Noir S, et al. Extensive molecular mapping of TCRalpha/delta- and TCRbeta-involved chromosomal translocations reveals distinct mechanisms of oncogene activation in T-ALL. Blood. 2012;120(16):3298–309.
55. Cauwelier B, et al. Molecular cytogenetic study of 126 unselected T-ALL cases reveals high incidence of TCRbeta locus rearrangements and putative new T-cell oncogenes. Leukemia. 2006;20(7):1238–44.
56. Mansour MR, et al. Oncogene regulation. An oncogenic super-enhancer formed through somatic mutation of a noncoding intergenic element. Science. 2014;346(6215):1373–7.
57. Thielemans N, et al. TAL1 cooperates with PI3K/AKT pathway activation in T-cell acute lymphoblastic leukemia. Haematologica. 2022;107(10):2304–17.
58. Muller J, et al. How T-lymphoblastic leukemia can be classified based on genetics using standard diagnostic techniques enhanced by whole genome sequencing. Leukemia. 2023;37(1):217–21.
59. Xia Y, et al. TAL2, a helix-loop-helix gene activated by the (7;9)(q34;q32) translocation in human T-cell leukemia. Proc Natl Acad Sci USA. 1991;88(24):11416–20.
60. Drieux F, et al. Detection of gene fusion transcripts in peripheral T-cell lymphoma using a multiplexed targeted sequencing assay. J Mol Diagn. 2021;23(8):929–40.

61. La Starza R, et al. Design of a comprehensive fluorescence in situ hybridization assay for genetic classification of T-cell acute lymphoblastic leukemia. J Mol Diagn. 2020;22(5):629–39.
62. Lato MW, et al. The new therapeutic strategies in pediatric T-cell acute lymphoblastic leukemia. Int J Mol Sci. 2021;22(9):4502.
63. Van Vlierberghe P, et al. PHF6 mutations in T-cell acute lymphoblastic leukemia. Nat Genet. 2010;42(4):338–42.
64. Pinton A, et al. PHF6-altered T-ALL harbor epigenetic repressive switch at bivalent promoters and respond to 5-azacitidine and venetoclax. Clin Cancer Res. 2024;30(1):94–105.
65. Vanden Bempt M, et al. Cooperative enhancer activation by TLX1 and STAT5 drives development of NUP214-ABL1/TLX1-positive T cell acute lymphoblastic leukemia. Cancer Cell. 2018;34(2):271–285.e7.
66. Van Vlierberghe P, et al. Cooperative genetic defects in TLX3 rearranged pediatric T-ALL. Leukemia. 2008;22(4):762–70.
67. Hansen-Hagge TE, et al. Disruption of the RanBP17/Hox11L2 region by recombination with the TCRdelta locus in acute lymphoblastic leukemias with t(5;14)(q34;q11). Leukemia. 2002;16(11):2205–12.
68. Su XY, et al. Various types of rearrangements target TLX3 locus in T-cell acute lymphoblastic leukemia. Genes Chromosom Cancer. 2004;41(3):243–9.
69. Attarbaschi A, et al. Prognostic relevance of TLX3 (HOX11L2) expression in childhood T-cell acute lymphoblastic leukaemia treated with Berlin-Frankfurt-Munster (BFM) protocols containing early and late re-intensification elements. Br J Haematol. 2010;148(2):293–300.
70. Gottardo NG, et al. Significance of HOX11L2/TLX3 expression in children with T-cell acute lymphoblastic leukemia treated on Children's Cancer Group protocols. Leukemia. 2005;19(9):1705–8.
71. Nagel S, et al. The cardiac homeobox gene NKX2-5 is deregulated by juxtaposition with BCL11B in pediatric T-ALL cell lines via a novel t(5;14)(q35.1;q32.2). Cancer Res. 2003;63(17):5329–34.
72. Delafoy M, et al. Oncogenomic profiling in infant-toddler T-ALL identifies NKX2 family genes as drivers linked to favorable outcomes. Hemasphere. 2025;9(5):e70154.
73. Sang M, et al. LIM-domain-only proteins: multifunctional nuclear transcription coregulators that interacts with diverse proteins. Mol Biol Rep. 2014;41(2):1067–73.
74. Van Vlierberghe P, et al. The cryptic chromosomal deletion del(11)(p12p13) as a new activation mechanism of LMO2 in pediatric T-cell acute lymphoblastic leukemia. Blood. 2006;108(10):3520–9.
75. Dai YT, et al. Transcriptome-wide subtyping of pediatric and adult T cell acute lymphoblastic leukemia in an international study of 707 cases. Proc Natl Acad Sci USA. 2022;119(15):e2120787119.
76. Tremblay M, et al. Modeling T-cell acute lymphoblastic leukemia induced by the SCL and LMO1 oncogenes. Genes Dev. 2010;24(11):1093–105.
77. Homminga I, et al. Characterization of a pediatric T-cell acute lymphoblastic leukemia patient with simultaneous LYL1 and LMO2 rearrangements. Haematologica. 2012;97(2):258–61.
78. Parvin S, et al. LMO2 confers synthetic lethality to PARP inhibition in DLBCL. Cancer Cell. 2019;36(3):237–249.e6.
79. Seki M, et al. Recurrent SPI1 (PU.1) fusions in high-risk pediatric T cell acute lymphoblastic leukemia. Nat Genet. 2017;49(8):1274–81.
80. Mellentin JD, Smith SD, Cleary ML. lyl-1, a novel gene altered by chromosomal translocation in T cell leukemia, codes for a protein with a helix-loop-helix DNA binding motif. Cell. 1989;58(1):77–83.
81. Souroullas GP, et al. Adult hematopoietic stem and progenitor cells require either Lyl1 or Scl for survival. Cell Stem Cell. 2009;4(2):180–6.
82. Giroux S, et al. lyl-1 and tal-1/scl, two genes encoding closely related bHLH transcription factors, display highly overlapping expression patterns during cardiovascular and hematopoietic ontogeny. Gene Expr Patterns. 2007;7(3):215–26.

83. Panagopoulos I, et al. Chromosome translocation t(14;21)(q11;q22) activates both OLIG1 and OLIG2 in pediatric T-cell lymphoblastic malignancies and may signify adverse prognosis. Cancer Genomics Proteomics. 2020;17(1):41–8.
84. Wang J, et al. The t(14;21)(q11.2;q22) chromosomal translocation associated with T-cell acute lymphoblastic leukemia activates the BHLHB1 gene. Proc Natl Acad Sci USA. 2000;97(7):3497–502.
85. Gutierrez A, et al. Inactivation of LEF1 in T-cell acute lymphoblastic leukemia. Blood. 2010;115(14):2845–51.
86. Zhang J, et al. The genetic basis of early T-cell precursor acute lymphoblastic leukaemia. Nature. 2012;481(7380):157–63.
87. Gutierrez A, et al. Absence of biallelic TCRgamma deletion predicts early treatment failure in pediatric T-cell acute lymphoblastic leukemia. J Clin Oncol. 2010;28(24):3816–23.

Prognostic and Predictive Biomarkers in Acute Myeloid Leukemia

15

Scott C. Smith, Priscilla Quach, Allison J. Kalinousky, Aravindh Nagarajan, Emily K. O'Donnell, John Herriges, and Lei Zhang

Introduction

Acute myeloid leukemia (AML) is a malignant hematological disorder characterized by the uncontrolled growth and blocked differentiation of myeloid lineage hematopoietic cells [1]. The overall incidence of AML in the pediatric population is about seven per million [2] with the highest rate for infants at 1.5 per 100,000 individuals. For those aged 1–4 years the incidence is 0.9 per 100,000 individuals, and for those aged 5–9 years it is 0.4 per 100,000 individuals [3]. It has long been recognized that AML is a genetically heterogeneous group of diseases. Over the past few decades, considerable progress has been made in identifying genetic and molecular markers [4–6]. The classification of AML has been restructured to emphasize breakthrough genetic findings in the 2022 updates by two systems: World Health Organization (WHO) and International Consensus Classification (ICC) [7, 8]. Studies also began to appreciate the genetic differences between pediatric and adult AML (pAML and aAML), although pAML and aAML have

S. C. Smith
Department of Pathology, SUNY Upstate Medical University, Syracuse, NY, USA

P. Quach
Department of Pathology, Nebraska Methodist Hospital, Omaha, NE, USA

A. J. Kalinousky · A. Nagarajan
Department of Pathology and Laboratory Medicine, Children's Mercy Kansas City, Kansas City, MO, USA

E. K. O'Donnell · J. Herriges · L. Zhang (✉)
Department of Pathology and Laboratory Medicine, Children's Mercy Kansas City, Kansas City, MO, USA

Departments of Pathology and Pediatrics, University of Missouri Kansas City—School of Medicine, Kansas City, MO, USA
e-mail: lzhang@cmh.edu

W. Li (ed.), *Laboratory Assessments of Pediatric Leukemia*,
https://doi.org/10.1007/978-3-032-26557-9_15

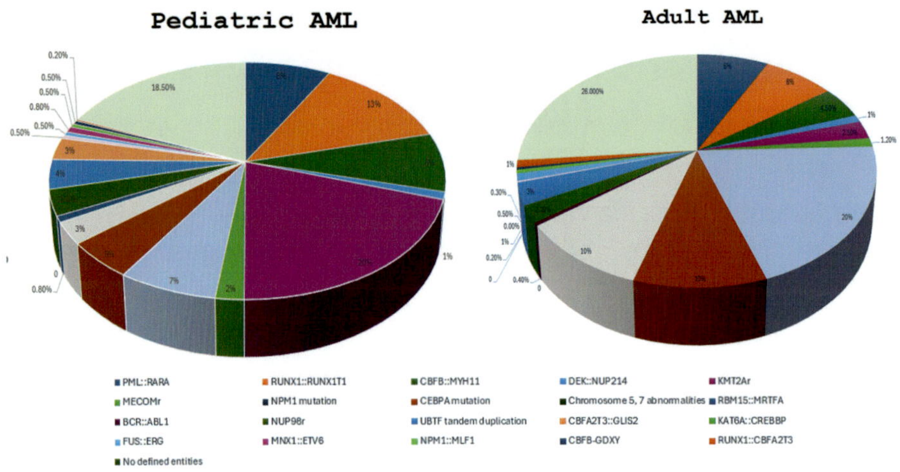

Fig. 15.1 Frequencies of defined entities for pediatric and adult AML

many shared clinical and pathological characteristics [9, 10]. Notably, *KMT2A* [9] and *NUP98* rearrangements [11] as well as *UBTF* tandem duplication [12] are more common in pAML, while aAML frequently harbors mutations in *DNMT3A* and splicing factor genes, and core binding factor (CBF) AMLs are common across all ages [9]. A new classification system and high-risk categories specific for pAML have been recently proposed [13].

Advancements in defining biomarkers has played a crucial role in risk stratification; for example, *NPM1, FLT3*-ITD, *WT1, CEBPA* mutations, and *KMT2A* rearrangements are important pAML prognostic markers [7, 8]. More accurate risk stratification has guided treatment and led to the development of targeted therapies that have significantly improved patient outcomes [14–16]. While the 5-year overall survival (OS) of pediatric patients with AML is approximately 70%, it is still quite lower than the 95% 5-year OS for pediatric acute lymphoblastic leukemia (ALL) [17–19], and survival at the individual level may be dependent on detected genomic abnormalities. Accurate and timely diagnoses can aid in risk-stratification or nominate targeted therapies based on the genetic background.

This chapter describes the various recurrent biomarkers in AML in the categories of favorable prognosis, intermediate prognosis, unfavorable prognosis, variable prognosis, and uncertain/potential prognosis. Each category will start with WHO- and ICC-defined entities with mutually exclusive abnormalities, followed by newly emerged potential genetic subtypes. The comparison of incidence for unique AML entities between pediatric and adult patients is shown in Fig. 15.1. The diagnostic, prognostic, and therapeutic value, as well as other associated genetic abnormalities will be discussed in each listed genetic entity. Characteristic genetic changes in Down syndrome AML will also be reviewed.

Diagnostic Approaches

The diagnostic approach for a heterogeneous disease like AML is complex and requires a high level of expertise. It involves the initial evaluation of blood and bone marrow with a combination of tests at all levels of cell, protein, and DNA; and potentially tests at the RNA level. Tests at the protein level include flow cytometry (FCM), immunohistochemistry, and cytochemistry, which are performed in pathology laboratories. Genetic testing specifically has played an important role in AML classification, risk stratification, and therapeutic guidance.

Clinical cytogenetics has been of paramount importance in hematological malignancies. It now includes technologies beyond chromosome analysis that are rooted in molecular biology, such as fluorescent in situ hybridization (FISH) and chromosomal microarray (CMA). Chromosomal analysis (karyotyping) and FISH have traditionally been the main tools in clinical cytogenetics laboratories for standard cytogenetic workup. Karyotyping, while cost-effective and broadly informative, is limited by low resolution (6–10 Mb) and is reliant on culturing live cells. Despite these constraints, its ability as a single-cell assay to provide a detailed look at clonal architecture is invaluable in cancer genetics. FISH was developed to complement the limitations of karyotyping. It offers better resolution and specificity, detecting chromosomal aberrations that karyotyping might miss. However, since FISH is designed to detect specific genetic abnormalities, it is a not genome-wide assay. The combination of karyotyping and FISH has been instrumental for understanding the genome, as well as aiding in accurate diagnosis and treatment, especially in complex cases like AML.

To counter the shortfalls of FISH and karyotyping, molecular methodologies have increasingly found their way into the diagnostic realm. CMA provides a quasi-genome-wide view in an attempt to compensate for chromosome resolution shortcomings and the continually increasing number of crucial aberrations that makes FISH impractical. CMA, which has a resolution of approximately 10–20 kilobases (kb) in comparison to 6–10 Mb in chromosome analysis [20], and has been incorporated into the AML workup in the past decade. Single nucleotide polymorphism (SNP) arrays can not only detect copy number variants but also regions of homozygosity (ROH)/loss of heterozygosity (LOH). Detecting ROH/LOH somatically can be especially useful as it suggests biallelic variants in the ROH/LOH region. One limitation of CMA is that it cannot detect balanced translocations. In recent years, another cutting-edge technology, optical genome mapping (OGM), has rapidly gained traction in the field of cytogenetic analysis. It can provide high-resolution copy number analysis of the whole genome and detect structural rearrangements, such as translocations, insertions, and inversions.

Approximately 15 years ago, molecular testing was incorporated into the AML diagnostic process after the recognition that AML patients with a normal karyotype frequently harbored somatic mutations [5, 21]. Technologies like polymerase chain reaction (PCR), Sanger sequencing, and multiplex ligation-dependent probe amplification (MLPA) have been employed to detect these somatic mutations. In addition, reverse transcriptase–PCR (RT-PCR) is frequently used to detect or monitor recurrent gene fusions, such as *RUNX1-RUNX1T1*, *CBFB-MYH11*, *MLLT3-MLL*, or *DEK-NUP214,* especially when chromosome morphology is poor or chromosome analysis is unavailable [22, 23]. In recent years, the evolution of next-generation sequencing (NGS) approaches has yielded a rapidly expanding understanding of genetic and epigenetic alterations in AML [10]. Accordingly, DNA-based whole or targeted genome/exome sequencing, RNA-based targeted fusion testing, and RNA-based whole transcriptome expression analysis have become first or second line tests [6, 24, 25].

Genetic Biomarkers with Favorable Prognosis

Acute Promyelocytic Leukemia (APL)—*RARA* Fusion

Acute promyelocytic leukemia (APL) is a unique entity in AML most often characterized by a t(15;17)(q24;q21) translocation that creates a *PML::RARA* gene fusion [26]. In the pediatric population, it accounts for only 5–10% of all AML, and is observed in less than 2% of infant AML [27]. While considered to have generally favorable outcomes, favorability depends greatly on the results of baseline coagulation tests and the actions taken thereafter, as disseminated intravascular coagulation (DIC) can be a presenting feature of the entity [28, 29]. Indeed, this coagulopathy creates an urgent situation for a patient with suspected APL, requiring immediate action. A white blood cell count at diagnosis has proven a most effective predictor of relapse outcomes with fewer than 10,000 cells/μL considered standard risk for relapse, and greater than 10,000 cells/μL considered high risk of relapse [30]. Although high-risk patients have a propensity to suffer higher rates of early death due to DIC or therapy complications, typically associated with pulmonary or intracranial hemorrhage, fatal bleeding is only observed in approximately 10% of cases [26].

The reciprocal translocation between chromosomes 15 and 17, t(15;17), is the cytogenetic hallmark of APL, and accounts for 95% of all cases. The *PML::RARA* fusion transcript generated by this juxtaposition is comprised of the promyelocytic leukemia (*PML*) gene at 15q24 and the retinoic acid receptor alpha (*RARA*) gene at 17q21 [26, 31–33]. FISH dual-color dual-fusion probes are employed in clinical cytogenetics laboratories to quickly identify the presence or absence of the *PML::RARA* fusion. The fusion gene represses RARα targets and inhibits promyelocyte differentiation. Over the last two decades, leukemogenesis via p53 altered activation, mediated by PML alterations, has been identified, leading to reduced apoptosis. This reduction in apoptotic signaling plus the inhibition of differentiation results in leukemogenesis [34, 35]. In the absence of a *PML::RARA* fusion, APL may also be diagnosed with an alternate *RARA* rearrangement. Variant *RARA* rearrangements account for approximately 2% of all APL and typically provide an additional complication in diagnosis and treatment, in part due to potential delays in diagnosis [36]. The most common *RARA* rearrangement partner other than *PML* is *ZBTB16* [t(11;17)(q23;q21)][t(11;17)(q221)], reported in approximately 1% of

APL cases. Other recurrent rearrangement partners include *BCOR* [t(X;17)(p11;q21)], *IRF2BP2* [t(1;17)(q42;q21)], *TBLR1* [t(3;17)(q26;q21)], *FIP1L1* [t(4;17)(q12;q21)], *NPM1* [t(5;17)(q35;q21)], *STAT5B* [t(17;17)(q21;q21)], and *PRKAR1A* [t(17;17)(q21;q24)] [36]. In many clinical cytogenetics laboratories *RARA* break-apart FISH probes are hybridized in parallel with the *PML::RARA* dual-color dual-fusion probes to check for an alternate rearrangement, saving time during diagnosis.

APLs with good prognosis possess *PML::RARA* rearrangements which are sensitive to all *trans* retinoic acid (ATRA) and arsenic trioxide (ATO), the standard of care in pediatric patients [26]. This therapeutic combination promotes promyelocyte differentiation and apoptosis, which may have a misleading effect on conventional cytogenetic testing as incomplete blast differentiation is commonly observed in APL for up to 28 days, and occasionally 50 days post-induction [32]. This will lead to the detection of a t(15;17) *PML::RARA* fusion by chromosomes and FISH if performed in this post-induction window. While event-free outcomes can exceed 90% following this regiment in *PML::RARA*-positive APL [26], variant APL with *RARA* or genes of other retinoic acid receptor isoforms have a much more limited response. Specifically, *ZBTB16::RARA* and *STAT5B::RARA* rearrangements are resistant to ATRA and ATO, but rearrangements involving *NPM1, IRF2BP2,* and *FIP1L1* are sensitive to ATRA [36].

Core-Binding Factor (CBF) AML

CBF AML accounts for approximately 25–30% of pAML and 15% of aAML [37]. The median age in children is about 9 years old with a range of 3–16 years. CBF is a hematopoietic transcription factor comprised of two subunits, CBF α and β (CBFB), and is involved in the transcriptional regulation of normal hematopoiesis. The α subunit binds to a consensus DNA sequence and the β subunit stabilizes the interaction between the α subunit and DNA but does not interact with DNA independently [38, 39]. CBFα is a member of the Runt-related transcription factor (*RUNX*) gene family (*RUNX1, RUNX2, RUNX3*). CBF AML is a subtype of AML associated with various chromosomal aberrations disrupting the α and β subunits of CBF with primary aberrations being the t(8;21)(q22;q22)–*RUNX1::RUNX1T1* fusion and inv(16)(p13.1q22) or t(16;16)(p13.1;q22)–*CBFB::MYH11* fusion [7]. The *RUNX1::RUNX1T1* fusion product lacks a C-terminal transactivation domain from *RUNX1*, thus disrupting normal hematopoiesis in a dominant-negative fashion [40]. The *CBFB::MYH11* fusion product forms large nuclear aggregates and sequesters the α subunit *RUNX1* in the cytoplasm [41, 42]. Both fusions result in a dominant inhibitory effect on native *RUNX1* and the repression of target gene transcription.

The t(8;21)(q22;q22.1)–*RUNX1::RUNX1T1* fusion accounts for 12–14% of pAML [43, 44]. This particular AML is known to have a phenotype of subtype M2 according to the French-American-British (FAB) classification. This fusion can also be seen in acute myelomonocytic leukemia (AMML) (FAB M4) and in therapy-related AML [45]. Variant three-way translocations have been reported in about 3% of cases [46]. Additional abnormalities have been reported in approximately 70% of cases including loss of a sex chromosome (53%), del(9q) (12%), del(7q) (9%), +8 (5%), +21, +6, copy neutral LOH (cnLOH) of 19p encompassing *ZBTB7A* (highly mutated in t(8;21) AML), focal gain confined to *CCDC26*, focal deletions involving *WT1, BXORL1, RAD21, NF1, IKZF1, ETV6, PDS5A, and MGA,* as well as gain of *MYB* and *CNOT4*. Most of the additional abnormalities do not appear to affect the favorable prognosis associated with t(8;21); however, gain of chromosome 6 may indicate a less favorable disease course [47, 48], and *ETV6* deletion has been associated with adverse outcomes [49]. In the context of CBF AML, one study showed that disease-free survival (DFS) of those with *ETV6* deletion was 0%, whereas those without had a DFS of 61% ($P = 0.009$) [49].

Although rare, other partners for *RUNX1* have been reported, including *CBFA2T2* and *CBFA2T3* (also known as *RUNX1T3*) [50, 51]. *RUNX1T1*, *CBFA2T2,* and *CBFA2T3* are members of the myeloid translocation gene (MTG) family [51]. *CBFA2T3* is a hematopoietic corepressor that plays roles in both normal and malignant hematopoiesis, including inhibiting terminal erythromegakaryocytic differentiation, maintaining stemness of long-term hematopoietic stem cells (HSCs), and promoting the expansion of leukemia stem cells [50]. *RUNX1::CBFA2T3,* resulting from t(16;21)(q24;q22), represents approximately 0.1–0.3% of pAML cases, with a median age of presentation of 7 years [52], and ~1% of aAML [53]. Patients with *RUNX1::CBFA2T3* fusion have a gene expression profile that is closely related to cases of *RUNX1::RUNX1T1* fusion; thus, they have been called a *RUNX1::RUNX1T1*-like subtype [52, 54]. *RUNX1::CBFA2T3* fusions in adults are primarily therapy related and are associated with a poor prognosis; whereas in pediatric patients this translocation tends to present in de novo AML and is associated with a favorable prognosis from limited studies [52, 55]. *RUNX1::CBFA2T3* pAML patients may benefit from a treatment protocol for standard risk AML without stem cell transplantation [54]. *RUNX1::CBFA2T2* has only been reported in a few cases with largely unknown clinicopathological features and genomic characterization [51].

Inv(16)(p13.1;q22) or t(16;16)(p13.1;q22)—*CBFB::MYH11* accounts for 7–9% of pAML [43, 44]. The morphologic characteristic of this AML is the presence of myelomonocytic blasts and atypical eosinophils. Patients with this fusion have a higher risk of central nervous system (CNS) involvement than patients with other types of AML [56]. FISH analysis of *CBFB::MYH11* is specifically helpful to aid in diagnosis since recognition of the chromosome abnormality can be challenging, especially when the chromosome morphology is not optimal. Additional abnormalities can be detected in about 30% of cases including +22 (13%), +8 (10%), del(7q) (12%), +21, focal deletion of *FOXP1* (5%), and focal gain confined to *CCDC26*. Additional abnormalities do not appear to affect the favorable prognosis associated with *CBFB::MYH11* fusion [48].

Although CBF AML has a high rate of complete remission after chemotherapy (85–98%) [44], 30–50% of patients relapse with a 5-year survival of 50% [57]. Recent studies have demonstrated that pediatric CBF AML is highly heterogeneous with a remarkably different spectrum of cooperating mutations in the tyrosine kinase pathway (including KIT, FLT3, and N/KRAS), epigenetic regulators, and cohesion [37, 58]. Among these, *KIT* mutations have gained special attention as a potential therapy target due to their association with unfavorable outcomes [58].

The *KIT* gene, located at 4q12, is a proto-oncogene comprised of 21 exons [59]. It encodes the KIT receptor tyrosine kinase (KIT RTK), which is a member of the type III RTK subfamily [60]. Approximately 20–45% of CBF AML patients have a *KIT* mutation [61] with higher detection rates in *RUNX1::RUNX1T1* fusion AML than in *CBFB::MYH11* fusion AML [61, 62]. Many types of *KIT* mutations have been identified, but three mutation hotspots in AML exist: exon 8, exon 10–11, and exon 17 [63, 64]. These mutations are more common in t(8;21) than in inv(16). Mutations in exon 17 of *KIT* are more common than mutations in exon 8, and are reported to be associated with inferior outcomes in pAML with *RUNX1::RUNX1T1* fusion. Patients with this mutation are responsive to the treatment of gemtuzumab ozogamicin (GO) and tyrosine kinase inhibitors (TKIs) [60, 65–67].

A new *CBFB*-involved abnormality, a nine base pair insertion in exon 3 of *CBFB* (NM_022845.3), was recently identified in approximately 0.4% of AML, and has an overlapping gene expression profile with *CBFB::MYH11* AML, despite its lack of a *CBFB::MYH11* fusion [52, 68]. At the protein level, all described insertions lead to replacement of four amino acids starting with aspartic acid at position 87 (D87) with either glycine, aspartic acid, serine, and tyrosine (GDSY), or glycine, aspartic acid, threonine, and tyrosine (GDTY). Thus, *CBFB*-GDXY has become the representative term for this type of AML. Compared to *CBFB::MYH11* AML, *CBFB*-GDXY AML frequently co-occurs with *FLT3* tyrosine kinase domain (TKD) mutations internal tandem duplications (ITDs) and mutations outside the TKD are also observed) and *BCORL1* mutations, and lacks *KIT* mutations. Recurrent chromosomal alterations in *CBFB*-GDXY AML include trisomy 6 and trisomy 22, whereas trisomy 8 is not observed. *CBFB*-GDXY AML also shows a stemness-related gene expression signature and appears to be enriched among adolescents and young adults with unclear outcomes, given the limited reports. One study suggested that these patients may not have the same favorable outcome as patients with *CBFB::MYH11* fusions [68], while another study observed a favorable outcome in the *CBFB*-GDXY group of patients [52].

NPM1 Variants

AML with mutated *NPM1* is one of the most common genetic subtypes of AML in adults, comprising approximately 30% of cases, and is often associated with a normal karyotype. In addition, there is a female predominance, and most cases are seen in patients approximately 40–50 years of age [69]. The frequency in the pediatric population, however, is much lower, comprising approximately 8% of pAML cases. There is also a female predominance, and a significant majority of the patients are greater than 3 years of age [70]. Morphologically, *NPM1*-mutated AML leukemic blasts may show a characteristic "cup-shaped" morphology. *NPM1* mutations are associated with a favorable prognosis [69].

NPM1 is a member of the Nucleophosmin/Nucleoplasmin family of proteins. This family of proteins is ubiquitous and can be further subclassified into four groups: NPM1, NPM2, NPM3, and NPM-like. The overall structure of NPM1 consists of a conserved N-terminal domain (a key feature of this protein family), a central unstructured domain, and a C-terminal domain. NPM1 predominantly resides in the nucleolus under normal circumstances, and has numerous functions that require shuttling between the nucleolus, the nucleus, and the cytoplasm. As such, it requires a nucleolar localization signal (NoLS) found in the C-terminal domain, a nuclear localization signal found in the central unstructured domain, and a nuclear export signal found in the N-terminal domain [69].

Permanent cytoplasmic localization of NPM1 is the key abnormality in *NPM1*-mutated AML. The *NPM1* gene is located on chromosome 5q35 and has 12 exons [1]. A frameshift mutation via a 4 bp insertion or duplication in exon 12 (C-terminal domain) leads to loss of either Tryptophan 288, Tryptophan 290, or both, thereby causing the NoLS to be lost and increasing the affinity for a nuclear export protein (Exportin1) [71]. Re-localization to the nucleus or degradation of the abnormal NPM1 protein has been shown to decrease HOX expression and promote differentiation of leukemic cells. The exact mechanism of upregulation, however, is still unclear [72].

There are many types of *NPM1* mutations described, with the most prevalent being mutations A, B, and D. Mutation A is caused by a TCTG insertion and is the most common in adults (approximately 70–80% of cases). Mutation B (approximately 10% of cases) and mutation D (approximately 5% of cases) have 4 bp insertions of CATG and CCTG, respectively [71]. Non-type A mutations are more common in children [73]. Notably, the mutated NPM1 protein can heterodimerize with the wild-type NPM1 protein also causing it to be abnormally localized in the cytoplasm. This leads to the invariable heterozygous state seen in this type of AML [69, 71].

Despite NPM1 having wide-reaching effects on the cell, an *NPM1* mutation alone is not sufficient to initiate leukemogenesis, rather it is considered a late event in disease progression, and other mutations are required first. The most common of these are mutations in *DNMT3A* and the *FLT3* internal tandem duplication (*FLT3*-ITD). These mutations not only aid in progression to overt leukemia but also have prognostic significance. *DNMT3A*, *IDH1/2*, and *TET2* are genes associated with epigenetic regulation. Of the three, *DNMT3A* mutations are the most common that co-occur in *NPM1*-mutated AML (60% of cases). *IDH1/2* and *TET2* mutations are seen in 25% and 20% of cases, respectively [74]. However, in patients older than 75 years of age, *TET2* and *SRSF2* mutations are more common [75]. Presence of a mutation in these epigenetic regulators are an unfavorable prognostic marker in patients with *NPM1*-mutated AML [74]. *FLT3*-ITD is also a common co-occurring mutation seen in *NPM1*-mutated AML. The combination of *DNMT3A*, *FLT3*-ITD, and *NPM1* mutations is the most frequent combination of mutations found in AML, conferring a poor prognosis [69]. *NRAS* mutations may also co-occur but are less common (approximately 20% of cases) and carry a favorable prognosis if co-occurring with a *DNMT3A* mutation [74].

Several modalities are available to detect *NPM1* mutations. PCR with fragment length analysis is the preferred method due to its ability to detect all insertion types. NGS can detect the insertion sequence as well as any co-occurring mutations, which may have prognostic significance. Immunohistochemistry directed against different *NPM1* domains (e.g., C-terminus, N-terminus) can be used to detect the presence of an abnormal protein based on the staining localization pattern and acts as a surrogate for detection of a *NPM1* mutation.

Overall, *NPM1*-mutated AML is a chemosensitive disease. Frontline chemotherapy induces remission in approximately 90% of cases. *NPM1*-mutated AML leukemic cells are known to have increased CD33 expression. Thus, an anti-CD33 immunotherapy agent (i.e., GO) can be added to frontline therapy. In addition, if a concurrent *FLT3* mutation is present, a *FLT3* inhibitor should also be added [76]. Despite having excellent remission rates, relapse rates are highly variable, with approximately 30–50% of patients relapsing after treatment [77]. Several other targeted treatment options are under investigation and include targeting the nuclear export of NPM1, HOX expression, the nucleolus, and the mutant NPM1 protein for immunotherapy [76].

CEBPA Variants

The *CEBPA* gene, located on chromosome 19q, encodes for a family of transcription factor CCAAT/enhancer-binding proteins (C/EBP) consisting of six members: C/EBPα, -β, -δ, -ε, -γ, and -ζ. All members have a conserved C-terminal basic-leucine zipper (bZIP) region and a N-terminal transactivation domain, which are more variable among family members. C/EBPα specifically is key in both activating myeloid hematopoietic stem cell differentiation by binding to the promoters or enhancers of myeloid-related genes (*CSF3R*, *IL-6R*, *CEBPE*, *GFI-1*, or *KLF5*) and suppressing non-myeloid-related genes [78].

AML with mutated *CEBPA* is an uncommon subtype of AML comprising approximately 10% of adult cases and 5% of pediatric cases [7]. There are three types of mutations: biallelic mutations (bi*CEBPA*), single mutation in the bZIP region (smbZIP-*CEBPA*), and single mutation in the N-terminal transactivation domain (TAD-*CEBPA*) [78]. bi*CEBPA* mutations usually consist of an out-of-frame mutation in the N-terminal region on one allele and an in-frame mutation in the C-terminal region containing the bZIP region on the other allele. Other combinations (i.e., both in the N-terminal or both in the C-terminal) are rare [78]. Approximately 80% of pediatric patients with *CEBPA* variants have bi*CEBPA* mutations, which are predictive of a favorable prognosis [79]. The single *CEBPA* variants in the bZIP C-terminal domain were recognized to have clinical characteristics and favorable outcomes similar to those of patients with double-variant *CEBPA* AML. They also have similar co-mutational profiles with *GATA2*, *WT1*, and *TET2* being reported as co-mutated genes [80]. In 5–10% of biCEBPA AML, germline CEBPA variants are detected. Therefore, germline testing should be considered in AML patients with biCEBPA [81].

TAD-*CEBPA* single mutations are extremely rare in pediatric patients but can be seen in older patients, with an average age of 60 years and a prognosis similar to that of AML with wildtype *CEBPA*. The most common co-occurring mutations are *NPM1* variants or mutations in epigenetic regulators (i.e., *DNMT3A*, *TET2*, *IDH1/2*) and RNA splicing genes (i.e., *SRSF2*, *SF3B1*) [80]. In pediatrics, there is also a high frequency of co-occurring *CSF3R* mutations, which is mutually exclusive with *GATA2* mutations. While relapse rates are increased with the presence of *CSF3R* mutations, overall survival is not affected due to the success of salvage therapy [81, 82].

AML with mutated *CEBPA* has an excellent response to standard chemotherapy treatment with remission rates post-induction greater than 90%. Relapse rates are still a problem, however, with most cases occurring within the first 2 years. Despite this, patients still do extremely well following a stem cell transplant or re-induction chemotherapy first, followed by stem cell transplant [83].

Genetic Biomarkers with Intermediate Prognosis

NPM1::MLF1 Fusion-t(3;5)(q25;q34)

AML with an *NPM1::MLF1* fusion [t(3;5)(q25;q34)] was first reported in 1996 [84]. Unlike AML with mutated *NPM1*, an *NPM1::MLF1* fusion is extremely rare and found in approximately 0.5% of cases, most of which occur in adolescents [85]. Cases with *NPM1::MLF1* fusion are associated with multilineage dysplasia, and blast morphology ranges from myelomonocytic to erythroleukemia with no characteristic immunophenotype [86]. This reciprocal translocation can be seen in both AML and myelodysplastic syndrome (MDS), and affects gene regulation via the enhanced recruitment of nucleosome remodeling and deacetylase (NuRD) to target genes, thereby promoting leukemogenesis. Interestingly, there is still cytoplasmic localization of NPM1, similar to AML with mutated *NPM1* [87].

NPM1::MLF1 fusion has been associated with an intermediate prognosis [88]. The prognosis depends on whether or not the *NPM1::MLF1* fusion is the sole chromosomal abnormality detected. In the young adult population this is usually the case, and the prognosis is more favorable with aggressive therapy to include stem cell transplant. In contrast, elderly patients may more frequently have concurrent trisomy 8, which is associated with a worse prognosis and aggressive clinical course. Although less common, a complex karyotype may also be seen in some cases, which carries a worse prognosis [86].

Genetic Biomarkers with Variable Prognosis

KMT2A Gene Rearrangement

AML with *KMT2A* rearrangement is seen in greater than 50% of infant cases (less than 1 year of age) and approximately 10% of adolescent cases. In adults, the frequency is much less at approximately 2–3% of cases. Clinical presentation at diagnosis is variable, although children more often than adults present with hyperleukocytosis [7]. Monocytic differentiation is commonly seen, but in children with *KMT2A::MLLT3* or *KMT2A::MLLT10* fusions, there is a preference for megakaryoblastic differentiation [89].

KMT2A is part of the lysine methyltransferase family 2 (KMT2), formerly known as mixed lineage leukemia (*MLL*). This family of genes is responsible for histone H3, lysine 4 (H3K4) methylation and is comprised of six members, *KMT2A* through *KMT2G,* with *KMT2A* having a significant impact on human disease. The KMT2A N-terminal region is responsible for chromatin interaction via a Menin-interaction domain, and the C-terminal is responsible for histone methylation of H3K4 via a SET domain. Menin, a scaffold protein encoded by the MEN1 gene, is an epigenetic cofactor in leukemogenesis. Regarding hematopoiesis, KMT2A regulates *HOX* genes, which control hematopoietic stem cell growth and differentiation. Thus, mutant KMT2A proteins cause an upregulation of *HOX* expression leading to leukemogenesis [7].

KMT2A rearrangements are a common abnormality identified, accounting for approximately 10% of hematologic malignancies. Rearrangements usually occur in the major breakpoint cluster region (BCR1) between exons 9 and 12, with fewer occurring in the minor breakpoint cluster region (BCR2) between exons 21 and 25 [90]. *KMT2A* is promiscuous, with over 100 identified gene fusion partners. The most common fusion is with *MLLT3* (*AF9*) on chromosome 9. Other common fusion partners include *AFF1* (*AF4/MLLT2*) on chromosome 4, *MLLT1* (*ENL*) and *ELL* on chromosome 19 (Fig. 15.2), *MLLT10* (*AF10*) on chromosome 10, and *AFDN* (*AF6/MLLT4*) on chromosome 6 [7]. The prognosis of *KMT2A* rearrangements varies with different partners but is commonly poor. In adult patients, a t(9;11) [*KMT2A::MLLT3*] fusion conveys an intermediate risk, whereas most other *KMT2A* rearrangements are associated with a poor prognosis [91]. In children, *KMT2A* fusion partners *ABI1, AFDN, AFF1, MLLT1,* and *MLLT10* have been associated with a high risk of relapse, while fusion partners *ELL, MLLT3, MLLT11,* and *SEPTIN6* are associated with a standard risk [92]. Breakpoint location has also been reported to affect prognosis. Breakpoints in intron 11 in the major region are associated with poor outcomes, and these are seen most often with *MLLT1* and *SEPTIN6* gene fusion partners [93].

Some co-mutations with prognostic impact have been identified in association with *KMT2A* rearranged AML in both adults and pediatrics. In adults, there are increased mutations in the RAS pathway (e.g., *KRAS, NRAS, PTPN11*) as well as *FLT3* mutations. *KRAS*, but not *NRAS* or *PTPN11,* mutations are associated with t(6;11) *KMT2A::AFDN,* and with worse overall outcomes. In pediatric AML, there

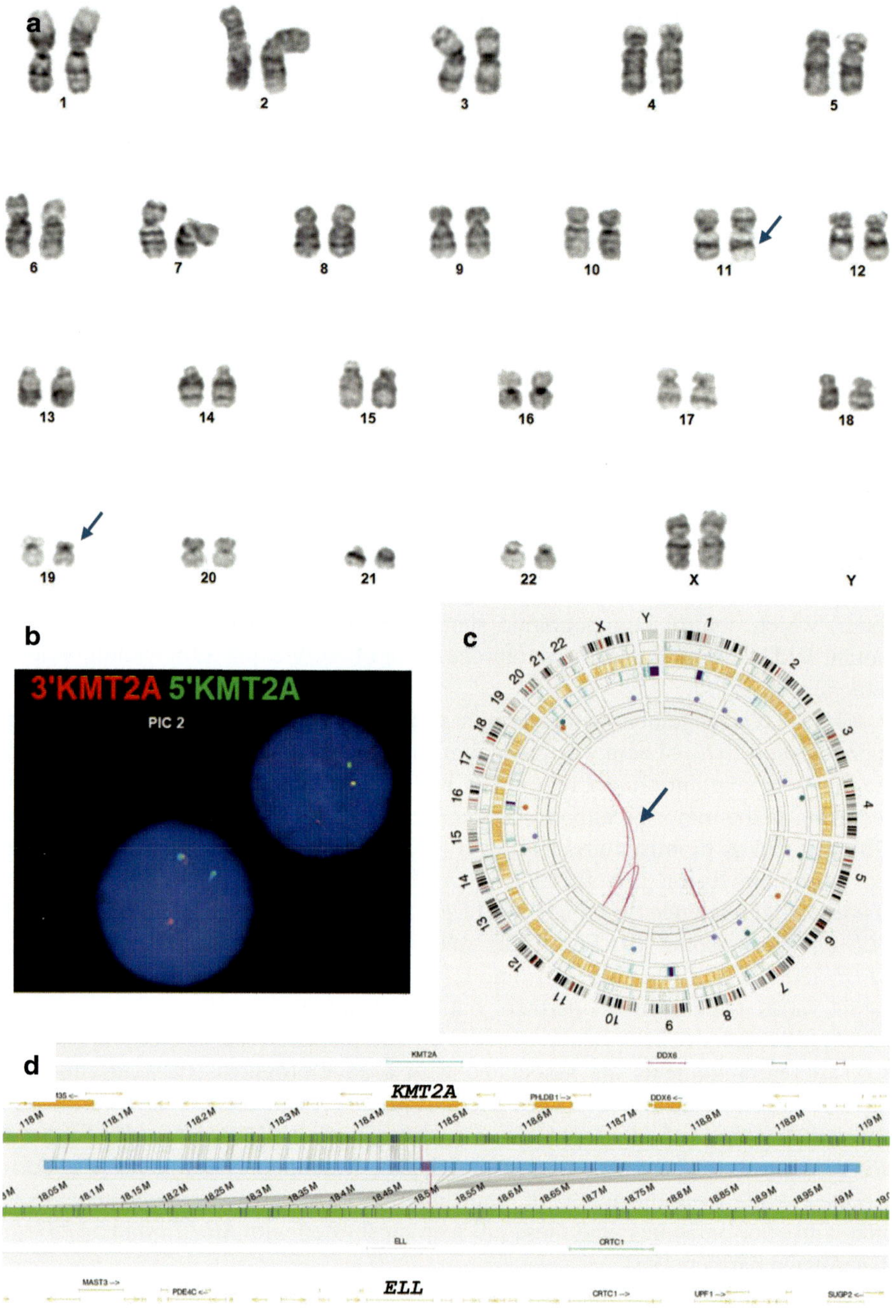

Fig. 15.2 A case with *KMT2A*::*ELL* fusion. (**a**) Chromosome analysis shows a complex rearrangement involving chromosomes 11 and 19. (**b**) FISH is positive for *KMT2A* rearrangement. Red: 3′*KMT2A* probe. Green: 5′*KMT2A* probe. (**c**) OGM Circos Plot View shows a complex rearrangement involving 11p, 11q, and 19p. (**d**) *KMT2A*::*ELL* fusion shown on genome browser analysis, resulting from the complex rearrangement

is an association with not only *RAS* pathway mutations but also *SETD2* mutations. In contrast to adults, *KRAS* mutations occur more commonly with a t(10;11) *KMT2A::MLLT10* fusion. *KRAS* mutations are a poor prognostic marker with decreased overall survival, and *SETD2* mutations are associated with increased relapse rates (approximately 80% in comparison to 40% in wild type *SETD2*) [94].

Currently, there is no targeted *KMT2A* rearrangement therapy. First-line treatment typically consists of chemotherapy, with remission rates varying from 40% to 80% depending on the specific gene fusion partner. In pediatric patients, treatment with conventional chemotherapy plus GO is associated with improved overall survival rates (60% vs. 50% without GO) and lower relapse rates (40% vs. 65% without GO) [95]. In relapse/refractory AML with *KMT2A* rearrangements, revumenib is an FDA-approved menin inhibitor with remission rates at approximately 30%. Further, hematopoietic stem cell transplant in this AML setting has had varying results [96].

KAT6A::CREBBP Fusion-t(8;16)(p11.2;p13.3)

AML with *KAT6A::CREBBP* fusion [t(8;16)(p11.2;p13.1)] is extremely rare and can be found in both adults and pediatrics. In the adult population, it is seen in less than 1% of cases and is more common in females with a median age of approximately 60 years. It can be seen in de novo AML or treatment-related AML, with the latter being more common [97]. In the pediatric population, the median age is approximately 1 year old with some congenital neonatal cases reported [98]. This AML entity is commonly associated with DIC and extramedullary disease, such as leukemia cutis and CNS involvement. Blasts have monocytic or monoblastic differentiation and frequently show erythrophagocytosis and cytoplasmic vacuoles [97, 99]. The exact leukemogenesis mechanism of the *KAT6A::CREBBP* fusion is unknown; however, it has been reported that the overexpression of *HOXA* genes is involved [98].

In patients with a *KAT6A::CREBBP* fusion, one study showed that the t(8;16) can been seen as the sole abnormality in approximately half of the cases, with the other half of cases having additional abnormalities or complex karyotypes [100]. Recurrent co-mutations have been reported in *ASXL1*, *FLT3*, *TP53*, *RUNX1*, and *TET2* [99]. Although the *KAT6A::CREBBP* fusion is associated with poor prognosis in adult patients, with a 5-year overall survival rate of 15–20% and a high relapse rate [99], the prognosis for the pediatric population is intermediate. Interestingly, there have been reports of neonatal congenital cases undergoing spontaneous and sustained remission; however, due to the high relapse rates, close follow-up is still recommended [98]. Intense induction therapy in combination with stem cell transplant has improved survival rates in de novo AML cases. Unfortunately, in patients with treatment-related AML, despite early stem cell transplant, prognosis continues to be poor due to the high relapse rates [99].

Genetic Biomarkers with Unfavorable Prognosis

BCR::ABL1 Fusion-t(9;22)(q34;q11.2)

The *BCR::ABL1* fusion, resulting from t(9;22)(q34;q11.2), defines a specific subtype for de novo AML in which the fusion is detected at diagnosis and no evidence of chronic myeloid leukemia (CML) can be established. AML with *BCR::ABL1* fusion is rare, accounting for <0.5% of all AML cases. It occurs mainly in adults with a male predominance [101], although it has been reported in pediatric patients [102, 103]. The t(9;22) may be the sole finding or occur with additional chromosomal abnormalities. Deletion of *IKZF1* and/or *CDKN2A/B* and mutations in *RUNX1* are common additional findings in AML with *BCR::ABL1*. The prognosis is poor with standard AML induction chemotherapy; however, survival after allogeneic transplantation appears similar to that for intermediate-risk AML [101]. The t(9;22) translocation results in a Philadelphia chromosome (Ph) and creates a fusion transcript involving the *ABL1* locus on chromosome 9 and the *BCR* locus on chromosome 22. This fusion can result in three different chimeric proteins: p190 (minor breakpoint), p210 (major breakpoint), or p230. The p210 *BCR::ABL1* fusion product, named after its approximate size (210 kD), is the cytogenetic hallmark of CML and the p190 fusion product can be observed in up to 5% of pediatric ALL [104]. In a multi-institutional study of adults with AML harboring a t(9;22) translocation, the vast majority of transcripts correlated with a p210 fusion transcript (10/12) [104]. In literature reviews spanning many reports, however, the *BCR::ABL1*-positive AML entity shows a more equal distribution between the p190 and p210 transcripts [105]. As the treatments differ vastly between t(9;22)-positive AML and CML in myeloid blast crisis (CML-MBC), it is extremely important to identify whether the leukemia bearing a t(9;22) is truely AML or CML-MBC. However, differentiating between the two entities can be very challenging in some cases.

Neither chromosome analysis studies nor molecular studies alone can determine whether the leukemia bearing a t(9;22) is AML or CML-MBC. While the p210 transcript is more commonly associated with CML, the p190 transcript as well as numerous rare transcripts can be found in CML [106, 107].

Since genetic findings can only make suggestions for classification, non-genetic findings can contribute a great deal. Splenomegaly, peripheral blood basophilia, and bone marrow basophilia are more prevalent in CML-MBC [104, 105], whereas bone marrow cellularity and myeloid to erythroid ratios are lower in AML. Aberrant co-expression of lymphoid markers has also been reported as a feature of t(9;22)-positive AML [105]. Despite these generalities, considerable overlap predominates between the two entities [104]. Following a thorough review of the literature over a period of approximately 40 years, Neuendorff et al proposed a clinical path to differentiate t(9;22)-positive AML from CML-MBC. The algorithm starts from blast count and detection of *BCR::ABL1* fusion and progresses to the consideration of *BCR::ABL1*-positive AML if there is a p190 transcript, fewer than 100% of metaphases bearing the t(9;22) fusion, and low level basophilia [105].

MLLT10 Gene Rearrangement-Non-*KMT2A::MLLT10* Fusions

MLLT10 (*AF10*) rearrangements account for approximately 6% of pAML and 1% of aAML cases [108, 109]. While *KMT2A* is the primary fusion partner found in approximately 80% of these cases, the remaining are equally distributed between *PICALM* (approximately 10%) and at least eight other fusion partners [108]. MLLT10 interacts with DOT1L, a histone methyltransferase transferase, and plays a crucial role in chromatin state control and the DNA damage response [110, 111]. The typical fusion combines the 3′ region of *MLLT10*, which contains the leucine zipper domain, with the 5′ region of the partner gene [111, 112]. The fusion protein blocks the differentiation and expansion of hematopoietic stem cells by upregulating *HOXA* cluster genes and other transcription factors [111, 113, 114].

In the pediatric population, the *PICALM::MLLT10* fusion is typically observed in older adolescents with a median age of 14 years [108, 115, 116]. *Non-KMT2A::MLLT10* rearrangements are also found in T-cell acute lymphoblastic leukemia/lymphoma (T-ALL) and mixed-phenotype acute leukemia (MPAL) cases [117–119]. The t(10;11)(p12.3;q14.2) translocation, leading to the *PICALM*::*MLLT10* fusion, can be identified with chromosome analysis but cryptic rearrangements have also been reported [108]. It can also be mistakenly reported as a t(10;11)(p12;q23) *KMT2A::MLLT10* fusion. Hence, FISH analysis using *MLLT10* break apart probes or other molecular techniques is recommended.

A Children's Oncology Group (COG) study found that non-*KMT2A*::*MLLT10* fusions had dismal outcomes, with 5-year event-free survival (EFS) and overall survival (OS) of 12.7% and 27.6%, respectively. These rates are even lower than outcomes for patients with the *KMT2A*::*MLLT10* fusion [108]. Another cohort specifically evaluating outcomes of *PICALM::MLLT10* fusion cases also found poor outcomes with a 5-year EFS of 22% and 5-year OS of 26% [115]. Hematopoietic stem cell transplantation (HSCT) was found to significantly improve outcomes for pediatric patients in both studies [108, 115]. Currently, there are no targeted therapies available and pAML cases involving *MLLT10* fusions are considered high risk associated with adverse outcomes [108].

MECOM Rearrangement–inv(3)(q21.3;q26.2)/t(3;3)(q21.3;q26.2) or t(3;21)(26.2;q22)

MECOM (MDS1 and EVI1 complex), located at 3q26.2, encodes for two transcription factors: EVI1 and MDS1-EVI1 [120]. EVI1 is a tightly regulated protein involved in hematopoietic stem/progenitor cell self-renewal, lineage differentiation, and proliferation [121, 122]. *GATA2* at 3q21.3 is a zinc-finger transcription factor essential for hematopoietic stem cell maintenance, endothelial development, and myelopoiesis [123, 124]. The recurrent inv(3)(q21.3;q26.2) inversion and t(3;3)(q21.3;q26.2) translocation had been originally considered to result in a *RPN1::EVI1* fusion, but later, it was clarified that these rearrangements result in hijacking of the *GATA2* enhancer by *MECOM* (without formation of a new oncogenic fusion transcript), leading to EVI1 overexpression and functional GATA2 haploinsufficiency [125, 126]. Increased EVI1 expression and GATA2 haploinsufficiency lead to progenitor self-renewal and survival [127, 128]. EVI1 overexpression, caused by fusion transcripts and other enhancer element collocation through fusion with *RUNX1* [(t(3;21)(q26.2;q22)], *ETV6* [t(3;12)(q26.2;p13)], and *MYC* [t(3;8)(q26.2;q24.2)], has also been reported [129–132].

MECOM rearrangements account for less than 1% of pAML and approximately 1% of de novo aAML cases [27, 43, 52, 133]. While the typical fusion caused by inv(3)/t(3;3) can be identified by chromosome analysis, other *MECOM* rearrangements can be cryptic. Hence, the use of MECOM break-apart FISH probes or other molecular techniques is recommended [132, 134–136]. In pediatric patients, common co-occurring genomic events in *MECOM*-rearranged AML include monosomy 7, 5q deletion, 11q abnormalities, karyotype complexity, and mutations in *SF3B1* and RAS-pathway genes [52, 137]. One study has shown that 61.8% of the patients with inv(3)/t(3;3) had the following molecular abnormalities, in descending frequency: *RAS* mutations, *RUNX1* mutations, *NF1* deletions, and *CBL* mutations [126].

While aAML patients with *MECOM* rearrangements have adverse prognostic outcomes [138–140], the prognostic significance in pediatric patients has yet to be established due to the low incidence rate [43, 141]. However, MECOM overexpression (as measured by transcript abundance across subtypes of AML) has been shown to have worse prognosis with increased relapse rates and poor event free and overall survival in pediatric patients [141, 142]. Hence, *MECOM* rearrangement in pAML is considered high risk and intensive chemotherapy followed by HSCT in the first complete remission is typically recommended [143, 144].

NUP98 **Gene Rearrangement**

NUP98 gene rearrangement is considered a specific genetic entity and accounts for approximately 3–10% of pediatric and 2–5% of adult AML cases [7, 52, 145–147]. *NUP98* encodes Nucleoporin 98, a core component of the nuclear pore complex which regulates the bidirectional transport of macromolecules between the nucleus and cytoplasm. Beyond its role in transportation, *NUP98* also contributes to transcriptional regulation and mitotic progression [148–150]. Structurally, the N-terminal portion of NUP98 consists of a series of intrinsically disordered phenylalanine-glycine (FG)/glycine-leucine-phenylalanine-glycine (GLFG) repeats and Gle2-binding-sequence (GLEBS) domain. In the majority of reported fusions, this N-terminal region of NUP98 (including FG/GLFG and GLEBS domains) fuses with the C-terminal portion of the fusion partner [149]. NUP98 fusion proteins act as an aberrant transcription factor and impair the normal development of progenitor cells [150]. Rearrangements are often karyotypically cryptic but can be detected by FISH or molecular techniques. Besides AML, *NUP98* rearrangements are also reported in CML in blast crisis phase, chronic myelomonocytic leukemia, MDS, ALL, and MPAL [150, 151].

The *NUP98::NSD1* [t(5;11)(q35;p15)] (Fig. 15.3) and *NUP98::KDM5A* [t(11;12)(p15;p13)] are the two most common fusions within this subtype, accounting for approximately 5% and 2% of pAML cases, respectively [7, 52, 145, 152]. At least 30 other *NUP98* fusion partners have been reported and account for about 1% of pAML cases [9, 52, 145, 153]. The *NUP98::KDM5A* fusion represents one of the most common recurrent cytogenetic aberrations in pediatric non-Down syndrome acute megakaryoblastic leukemia (AMKL), although it has also been identified across other FAB classification subtypes. The *NUP98::NSD1* fusion is predominantly linked to acute monocytic leukemia [7, 153] and is most prevalent in older children (median age of ~10 years), whereas *NUP98::KDM5A* fusions typically occur at a younger age (median age of ~3 years) [9, 147, 154, 155]. *FLT3-ITD, WT1* mutations, and trisomy 8 are common co-occurring genetic findings in *NUP98::NSD1* fusions. Loss of *RB1*, other chromosome 13 abnormalities, and trisomy 21 are the most common co-occurring findings in *NUP98::KDM5A* fusions [145, 149]. Other recurrent molecular alterations concurrent with *NUP98* rearrangement include mutations in *NBPF14, BCR, ODF1, NRAS, KRAS, MYC, KIT, ASXL1*, and *CEBPA* [149, 155].

Irrespective of the fusion partner, *NUP98* fusions are typically associated with poor outcomes [145, 149, 156] with the presence of *FLT3-ITD* further worsening the prognosis [149]. Patients with *NUP98::NSD1* and *NUP98::KDM5A* have inferior overall survival and event-free survival compared to those without a *NUP98* fusion, as well as a higher 5-year relapse risk [145, 156]. Currently, *NUP98* fusions are recognized as a high-risk subtype of leukemia and often require HSCT during the first complete molecular remission as no targeted therapy is available [149].

DEK::NUP214-t(6;9)(p23;q34.1)

AML with *DEK::NUP214* fusion is a rare subtype that is present in approximately 1–2% of AML patients and is associated with poor prognosis [7]. *DEK* encodes a DNA binding and chromatin remodeling protein involved with posttranslational histone modification, while NUP214 is part of the nuclear pore complex which helps to regulate molecular transport [157, 158]. The fusion creates a chimeric protein containing the 5′ end of *DEK* and the 3′ portion of *NUP214*. Studies support that the chimeric protein results in an increased sensitivity to cytokines which regulate proliferation and differentiation [159]. The fusion protein is thought to function in part by interfering with normal DEK and NUP214 protein activity [160].

This fusion is most often seen in de novo AML, but has been associated with relapsed, secondary AML, and MDS [161, 162]. The pathology findings observed in these patients include bilinear dysplasia, basophilia, and the presence of Auer rods. This rearrangement is more common in younger patients, with a median age of 23 years; however, in the pediatric population it is typically observed in adolescence. Individuals with this rearrangement typically do not have complex karyotypes, with the fusion being reported as the sole cytogenetic finding in over 70% of patients [161, 162]. Approximately 40% of patients with this fusion are also positive

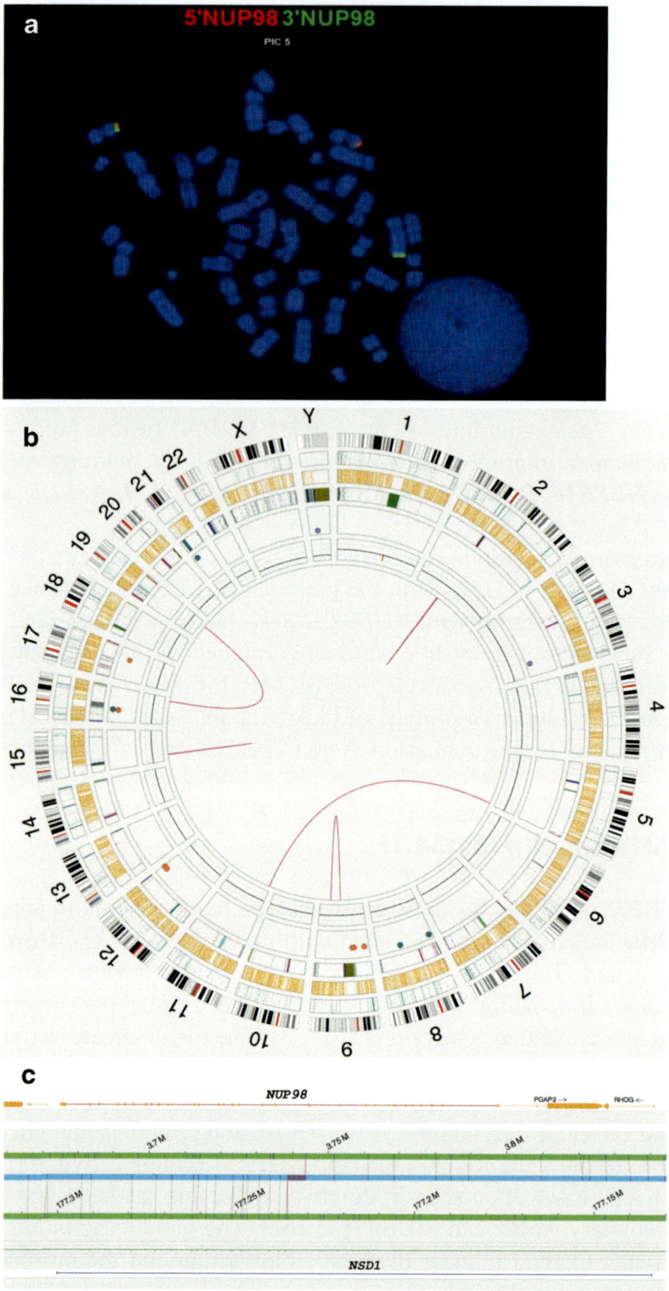

Fig. 15.3 A case with *NUP98::NSD1* fusion. (**a**) Metaphase FISH using a *NUP98* break apart probe shows rearrangement of the NUP98 locus at 11p15.4. Red: 5′*NUP98* probe. Green: 3′*NUP98* prob. (**b**) OGM Circos Plot View confirms the rearrangement between chromosomes 11 and 19. (**c**) OGM identified a fusion between *NUP98* and *NSD1* that was the result of a cytogenetically cryptic translocation

for *FLT3*-ITD, though this has not been shown to impact outcome [163]. Studies have suggested that treatment with HSCT results in a more favorable prognosis [162, 164].

FUS::ERG Fusion-t(16;21)(p11;q22)

The *FUS::ERG* fusion [t(16;21)(p11;q22)] (Fig. 15.4) is a rare but recurrent rearrangement in AML, which has been observed in all age groups with a predominance in young adults. It constitutes approximately 0.5% of pAML and has only been reported in patients aged more than 2 years [54, 165]. Data from limited studies showed that a *FUS::ERG* fusion is a poor prognostic factor associated with high risk disease [54, 166]. The *FUS* gene, located on 16p11, encodes an RNA-binding protein. The *ERG* gene, located at 21q22, belongs to the ETS oncogene family and functions as a transcription activator [165]. The *FUS::ERG* fusion product affects both gene transcription and RNA splicing, interfering with hematopoietic differentiation [167]. AMLs with *FUS::ERG* fusion produce a gene expression profile that clusters separately from other cytogenetic subgroups [54].

The *FUS::ERG* fusion is not associated with a particular FAB class or immunophenotype. In about one third of cases, this translocation is part of a complex karyotype, and it can be overlooked with conventional cytogenetics [54, 168]. Co-mutations have been reported in *RUNX1*, *DNMT3A*, *ASXL1*, and *BCOR* genes [169, 170].

inv(16)(p13.3;q24.3)-*CBFA2T3::GLIS2*

Acute megakaryoblastic leukemia (AMKL) is a subtype of AML that is characterized by the uncontrolled growth of immature megakaryocytes, and accounts for approximately 10% of childhood AML. Typically, AMKL is classified into three subgroups: AMKL arising in children with Down syndrome (DS), AMKL arising in children without DS (non-DS-AMKL), and AMKL arising in adults (typically without DS) [171]. A recurrent cryptic inversion on chromosome 16, inv(16)(p13.3q24.3), which results in the joining of the genes *CBFA2T3* (CBFA2/RUNX1 partner transcriptional co-repressor 3) and *GLIS2* (GLIS family zinc finger 2), is the most prevalent chromosomal aberration in non-DS-AMKL pediatric patients, accounting for approximately 20% of non-DS-AMKL patients and approximately 3% of pAML patients [172]. This fusion is not typically seen in adult populations. *CBFA2T3* (gene located at 16q24.3) is a hematopoietic corepressor that plays roles in both normal and malignant hematopoiesis, including inhibiting terminal erythromegakaryocytic differentiation, maintaining stemness of long-term hematopoietic stem cells, and promoting the expansion of leukemia stem cells, leading to AML relapse [173]. *GLIS2* (located at 16p13.3) encodes a nuclear transcription factor which is thought to support the pluripotent stem cell state, since its contribution to normal hematopoietic stem cell biology is mostly unknown [174]. *CBFA2T3::GLIS2* results from the inversion of the telomeric region of chromosome 16, fusing the 5′ portion

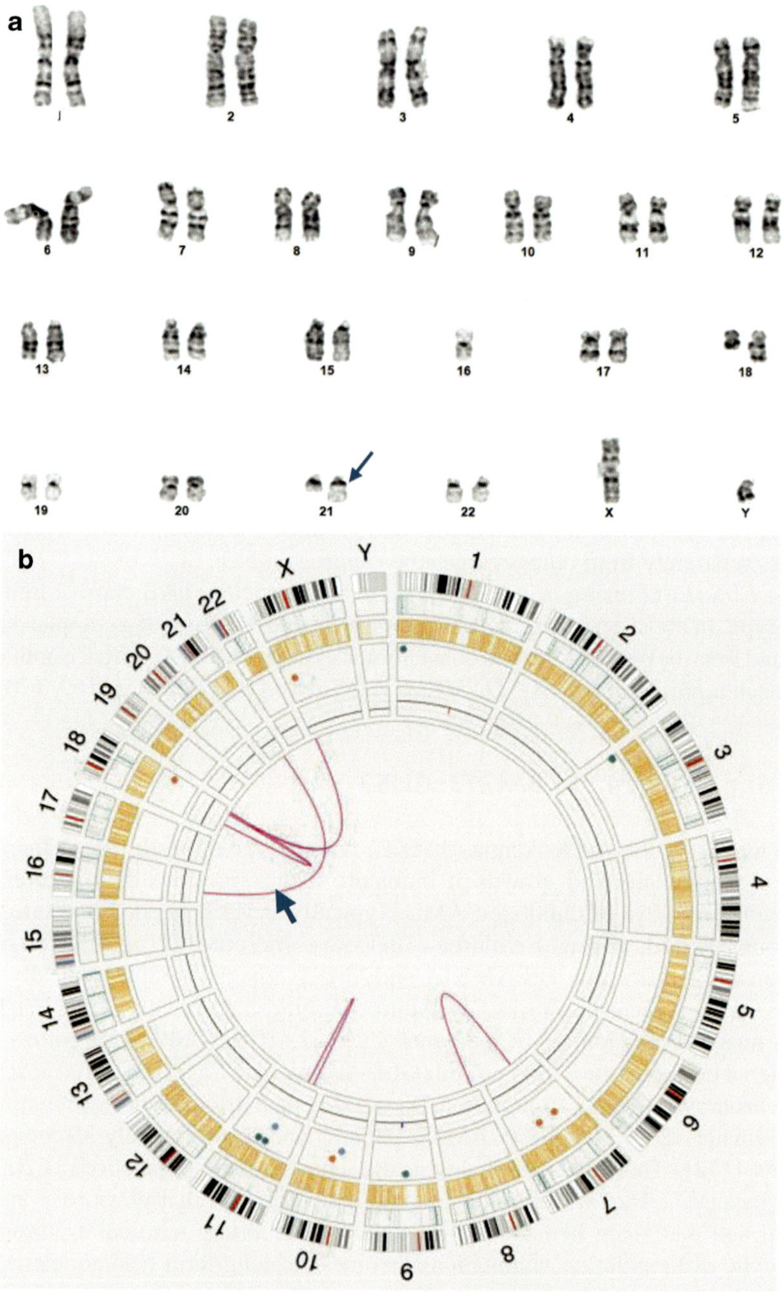

Fig. 15.4 A case with *FUS::ERG* fusion. (**a**) Chromosome analysis identified a complex karyotype with an unbalanced translocation between chromosomes 16 and 21, der(21)t(16;21) (arrow). (**b**) OGM Circos Plot View confirms the rearrangement between chromosomes 16 and 21. (**c**) OGM identified that the unbalanced translocation between chromosomes 16 and 21 results in a *FUS::ERG* fusion

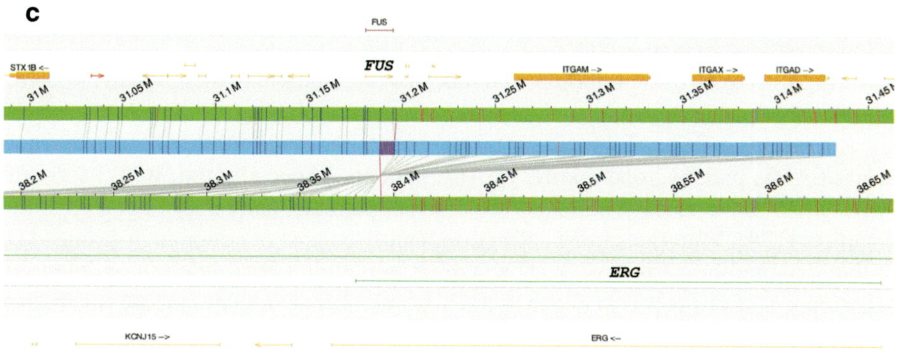

Fig. 15.4 (continued)

of *CBFA2T3* in frame with the 3′ region of *GLIS2*. The most common chimeric *CBFA2T3::GLIS2* transcript lies between exon 11 of *CBFA2T3* and exon 3 of *GLIS2* [175]. This fusion can be detected by FISH analysis utilizing *CBFA2T3::GLIS2* dual fusion probe [172]. Accompanying cytogenetic abnormalities are relatively rare, with the total burden of somatic mutations associated with *CBFA2T3::GLIS2* fusions significantly lower than that found in other subgroups of AMKL. Cooperating mutations that are seen in *CBFA2T3::GLIS2* positive AML include *FLT3* (17%), *JAK/STAT* (13–23%), *RAS* (6%), *GATA1* (17%), and *KIT* (8%) [176].

CBFA2T3::GLIS2 AML is highly enriched in younger AML populations (under 3 years of age), with nearly 12% of 1-year old infants with AML harboring this fusion [177]. Leukemia cells with *CBFA2T3::GLIS2* fusion have a distinct immunophenotype referred to as the RAM phenotype, consisting of high CD56, dim or negative expression of CD45 and CD38, and lack of HLA-DR expression [178]. *CBFA2T3::GLIS2* is considered the most aggressive of the fusions frequently found in non-DS AMKL, giving patients a poor prognosis and low response to conventional chemotherapy. Overall survival rates range between 15% and 30% [175]. In a large cohort study, approximately 94% of patients with *CBFA2T3::GLIS2* AML had detectable residual disease after induction 1 of chemotherapy and had an event-free survival at 5 years from study entry (event being death, relapse, or induction failure) of approximately 19% [177]. Allogenic HSCT (allo-HSCT) in first complete remission is generally considered, despite a lack of evidence that allo-HSCT improves outcomes. Preclinical studies targeting FOLR1 (folate receptor alpha), which is specifically expressed on the cell surface of leukemia cells with *CBFA2T3::GLIS2* fusion, using drug-conjugated antibodies or chimeric antigen receptor (CAR) T cells showed promising results. Additionally, drugs targeting the BCL families (i.e., navitoclax or DT2216) are also thought to be effective for this subtype [13].

FLT3 Mutations

FLT3 (FMS-like tyrosine kinase 3) is a receptor tyrosine kinase that, when mutated, causes constitutive activation of several pathways including RAS/MAPK, PI3K/AKT, and JAK/STAT. *FLT3* mutations have been observed in approximately one-third of AML patients, one-quarter of APL patients (especially the BCR-3 form of *PML::RARA*), 5% of ALL patients, 1% of MDS patients, and rarely in eosinophilic disorders [179]. Mutations in *FLT3* predominantly consist of either an in-frame ITD of the juxtamembrane region or a TKD point mutation. Other deletion or deletion/insertion mutations can also occur in the juxtamembrane domain but are much less common [180]. *FLT3*-ITD mutations are the most common *FLT3* mutation, accounting for approximately 25–30% of AML cases. Point mutations in the TKD of *FLT3* are less common, occurring in about 5–10% of AML cases [181]. The frequency of *FLT3*-ITD mutations in pAML is lower than that observed in adults, especially for children younger than 10 years, and ranges from 5% to 10% (compared with approximately 30% in adults) [182].

Although *FLT3* mutations are a known poor prognostic factor in both the adult and pediatric populations [181], there are other variables, such as of the presence of co-occurring mutations and cytogenetic abnormalities, the type of mutation, the allelic ratio (AR), variant allele fraction (VAF), and length of internal tandem duplication which can modify overall patient outcomes and impact prognosis [183]. The length of the duplication can range from 3 to >1000 nucleotides and are always in-frame. AR is measured using PCR and can be divided into low (*FLT3*-ITD^{Low}) and high (*FLT3*-ITD^{High}), which has historically been defined as an AR of ≥0.5. VAF is another way to quantitate *FLT3*-ITD mutations and is reported in NGS studies [184]. A larger length duplication, a high AR, and a VAF > 30% are associated with higher WBC counts and higher blast counts at presentation, and in turn, shorter overall survival [185].

While a normal karyotype is associated with 30–40% of *FLT3* mutated AML cases, there are also associated cytogenetic abnormalities including t(15;17)—*PML::RARA* fusion, the CBF AMLs with t(8;21)-*RUNX1::RUNX1T1* fusion and inv(16)–*MYH11::CBFB* fusion, and t(6;9)—*DEK::NUP214* fusion [186]. Mutated genes frequently cooccurring with *FLT3*-ITD include *NPM1, CEPBP*, and *WT1* [183]. Studies have shown evidence that these cooccurring genetic lesions can further influence the prognostic impact from *FLT3*-ITD [183, 187]. *NPM1* mutations with *FLT3*-ITD negative/*FLT3*-ITD^{Low} have a favorable prognosis, while *NPM1* wild type with *FLT3*-ITD^{High} has a poor prognosis. *NPM1* wild type with *FLT3*-ITD negative/*FLT3*-ITD^{Low} has an intermediate prognosis. In the pediatric/young adult population specifically, a favorable prognosis is seen not only with *NPM1* mutations, t(8;21), and inv(16), but also with *CEBPA* mutations. Conversely, a poor prognosis is seen with co-occurring *WT1* mutation, *UBTF* mutation, and *NUP98::NSD1* fusion. The latter is especially important because even with therapy intensification, patients with *NUP98::NSD1* fusion have poor outcomes [183].

Treatment options include the standard chemotherapy regimen in combination with FLT3 inhibitors. FLT3 inhibitors can be categorized as first and second generation and as Type 1 and Type 2. Type 1 inhibitors (e.g., midostaurin, gilteritinib, lestaurtinib, crenolanib) bind and inhibit FLT3 when in the active conformation, while Type 2 (e.g., quizartinib, sorafenib) inhibits FLT3 when in the inactive conformation. Unfortunately, like all treatments, resistance can develop due to various mechanisms including secondary *FLT3* mutations, mutations in parallel/downstream pathways, altered medication metabolism, or changes in the bone marrow microenvironment [184].

Determining *FLT3* mutation status can be done using PCR or NGS. While PCR has faster turnaround times, it has lower sensitivity compared to NGS. NGS can sometimes miss longer length ITDs, but that limitation is being addressed with new bioinformatic approaches. NGS is also the preferred method for monitoring *FLT3* minimal residual disease (MRD) status [184].

ETV6 Fusion

The *ETV6* gene (ETS variant transcription factor 6), formerly *TEL* (translocation, ETS, leukemia), is a sequence-specific DNA binding transcription factor which binds to a core recognition sequence of GGAA/T and plays a specific role in hematopoiesis within the bone marrow. The structure of ETV6 resembles that of many other ETS factors, with a DNA binding ETS domain located in the C-terminal half of the protein, while additional domains associated with protein–protein interactions are found in the N-terminal portion [188, 189]. *ETV6* fusions with a number of tyrosine kinase (TK) genes have been reported in AML, including *ABL1, ABL2, JAK2, FGFR3, SYK, FRK, LYN, NTRK3, PDGFRA, PDGFRB,* and *FLT3*, with many of the fusions showing distinct clinical features such as eosinophilia and a high risk of relapse. Tyrosine kinase inhibitors are potential treatments for these kind of fusions [190–192].

Several *ETV6* rearrangements in pAML may have additional mechanisms beyond TK activation in the development of AML. The recurrent rearrangements between *ETV6* and *MNX1* (motor neuron and pancreas homeobox 1; previously *HLXB9*), resulting from t(7;12)(q36;p13) translocations, occur in approximately 1% of pAML cases, and are virtually exclusively seen in children younger than 2 years, with a median age of diagnosis of 6 months [193]. It is associated with a dismal prognosis with extremely poor survival rates and ineffective treatment by HSCT [194]. The t(7;12) rearrangements are structurally diverse with the breakpoint on chromosome 7 exhibiting considerable heterogeneity, in which some translocations result in *MNX1::ETV6* fusion product, while others relocate the entire *MNX1* gene within the *ETV6* locus [195, 196]. A common feature in all such rearrangements appears to be MNX1 overexpression, which may become a therapy target [194]. The mechanisms of t(7;12) leukemogenesis remain poorly understood, but are likely attributed to the activity of *ETV6* locus regulatory elements and/or the topological repositioning of the *MNX1* gene to euchromatic nuclear compartments [192]. Of note, a significant portion of t(7;12) cases are reported in conjunction with specific aneusomies. The presence of one or more extra copies of chromosomes 8,

19, or 22 has been consistently observed, with trisomy 19 being particularly prevalent in over 70% of cases [194, 196].

Like *MNX1::ETV6* rearrangements, AMLs with rearrangement between *ETV6* and *MN1* (Meningioma-1) also have a mix of gene fusion and non-fusion products leading to universal MN1 overexpression [197]. In addition, enhancer hijacking has been recognized as the mechanism of partner gene overexpression when rearranged with an *ETV6* locus, for example, *GSX2 (GSH2), IL3,* and *CSF2* [198].

Abnormalities of Chromosome 5, 7, and Others

Chromosome 5 and 7 abnormalities are present in approximately 2% and 4% of pAML cases, respectively [199, 200], and up to 15% of de novo aAML cases [201]. The abnormalities include monosomy, deletion, or unbalanced rearrangements resulting in loss of material from either chromosome. Despite an intensive effort, no somatic mutations of single candidate tumor suppressor genes have been identified [202]. The genes on 5q exhibiting haploinsufficiency in AML have been involved in signal transduction, DNA repair, and cell cycle control [203]; while the genes on 7q in myeloid malignancies were reported to be critical for the DNA damage response, DNA replication, and chromatin regulation [204]. Chromosome 5 and 7 abnormalities are associated with a poor prognosis in children [43, 201], but appear to lack prognostic significance in AML patients with Down syndrome who are aged 4 years and younger [205].

Chromosome 7 deletions are commonly implicated in bone marrow failure syndromes, such as Fanconi anemia, severe congenital neutropenia, Shwachman–Diamond syndrome, and aplastic anemia [206, 207]. Germline *SAMD9, SAMD9L,* and *GATA2* mutations have been reported in pediatric MDS with monosomy 7 [208]. Cases associated with an underlying *RUNX1*-altered familial platelet disorder, telomere biology disorder, and germline *ERCC6L2* pathogenic variants have also been reported to have monosomy 7 [209]. Germline testing should be considered when monosomy 7 disease is identified.

The 5q- and 7q- or monosomy 7, in association with a complex karyotype, is the most common recurrent finding in AML-myelodysplasia related (AML-MR), as defined by the 5th edition of the WHO [210, 211]. AML-MR is a myeloid neoplasm harboring specific cytogenetic and/or molecular abnormalities associated with myelodysplastic neoplasia, arising de novo or after a known diagnosis of MDS or myelodysplastic/myeloproliferative neoplasm (MDS/MPN) [211]. Although monosomy 5 can be found, bona fide loss of chromosome 5 is uncommon, as remnant 5p material is often detected on ring or marker chromosomes. Other recurrent chromosome abnormalities in AML-MR include deletion of 11q, 12p, 17p, isochromosome 17q, monosomy 13 or 13q-, and isochromosome X [idic(X)(q13)] [211].

UBTF Tandem Duplication

UBTF is located at 17q21 and encodes a ubiquitously expressed nucleolar protein that interacts with ribosomal DNA to mediate RNA polymerase 1 ribosomal RNA transcription. Heterozygous somatic variants resulting in in-frame tandem duplications (TD) in exon 13 of *UBTF* are a major subtype-defining genomic alteration in pAML, accounting for 4% of newly diagnosed cases and 9% of relapse cases [12, 13]. These recurrent *UBTF*-TDs have recently been studied in adults and account for ~3% of aAML patients aged 18–60 years old [212, 213]. The mechanism in which *UBTF*-TDs promote leukemogenesis remains poorly understood. In pAML, *UBTF*-TDs frequently co-occur with *FLT3*-ITDs (two-thirds of cases with *UBTF*-TDs), *WT1* mutations (40% of cases with *UBTF*-TDs), normal karyotype or isolated trisomy 8, and activation of the *HOXA/HOXB* cluster genes [213]. *UBTF*-TDs are associated with high-risk pAML, with patients typically having poor outcome and MRD positivity after induction chemotherapy. In the AAML1031 clinical trial which included 1035 pAML patients, EFS and OS rates for patients with *UBTF*-TD were 30% and 44%, respectively, which were similar to that for patients with *KMT2A* rearrangements. Additionally, co-occurrence of *UBTF*-TD with either *FLT3*-ITD or *WT1* variants was associated with an inferior prognosis, compared with patients with *UBTF*-TD alone [12, 214]. Emerging data has found that *UBTF*-TD AMLs may benefit from the use of menin inhibitors [212].

Genetic Biomarkers with Potential Prognostic Impact

t(1;22)(p13;q13)-*RBM15::MRTFA*

RBM15::MRTFA fusions are typically restricted to AMKL patients (10–20% of pAMKL patients in comparison to 0.8% of pAML patients). This fusion is rarely seen in aAML patients, with only a few cases reported to date [215, 216]. *MRTFA* (previously known as *MKL1*, gene located at cytogenetic band 22q13.1q13.2) encodes a transcription factor that activates serum response factor, which is critical for megakaryocyte maturation [217]. *RBM15* (gene located at 1p13.3) plays a critical role in hematopoiesis, regulating hematopoietic cell differentiation, maintaining the quiescent state of HSCs, and influencing cell fate decisions. In most cases, *RBM15* functions as an oncogene [218]. For *RBM15::MKL1* fusions, the breakpoint on chromosome 1 is located within a 4-kb intron of *RBM15* downstream of the exon encoding the C-terminal SPOC domain, and generates an in-frame fusion with *MRTFA* that contains nearly the full-length coding regions of both *RBM15* and *MRTFA* [219]. This fusion protein disrupts RNA processing and the HOX and RAS/MAPK signaling pathways, leading to alterations in megakaryocyte proliferation and differentiation, which, in turn, promotes leukemia development [218]. This translocation can be detected by karyotyping, FISH (using *RBM15::MRTFA* dual fusion probes), and RT-PCR. Most cases have this fusion as the sole karyotype abnormality at diagnosis. Less frequently, and typically in older infants (aged

>6 months), a hyperdiploid karyotype with t(1;22) and +der(1)t(1;22) can be observed [220].

RBM15::MRTFA patients are amongst the youngest with AMKL, with an average age of 0.91 years. Cases with detectable *RBM15::MKL1* fusion transcripts in the absence of t(1;22) have also been reported because these young patients usually have hypoplastic bone marrow [221]. The prognostic significance of *RBM15::MRTFA* fusions in AMKL has not reached a consensus, with studies published to support better outcomes, worse outcomes, and similar outcomes to AMKL patients without fusions. COG published a study of 21 patients with AMKL with *RBM15::MRTFA* fusions (split into two cohorts; $n = 7$ and $n = 14$) and found 5-year EFS and 5-year OS ranges from approximately 50% in one cohort ($n = 14$) to approximately 86% in the other cohort ($n = 7$). Five-year relapse risk was 0% in one cohort ($n = 7$), and 38% in the larger cohort [153]. In another international study, the 4-year EFS rate for patients with *RBM15::MRTFA* AMKL was 59% and the OS rate was 70%, significantly better than for AMKL patients with other specific genetic abnormalities (*CBFA2T3::GUS2* fusions, *NUP98::KDM5A* fusions, *KMT2A* rearrangements, monosomy 7) [222].

HOX Rearrangements

The homeobox (*HOX*) genes (39 genes in humans) contain a highly conserved nucleotide sequence (homeodomain) and encodes a large family of transcription factors. These genes are organized into four genomic clusters, referred to as the *HOX A, B, C,* and *D* clusters, which share enhancers. *HOX A* (located at 7p15) and *HOX B* (located at 17q21) specifically are critical for hematopoietic lineage development [223]. Expression of *HOXA/B* and the *HOXA* cofactor *MEIS1* (myeloid ecotropic virus insertion site 1) is high in immature stem cell populations in bone marrow and decreases during maturation and differentiation [224]. The *HOX* genes can function as proto-oncogenes or tumor suppressors depending on the cellular context. *HOX* genes can promote the development of AML by forming chimeric fusions with other genes or by overexpression due to upstream binding of proteins such as CDX [223].

Cases with a gene fusion involving a *HOX* cluster gene occur in approximately 15% of pAML cases [225]. A common fusion partner is *NUP98*, which results from the fusion of the 5′ end of *NUP98* (located at 11p15) to the 3′ end of the *HOX* gene. *NUP98* fusions are seen in approximately 10% of pAML patients [226]. Rearranged *NUP98* AML is associated with poor prognosis, treatment failure, and high relapse rates. *NUP98* translocations can occur at any age but are more commonly observed in children, adolescents, and young adults, with a higher incidence in males [226]. Other genes fused with *HOX* genes may have a relatively favorable prognosis; however, this has not been studied in large cohorts [225]. Stem cell like expression of *HOXA* and *MEIS1* is also seen in pAML patients with *KMT2A* and *NPM1* rearrangements [224].

The *CDX* gene has been shown to influence organogenesis and hematopoiesis through regulation of *HOX* gene expression. Three CDX homologs (CDX1, CDX2, and CDX4) have consensus binding sites in the promoters of multiple *HOX* genes, leading to dysregulation of *HOX* expression [223]. This widespread dysregulated expression of multiple HOX family members is typically associated with a poor prognosis in AML [227].

RAS-Pathway Mutations in AML

RAS-pathway mutations occur in 20–25% of pAML [228, 229]. RAS proteins—KRAS, NRAS, and HRAS—are small GTPases that function as molecular switches, cycling between active GTP-bound and inactive GDP-bound states. Oncogenic mutations, particularly at codons 12, 13, and 61, lock RAS in its active state, leading to constitutive activation of downstream pathways such as RAF-MEK-ERK and PI3K-AKT-mTOR [230, 231]. *PTPN11* is also among the family of RAS pathway genes, with mutations reported in up to 3–4% of pAMLs [232]. The RAS signaling pathway plays a pivotal role in the molecular pathogenesis of AML, initiating key downstream hyper-proliferative signal transduction and promoting cell survival. *RAS*-pathway mutations are often subclonal in the context of pAML, and *NRAS* mutations are more commonly observed than *KRAS* mutations. In addition, *NRAS* mutations have been found to be more prevalent in patients with low-risk disease [229].

The prognostic significance of these variants in AML is not yet clearly defined. Some studies have linked *RAS* mutations to inferior outcomes in AML, while other studies have reported no survival difference [233, 234]. Still other reports have suggested that the presence of a *RAS* mutation may improve survival and/or response to therapy [235]. For example, a study in a large aAML cohort found that *RAS*-pathway alterations were associated with an improved OS compared to AML without *RAS* mutations; however, mutations in *KRAS* were noted to be less favorable than other *RAS* pathway alterations [236]. A different study in a pAML cohort found that *RAS*-mutated and non-*RAS*-mutated AML achieved similar complete remission rates; however, increased treatment-related mortality was observed in patients with *RAS* mutations [229]. A recent well-powered study in pML patients found that *PTPN11* mutations conferred an inferior EFS but not OS [5, 232].

Regarding therapeutics, at the time of this writing there are not currently any FDA-approved targeted therapies for RAS-pathway mutations in AML. However, there are FDA-approved *KRAS* p.G12C inhibitors which can be used for locally advanced or metastatic non-small cell lung carcinoma and colorectal carcinoma harboring the p.G12C variant, although this particular mutation is rare in AML. Additionally, other targeted inhibitors, such as MEK1/2 inhibitors, are actively being investigated in some solid tumors with oncogenic *RAS* mutations.

RUNX1 Mutations

RUNX1 on chromosome 21q22.3 encodes a transcription factor that is widely considered the master regulator of hematopoietic stem cell differentitation. Intragenic mutations, typically frameshift and missense mutations, of *RUNX1* have primarily been reported in MDS, secondary and therapy-related AML, radiation exposed MDS, and AML. *RUNX1*-mutated AML falls into the category of AML with other defined genetic alterations [7]. AML with *RUNX1* mutations is more commonly found in adults than in children, with an estimated prevalence of 5–16% in aAML [237, 238] and 3–5% of pAML [239]. In aAML, *RUNX1* mutations are typically associated with high-risk disease [240]; however, it is unclear in pAML if *RUNX1* mutations affect response or outcome, with studies showing conflicting evidence [239, 241]. *RUNX1* mutations in pAML are typically associated with an older age and increased prevalence in males. *FLT3*-ITD is a commonly occurring co-mutation seen in pAML, suggesting that *RUNX1* mutations preferably contributes to leukemogenesis by cooperating with the activating *FLT3*-ITD, instead of other activating pathways [239].

Germline *RUNX1* variants have been found to cause familial platelet disorder (FPD) which predisposes to the development of MDS and AML [239].

WT1 Mutations

WT1 mutations are present in approximately 10% of pAMLs [9, 242, 243]. The *WT1* gene encodes a transcription factor with four zinc finger motifs and a proline/glutamine-rich DNA-binding domain, playing a pivotal role in both normal development and cancer biology. *WT1* exhibits a dual role in cancer, initially identified as a tumor suppressor in Wilms' tumor, and functioning as an oncogene in other malignancies [244–246]. *WT1* binds DNA and regulates genes involved in cell proliferation, differentiation, and apoptosis. It interacts with key proteins like p53 and TET2, modulating gene expression through epigenetic mechanisms such as DNA methylation and hydroxymethylation [247].

WT1 mutations can be found in 25% of pAML cases with a normal karyotype and frequently co-occur with *FLT3*-ITD [248]. AML cases harboring *NUP98::NSD1* fusions frequently co-occur with both *FLT3* ITD and *WT1* mutations, with *WT1* mutations occurring in approximately 30–50% [147, 149]. While studies suggest that *WT1* mutations are associated with inferior outcomes in pAML, their independent prognostic significance requires further investigation as they have a strong correlation with *FLT3*-ITD and *NUP98::NSD1* fusions, both of which hold a poor prognosis. The most comprehensive study to date examining *WT1* mutations in pAML found that patients with *WT1* mutations in the absence of *FLT3*-ITD had outcomes comparable to those without *WT1* alterations [1]. In contrast, several studies have found that patients harboring both *WT1* mutations and *FLT3*-ITD exhibit markedly poor survival [183, 242, 243]. A recent study regarding the order of mutations in AML found that *WT1* mutations appeared both before and after mutations that occur typically early (e.g., *DNMT3A*) or late (e.g., *FLT3*). The *WT1*-first cases had small single-mutant clones when co-occurring with *NPM1* mutations, and were associated with age and higher neutrophil and monocyte counts [249].

Epigenetic Dysregulation

Epigenetic dysregulation, including abnormal DNA methylation patterns, dysregulated histone modification, and disrupted chromatin architecture, has emerged as a pivotal driver of leukemogenesis, with nearly half of AML cases harboring mutations in genes regulating DNA methylation (i.e., *DNMT3A, TET2, IDH1, IDH2*), and approximately one-third of AML cases with mutations that directly or indirectly modify chromatin (i.e., *KMT2A, ASXL1, EZH2*). These mutations silence key differentiation genes and sustain self-renewal pathways, contributing to the developmental arrest and hyper-proliferation that are the hallmarks of AML [250].

DNA-methyltransferase 3A (DNMT3A) is an enzyme responsible for de novo methylation, behaving as an oncogene in human cancers. Mutations in *DNMT3A* are found in approximately 20–25% of aAML patients and in 1–2% of pAML patients. Mutations predominantly involve an Arginine substitution at codon 882, seen in approximately 60% of AML with mutated *DNMT3A*. This mutation typically results in hypomorphic methylation activity of the methyltransferase, which then leads to hypomethylation at specific gene regions. *DNMT3A* mutations have been linked to increased chemotherapy resistance and increased risk of relapse. DNMT inhibitors (DNMTi), which alter DNA methylation patterns, and subsequently promote the expression of tumor suppressors and increase apoptosis, are used in aAML and have been shown to prolong overall survival compared to standard treatment. Investigation into the use of DNMTi for pAML preliminarily shows it is well-tolerated in newly diagnosed AML before standard combination chemotherapy as well as in sequence with intensive chemotherapy in relapsed/refractory AML [251].

IDH1 and IDH2 (isocitrate dehydrogenase 1 and 2) are enzymes that catalyze the oxidative decarboxylation of isocitrate to α-ketoglutarate (α-KG), which is used by numerous α-KG dioxygenases (i.e., TET (ten-eleven translocation) DNA hydroxylases). TET proteins are key catalytic proteins that mediate DNA demethylation [252]. Mutations within *IDH1/2* cause the processing of α-KG to the oncometabolite 2-hydroxyglutarate (2HG), which acts as a competitive inhibitor of α-KG dioxygenases due to the similar structure to α-KG. In AML cells with *IDH1/2* mutations, accumulation of 2HG impairs TET2 function, leading to a buildup of DNA methylation marks specifically at promoters of myeloid differentiation genes, which prevents expression, thus trapping cells in an immature, proliferative state [250]. *IDH1* mutations typically occur exclusively in codon 132 and *IDH2* mutations frequently occur at codon 140, both resulting in the replacement of an arginine [253]. Mutations in *IDH1/2* are seen in approximately 5–33% of aAML patients and in approximately 1–4% of pAML patients [251]. The prognostic impact of *IDH* mutations remains indeterminate but is hypothesized to cause inferior outcomes in aAML with

IDH1 mutations, whereas *IDH2* mutations seem to have a relatively favorable prognosis with standard intensive chemotherapy [254]. The use of IDH1 and IDH2 inhibitors, ivosidenib and enasidenib, are common therapies for treating relapsed/refractory AML [255].

Colony stimulating factor 3 receptor (CSF3R) plays an important role in driving the differentiation, growth, and survival of neutrophils through the binding of granulocyte colony stimulating factor (GCSF) leading to the subsequent activation of signal transduction pathways such as JAK/STAT, MAPK/ERK, and PI3K/AKT. *CSF3R* has been found as a germline predisposition gene for both myeloid and lymphoid neoplasms. *CSF3R* mutations are found in 0.5–1% of aAML cases and approximately 2% of pAML cases with T618I being a common mutation. *CSF3R* mutations are commonly found co-occurring with additional mutations. Specifically in pAML, *CSF3R* mutations frequently co-occur with t(8;21) or *CEBPA* mutations, with *CSF3R+/CEBPA* patients having a worse EFS (25%) and higher relapse rates (75%) in comparison to *CSF3R*+/t(8;21) cases (83% and 15%, respectively) [256].

ASXL proteins function as epigenetic scaffolds that assemble chromatin modification complexes and transcription factors [257]. Loss-of-function mutations in *ASXL1* lead to a reduction in global H3K27me3, which causes changes in chromatin accessibility [250]. *ASXL1* is mutated in approximately 3–15% of aAML cases, with the highest frequency in the elderly and secondary AML/MDS, and in approximately 1–9% of pAML cases [251]. *ASXL1* mutations are associated with a negative prognosis [255].

Down Syndrome AML (DS-AML)

There are two clonally related myeloproliferative conditions associated with DS: transient abnormal myelopoiesis (TAM) and myeloid leukemia [258]. Both have somatic *GATA1* mutations in addition to germline trisomy 21 in nearly all cases [259]. TAM is a transient newborn and young-infant version with most cases coming to clinical attention within 7 days of birth and with more than 90% of cases resolving spontaneously in 2–3 months without treatment [260, 261]. All symptomatic cases have increased blast cells in peripheral blood. Approximately 20% of TAM patients later develop DS-AML [260, 261]. TAM is generally not characterized by cytogenetic abnormalities other than trisomy 21; however, the presence of additional cytogenetic findings may predict an increased risk of developing subsequent AML [262].

DS-AML is an unremitting but chemosensitive version that appears later [258]. The median age of onset of DS-AML is 1.6 years with the vast majority of patients presenting within the first 4 years of life [263, 264]. The risk of developing AML in children with DS is 150-fold that of an individual without DS. Compared to an up to 20-fold increased risk of developing ALL, AML is the predominate form of leukemia in children with DS younger than 4 years of age [265], and at least one-third of patients have a history of antecedent TAM [263, 264]. The majority of DS-AML cases have M7 morphology (FAB classification); thus, they are also called AMKL cases. Recurrent somatic abnormalities in DS-AML children frequently include +8, +11, +19, dup(1p), del(6q), del(7p), dup(7q), and del(16q). Conversely, the typical favorable translocations associated with non-DS AML [e.g., t(8;21); t(15;17); inv(16), 11q23 rearrangements] are rarely seen in DS-AML patients [266]. In addition to the somatic *GATA1* variants, mutations predominantly affecting chromatin (e.g., the cohesin complex), epigenetic regulators (e.g., *ASXL1*, *BCOR*, and *DNMT1*), *RAS*, and signaling mediators other than the ones on chromosome 21 have been reported [267].

Despite significant progress in this area, pathogenesis of DS-AML is still not fully understood, and there are no targeted therapies. A multistep clonal evolution process has been proposed [268, 269]. Trisomy 21 represents a "primary hit," which results in genome-wide transcriptional perturbation, including genes encoding transcription factors, pro-inflammatory cytokines, and various microRNA in fetal hematopoietic stem and progenitor cells and in stromal cells; thus, it alters hematopoiesis during embryonic development. Acquisition of somatic *GATA1* mutations represents a "secondary hit." *GATA1* is located at Xp11.23 and encodes a transcription factor that is required for normal development of erythroid cells, megakaryocytes, eosinophils, and mast cells. These mutations generally occur within exon 2 and include nonsense, missense, insertion, and deletion mutations and result in alternative splicing of the exon or cause expression of the gene from an alternative downstream translation start site. These alterations uniformly lead to exclusive production of a short isoform termed GATA1s which lacks the N-terminal transactivation domain and has decreased activity resulting in fetal blood cell development disruption [171, 268]. The full development of DS-AML requires acquisition and selection of clones with additional somatic mutations and chromosomal structural abnormalities [267–269]. There is evidence that DS-AML evolves from a subclone of TAM after the acquisition of additional mutations [270]. Of note, *GATA1*-truncating variants have also been reported in approximately 10% of non-DS AMKL, arising in young children (median age of 1–2 years) and are associated with amplification of the *RCAN1* gene on chromosome 21. Although the sample size was small, these patients appeared to have a favorable outcome if there were no prognostically unfavorable co-occurring gene fusions [24, 225].

Age and WBC count are recognized prognostic factors in DS-AML with older age (> 3-years-old) and high WBC counts predicting a poor prognosis [271]. DS-AML cases presenting in patients over 4 years of age have been shown to lack *GATA1* mutations and are more akin to sporadic AML in terms of cytogenetic abnormalities and risk of relapse [272]. In addition, DS-AML patients with a history of transient myeloproliferative disease (TMD) have a significantly better outcome than children with DS-AML without documented TMD [261]. There has been controversial data on the impact of acquired chromosomal abnormalities [205, 273], however, gain of chromosome 8 has been associated with poor prognosis [264] and distal 1q gain may have adverse outcome [274, 275].

The prognosis of DS-AML is significantly better than that for AML in children without DS with EFS of 87–89% versus 47–53% and OS of 89–93% versus 63–69%

[16, 263, 264] due to increased sensitivity to chemotherapeutic agents [276]. In older children with megakaryocytic AML, it is important to rule out the presence of co-existing trisomy 21 and *GATA1* mutations as these children may be successfully treated with the lower-intensity chemotherapy regimens [225]. Of note, although initial diagnosis of DS-AML has a favorable prognosis, refractory and relapsed disease can be difficult to treat as high-dose chemotherapy causes unacceptable toxicity in DS children [264].

Summary

Conventional cytogenetic abnormalities (karyotype and FISH) laid the foundation for earlier versions of the WHO classification system for AML subtypes [277, 278]. With the implementation of advanced diagnostic technologies, including microarray, NGS, and RNA transcriptome sequencing, many new entities have been discovered, which lead to the revision of the WHO subtype/risk group classification the ICC, as well as the European LeukemiaNet (ELN) classification in 2022 [7, 8, 279]. Thissubtype list is still expanding today. In this chapter, we described more than 20 biomarkers for de novo AML, including both well-established and newly-recognized abnormalities (Tables 15.1 and 15.2). Each of the markers has one or more values in the diagnostic, prognostic, and predictive process. The discovery of these biomarkers has driven exciting progress in precision medicine therapeutics, for example, FLT3 inhibitors, menin inhibitors, BCL-2 inhibitors, and CD33-targeted immunotherapies [280]. Despite significant progress, various challenges remain pertinent, such as relatively high rates (~30%) [281]. Therefore, further exploration is needed to improve pAML treatment results. Novel biomarkers, multi-omics integration, and technologies like machine learning and deep learning may offer promising insights into disease mechanisms, prognosis assessment, and combined treatment strategies in this modern era of precision medicine-based therapy [282].

Table 15.1 Well-recognized biomarkers in pediatric acute myeloid leukemia

Biomarkers	Incidence in pAML	Prognosis	Alteration	Function	Targeted therapy	Co-occurring genetic aberrations	Comments
t(15;17)(q22;q21) *PML::RARA* (APL)	5–10% <2% in infants	Good	Translocation	Impairie myeloid differentiation	All-trans retinoic acid	7q-, +8, mutations in *FLT3*, *WT1*, *NRAS*, *USP9X*, *ARID1A*, *EED*, *KRAS*	N/A
t(8;21)(q22;q22.1) *RUNX1::RUNX1T1*	12–14%	Good	Translocation	Inhibit core binding factor function	N/A	*KIT* mutations RAS pathway gene mutations Loss of X/Y, del(9q), del(7q), +8, 19p cnLOH Deletions in *WT1*, *BXORL1*, *RAD21*, *NF1*,*IKZF1*, *ETV6*	Gemtuzumab ozogamicin (GO) and tyrosine kinase inhibitors (TKIs) can be applied if with *KIT* mutation
inv(16)(p13.1;q22) or t(16;16)(p13.1;q22) *CBFB::MYH11*	7–9%	Good	Translocation	Inhibit core binding factor function	N/A	*KIT* mutations RAS pathway gene mutations Gain 22, 8, and 21; del (7q), focal deletion of *FOXP1*	GO and TKIs can be applied if with *KIT* mutation
NPM1 mutation	8%	Good	Frameshift	Cytoplasmic NPM1 upregulating homeobox (*HOX*) genes	N/A	Mutations in *FLT3*, *DNMT3A*, *IDH1/2*, *TET2*	FLT3-inhibitor can be used if *FLT3* mutation is present
CEBPA mutation	5%	Good	Out-of-frame or in-frame variants	Deregulate myeloid differentiation	N/A	Mutations in *GATA2*, *WT1*, *TET2*, *CSF3R*	Good prognosis only if bi-allelic mutations or single mutation in bZIP region

(continued)

Table 15.1 (continued)

Biomarkers	Incidence in pAML	Prognosis	Alteration	Function	Targeted therapy	Co-occurring genetic aberrations	Comments
FLT3-ITD FLT3D385	10–30%	Poor	In-frame internal tandem duplication; Point mutation	Constitutive activation of several pathways including RAS/MAPK, PI3K/AKT, and JAK/STAT	1st and 2nd generation FLT3 inhibitors	t(15;17) PML::RARA, the core binding factor AMLs t(8;21) and inv(16), t(6;9) *DEK::NUP214*, *NUP98::NSD1*, mutations in *NPM1, CEBPA, WT1, UBTF*	Prognosis can be influenced by co-occurring mutations
KMT2A rearrangements	>50% in infants, 10% in adolescents	Poor/ intermediate	Translocation	Upregulation of HOX expression	Menin-KMT2A inhibitor	Mutations in RAS pathway, *SETD2*	*KMT2A::MLLT3*—intermediate prognosis. Other fusions-poor
HOX rearrangements	15%	Poor	Translocations	Chimeric fusions or overexpression due to upstream binding of proteins	N/A	No pattern	Can function as proto-oncogenes or tumor suppressors depending on the cellular context
NUP98 rearrangements	3–10%	Poor	Translocation	Transcriptional regulation and mitotic progression	N/A	*NUP98::NSD1—WT1* mutation and +8; *NUP98::KDM5A—RB1* loss, chromosome 13 alteration, +21	At least 30 different partner—poor outcome irrespective of the partner
inv(3) (q21.3;q26.2)/t(3;3) (q21.3;q26.2) MECOM rearrangement	~1%	Poor	Enhancer hijacking (MECOM)	Hematopoietic stem/progenitor cell self-renewal, lineage differentiation and proliferation	N/A	No pattern	Mechanisms other than classic inv(3;3)/t(3;3) have been reported—including fusion proteins and other enhancer hijacking

inv(16)(p13.3;q24.3) *CBFA2T3::GLIS2*	~3%	Poor	Translocation	Fusion product blocks in differentiation and increased self-renewal	N/A	No pattern	Distinct immunophenotype referred to as the RAM phenotype
t(1;22)(p13;q13) *RBM15::MRTFA*	~0.8%	Uncertain	Translocation	Disrupts RNA processing and the HOX and RAS/MAPK signaling pathways	N/A	No pattern	Present commonly in AMKL. Some studies support better outcomes, worse outcomes, and similar outcomes to AMKL patients without fusions.
t(6;9)(p22.3;q34.1) *DEK::NUP214*	0.6–1.7%	Poor	Translocation	Not fully elucidated	N/A	*FLT3* ITD in 55–80%; Mutations in RAS pathway	Usually as a sole abnormality cytogenetically
t(16;21)(p11;q22) *FUS::ERG*	~0.5%	Poor	Translocation	Affects gene transcription and RNA splicing	N/A	Mutations in *RUNX1*, *DNMT3A*, *ASXL1*, *BCOR;* +8, +10, complex karyotype	All reported patients older than 2 years
t(9;22)(q34;q11.2) *BCR::ABL1*	Extremely rare in children	Poor	Translocation	Constitutively active tyrosine kinase	Tyrosine kinase inhibitor	Deletion of *IKZF1* and/or *CDKN2A/B;* mutation in *RUNX1*	N/A
Chromosome 5, 7 abnormalities	2–4% (15% in adult)	Poor	Loss	Impact DNA damage response, DNA replication, and chromatin regulation	N/A	Complex karyotype	N/A

(continued)

Table 15.1 (continued)

Biomarkers	Incidence in pAML	Prognosis	Alteration	Function	Targeted therapy	Co-occurring genetic aberrations	Comments
RAS mutations	20–25%	Uncertain	Gain of function	RAF/MEK/ERK and PI3K/AKT/mTOR pathways	N/A	*KMT2A* rearrangement, inv(16), t(8;21)	N/A
WT1 mutations	10%	Poor/depend on co-mutations	Loss of function	Transcription factor	N/A	*FLT3*-ITD and *NUP98::NSD1* fusions	Independent prognostic significance requires further investigation as they have a strong correlation with *FLT3*-ITD and *NUP98::NSD1* fusions, which both herald a poor prognosis.
RUNX1 mutations	3–5%	Uncertain	Missense and frameshift mutations	Regulator of the differentiation of hematopoietic stem cells into mature blood cells	N/A	*FLT3*-ITD	N/A

Table 15.2 Selected newly recognized biomarkers in pediatric acute myeloid leukemia

Biomarkers	Incidence in pAML	Prognosis	Alteration	Function	Targeted therapy	Co-occurring genetic aberrations	Comments
Non-*KMT2A::MLLT10* fusions	~1%	Poor	Translocation	Interacts with *DOT1L*, a histone methyltransferase transferase	N/A	No pattern	N/A
t(7;12)(q36;p13) *ETV6::MNX1*	~1%	Poor	Translocation	MNX1 overexpression	N/A	+19, +8, +22	Exclusively in children <2 years
t(16;21)(q24;q22) *RUNX1::CBFA2T3*	0.1–0.3%	Good/poor	Translocation	Regulation of hematopoietic-specific genes	N/A	No pattern	Poor prognosis in adult AML
UBTF tandem duplication	~4%	Poor	In frame tandem duplications	Interacts with ribosomal DNA to mediate RNA polymerase 1 ribosomal RNA transcription	Menin inhibitors	*FLT3*-ITD, *WT1* mutations, normal karyotype or isolated trisomy 8, activation of the *HOXA/HOXB* genes	Co-occurrence either *FLT3*-ITD or *WT1* mutations was associated with an inferior prognosis, compared with patients with *UBTF* tandem duplication alone
CBFB-GDXY	0.4%	Good	Insertion	Causes loss of regular CBFB function, impairing the core banding factor's ability to promote normal hematopoietic cell growth	N/A	*Mutations in FLT3, BCORE, +6, +22*	Lack *KIT* mutations and +8
DNMT2A mutations	1–2%	Poor	Missense mutation	Responsible for de novo methylation, behaving as an oncogene	DNMT inhibitors	No pattern	N/A

(continued)

Table 15.2 (continued)

Biomarkers	Incidence in pAML	Prognosis	Alteration	Function	Targeted therapy	Co-occurring genetic aberrations	Comments
IDH1/IDH2 mutations	1–4%	Poor/good	Missense mutation	DNA demethylation	IDH1/IDH2 inhibitors	No pattern	In a AML *IDH1* mutations have an inferior outcome whereas *IDH2* mutations have a relatively favorable prognosis; remains debated for pAML
CSF3R mutations	~2%	Poor	Missense mutation	Activation of signal transduction pathways	N/A	t(8;21) or *CEBPA* mutations	N/A
ASXL1 mutations	~1–9%	Poor	Loss of function mutations	Epigenetic scaffolds that assemble chromatin modification complexes and transcription factors	N/A	No pattern	N/A
t(3;5)(q25;q34) *NPM1::MFL1*	Extremely rare	Favorable as sole abnormality	Translocation	Enhanced recruitment of nucleosome remodeling and deacetylase (NuRD) to target genes	N/A	Trisomy 8, complex karyotype	Worse prognosis if concurrent with trisomy 8 or complex karyotype
t(8;16)(p11.2;p13.3) *KAT6A::CREBBP*	Extremely rare	Intermediate	Translocation	Upregulation of HOXA expression	N/A	CHIP family mutations or MDS-related mutations	Poor prognosis in adults with treatment-related AML. Some neonatal congenital cases with spontaneous and sustained remission

References

1. Yamashita M, Dellorusso PV, Olson OC, Passegue E. Dysregulated haematopoietic stem cell behaviour in myeloid leukaemogenesis. Nat Rev Cancer. 2020;20(7):365–82.
2. Reinhardt D, Antoniou E, Waack K. Pediatric acute myeloid leukemia-past, present, and future. J Clin Med. 2022;11(3):504.
3. de Rooij JD, Zwaan CM, van den Heuvel-Eibrink M. Pediatric AML: from biology to clinical management. J Clin Med. 2015;4(1):127–49.
4. Iwai T, Yokota S, Nakao M, Okamoto T, Taniwaki M, Onodera N, et al. Internal tandem duplication of the FLT3 gene and clinical evaluation in childhood acute myeloid leukemia. The Children's Cancer and Leukemia Study Group, Japan. Leukemia. 1999;13(1):38–43.
5. Schlenk RF, Dohner K, Krauter J, Frohling S, Corbacioglu A, Bullinger L, et al. Mutations and treatment outcome in cytogenetically normal acute myeloid leukemia. N Engl J Med. 2008;358(18):1909–18.
6. Hoffmeister LM, Suttorp J, Walter C, Antoniou E, Behrens YL, Gohring G, et al. Panel-based RNA fusion sequencing improves diagnostics of pediatric acute myeloid leukemia. Leukemia. 2024;38(3):538–44.
7. Khoury JD, Solary E, Abla O, Akkari Y, Alaggio R, Apperley JF, et al. The 5th edition of the World Health Organization classification of haematolymphoid tumours: myeloid and histiocytic/dendritic neoplasms. Leukemia. 2022;36(7):1703–19.
8. Arber DA, Orazi A, Hasserjian RP, Borowitz MJ, Calvo KR, Kvasnicka HM, et al. International Consensus Classification of Myeloid Neoplasms and Acute Leukemias: integrating morphologic, clinical, and genomic data. Blood. 2022;140(11):1200–28.
9. Bolouri H, Farrar JE, Triche T Jr, Ries RE, Lim EL, Alonzo TA, et al. The molecular landscape of pediatric acute myeloid leukemia reveals recurrent structural alterations and age-specific mutational interactions. Nat Med. 2018;24(1):103–12.
10. Cancer Genome Atlas Research N, Ley TJ, Miller C, Ding L, Raphael BJ, Mungall AJ, et al. Genomic and epigenomic landscapes of adult de novo acute myeloid leukemia. N Engl J Med. 2013;368(22):2059–74.
11. Jaju RJ, Fidler C, Haas OA, Strickson AJ, Watkins F, Clark K, et al. A novel gene, NSD1, is fused to NUP98 in the t(5;11)(q35;p15.5) in de novo childhood acute myeloid leukemia. Blood. 2001;98(4):1264–7.
12. Umeda M, Ma J, Huang BJ, Hagiwara K, Westover T, Abdelhamed S, et al. Integrated genomic analysis identifies UBTF tandem duplications as a recurrent lesion in pediatric acute myeloid leukemia. Blood Cancer Discov. 2022;3(3):194–207.
13. Umeda M, Liu YC, Karol SE, Klco JM. Novel classification system and high-risk categories of pediatric acute myeloid leukemia. Haematologica. 2025;110(9):1962–73.
14. Stankiewicz J, Styczynski J. Improved outcome in pediatric acute myeloid leukemia: progress with hematopoietic cell transplantation. Anticancer Res. 2022;42(9):4499–504.
15. Tomizawa D, Tsujimoto SI. Risk-stratified therapy for pediatric acute myeloid leukemia. Cancers (Basel). 2023;15(16):4171.
16. Gamis AS, Alonzo TA, Meshinchi S, Sung L, Gerbing RB, Raimondi SC, et al. Gemtuzumab ozogamicin in children and adolescents with de novo acute myeloid leukemia improves event-free survival by reducing relapse risk: results from the randomized phase III Children's Oncology Group trial AAML0531. J Clin Oncol. 2014;32(27):3021–32.
17. Pollard JA, Alonzo TA, Gerbing R, Brown P, Fox E, Choi J, et al. Sorafenib in combination with standard chemotherapy for children with high allelic ratio FLT3/ITD+ acute myeloid leukemia: a report from the Children's Oncology Group protocol AAML1031. J Clin Oncol. 2022;40(18):2023–35.
18. Rubnitz JE, Lacayo NJ, Inaba H, Heym K, Ribeiro RC, Taub J, et al. Clofarabine can replace anthracyclines and etoposide in remission induction therapy for childhood acute myeloid leukemia: the AML08 multicenter, randomized phase III trial. J Clin Oncol. 2019;37(23):2072–81.

19. Inaba H, Pui CH. Advances in the diagnosis and treatment of pediatric acute lymphoblastic leukemia. J Clin Med. 2021;10(9):1926.
20. Shao L, Akkari Y, Cooley LD, Miller DT, Seifert BA, Wolff DJ, et al. Chromosomal microarray analysis, including constitutional and neoplastic disease applications, 2021 revision: a technical standard of the American College of Medical Genetics and Genomics (ACMG). Genet Med. 2021;23(10):1818–29.
21. Dohner H, Estey EH, Amadori S, Appelbaum FR, Buchner T, Burnett AK, et al. Diagnosis and management of acute myeloid leukemia in adults: recommendations from an international expert panel, on behalf of the European LeukemiaNet. Blood. 2010;115(3):453–74.
22. van Dongen JJ, Macintyre EA, Gabert JA, Delabesse E, Rossi V, Saglio G, et al. Standardized RT-PCR analysis of fusion gene transcripts from chromosome aberrations in acute leukemia for detection of minimal residual disease. Report of the BIOMED-1 Concerted Action: investigation of minimal residual disease in acute leukemia. Leukemia. 1999;13(12):1901–28.
23. Mrozek K, Prior TW, Edwards C, Marcucci G, Carroll AJ, Snyder PJ, et al. Comparison of cytogenetic and molecular genetic detection of t(8;21) and inv(16) in a prospective series of adults with de novo acute myeloid leukemia: a Cancer and Leukemia Group B Study. J Clin Oncol. 2001;19(9):2482–92.
24. Meena JP, Pathak N, Gupta AK, Bakhshi S, Gupta R, Makkar H, et al. Molecular evaluation of gene mutation profiles and copy number variations in pediatric acute myeloid leukemia. Leuk Res. 2022;122:106954.
25. Hu Z, Kovach AE, Yellapantula V, Ostrow D, Doan A, Ji J, et al. Transcriptome sequencing allows comprehensive genomic characterization of pediatric B-acute lymphoblastic leukemia in an academic clinical laboratory. J Mol Diagn. 2024;26(1):49–60.
26. Conneely SE, Stevens AM. Advances in pediatric acute promyelocytic leukemia. Children (Basel). 2020;7(2):11.
27. Creutzig U, Zimmermann M, Reinhardt D, Rasche M, von Neuhoff C, Alpermann T, et al. Changes in cytogenetics and molecular genetics in acute myeloid leukemia from childhood to adult age groups. Cancer. 2016;122(24):3821–30.
28. Breen KA, Grimwade D, Hunt BJ. The pathogenesis and management of the coagulopathy of acute promyelocytic leukaemia. Br J Haematol. 2012;156(1):24–36.
29. Sanz MA, Montesinos P. Advances in the management of coagulopathy in acute promyelocytic leukemia. Thromb Res. 2020;191(Suppl 1):S63–S7.
30. Sanz MA, Lo Coco F, Martin G, Avvisati G, Rayon C, Barbui T, et al. Definition of relapse risk and role of nonanthracycline drugs for consolidation in patients with acute promyelocytic leukemia: a joint study of the PETHEMA and GIMEMA cooperative groups. Blood. 2000;96(4):1247–53.
31. Fan Z, Yang LC, Chen YQ, Wan WQ, Zhou DH, Mai HR, et al. Prognostic significance of MRD and its correlation with arsenic concentration in pediatric acute promyelocytic leukemia: a retrospective study by SCCLG-APL group. Ther Adv Hematol. 2025;16:20406207241311774.
32. Sanz MA, Fenaux P, Tallman MS, Estey EH, Lowenberg B, Naoe T, et al. Management of acute promyelocytic leukemia: updated recommendations from an expert panel of the European LeukemiaNet. Blood. 2019;133(15):1630–43.
33. Zhang L, Samad A, Pombo-de-Oliveira MS, Scelo G, Smith MT, Feusner J, et al. Global characteristics of childhood acute promyelocytic leukemia. Blood Rev. 2015;29(2):101–25.
34. Bellodi C, Kindle K, Bernassola F, Cossarizza A, Dinsdale D, Melino G, et al. A cytoplasmic PML mutant inhibits p53 function. Cell Cycle. 2006;5(22):2688–92.
35. Guo A, Salomoni P, Luo J, Shih A, Zhong S, Gu W, et al. The function of PML in p53-dependent apoptosis. Nat Cell Biol. 2000;2(10):730–6.
36. Guarnera L, Ottone T, Fabiani E, Divona M, Savi A, Travaglini S, et al. Atypical rearrangements in APL-like acute myeloid leukemias: molecular characterization and prognosis. Front Oncol. 2022;12:871590.
37. Qiu KY, Liao XY, Li Y, Huang K, Xu HG, Fang JP, et al. Outcome and prognostic factors of CBF pediatric AML patients with t(8;21) differ from patients with inv(16). BMC Cancer. 2023;23(1):476.

38. Link KA, Chou FS, Mulloy JC. Core binding factor at the crossroads: determining the fate of the HSC. J Cell Physiol. 2010;222(1):50–6.
39. Sinha C, Cunningham LC, Liu PP. Core binding factor acute myeloid leukemia: new prognostic categories and therapeutic opportunities. Semin Hematol. 2015;52(3):215–22.
40. Marcucci G, Caligiuri MA, Bloomfield CD. Molecular and clinical advances in core binding factor primary acute myeloid leukemia: a paradigm for translational research in malignant hematology. Cancer Investig. 2000;18(8):768–80.
41. Wijmenga C, Gregory PE, Hajra A, Schrock E, Ried T, Eils R, et al. Core binding factor beta-smooth muscle myosin heavy chain chimeric protein involved in acute myeloid leukemia forms unusual nuclear rod-like structures in transformed NIH 3T3 cells. Proc Natl Acad Sci USA. 1996;93(4):1630–5.
42. Adya N, Stacy T, Speck NA, Liu PP. The leukemic protein core binding factor beta (CBFbeta)-smooth-muscle myosin heavy chain sequesters CBFalpha2 into cytoskeletal filaments and aggregates. Mol Cell Biol. 1998;18(12):7432–43.
43. Harrison CJ, Hills RK, Moorman AV, Grimwade DJ, Hann I, Webb DK, et al. Cytogenetics of childhood acute myeloid leukemia: United Kingdom Medical Research Council Treatment trials AML 10 and 12. J Clin Oncol. 2010;28(16):2674–81.
44. Creutzig U, Zimmermann M, Bourquin JP, Dworzak MN, von Neuhoff C, Sander A, et al. Second induction with high-dose cytarabine and mitoxantrone: different impact on pediatric AML patients with t(8;21) and with inv(16). Blood. 2011;118(20):5409–15.
45. Klaus M, Haferlach T, Schnittger S, Kern W, Hiddemann W, Schoch C. Cytogenetic profile in de novo acute myeloid leukemia with FAB subtypes M0, M1, and M2: a study based on 652 cases analyzed with morphology, cytogenetics, and fluorescence in situ hybridization. Cancer Genet Cytogenet. 2004;155(1):47–56.
46. Bae SY, Kim JS, Ryeu BJ, Lee KN, Lee CK, Kim YK, et al. Acute myeloid leukemia (AML-M2) associated with variant t(8;21): report of three cases. Cancer Genet Cytogenet. 2010;199(1):31–7.
47. Choi J, Song J, Kim SJ, Choi JR, Kim SJ, Min YH, et al. Prognostic significance of trisomy 6 in an adult acute myeloid leukemia with t(8;21). Cancer Genet Cytogenet. 2010;202(2):141–3.
48. Duployez N, Boudry-Labis E, Roumier C, Boissel N, Petit A, Geffroy S, et al. SNP-array lesions in core binding factor acute myeloid leukemia. Oncotarget. 2018;9(5):6478–89.
49. Helton HL, Ries RE, Alonzo TA, et al. Clinically significant mutations, deletions and translocations involving ETV6 identified by whole genome and whole exome sequencing; report from NCI/COG target AML initiative [Abstract]. Blood. 2012;120(21):125. https://ashpublications.org/blood/article/120/21/125/89569/Clinically-Significant-Mutations-Deletions-and
50. Ottone T, Hasan SK, Montefusco E, Curzi P, Mays AN, Chessa L, et al. Identification of a potential "hotspot" DNA region in the RUNX1 gene targeted by mitoxantrone in therapy-related acute myeloid leukemia with t(16;21) translocation. Genes Chromosom Cancer. 2009;48(3):213–21.
51. Han L, Koduru P, Cantu M, Fuda F, Chen W. RUNX1::CBFA2T2 rearranged acute myeloid leukemia transformed from JAK2 V617F mutated primary myelofibrosis. EJHaem. 2024;5(6):1330–4.
52. Umeda M, Ma J, Westover T, Ni Y, Song G, Maciaszek JL, et al. A new genomic framework to categorize pediatric acute myeloid leukemia. Nat Genet. 2024;56(2):281–93.
53. Liu H, Wang SA, Schlette EJ, Xu J, Jorgensen JL, Cameron Yin C, et al. Myeloid neoplasms with t(16;21)(q24;q22)/RUNX1-RUNX1T3 mimics acute myeloid leukemia with RUNX1-RUNX1T1. Ann Hematol. 2018;97(10):1775–83.
54. Noort S, Zimmermann M, Reinhardt D, Cuccuini W, Pigazzi M, Smith J, et al. Prognostic impact of t(16;21)(p11;q22) and t(16;21)(q24;q22) in pediatric AML: a retrospective study by the I-BFM Study Group. Blood. 2018;132(15):1584–92.
55. Kawashima N, Shimada A, Taketani T, Hayashi Y, Yoshida N, Matsumoto K, et al. Childhood acute myeloid leukemia with bone marrow eosinophilia caused by t(16;21)(q24;q22). Int J Hematol. 2012;95(5):577–80.
56. Paschka P. Core binding factor acute myeloid leukemia. Semin Oncol. 2008;35(4):410–7.

57. Solh M, Yohe S, Weisdorf D, Ustun C. Core-binding factor acute myeloid leukemia: heterogeneity, monitoring, and therapy. Am J Hematol. 2014;89(12):1121–31.
58. Hu Z, Tang X, Chen F, Li T, Liu Y, Zhou G, et al. Molecular genetics profiling of core-binding factor acute myeloid leukemia in pediatrics. Ther Adv Hematol. 2025;16:20406207251330064.
59. Lennartsson J, Ronnstrand L. Stem cell factor receptor/c-Kit: from basic science to clinical implications. Physiol Rev. 2012;92(4):1619–49.
60. Katagiri S, Chi S, Minami Y, Fukushima K, Shibayama H, Hosono N, et al. Mutated KIT tyrosine kinase as a novel molecular target in acute myeloid leukemia. Int J Mol Sci. 2022;23(9):4694.
61. Duan W, Liu X, Zhao X, Jia J, Wang J, Gong L, et al. Both the subtypes of KIT mutation and minimal residual disease are associated with prognosis in core binding factor acute myeloid leukemia: a retrospective clinical cohort study in single center. Ann Hematol. 2021;100(5):1203–12.
62. Ishikawa Y, Kawashima N, Atsuta Y, Sugiura I, Sawa M, Dobashi N, et al. Prospective evaluation of prognostic impact of KIT mutations on acute myeloid leukemia with RUNX1-RUNX1T1 and CBFB-MYH11. Blood Adv. 2020;4(1):66–75.
63. Paschka P, Du J, Schlenk RF, Gaidzik VI, Bullinger L, Corbacioglu A, et al. Secondary genetic lesions in acute myeloid leukemia with inv(16) or t(16;16): a study of the German-Austrian AML Study Group (AMLSG). Blood. 2013;121(1):170–7.
64. Cairoli R, Beghini A, Grillo G, Nadali G, Elice F, Ripamonti CB, et al. Prognostic impact of c-KIT mutations in core binding factor leukemias: an Italian retrospective study. Blood. 2006;107(9):3463–8.
65. Tarlock K, Alonzo TA, Wang YC, Gerbing RB, Ries R, Loken MR, et al. Functional properties of KIT mutations are associated with differential clinical outcomes and response to targeted therapeutics in CBF acute myeloid leukemia. Clin Cancer Res. 2019;25(16):5038–48.
66. Shafik NF, Ibraheem D, Selim MM, Allam RM, Fathalla LA. The prognostic significance of c-KIT mutations in core binding factor acute myeloid leukemia. Clin Lymphoma Myeloma Leuk. 2022;22(6):e363–e75.
67. Srinivasan S, Dhamne C, Patkar N, Chatterjee G, Moulik NR, Chichra A, et al. KIT exon 17 mutations are predictive of inferior outcome in pediatric acute myeloid leukemia with RUNX1::RUNX1T1. Pediatr Blood Cancer. 2024;71(2):e30791.
68. Ryland GL, Umeda M, Holmfeldt L, Lehmann S, Herlin MK, Ma J, et al. Description of a novel subtype of acute myeloid leukemia defined by recurrent CBFB insertions. Blood. 2023;141(7):800–5.
69. Zarka J, Short NJ, Kanagal-Shamanna R, Issa GC. Nucleophosmin 1 mutations in acute myeloid leukemia. Genes (Basel). 2020;11(6):649.
70. Brown P, McIntyre E, Rau R, Meshinchi S, Lacayo N, Dahl G, et al. The incidence and clinical significance of nucleophosmin mutations in childhood AML. Blood. 2007;110(3):979–85.
71. Federici L, Falini B. Nucleophosmin mutations in acute myeloid leukemia: a tale of protein unfolding and mislocalization. Protein Sci. 2013;22(5):545–56.
72. Brunetti L, Gundry MC, Sorcini D, Guzman AG, Huang YH, Ramabadran R, et al. Mutant NPM1 maintains the leukemic state through HOX expression. Cancer Cell. 2018;34(3):499–512 e9.
73. Thiede C, Creutzig E, Reinhardt D, Ehninger G, Creutzig U. Different types of NPM1 mutations in children and adults: evidence for an effect of patient age on the prevalence of the TCTG-tandem duplication in NPM1-exon 12. Leukemia. 2007;21(2):366–7.
74. Sharma N, Liesveld JL. NPM 1 mutations in AML—the landscape in 2023. Cancers (Basel). 2023;15(4):1177.
75. Pettersson L, Holmgren B, Juliusson G, Lazarevic VL, Ehinger M. Mutational spectrum of de novo NPM1-mutated acute myeloid leukemia patients older than 75 years. Leuk Lymphoma. 2021;62(8):1958–66.
76. Falini B, Brunetti L, Sportoletti P, Martelli MP. NPM1-mutated acute myeloid leukemia: from bench to bedside. Blood. 2020;136(15):1707–21.

77. Braune J, Rieger K, Blau O, Keller U, Bullinger L, Kronke J. Relapse of NPM1-mutated AML with extramedullary manifestation 17 years after allogeneic hematopoietic stem cell transplantation. Case Rep Hematol. 2022;2022:3317936.
78. Avellino R, Delwel R. Expression and regulation of C/EBPalpha in normal myelopoiesis and in malignant transformation. Blood. 2017;129(15):2083–91.
79. Hollink IH, van den Heuvel-Eibrink MM, Arentsen-Peters ST, Zimmermann M, Peeters JK, Valk PJ, et al. Characterization of CEBPA mutations and promoter hypermethylation in pediatric acute myeloid leukemia. Haematologica. 2011;96(3):384–92.
80. Taube F, Georgi JA, Kramer M, Stasik S, Middeke JM, Rollig C, et al. CEBPA mutations in 4708 patients with acute myeloid leukemia: differential impact of bZIP and TAD mutations on outcome. Blood. 2022;139(1):87–103.
81. Tawana K, Wang J, Renneville A, Bodor C, Hills R, Loveday C, et al. Disease evolution and outcomes in familial AML with germline CEBPA mutations. Blood. 2015;126(10):1214–23.
82. Tarlock K, Lamble AJ, Wang YC, Gerbing RB, Ries RE, Loken MR, et al. CEBPA-bZip mutations are associated with favorable prognosis in de novo AML: a report from the Children's Oncology Group. Blood. 2021;138(13):1137–47.
83. Schlenk RF, Taskesen E, van Norden Y, Krauter J, Ganser A, Bullinger L, et al. The value of allogeneic and autologous hematopoietic stem cell transplantation in prognostically favorable acute myeloid leukemia with double mutant CEBPA. Blood. 2013;122(9):1576–82.
84. Yoneda-Kato N, Look AT, Kirstein MN, Valentine MB, Raimondi SC, Cohen KJ, et al. The t(3;5)(q25.1;q34) of myelodysplastic syndrome and acute myeloid leukemia produces a novel fusion gene, NPM-MLF1. Oncogene. 1996;12(2):265–75.
85. Lim G, Choi JR, Kim MJ, Kim SY, Lee HJ, Suh JT, et al. Detection of t(3;5) and NPM1/MLF1 rearrangement in an elderly patient with acute myeloid leukemia: clinical and laboratory study with review of the literature. Cancer Genet Cytogenet. 2010;199(2):101–9.
86. Arber DA, Chang KL, Lyda MH, Bedell V, Spielberger R, Slovak ML. Detection of NPM/MLF1 fusion in t(3;5)-positive acute myeloid leukemia and myelodysplasia. Hum Pathol. 2003;34(8):809–13.
87. Darracq A, Pak H, Bourgoin V, Zmiri F, Dellaire G, Affar EB, et al. NPM and NPM-MLF1 interact with chromatin remodeling complexes and influence their recruitment to specific genes. PLoS Genet. 2019;15(11):e1008463.
88. Dumezy F, Renneville A, Mayeur-Rousse C, Nibourel O, Labis E, Preudhomme C. Acute myeloid leukemia with translocation t(3;5): new molecular insights. Haematologica. 2013;98(4):e52–4.
89. Nomdedeu J, Bussaglia E, Villamor N, Martinez C, Esteve J, Tormo M, et al. Immunophenotype of acute myeloid leukemia with NPM mutations: prognostic impact of the leukemic compartment size. Leuk Res. 2011;35(2):163–8.
90. Meyer C, Larghero P, Lopes BA, Marschalek R. The KMT2A/MLL consensus gene structure: a comprehensive update for research and diagnostic implications. Leukemia. 2024;38(6):1403–6.
91. Khoury JD, et al. Acute myeloid leukaemia with KMT2A rearrangement. In: WHO Classification of Tumours Editorial Board. Haematolymphoid tumours [Internet]. Lyon: International Agency for Research on Cancer; 2024 [cited 05 Nov 2025] (WHO classification of tumours series, 5th ed., vol. 11). Available from: https://tumourclassification.iarc.who.int/chaptercontent/63/41
92. Balgobind BV, Raimondi SC, Harbott J, Zimmermann M, Alonzo TA, Auvrignon A, et al. Novel prognostic subgroups in childhood 11q23/MLL-rearranged acute myeloid leukemia: results of an international retrospective study. Blood. 2009;114(12):2489–96.
93. Meyer C, Larghero P, Almeida Lopes B, Burmeister T, Groger D, Sutton R, et al. The KMT2A recombinome of acute leukemias in 2023. Leukemia. 2023;37(5):988–1005.
94. Yuen KY, Liu Y, Zhou YZ, Wang Y, Zhou DH, Fang JP, et al. Mutational landscape and clinical outcome of pediatric acute myeloid leukemia with 11q23/KMT2A rearrangements. Cancer Med. 2023;12(2):1418–30.

95. Pollard JA, Guest E, Alonzo TA, Gerbing RB, Loken MR, Brodersen LE, et al. Gemtuzumab ozogamicin improves event-free survival and reduces relapse in pediatric KMT2A-rearranged AML: results from the phase III Children's Oncology Group trial AAML0531. J Clin Oncol. 2021;39(28):3149–60.
96. Zhang RX, Huang HH, Zhang Y, Xia Y, Huang JY, Jiang CH, et al. Outcomes of acute myeloid leukemia with KMT2A (MLL) rearrangement: a multicenter study of TROPHY group. Blood Cancer J. 2025;15(1):84.
97. Gervais C, Murati A, Helias C, Struski S, Eischen A, Lippert E, et al. Acute myeloid leukaemia with 8p11 (MYST3) rearrangement: an integrated cytologic, cytogenetic and molecular study by the groupe francophone de cytogenetique hematologique. Leukemia. 2008;22(8):1567–75.
98. Coenen EA, Zwaan CM, Reinhardt D, Harrison CJ, Haas OA, de Haas V, et al. Pediatric acute myeloid leukemia with t(8;16)(p11;p13), a distinct clinical and biological entity: a collaborative study by the International-Berlin-Frankfurt-Munster AML-study group. Blood. 2013;122(15):2704–13.
99. Kayser S, Hills RK, Langova R, Kramer M, Guijarro F, Sustkova Z, et al. Characteristics and outcome of patients with acute myeloid leukaemia and t(8;16)(p11;p13): results from an International Collaborative Study. Br J Haematol. 2021;192(5):832–42.
100. Xie W, Hu S, Xu J, Chen Z, Medeiros LJ, Tang G. Acute myeloid leukemia with t(8;16)(p11.2;p13.3)/KAT6A-CREBBP in adults. Ann Hematol. 2019;98(5):1149–57.
101. Hu S, et al. Acute myeloid leukaemia with BCR::ABL1 fusion. In: WHO Classification of Tumours Editorial Board, editor. Haematolymphoid tumours [Internet], WHO classification of tumours series, vol. 11. 5th ed. Lyon: International Agency for Research on Cancer; 2024. Available from: https://tumourclassification.iarc.who.int/chaptercontent/63/45.
102. Alamri RM, Alanazi M, AlRajeh RK, Tashkandi SA, Alswayyed AF, Samman MA, et al. A rare presentation of BCR-ABL1 and RUNX1-MECOM rearrangement in a pediatric patient with acute myeloid leukemia. Clin Case Reports. 2024;12(5):e8917.
103. Sepúlveda-Robles O, Jiménez-Hernández E, Domínguez-Catzín V, Gómez-Flores E, Martín-Trejo JA, Flores-Lujano J, et al. Analytical study of RUNX1-RUNXT1, PML-RARA, CBFB-MYH11, BCR-ABL1^{p210}, and KMT2-MLLT3 in Mexican children with acute myeloid leukemia: a multicenter study of the Mexican interinstitutional group for the identification of the causes of childhood leukemia (MIGICCL). Front Pediatr. 2022;10:946690.
104. Soupir CP, Vergilio JA, Dal Cin P, Muzikansky A, Kantarjian H, Jones D, et al. Philadelphia chromosome-positive acute myeloid leukemia: a rare aggressive leukemia with clinicopathologic features distinct from chronic myeloid leukemia in myeloid blast crisis. Am J Clin Pathol. 2007;127(4):642–50.
105. Neuendorff NR, Burmeister T, Dorken B, Westermann J. BCR-ABL-positive acute myeloid leukemia: a new entity? Analysis of clinical and molecular features. Ann Hematol. 2016;95(8):1211–21.
106. Xue M, Wang Q, Huo L, Wen L, Yang X, Wu Q, et al. Clinical characteristics and prognostic significance of chronic myeloid leukemia with rare BCR-ABL1 transcripts. Leuk Lymphoma. 2019;60(12):3051–7.
107. Arun AK, Senthamizhselvi A, Mani S, Vinodhini K, Janet NB, Lakshmi KM, et al. Frequency of rare BCR-ABL1 fusion transcripts in chronic myeloid leukemia patients. Int J Lab Hematol. 2017;39(3):235–42.
108. Abla O, Ries RE, Triche T Jr, Gerbing RB, Hirsch B, Raimondi S, et al. Structural variants involving MLLT10 fusion are associated with adverse outcomes in pediatric acute myeloid leukemia. Blood Adv. 2024;8(8):2005–17.
109. Forgione MO, McClure BJ, Yeung DT, Eadie LN, White DL. MLLT10 rearranged acute leukemia: incidence, prognosis, and possible therapeutic strategies. Genes Chromosom Cancer. 2020; https://doi.org/10.1002/gcc.22887.
110. Okada Y, Feng Q, Lin Y, Jiang Q, Li Y, Coffield VM, et al. hDOT1L links histone methylation to leukemogenesis. Cell. 2005;121(2):167–78.

111. Deutsch JL, Heath JL. MLLT10 in benign and malignant hematopoiesis. Exp Hematol. 2020;87:1–12.
112. Deshpande AJ, Rouhi A, Lin Y, Stadler C, Greif PA, Arseni N, et al. The clathrin-binding domain of CALM and the OM-LZ domain of AF10 are sufficient to induce acute myeloid leukemia in mice. Leukemia. 2011;25(11):1718–27.
113. Conway AE, Haldeman JM, Wechsler DS, Lavau CP. A critical role for CRM1 in regulating HOXA gene transcription in CALM-AF10 leukemias. Leukemia. 2015;29(2):423–32.
114. Caudell D, Zhang Z, Chung YJ, Aplan PD. Expression of a CALM-AF10 fusion gene leads to Hoxa cluster overexpression and acute leukemia in transgenic mice. Cancer Res. 2007;67(17):8022–31.
115. Mark C, Meshinchi S, Joyce B, Gibson B, Harrison C, Bergmann AK, et al. Treatment outcomes of childhood PICALM::MLLT10 acute leukaemias. Br J Haematol. 2024;204(2):576–84.
116. Ma J, Liu YC, Voss RK, Ma J, Palagani A, Caldwell E, et al. Genomic and global gene expression profiling in pediatric and young adult acute leukemia with PICALM::MLLT10 Fusion. Leukemia. 2024;38(5):981–90.
117. Ben Abdelali R, Asnafi V, Petit A, Micol JB, Callens C, Villarese P, et al. The prognosis of CALM-AF10-positive adult T-cell acute lymphoblastic leukemias depends on the stage of maturation arrest. Haematologica. 2013;98(11):1711–7.
118. Asnafi V, Radford-Weiss I, Dastugue N, Bayle C, Leboeuf D, Charrin C, et al. CALM-AF10 is a common fusion transcript in T-ALL and is specific to the TCRgammadelta lineage. Blood. 2003;102(3):1000–6.
119. Sun H, Zhu Y, Li J, Zhao L, Yang G, Yan Z, et al. PICALM::MLLT10 may indicate a new subgroup of acute leukemias with miscellaneous immunophenotype and poor initial treatment response but showing sensitivity to venetoclax. EJHaem. 2024;5(3):565–72.
120. Bordereaux D, Fichelson S, Tambourin P, Gisselbrecht S. Alternative splicing of the Evi-1 zinc finger gene generates mRNAs which differ by the number of zinc finger motifs. Oncogene. 1990;5(6):925–7.
121. Kataoka K, Sato T, Yoshimi A, Goyama S, Tsuruta T, Kobayashi H, et al. Evi1 is essential for hematopoietic stem cell self-renewal, and its expression marks hematopoietic cells with long-term multilineage repopulating activity. J Exp Med. 2011;208(12):2403–16.
122. Goyama S, Yamamoto G, Shimabe M, Sato T, Ichikawa M, Ogawa S, et al. Evi-1 is a critical regulator for hematopoietic stem cells and transformed leukemic cells. Cell Stem Cell. 2008;3(2):207–20.
123. Castaño J, Aranda S, Bueno C, Calero-Nieto FJ, Mejia-Ramirez E, Mosquera JL, et al. GATA2 promotes hematopoietic development and represses cardiac differentiation of human mesoderm. Stem Cell Rep. 2019;13(3):515–29.
124. Vicente C, Conchillo A, García-Sánchez MA, Odero MD. The role of the GATA2 transcription factor in normal and malignant hematopoiesis. Crit Rev Oncol Hematol. 2012;82(1):1–17.
125. Yamazaki H, Suzuki M, Otsuki A, Shimizu R, Bresnick EH, Engel JD, et al. A remote GATA2 hematopoietic enhancer drives leukemogenesis in inv(3)(q21;q26) by activating EVI1 expression. Cancer Cell. 2014;25(4):415–27.
126. Wang HY, Rashidi HH. The new clinicopathologic and molecular findings in myeloid neoplasms with inv(3)(q21q26)/t(3;3)(q21;q26.2). Arch Pathol Lab Med. 2016;140(12):1404–10.
127. Morishita K, Parker DS, Mucenski ML, Jenkins NA, Copeland NG, Ihle JN. Retroviral activation of a novel gene encoding a zinc finger protein in IL-3-dependent myeloid leukemia cell lines. Cell. 1988;54(6):831–40.
128. Gröschel S, Sanders MA, Hoogenboezem R, de Wit E, Bouwman BAM, Erpelinck C, et al. A single oncogenic enhancer rearrangement causes concomitant EVI1 and GATA2 deregulation in leukemia. Cell. 2014;157(2):369–81.
129. D'Angiò M, Fazio G, Grioni A, Palamini S, Sala S, Galbiati M, et al. High EVI1 expression due to NRIP1/EVI1 fusion in therapy-related acute myeloid leukemia: description of the first pediatric case. Hema. 2020;4(5):e471.

130. Tang Z, Wang W, Yang S, El Achi H, Fang H, Nahmod KA, et al. 3q26.2/MECOM rearrangements by pericentric Inv(3): diagnostic challenges and clinicopathologic features. Cancers (Basel). 2023;15(2):458.
131. Yang JJ, Cho SY, Suh JT, Lee HJ, Lee WI, Yoon HJ, et al. Detection of RUNX1-MECOM fusion gene and t(3;21) in a very elderly patient having acute myeloid leukemia with myelodysplasia-related changes. Ann Lab Med. 2012;32(5):362–5.
132. Tang Z, Tang G, Hu S, Patel KP, Yin CC, Wang W, et al. Deciphering the complexities of MECOM rearrangement-driven chromosomal aberrations. Cancer Genet. 2019;233–234:21–31.
133. Conneely SE, Rau RE. The genomics of acute myeloid leukemia in children. Cancer Metastasis Rev. 2020;39(1):189–209.
134. Haferlach C, Bacher U, Grossmann V, Schindela S, Zenger M, Kohlmann A, et al. Three novel cytogenetically cryptic EVI1 rearrangements associated with increased EVI1 expression and poor prognosis identified in 27 acute myeloid leukemia cases. Genes Chromosom Cancer. 2012;51(12):1079–85.
135. Döhner H, Estey E, Grimwade D, Amadori S, Appelbaum FR, Büchner T, et al. Diagnosis and management of AML in adults: 2017 ELN recommendations from an international expert panel. Blood. 2017;129(4):424–47.
136. Rack KA, van den Berg E, Haferlach C, Beverloo HB, Costa D, Espinet B, et al. European recommendations and quality assurance for cytogenomic analysis of haematological neoplasms. Leukemia. 2019;33(8):1851–67.
137. Richard-Carpentier G, Rausch CR, Sasaki K, Hammond D, Morita K, Takahashi K, et al. Characteristics and clinical outcomes of patients with acute myeloid leukemia with inv(3)(q21q26.2) or t(3;3)(q21;q26.2). Haematologica. 2023;108(9):2331–42.
138. Rogers HJ, Vardiman JW, Anastasi J, Raca G, Savage NM, Cherry AM, et al. Complex or monosomal karyotype and not blast percentage is associated with poor survival in acute myeloid leukemia and myelodysplastic syndrome patients with inv(3)(q21q26.2)/t(3;3)(q21;q26.2): a Bone Marrow Pathology Group study. Haematologica. 2014;99(5):821–9.
139. Summerer I, Haferlach C, Meggendorfer M, Kern W, Haferlach T, Stengel A. Prognosis of MECOM (EVI1)-rearranged MDS and AML patients rather depends on accompanying molecular mutations than on blast count. Leuk Lymphoma. 2020;61(7):1756–9.
140. Lugthart S, van Drunen E, van Norden Y, van Hoven A, Erpelinck CA, Valk PJ, et al. High EVI1 levels predict adverse outcome in acute myeloid leukemia: prevalence of EVI1 overexpression and chromosome 3q26 abnormalities underestimated. Blood. 2008;111(8):4329–37.
141. Ho PA, Alonzo TA, Gerbing RB, Pollard JA, Hirsch B, Raimondi SC, et al. High EVI 1 expression is associated with MLL rearrangements and predicts decreased survival in paediatric acute myeloid leukaemia: a report from the Children's Oncology Group. Br J Haematol. 2013;162(5):670–7.
142. Elsherif M, Hammad M, Hafez H, Yassin D, Ashraf M, Yasser N, et al. MECOM gene overexpression in pediatric patients with acute myeloid leukemia. Acta Oncol. 2022;61(4):516–22.
143. Kim H. Treatments for children and adolescents with AML. Blood Res. 2020;55(S1):S5–s13.
144. Nagarajan R, Gerbing R, Alonzo T, Johnston DL, Aplenc R, Kolb EA, et al. Quality of life in pediatric acute myeloid leukemia: report from the Children's Oncology Group. Cancer Med. 2019;8(9):4454–64.
145. Bertrums EJM, Smith JL, Harmon L, Ries RE, Wang YJ, Alonzo TA, et al. Comprehensive molecular and clinical characterization of NUP98 fusions in pediatric acute myeloid leukemia. Haematologica. 2023;108(8):2044–58.
146. Kim N, Choi YJ, Cho H, Jang JE, Lee ST, Song J, et al. NUP98 is rearranged in 5.0% of adult East Asian patients with AML. Blood Adv. 2024;8(19):5122–5.
147. Hollink IH, van den Heuvel-Eibrink MM, Arentsen-Peters ST, Pratcorona M, Abbas S, Kuipers JE, et al. NUP98/NSD1 characterizes a novel poor prognostic group in acute myeloid leukemia with a distinct HOX gene expression pattern. Blood. 2011;118(13):3645–56.
148. Chatel G, Desai SH, Mattheyses AL, Powers MA, Fahrenkrog B. Domain topology of nucleoporin Nup98 within the nuclear pore complex. J Struct Biol. 2012;177(1):81–9.

149. Michmerhuizen NL, Klco JM, Mullighan CG. Mechanistic insights and potential therapeutic approaches for NUP98-rearranged hematologic malignancies. Blood. 2020;136(20):2275–89.
150. Gough SM, Slape CI, Aplan PD. NUP98 gene fusions and hematopoietic malignancies: common themes and new biologic insights. Blood. 2011;118(24):6247–57.
151. Tian J, Zhu Y, Li J, Yang G, Weng X, Huang T, et al. The landscape of NUP98 rearrangements clinical characteristics and treatment response from 1491 acute leukemia patients. Blood Cancer J. 2024;14(1):81.
152. Xiao W, Nardi V, Stein E, Hasserjian RP. A practical approach on the classifications of myeloid neoplasms and acute leukemia: WHO and ICC. J Hematol Oncol. 2024;17(1):56.
153. Chisholm KM, Smith J, Heerema-McKenney AE, Choi JK, Ries RE, Hirsch BA, et al. Pathologic, cytogenetic, and molecular features of acute myeloid leukemia with megakaryocytic differentiation: a report from the Children's Oncology Group. Pediatr Blood Cancer. 2023;70(5):e30251.
154. Noort S, Wander P, Alonzo TA, Smith J, Ries RE, Gerbing RB, et al. The clinical and biological characteristics of NUP98-KDM5A in pediatric acute myeloid leukemia. Haematologica. 2021;106(2):630–4.
155. Struski S, Lagarde S, Bories P, Puiseux C, Prade N, Cuccuini W, et al. NUP98 is rearranged in 3.8% of pediatric AML forming a clinical and molecular homogenous group with a poor prognosis. Leukemia. 2017;31(3):565–72.
156. Sheikhi M, Siyadat P, Rostami M, Sadeghian MH, Zahiri E, Ghorbani M, et al. Prognostic importance of NUP98-rearrangements in acute myeloid leukemia: a systematic review and meta-analysis. Caspian J Intern Med. 2024;15(4):579–88.
157. Wilcher KE, Page ERH, Privette Vinnedge LM. The impact of the chromatin binding DEK protein in hematopoiesis and acute myeloid leukemia. Exp Hematol. 2023;123:18–27.
158. Bruserud O, Reikvam H. NUP214 in acute myeloid leukemia. Cells. 2025;14(18):1461.
159. Matsushima T, Saitoh T, Karasawa M, Takizawa M, Miyawaki S, Nojima Y, et al. Effect of cytokines on growth and differentiation of leukaemic cells with translocation t(6;9)(p23;q34). Br J Haematol. 2001;115(4):812–6.
160. Chiriches C, Nicolaisen N, Wieske M, Elhaddad H, Mehmetbeyoglu E, Alvares C, et al. Understanding a high-risk acute myeloid leukemia by analyzing the interactome of its major driver mutation. PLoS Genet. 2022;18(10):e1010463.
161. Slovak ML, Gundacker H, Bloomfield CD, Dewald G, Appelbaum FR, Larson RA, et al. A retrospective study of 69 patients with t(6;9)(p23;q34) AML emphasizes the need for a prospective, multicenter initiative for rare 'poor prognosis' myeloid malignancies. Leukemia. 2006;20(7):1295–7.
162. Sandahl JD, Coenen EA, Forestier E, Harbott J, Johansson B, Kerndrup G, et al. t(6;9)(p22;q34)/DEK-NUP214-rearranged pediatric myeloid leukemia: an international study of 62 patients. Haematologica. 2014;99(5):865–72.
163. Tarlock K, Alonzo TA, Moraleda PP, Gerbing RB, Raimondi SC, Hirsch BA, et al. Acute myeloid leukaemia (AML) with t(6;9)(p23;q34) is associated with poor outcome in childhood AML regardless of FLT3-ITD status: a report from the Children's Oncology Group. Br J Haematol. 2014;166(2):254–9.
164. Ishiyama K, Takami A, Kanda Y, Nakao S, Hidaka M, Maeda T, et al. Prognostic factors for acute myeloid leukemia patients with t(6;9)(p23;q34) who underwent an allogeneic hematopoietic stem cell transplant. Leukemia. 2012;26(6):1416–9.
165. Zhang H, Zhan Q, Wang X, Gao F, Yu J, Wang J, et al. TLS/FUS-ERG fusion gene in acute leukemia and myelodysplastic syndrome evolved to acute leukemia: report of six cases and a literature review. Ann Hematol. 2022;101(12):2583–600.
166. Tomizawa D, Yoshida M, Kondo T, Miyamura T, Taga T, Adachi S, et al. Allogeneic hematopoietic stem cell transplantation for children and adolescents with high-risk cytogenetic AML: distinctly poor outcomes of FUS-ERG-positive cases. Bone Marrow Transplant. 2019;54(3):393–401.
167. Sotoca AM, Prange KH, Reijnders B, Mandoli A, Nguyen LN, Stunnenberg HG, et al. The oncofusion protein FUS-ERG targets key hematopoietic regulators and modulates the

all-trans retinoic acid signaling pathway in t(16;21) acute myeloid leukemia. Oncogene. 2016;35(15):1965–76.
168. Kong XT, Ida K, Ichikawa H, Shimizu K, Ohki M, Maseki N, et al. Consistent detection of TLS/FUS-ERG chimeric transcripts in acute myeloid leukemia with t(16;21)(p11;q22) and identification of a novel transcript. Blood. 1997;90(3):1192–9.
169. Ismael O, Shimada A, Elmahdi S, Elshazley M, Muramatsu H, Hama A, et al. RUNX1 mutation associated with clonal evolution in relapsed pediatric acute myeloid leukemia with t(16;21)(p11;q22). Int J Hematol. 2014;99(2):169–74.
170. Zerkalenkova E, Panfyorova A, Kazakova A, Baryshev P, Shelihova L, Kalinina I, et al. Molecular characteristic of acute leukemias with t(16;21)/FUS-ERG. Ann Hematol. 2018;97(6):977–88.
171. McNulty M, Crispino JD. Acute megakaryocytic leukemia. Cold Spring Harb Perspect Med. 2020;10(2)
172. Gruber TA, Larson Gedman A, Zhang J, Koss CS, Marada S, Ta HQ, et al. An Inv(16)(p13.3q24.3)-encoded CBFA2T3-GLIS2 fusion protein defines an aggressive subtype of pediatric acute megakaryoblastic leukemia. Cancer Cell. 2012;22(5):683–97.
173. Steinauer N, Guo C, Zhang J. The transcriptional corepressor CBFA2T3 inhibits all-trans-retinoic acid-induced myeloid gene expression and differentiation in acute myeloid leukemia. J Biol Chem. 2020;295(27):8887–900.
174. Thirant C, Ignacimouttou C, Lopez CK, Diop M, Le Mouel L, Thiollier C, et al. ETO2-GLIS2 hijacks transcriptional complexes to drive cellular identity and self-renewal in pediatric acute megakaryoblastic leukemia. Cancer Cell. 2017;31(3):452–65.
175. Masetti R, Bertuccio SN, Pession A, Locatelli F. CBFA2T3-GLIS2-positive acute myeloid leukaemia. A peculiar paediatric entity. Br J Haematol. 2019;184(3):337–47.
176. Khoury JD, et al. Acute myeloid leukaemia with other defined genetic alterations. In: WHO Classification of Tumours Editorial Board. Haematolymphoid tumours [Internet]. Lyon: International Agency for Research on Cancer; 2024 [cited 03 Nov 2025]. (WHO classification of tumours series, 5th ed., vol. 11). Available from: https://tumourclassification.iarc.who.int/chaptercontent/63/47
177. Smith JL, Ries RE, Hylkema T, Alonzo TA, Gerbing RB, Santaguida MT, et al. Comprehensive transcriptome profiling of cryptic CBFA2T3-GLIS2 fusion-positive AML defines novel therapeutic options: a COG and TARGET pediatric AML study. Clin Cancer Res. 2020;26(3):726–37.
178. Eidenschink Brodersen L, Alonzo TA, Menssen AJ, Gerbing RB, Pardo L, Voigt AP, et al. A recurrent immunophenotype at diagnosis independently identifies high-risk pediatric acute myeloid leukemia: a report from Children's Oncology Group. Leukemia. 2016;30(10):2077–80.
179. Ruglioni M, Crucitta S, Luculli GI, Tancredi G, Del Giudice ML, Mechelli S, et al. Understanding mechanisms of resistance to FLT3 inhibitors in adult FLT3-mutated acute myeloid leukemia to guide treatment strategy. Crit Rev Oncol Hematol. 2024;201:104424.
180. Small D. FLT3 mutations: biology and treatment. Hematology Am Soc Hematol Educ Program. 2006;2006:178–84.
181. Jalte M, Abbassi M, El Mouhi H, Daha Belghiti H, Ahakoud M, Bekkari H. FLT3 mutations in acute myeloid leukemia: unraveling the molecular mechanisms and implications for targeted therapies. Cureus. 2023;15(9):e45765.
182. Zwaan CM, Meshinchi S, Radich JP, Veerman AJ, Huismans DR, Munske L, et al. FLT3 internal tandem duplication in 234 children with acute myeloid leukemia: prognostic significance and relation to cellular drug resistance. Blood. 2003;102(7):2387–94.
183. Tarlock K, Gerbing RB, Ries RE, Smith JL, Leonti A, Huang BJ, et al. Prognostic impact of cooccurring mutations in FLT3-ITD pediatric acute myeloid leukemia. Blood Adv. 2024;8(9):2094–103.
184. Kennedy VE, Smith CC. FLT3 mutations in acute myeloid leukemia: key concepts and emerging controversies. Front Oncol. 2020;10:612880.

185. Zhang KN, Ma XH, Lu XX, Ruan GR, Wei FF, Jiang H, et al. Impact of FLT3-ITD molecular characteristics on the prognosis of patients with de novo acute myeloid leukemia. Blood. 2024;144:5940–1.
186. Patnaik MM. The importance of FLT3 mutational analysis in acute myeloid leukemia. Leuk Lymphoma. 2018;59(10):2273–86.
187. Xu LH, Fang JP, Liu YC, Jones AI, Chai L. Nucleophosmin mutations confer an independent favorable prognostic impact in 869 pediatric patients with acute myeloid leukemia. Blood Cancer J. 2020;10(1):1.
188. Hock H, Shimamura A. ETV6 in hematopoiesis and leukemia predisposition. Semin Hematol. 2017;54(2):98–104.
189. Baens M, Peeters P, Guo C, Aerssens J, Marynen P. Genomic organization of TEL: the human ETS-variant gene 6. Genome Res. 1996;6(5):404–13.
190. Biswas A, Rajesh Y, Mitra P, Mandal M. ETV6 gene aberrations in non-haematological malignancies: a review highlighting ETV6 associated fusion genes in solid tumors. Biochim Biophys Acta Rev Cancer. 2020;1874(1):188389.
191. Xue S, Sun HP, Huang XB, Chen X, Wang T, Ma W, et al. Characteristics and literature review of ETV6::ABL1 fusion gene-positive acute myeloid leukemia. Int J Hematol. 2024;119(5):564–72.
192. Monovich AC, Gurumurthy A, Ryan RJH. The diverse roles of ETV6 alterations in B-lymphoblastic leukemia and other hematopoietic cancers. Adv Exp Med Biol. 2024;1459:291–320.
193. Espersen ADL, Noren-Nystrom U, Abrahamsson J, Ha SY, Pronk CJ, Jahnukainen K, et al. Acute myeloid leukemia (AML) with t(7;12)(q36;p13) is associated with infancy and trisomy 19: data from Nordic Society for Pediatric Hematology and Oncology (NOPHO-AML) and review of the literature. Genes Chromosom Cancer. 2018;57(7):359–65.
194. Tosi S, Mostafa Kamel Y, Owoka T, Federico C, Truong TH, Saccone S. Paediatric acute myeloid leukaemia with the t(7;12)(q36;p13) rearrangement: a review of the biological and clinical management aspects. Biomark Res. 2015;3:21.
195. Ostlund A, Waraky A, Staffas A, Sjogren H, De Moerloose B, Arad-Cohen N, et al. Characterization of pediatric acute myeloid leukemia with t(7;12)(q36;p13). Genes Chromosom Cancer. 2024;63(11):e70003.
196. Ragusa D, Dijkhuis L, Pina C, Tosi S. Mechanisms associated with t(7;12) acute myeloid leukaemia: from genetics to potential treatment targets. Biosci Rep. 2023;43(1):BSR20220489.
197. Wang T, Chen X, Hui S, Ni J, Yin Y, Cao W, et al. Ectopia associated MN1 fusions and aberrant activation in myeloid neoplasms with t(12;22)(p13;q12). Cancer Gene Ther. 2020;27(10–11):810–8.
198. Cools J, Mentens N, Odero MD, Peeters P, Wlodarska I, Delforge M, et al. Evidence for position effects as a variant ETV6-mediated leukemogenic mechanism in myeloid leukemias with a t(4;12)(q11-q12;p13) or t(5;12)(q31;p13). Blood. 2002;99(5):1776–84.
199. Johnston DL, Alonzo TA, Gerbing RB, Hirsch B, Heerema NA, Ravindranath Y, et al. Outcome of pediatric patients with acute myeloid leukemia (AML) and -5/5q- abnormalities from five pediatric AML treatment protocols: a report from the Children's Oncology Group. Pediatr Blood Cancer. 2013;60(12):2073–8.
200. Hasle H, Alonzo TA, Auvrignon A, Behar C, Chang M, Creutzig U, et al. Monosomy 7 and deletion 7q in children and adolescents with acute myeloid leukemia: an international retrospective study. Blood. 2007;109(11):4641–7.
201. Kendrick TS, Buic D, Fuller KA, Erber WN. Abnormalities in chromosomes 5 and 7 in myelodysplastic syndrome and acute myeloid leukemia. Ann Lab Med. 2025;45(2):133–45.
202. Lai F, Godley LA, Joslin J, Fernald AA, Liu J, Espinosa R 3rd, et al. Transcript map and comparative analysis of the 1.5-Mb commonly deleted segment of human 5q31 in malignant myeloid diseases with a del(5q). Genomics. 2001;71(2):235–45.
203. Barlow JL, Drynan LF, Trim NL, Erber WN, Warren AJ, McKenzie AN. New insights into 5q- syndrome as a ribosomopathy. Cell Cycle. 2010;9(21):4286–93.

204. Mori M, Kubota Y, Durmaz A, Gurnari C, Goodings C, Adema V, et al. Genomics of deletion 7 and 7q in myeloid neoplasm: from pathogenic culprits to potential synthetic lethal therapeutic targets. Leukemia. 2023;37(10):2082–93.
205. Blink M, Zimmermann M, von Neuhoff C, Reinhardt D, de Haas V, Hasle H, et al. Normal karyotype is a poor prognostic factor in myeloid leukemia of Down syndrome: a retrospective, international study. Haematologica. 2014;99(2):299–307.
206. Kalra R, Dale D, Freedman M, Bonilla MA, Weinblatt M, Ganser A, et al. Monosomy 7 and activating RAS mutations accompany malignant transformation in patients with congenital neutropenia. Blood. 1995;86(12):4579–86.
207. Pezeshki A, Podder S, Kamel R, Corey SJ. Monosomy 7/del (7q) in inherited bone marrow failure syndromes: a systematic review. Pediatr Blood Cancer. 2017;64(12):10.1002/pbc.26714.
208. Sahoo SS, Pastor VB, Goodings C, Voss RK, Kozyra EJ, Szvetnik A, et al. Clinical evolution, genetic landscape and trajectories of clonal hematopoiesis in SAMD9/SAMD9L syndromes. Nat Med. 2021;27(10):1806–17.
209. Wlodarski MW, Sahoo SS, Niemeyer CM. Monosomy 7 in pediatric myelodysplastic syndromes. Hematol Oncol Clin North Am. 2018;32(4):729–43.
210. Alaggio R, Amador C, Anagnostopoulos I, Attygalle AD, Araujo IBO, Berti E, et al. The 5th edition of the World Health Organization classification of haematolymphoid tumours: lymphoid neoplasms. Leukemia. 2022;36(7):1720–48.
211. Haferlach T, et al. Acute myeloid leukaemia, myelodysplasia-related. In: WHO Classification of Tumours Editorial Board. Haematolymphoid tumours [Internet]. Lyon: International Agency for Research on Cancer; 2024 [cited 02 Nov 2025]. (WHO classification of tumours series, 5th ed., vol. 11). Available from: https://tumourclassification.iarc.who.int/chaptercontent/63/47.
212. Barajas JM, Rasouli M, Umeda M, Hiltenbrand R, Abdelhamed S, Mohnani R, et al. Acute myeloid leukemias with UBTF tandem duplications are sensitive to menin inhibitors. Blood. 2024;143(7):619–30.
213. Duployez N, Vasseur L, Kim R, Largeaud L, Passet M, L'Haridon A, et al. UBTF tandem duplications define a distinct subtype of adult de novo acute myeloid leukemia. Leukemia. 2023;37(6):1245–53.
214. Aplenc R, Meshinchi S, Sung L, Alonzo T, Choi J, Fisher B, et al. Bortezomib with standard chemotherapy for children with acute myeloid leukemia does not improve treatment outcomes: a report from the Children's Oncology Group. Haematologica. 2020;105(7):1879–86.
215. Hsiao HH, Yang MY, Liu YC, Hsiao HP, Tseng SB, Chao MC, et al. RBM15-MKL1 (OTT-MAL) fusion transcript in an adult acute myeloid leukemia patient. Am J Hematol. 2005;79(1):43–5.
216. Saito Y, Makita S, Chinen S, Kito M, Fujino T, Ida H, et al. Acute megakaryoblastic leukaemia with t(1;22)(p13.3;q13.1)/RBM15-MKL1 in an adult patient following a non-mediastinal germ cell tumour. Br J Haematol. 2020;190(6):e329–e32.
217. Rahman NT, Schulz VP, Wang L, Gallagher PG, Denisenko O, Gualdrini F, et al. MRTFA augments megakaryocyte maturation by enhancing the SRF regulatory axis. Blood Adv. 2018;2(20):2691–703.
218. Long X, Hu B, Zhu S, Wu Y, Wang T. RNA binding motif protein 15 (RBM15): structure, function and its research progress in tumors. Int J Gen Med. 2025;18:3635–49.
219. Ma X, Renda MJ, Wang L, Cheng EC, Niu C, Morris SW, et al. Rbm15 modulates Notch-induced transcriptional activation and affects myeloid differentiation. Mol Cell Biol. 2007;27(8):3056–64.
220. Carroll A, Civin C, Schneider N, Dahl G, Pappo A, Bowman P, et al. The t(1;22) (p13;q13) is nonrandom and restricted to infants with acute megakaryoblastic leukemia: a Pediatric Oncology Group Study. Blood. 1991;78(3):748–52.
221. Duchayne E, Fenneteau O, Pages MP, Sainty D, Arnoulet C, Dastugue N, et al. Acute megakaryoblastic leukaemia: a national clinical and biological study of 53 adult and child-

hood cases by the Groupe Francais d'Hematologie Cellulaire (GFHC). Leuk Lymphoma. 2003;44(1):49–58.
222. de Rooij JD, Masetti R, van den Heuvel-Eibrink MM, Cayuela JM, Trka J, Reinhardt D, et al. Recurrent abnormalities can be used for risk group stratification in pediatric AMKL: a retrospective intergroup study. Blood. 2016;127(26):3424–30.
223. Khan I, Amin MA, Eklund EA, Gartel AL. Regulation of HOX gene expression in AML. Blood Cancer J. 2024;14(1):42.
224. Juul-Dam KL, Shukla NN, Cooper TM, Cuglievan B, Heidenreich O, Kolb EA, et al. Therapeutic targeting in pediatric acute myeloid leukemia with aberrant HOX/MEIS1 expression. Eur J Med Genet. 2023;66(12):104869.
225. de Rooij JD, Branstetter C, Ma J, Li Y, Walsh MP, Cheng J, et al. Pediatric non-Down syndrome acute megakaryoblastic leukemia is characterized by distinct genomic subsets with varying outcomes. Nat Genet. 2017;49(3):451–6.
226. Rasouli M, Troester S, Grebien F, Goemans BF, Zwaan CM, Heidenreich O. NUP98 oncofusions in myeloid malignancies: an update on molecular mechanisms and therapeutic opportunities. Hema. 2024;8(9):e70013.
227. Bansal D, Scholl C, Frohling S, McDowell E, Lee BH, Dohner K, et al. Cdx4 dysregulates Hox gene expression and generates acute myeloid leukemia alone and in cooperation with Meis1a in a murine model. Proc Natl Acad Sci USA. 2006;103(45):16924–9.
228. Balgobind BV, Hollink IH, Arentsen-Peters ST, Zimmermann M, Harbott J, Beverloo HB, et al. Integrative analysis of type-I and type-II aberrations underscores the genetic heterogeneity of pediatric acute myeloid leukemia. Haematologica. 2011;96(10):1478–87.
229. Berman JN, Gerbing RB, Alonzo TA, Ho PA, Miller K, Hurwitz C, et al. Prevalence and clinical implications of NRAS mutations in childhood AML: a report from the Children's Oncology Group. Leukemia. 2011;25(6):1039–42.
230. Chen Y, Yin Z, Westover KD, Zhou Z, Shu L. Advances and challenges in RAS signaling targeted therapy in leukemia. Mol Cancer Ther. 2025;24(1):33–46.
231. Alawieh D, Cysique-Foinlan L, Willekens C, Renneville A. RAS mutations in myeloid malignancies: revisiting old questions with novel insights and therapeutic perspectives. Blood Cancer J. 2024;14(1):72.
232. Kaburagi T, Yamato G, Shiba N, Yoshida K, Hara Y, Tabuchi K, et al. Clinical significance of RAS pathway alterations in pediatric acute myeloid leukemia. Haematologica. 2022;107(3):583–92.
233. Paquette RL, Landaw EM, Pierre RV, Kahan J, Lubbert M, Lazcano O, et al. N-ras mutations are associated with poor prognosis and increased risk of leukemia in myelodysplastic syndrome. Blood. 1993;82(2):590–9.
234. Bowen DT, Frew ME, Hills R, Gale RE, Wheatley K, Groves MJ, et al. RAS mutation in acute myeloid leukemia is associated with distinct cytogenetic subgroups but does not influence outcome in patients younger than 60 years. Blood. 2005;106(6):2113–9.
235. Bacher U, Haferlach T, Schoch C, Kern W, Schnittger S. Implications of NRAS mutations in AML: a study of 2502 patients. Blood. 2006;107(10):3847–53.
236. Rivera D, Kim K, Kanagal-Shamanna R, Borthakur G, Montalban-Bravo G, Daver N, et al. Implications of RAS mutational status in subsets of patients with newly diagnosed acute myeloid leukemia across therapy subtypes. Am J Hematol. 2022;97(12):1599–606.
237. Gaidzik VI, Bullinger L, Schlenk RF, Zimmermann AS, Rock J, Paschka P, et al. RUNX1 mutations in acute myeloid leukemia: results from a comprehensive genetic and clinical analysis from the AML study group. J Clin Oncol. 2011;29(10):1364–72.
238. Greif PA, Konstandin NP, Metzeler KH, Herold T, Pasalic Z, Ksienzyk B, et al. RUNX1 mutations in cytogenetically normal acute myeloid leukemia are associated with a poor prognosis and up-regulation of lymphoid genes. Haematologica. 2012;97(12):1909–15.
239. Sendker S, Awada A, Domagalla S, Sendker M, Orhan E, Hoffmeister LM, et al. RUNX1 mutation has no prognostic significance in paediatric AML: a retrospective study of the AML-BFM study group. Leukemia. 2023;37(7):1435–43.

240. Rungjirajittranon T, Siriwannangkul T, Kungwankiattichai S, Leelakanok N, Rotchanapanya W, Vittayawacharin P, et al. Clinical outcomes of acute myeloid leukemia patients harboring the RUNX1 mutation: is it still an unfavorable prognosis? A cohort study and meta-analysis. Cancers (Basel). 2022;14(21):5239.
241. Yamato G, Shiba N, Yoshida K, Hara Y, Shiraishi Y, Ohki K, et al. RUNX1 mutations in pediatric acute myeloid leukemia are associated with distinct genetic features and an inferior prognosis. Blood. 2018;131(20):2266–70.
242. Ho PA, Zeng R, Alonzo TA, Gerbing RB, Miller KL, Pollard JA, et al. Prevalence and prognostic implications of WT1 mutations in pediatric acute myeloid leukemia (AML): a report from the Children's Oncology Group. Blood. 2010;116(5):702–10.
243. Hollink IH, van den Heuvel-Eibrink MM, Zimmermann M, Balgobind BV, Arentsen-Peters ST, Alders M, et al. Clinical relevance of Wilms tumor 1 gene mutations in childhood acute myeloid leukemia. Blood. 2009;113(23):5951–60.
244. Owen C, Fitzgibbon J, Paschka P. The clinical relevance of Wilms Tumour 1 (WT1) gene mutations in acute leukaemia. Hematol Oncol. 2010;28(1):13–9.
245. Yang L, Han Y, Suarez Saiz F, Minden MD. A tumor suppressor and oncogene: the WT1 story. Leukemia. 2007;21(5):868–76.
246. Ariyaratana S, Loeb DM. The role of the Wilms tumour gene (WT1) in normal and malignant haematopoiesis. Expert Rev Mol Med. 2007;9(14):1–17.
247. Rampal R, Alkalin A, Madzo J, Vasanthakumar A, Pronier E, Patel J, et al. DNA hydroxymethylation profiling reveals that WT1 mutations result in loss of TET2 function in acute myeloid leukemia. Cell Rep. 2014;9(5):1841–55.
248. Herlin MK, Kjeldsen E, Abrahamsson J, Arad-Cohen N, Cheuk D, De Moerloose B, et al. Characteristics and prognosis of paediatric normal karyotype acute myeloid leukaemia: a NOPHO-DBH AML study. Br J Haematol. 2025;207(4):1454–63.
249. Schwede M, Jahn K, Kuipers J, Miles LA, Bowman RL, Robinson T, et al. Mutation order in acute myeloid leukemia identifies uncommon patterns of evolution and illuminates phenotypic heterogeneity. Leukemia. 2024;38(7):1501–10.
250. Schrezenmeier J, Huntly BJP. Epigenetic dysregulation in acute myeloid leukemia. Semin Hematol. 2025;62(3):177–86.
251. Xu H, Wen Y, Jin R, Chen H. Epigenetic modifications and targeted therapy in pediatric acute myeloid leukemia. Front Pediatr. 2022;10:975819.
252. Liu W, Wu G, Xiong F, Chen Y. Advances in the DNA methylation hydroxylase TET1. Biomark Res. 2021;9(1):76.
253. Andersson AK, Miller DW, Lynch JA, Lemoff AS, Cai Z, Pounds SB, et al. IDH1 and IDH2 mutations in pediatric acute leukemia. Leukemia. 2011;25(10):1570–7.
254. Issa GC, DiNardo CD. Acute myeloid leukemia with IDH1 and IDH2 mutations: 2021 treatment algorithm. Blood Cancer J. 2021;11(6):107.
255. Zhao X, Liu HQ, Wang LN, Yang L, Liu XL. Current and emerging molecular and epigenetic disease entities in acute myeloid leukemia and a critical assessment of their therapeutic modalities. Semin Cancer Biol. 2022;83:121–35.
256. Wang N, Li X, She C, Zhang J. Research progress on the mechanisms of CSF3R mutations in leukemogenesis and treatment strategies. Cancer Cell Int. 2025;25(1):304.
257. Medina EA, Delma CR, Yang FC. ASXL1/2 mutations and myeloid malignancies. J Hematol Oncol. 2022;15(1):127.
258. Roberts I.A.G and Hitzler JK. Myeloid proliferations associated with Down syndrome. In: WHO Classification of Tumours Editorial Board. Haematolymphoid tumours [Internet]. Lyon: International Agency for Research on Cancer; 2024 [cited 19 Oct 2025]. (WHO classification of tumours series, 5th ed., vol. 11). Available from: https://tumourclassification.iarc.who.int/chaptercontent/44/10
259. Greene ME, Mundschau G, Wechsler J, McDevitt M, Gamis A, Karp J, et al. Mutations in GATA1 in both transient myeloproliferative disorder and acute megakaryoblastic leukemia of Down syndrome. Blood Cells Mol Dis. 2003;31(3):351–6.

260. Gamis AS, Alonzo TA, Gerbing RB, Hilden JM, Sorrell AD, Sharma M, et al. Natural history of transient myeloproliferative disorder clinically diagnosed in Down syndrome neonates: a report from the Children's Oncology Group Study A2971. Blood. 2011;118(26):6752–9. quiz 996
261. Klusmann JH, Creutzig U, Zimmermann M, Dworzak M, Jorch N, Langebrake C, et al. Treatment and prognostic impact of transient leukemia in neonates with Down syndrome. Blood. 2008;111(6):2991–8.
262. Massey GV, Zipursky A, Chang MN, Doyle JJ, Nasim S, Taub JW, et al. A prospective study of the natural history of transient leukemia (TL) in neonates with Down syndrome (DS): Children's Oncology Group (COG) study POG-9481. Blood. 2006;107(12):4606–13.
263. Taub JW, Berman JN, Hitzler JK, Sorrell AD, Lacayo NJ, Mast K, et al. Improved outcomes for myeloid leukemia of Down syndrome: a report from the Children's Oncology Group AAML0431 trial. Blood. 2017;129(25):3304–13.
264. Uffmann M, Rasche M, Zimmermann M, von Neuhoff C, Creutzig U, Dworzak M, et al. Therapy reduction in patients with Down syndrome and myeloid leukemia: the international ML-DS 2006 trial. Blood. 2017;129(25):3314–21.
265. Lange BJ, Kobrinsky N, Barnard DR, Arthur DC, Buckley JD, Howells WB, et al. Distinctive demography, biology, and outcome of acute myeloid leukemia and myelodysplastic syndrome in children with Down syndrome: Children's Cancer Group Studies 2861 and 2891. Blood. 1998;91(2):608–15.
266. Forestier E, Izraeli S, Beverloo B, Haas O, Pession A, Michalova K, et al. Cytogenetic features of acute lymphoblastic and myeloid leukemias in pediatric patients with Down syndrome: an iBFM-SG study. Blood. 2008;111(3):1575–83.
267. Li J, Kalev-Zylinska ML. Advances in molecular characterization of myeloid proliferations associated with Down syndrome. Front Genet. 2022;13:891214.
268. Baruchel A, Bourquin JP, Crispino J, Cuartero S, Hasle H, Hitzler J, et al. Down syndrome and leukemia: from basic mechanisms to clinical advances. Haematologica. 2023;108(10):2570–81.
269. Kosmidou A, Tragiannidis A, Gavriilaki E. Myeloid leukemia of Down syndrome. Cancers (Basel). 2023;15(13):3265.
270. Yoshida K, Toki T, Okuno Y, Kanezaki R, Shiraishi Y, Sato-Otsubo A, et al. The landscape of somatic mutations in Down syndrome-related myeloid disorders. Nat Genet. 2013;45(11):1293–9.
271. Wechsler J, Greene M, McDevitt MA, Anastasi J, Karp JE, Le Beau MM, et al. Acquired mutations in GATA1 in the megakaryoblastic leukemia of Down syndrome. Nat Genet. 2002;32(1):148–52.
272. Hasle H, Abrahamsson J, Arola M, Karow A, O'Marcaigh A, Reinhardt D, et al. Myeloid leukemia in children 4 years or older with Down syndrome often lacks GATA1 mutation and cytogenetics and risk of relapse are more akin to sporadic AML. Leukemia. 2008;22(7):1428–30.
273. Picos Cardenas VJ, Meza Espinoza JP, Garibaldi Covarrubias RF, Barajas Torres RL, Gonzalez Garcia JR. Transient myeloproliferative disorder progression and acquired chromosomal abnormalities in children with Down syndrome. Pediatr Blood Cancer. 2012;59(5):962–3.
274. Moassass F, Wafa A, Liehr T, Al-Ablog A, Al Achkar W. Down syndrome associated childhood myeloid leukemia with yet unreported acquired chromosomal abnormalities and a new potential adverse marker: dup(1)(q25q44). Mol Cytogenet. 2018;11:22.
275. de Souza DC, de Figueiredo AF, Ney Garcia DR, da Costa ES, Othman MAK, Liehr T, et al. A unique set of complex chromosomal abnormalities in an infant with myeloid leukemia associated with Down syndrome. Mol Cytogenet. 2017;10:35.
276. Zwaan CM, Kaspers GJ, Pieters R, Hahlen K, Janka-Schaub GE, van Zantwijk CH, et al. Different drug sensitivity profiles of acute myeloid and lymphoblastic leukemia and normal peripheral blood mononuclear cells in children with and without Down syndrome. Blood. 2002;99(1):245–51.

277. Vardiman JW, Thiele J, Arber DA, Brunning RD, Borowitz MJ, Porwit A, et al. The 2008 revision of the World Health Organization (WHO) classification of myeloid neoplasms and acute leukemia: rationale and important changes. Blood. 2009;114(5):937–51.
278. Vardiman JW, Harris NL, Brunning RD. The World Health Organization (WHO) classification of the myeloid neoplasms. Blood. 2002;100(7):2292–302.
279. Döhner H, Wei AH, Appelbaum FR, Craddock C, DiNardo CD, Dombret H, et al. Diagnosis and management of AML in adults: 2022 recommendations from an international expert panel on behalf of the ELN. Blood. 2022;140(12):1345–77.
280. Egan G, Tasian SK. Precision medicine for high-risk gene fusions in pediatric AML: a focus on KMT2A, NUP98, and GLIS2 rearrangements. Blood. 2025;145(22):2574–86.
281. van de Pol JJ, Schulpen M, Goemans BF, Kaspers G, Karim-Kos HE, Zwaan CM. Outcome of children with relapsed acute myeloid leukemia improved over time in the Netherlands between 1998 and 2018. Ejc Paediatr Oncol. 2023;1:100010.
282. Rao M, Luo W, Luo C, Wu B, Xu T, Wei Z, et al. Prognostic factors and outcomes in pediatric acute myeloid leukemia: a comprehensive bibliometric analysis of global research trends. Front Oncol. 2025;15:1466818.

CAR T-Cell Analysis

16

Weijie Li

Introduction

Chimeric antigen receptor T-cell (CAR-T) therapy is one of the most successful examples of applying innovative research achievements to the treatment of leukemia and other malignancies in the field of oncology. Most of the CAR-Ts are autologous, that is, generated from patients' own T cells. The process of CAR-T treatments starts with collecting T cells from patients through leukapheresis. The collected T cells are then genetically modified ex vivo, with gene constructs coding for CARs transduced by a viral vector. The CAR-Ts expressing tumor antigen-specific CAR are expanded ex vivo and then infused into patients to attack and kill tumor cells in vivo (Fig. 16.1). The key element of CAR-T therapy is CAR, a synthetic immunoreceptor that directs T cells to recognize the tumor antigen, activate, proliferate, and attack tumor cells [1]. The basic structure of a CAR consists of three main components: (1) the extracellular single-chain antibody variable fragment (scFv) specific to tumor antigen and a hinge, (2) the transmembrane domain, and (3) the intracellular signaling domain (Fig. 16.2). Although this basic structural frame remains the same, the intracellular domain has evolved with the progress in CAR development. First-generation CARs contain a single CD3-zeta chain. Second-generation CARs include an additional costimulatory domain, such as CD28 or 4-1BB, and third-generation CARs contain two costimulatory molecules [2–4]. Fourth-generation CARs include additional genetic modifications adding features such as constitutive or inducible cytokine secretion and surface costimulatory receptors to improve their performance [4].

W. Li (✉)
Department of Pathology and Laboratory Medicine, Children's Mercy Kansas City, Kansas City, Missouri, USA

University of Missouri–Kansas City School of Medicine, Kansas City, Missouri, USA
e-mail: wli@cmh.edu

W. Li (ed.), *Laboratory Assessments of Pediatric Leukemia*,
https://doi.org/10.1007/978-3-032-26557-9_16

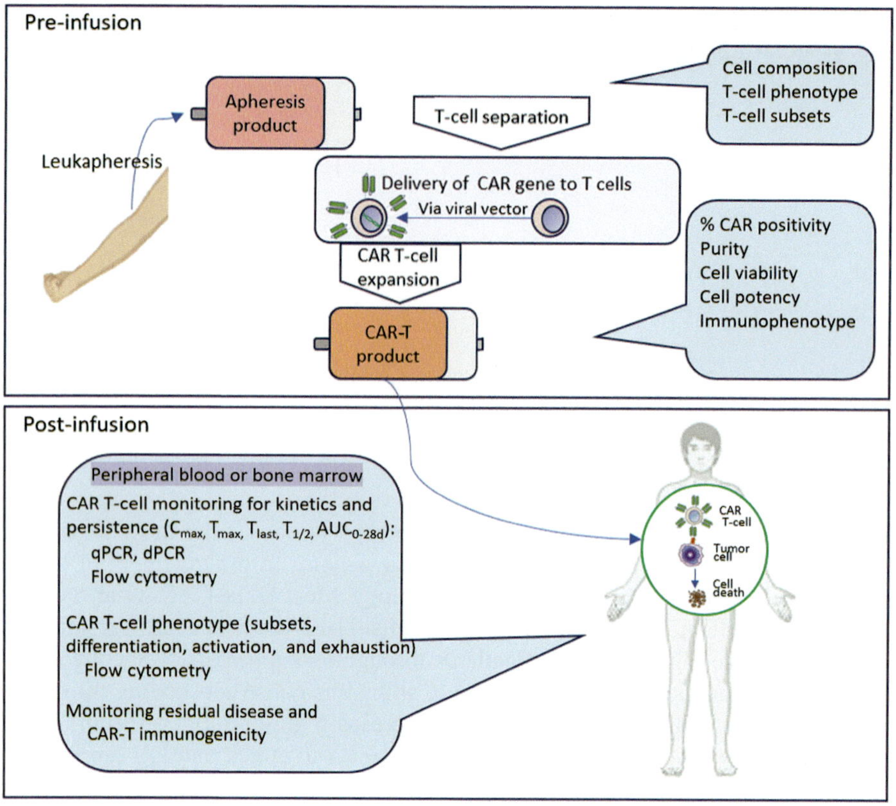

Fig. 16.1 Process of CAR T-cell therapy and related laboratory assessments. The patient's T-cells are collected through a leukapheresis process. The apheresis product is assessed for cell composition, T-cell count, and T-cell phenotype/subsets. The separated T-cells are modified ex vivo by introducing a CAR-coding gene construct via a viral vector. The CAR T-cell product is accessed for transduction efficiency, purity, viability, potency, and phenotypic characterization. After being infused back into patients, the CAR T-cells are monitored for cellular kinetics and persistence by quantitative PCR/digital PCR and/or a flow cytometry method. Phenotypic features and subsets of the CAR T-cells are assessed by flow cytometry. Also monitored are residual disease and CAR T-cell immunogenicity

Many CAR-T therapies have been developed and extensively studied in clinical trials worldwide. Promising therapeutic outcomes have been observed in CAR-T treatments for hematologic malignancies [5–7], leading to the approval of seven CAR-T therapies by the US Food and Drug Administration (FDA). Of these FDA-approved CAR-T products, five are anti-CD19 CAR-T therapies designed for treating relapsed or refractory B-cell leukemias or lymphomas, including tisagenlecleucel, lisocabtagene maraleucel, axicabtagene ciloleucel, obecabtagene autoleucel, and brexucabtagene autoleucel. Two are anti-B-cell maturation antigen (BCMA) CAR-T therapies, ciltacabtagene autoleucel and idecabtagene vicleucel, for the treatment of relapsed or refractory multiple myeloma. Many more are expected to be approved

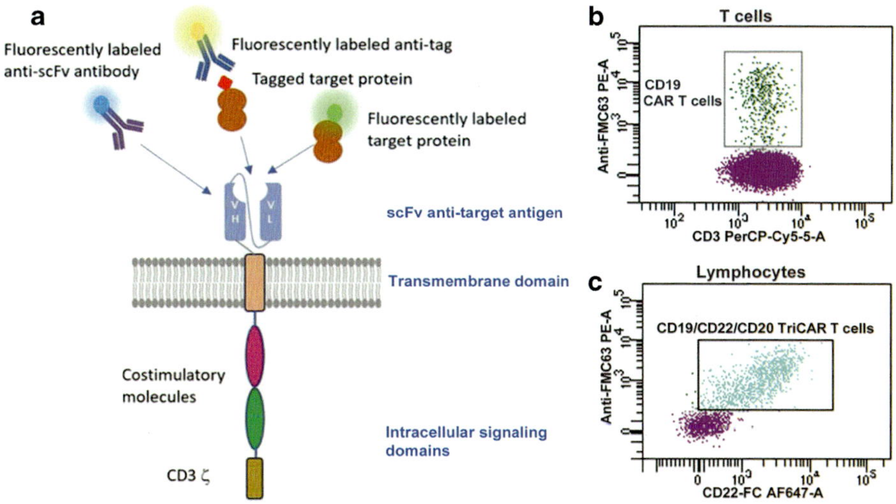

Fig. 16.2 CAR T-cell detection by flow cytometry. (**a**) Basic CAR structure and commonly used CAR-staining agents. (**b**) Dot plot of flow cytometry detection of anti-CD19 CAR T-cells by PE-conjugated monoclonal antibody against FMC63 scFv. (**c**) Dot plot of flow cytometry detection of CD19/CD22/CD20 TriCAR T-cells by PE-conjugated anti-FMC63 antibody and AF647-conjugated human CD22-FC protein

in the future. However, not all patients respond well to CAR-T therapies, and there are safety concerns related to their use, including potential toxicities such as cytokine release syndrome (CRS) and immune effector cell-associated neurotoxicity syndrome (ICANS) [8].

Laboratory assessments are critically important to the success of CAR-T therapy, and indeed, every step of the treatment needs proper laboratory tests (Fig. 16.1). Before the procedure begins, the selected patients are tested for complete blood counts, lymphocyte subset composition, and T-cell count. Based on the estimated T-cell number, a proposed volume of apheresis sample is aimed to obtain enough T cells for the treatment. The apheresis sample is analyzed for cell composition, T-cell count, T-cell subsets, and potential phenotypes prior to the experiment of CAR gene incorporation. The genetically modified T cells (CAR-T products) are evaluated for transduction efficiency, purity, cell viability, cell potency, and phenotypic characterization. After infusion, the CAR-Ts are monitored via polymerase chain reaction (PCR)-based and/or flow cytometry (FCM) assays for cellular kinetics and persistence in vivo. The post-infusion CAR-Ts are also phenotypically characterized by FCM to illustrate the subset composition of CAR-Ts and their activation and exhaustion status. Additionally, tests are also needed to monitor measurable residual disease (MRD), cytotoxicity, and CAR-T immunogenicity. For details on the methods and clinical significance of MRD detection, please refer to Chaps. 8, 9 and 10. This chapter provides an overview of laboratory assessments of CAR-T therapies with an emphasis on CAR-T detection assays.

CAR T-Cell Detection

It is important to evaluate CAR-Ts in CAR-T products to ensure they meet the required quality standards, which is usually done by the manufacturers before they release the products. Monitoring CAR-Ts in vivo after infusion also offers significant clinical relevance. The CAR-T cellular kinetics and phenotypic features are important factors in predicting therapeutic response and durability. There are a variety of CAR-T detection methods described in published research studies or clinical trials [9]. Among them, FCM and quantitative polymerase chain reaction (qPCR) are the two most useful techniques because they are well established and widely available [5, 10–12]. The two methods correlate well with each other for the quantification of CAR-Ts [12–17]. Occasional specimens are positive by qPCR but negative or at a much lower level by FCM. These discordances are likely related to the lower sensitivity of FCM methods. A relatively newer PCR technique, digital PCR (dPCR), has been applied in CAR-T detection recently due to its several advantages. The PCR-based assays measure CAR transgene on a genomic level, while the FCM approaches detect CAR expression on the cell surface. The key features, advantages, and disadvantages of these CAR-T detection methods are listed in Table 16.1.

CAR T-Cell Detection by Flow Cytometry

FCM is a powerful technique capable of providing rapid multi-parameter analysis of single cells. FCM CAR-T assays allow for the assessment of CAR expression at a cellular level, and they offer the benefits of absolute CAR-T cell counting and simultaneous phenotypic characterization of CAR-Ts. Moreover, FCM is fast,

Table 16.1 Key features, advantages, and disadvantages of the CAR T-cell detection methods

Method	Flow cytometry	Quantitative PCR	Digital PCR
Key features	Measure CAR expression at the cellular level Single-cell analysis using specific anti-CAR antibody or recombinant CAR-targeted protein LLOQ can reach 0.01% of total T cells [18]	Detect CAR transgene at the genomic level Singleplex or duplex real-time PCR using specific primers and probes targeting CAR transgene and a reference gene Calculate CAR TCN based on Ct and standard curve LLOQ can reach 2 TCN/ug gDNA, and 100 TCN/mL blood [19]	Partition gDNA sample into many tiny droplets Run PCR in each droplet and read the endpoint result as positive or negative Calculate TCN by Poisson statistical analysis LLOQ can reach 0.1 TCN/ug gDNA [20]

(continued)

Table 16.1 (continued)

Method	Flow cytometry	Quantitative PCR	Digital PCR
Advantages	Measure functional CAR (expression) level Fast turnaround time Widely available Simultaneous phenotypic analysis	Sensitive Easy standardization Wide analytic range	Sensitive and accurate Absolute quantitation No need for standard curve Less affected by PCR inhibitors Improved PCR efficiency and precision
Limitations	Need fresh/viable samples Require high level of expertise Limited sensitivity Limited standardization Interference from monoclonal antibody therapies	Unable to assess CAR expression Need calibrating curve Matrix interference	Unable to assess CAR expression Smaller analytic range More expensive Longer running time

Abbreviations: *CAR* chimeric antigen receptor, *LLOQ* lower limit of quantitation, *gDNA* genomic DNA, *TCN* transgene copy number, *Ct* cycle threshold

widely available, and relatively sensitive. The drawbacks of FCM assays include difficulty in standardization, the requirement of fresh viable samples, and a high level of expertise. The method development and validation of FCM assays should follow the Clinical and Laboratory Standards Institute (CLSI) guideline [21], general recommendations for FCM assays [22, 23], and specific recommendations for FCM CAR-T analysis [24].

Critical Reagents

The critical reagents for developing FCM CAR-T assays are the CAR-staining agents, which determine the assay specificity and sensitivity. Multiple reagents have been used for this purpose in published research or clinical studies, and many of them or similar products are commercially available now [4, 9, 24]. Generic immunoglobulin (Ig)-binding agents such as protein-L and polyclonal anti-IgG antibodies have been used in some CAR-T studies [25, 26], though they are not ideal for monitoring CAR-T cellular kinetics because of their high levels of nonspecific staining and limited sensitivity [12]. Anti-idiotype antibodies and antigen-based reagents (target proteins) are the two types of CAR-specific staining agents most useful for monitoring in vivo CAR-T expansion and persistence (Fig. 16.2).

Most anti-idiotype antibodies for CAR-T assays bind the variable region of the scFv of a CAR and exhibit high specificity with low nonspecific binding. The monoclonal antibody against anti-CD19 CAR FMC63 (Fig. 16.2b) has been commonly used to detect anti-CD19 CAR-Ts in preclinical and clinical studies [10], and the limit of detection (LOD) can reach 0.1–0.01% of total T cells [18, 27]. The advantages of anti-idiotype antibodies include high reagent stability, low nonspecific staining, flexibility in panel design, and compatibility with staining methods other than FCM. Nevertheless, the generation of antibodies is complicated and time-consuming, and very limited anti-CAR antibodies are available commercially.

A biosynthetic target protein can bind the CAR specifically and be used as a CAR-staining agent (Fig. 16.2a, c). Most are chimeric proteins with an N-terminal target antigen fused to an Fc C-terminal fragment. Antigen-Fc can be labeled by a protein tag, such as biotin or histidine, and the assay is completed by a second staining step [14, 15]. Alternatively, the antigen-Fc can be directly conjugated to a fluorochrome, and save the secondary staining step (Fig. 16.2c). The two-step staining assay for anti-CD19 CAR-Ts has been reported to have better sensitivity and specificity than the one-step direct staining assay [15]. Antigen-Fc can show functional CAR binding, is flexible in panel design for FCM assays, and is especially useful in independently measuring the expression of each CAR in dual CAR-Ts [28]. The disadvantages of antigen-Fc include being relatively expensive, likely less stable in solution than antibodies, possible incompatibility with Fc receptor blocking solution, and possible nonspecific binding to Fc receptors of cells. Some antigen-Fcs may not work in TransFix-treated samples [29].

Panels

The panel of an FCM CAR-T assay is designed based on the intended use. FCM CAR-T assays are primarily intended for two purposes: to evaluate CAR-T products (pre-infusion) and to assess CAR-T cellular kinetics (post-infusion). The assays for the first purpose are primarily performed at manufacturers' or GMP facilities, whereas reference labs or local clinical labs conduct the assays mainly for the second purpose. The assays used to evaluate CAR-T products should be able to measure important product features such as purity, viability, stability, potency, and immunophenotype. The assay should also be able to distinguish CAR-expressing T cells from other unwanted CAR-expressing cell types [30]. The panel for this purpose should include a viability dye, the CAR staining agent, CD3, CD4, CD8, and markers for other cell types such as CD19, CD14, and CD56. The assays intended for CAR-T cellular kinetics should have the ability to detect and quantify circulating CAR-Ts at low levels and characterize the phenotype of these cells. The assay should be designed for rare-event detection. The basic panel should include a viability dye, CAR-staining agent, CD3, CD19, and CD45. Using FMO for the CAR-staining agent is recommended to facilitate the gating strategy. The expanded panel can include additional markers to assess CAR-T subset composition and differentiation status (helper/cytotoxic: CD4, CD8; naïve/memory: CD27, CD45RA, CD45RO, CD62L; and proliferation/activation/exhaustion markers such as CD25, CD279, CD223, BTLA), and other cell type-specific markers. Given the possible presence of a limited quantity of the specimen, the panel including markers for simultaneous detection of residual disease is also beneficial. Given the possibility of downregulation or loss of the targeted antigen in leukemia cells, it is crucial to design a panel capable of capturing leukemia cells with these changes for residual disease detection. The CAR staining agents should be conjugated to a bright fluorochrome if possible and properly titrated to ensure optimal resolution. Panel design should follow the guidelines and recommendations for the current best practices for FCM assays [18, 21].

Specimen Stability and Controls

For CAR-T product analysis, the samples are usually tested within several hours after production, and there is no need for stability assessment. For CAR-T cellular kinetic assays, the specimens may require long-distance delivery, delaying testing by 1 or 2 days after collection, and thus, specimen stability should be evaluated. The most common specimen for CAR-T kinetic assay is peripheral blood (PB). Bone marrow (BM) and cerebrospinal fluid (CSF) may also be collected for this test. Lymph nodes or other tissue specimens may be collected on rare occasions. Spiked samples, as used frequently in method development and validation, are not recommended for stability assessment because the stability of spiked CAR-Ts does not represent that of circulating CAR-Ts [18].

Two types of samples are typically used as positive controls for FCM CAR-T assays: transduced cell lines with stable CAR expression and CAR-T products generated from patients. CAR-expressing cell lines are commercially available and useful for early assay optimization, including titration of the reagents and assessment of the specificity. However, their use as a control is limited in developing appropriate gating and/or quantification strategies and assay validation because of their different biological matrices and lack of T-cell antigen expression profiles. CAR-T products and/or their spiked samples should be used as better quality controls.

Quantitation, Reporting Units, and Sensitivity

The values of CAR-Ts are commonly expressed as the percentage of total T cells by FCM CAR-T assays. Absolute numeration of CAR-Ts and reporting the results by the number of CAR-Ts per milliliter of blood are also possible when analyzing blood specimens. The enumeration can be performed through a single platform by using quantification beads or a two-platform approach by using the percentages of CAR-Ts and lymphocytes and the white blood cell (WBC) count from the hematology analyzer or other cell counters. Given that lymphopenia is commonly seen in CAR-T-treated patients, the unit of CAR-T number per milliliter of blood likely more accurately reflects the dynamic changes of CAR-T levels in vivo.

Since this assay is designed to quantitate CAR-Ts, the analytical sensitivity should be determined, and it should include the limit of blank (LOB), the limit of detection (LOD), and the lower limit of quantification (LLOQ). LOB means the highest signal that could be detected in the blank samples. LOD is the lowest concentration that can be distinguished from the background, while LLOQ refers to the lowest concentration at which the assay can quantify the analyte at accepted levels of precision and accuracy. LOD and LOB are determined by running the blank specimens from healthy donors or patients, and a minimum of 10–20 samples in triplicate from at least three different donors/patients are recommended to run [18]. The LOB can be calculated by adding 1.645SD to the mean value of the blank specimens. The LOD can be determined using the mean value of blank specimens plus 3SD [23]. At least three blank specimens spiked with CAR-Ts at ≥5 concentrations are recommended to run in triplicate for LLOQ evaluation [18, 21, 23]. The LLOQ of a CAR-T assay is defined as the lowest concentration at which CAR expression is detected in all triplicates with a coefficient of variation (CV) <30–35% [18]. Both the frequency of the population (% of total T cells) and the number of target events need evaluation for LLOQ.

Assay sensitivity is influenced by the frequency of the cell population of interest, the overall assay specificity, and the system background [23]. For rare event assays, analytical sensitivity is proportional to the total number of cells/events acquired. Since patients receiving CAR-T treatments typically have lymphopenia, the assay optimization should establish the target and minimal numbers of cells to be acquired.

Accuracy, Specificity, and Selectivity

Accuracy is the degree of closeness of a measured value to the true value of the analyte. The accuracy of a CAR-T assay can be assessed by comparing the results with the expected values of a series of dilutional samples. The comparison of the results to those of an alternative method, such as qPCR or those from another laboratory, should also be performed, if possible. The tests should include at least three samples with low, medium, and high concentrations for comparison, and the samples should be split and tested in parallel by different assays. The degree of agreement between the assays can be assessed using nonparametric analysis since the readouts from different platforms can be quite different, and linear regression analysis should also be performed. The acceptance criteria depend on the alternative methods used. The specificity of an FCM CAR-T assay refers to its ability to measure CAR-Ts specifically. Selectivity refers to the ability of the assay to correctly identify CAR-Ts without interference by other substances present in the sample or disease states. The selectivity and specificity should be assessed in the assay development stage, and their assessment can use the accuracy experiment data [18].

Precision

The precision of CAR-T assays should be assessed at different levels across the analytic range following published guidelines and recommendations [21–23]. The assessment should include intra-assay precision (within-run precision, repeatability), inter-assay precision (between-run precision, reproducibility), inter-operator, and inter-instrument variation. The tests should include three to six negative PB and/or BM samples spiked with CAR-Ts with concentrations spanning the expected range. The results from the experiments for sensitivity and accuracy evaluation can be used for precision evaluation. The target acceptable assay imprecision is a CV < 10–25%, and it can be adjusted based on intended use [18, 21].

Assay Validation

The extent of the validation process depends on the intended use (CAR-T product characterization vs CAR-T cellular kinetics analysis), the regulatory requirements, the regulatory setting, and the risk to patient care [21, 31]. The laboratory director should determine what validation parameters should be evaluated and what acceptance criteria should be followed. The validation should include at least accuracy, precision, specificity, sensitivity, and specimen stability.

CAR T-Cell Detection by qPCR

The real-time qPCR technique amplifies and quantifies a gene sequence using target-specific primers and fluorescent probes. Based on the amplicon fluorescence signal at the end of each PCR cycle, the absolute copy number of the target (compared to a standard curve) or relative copy number (compared to the reference gene) can be measured (Fig. 16.3a). qPCR can measure transgene copy number (TCN) in CAR-T products to assess transduction efficiency, or in patients' post-infusion specimens for CAR-T cellular kinetic analysis. With good method design and optimization, the qPCR CAR detection assay is sensitive and easy to perform with a fast turnaround time, a wide analytic range, good accuracy, and precision. However, qPCR cannot tell whether the CAR is expressed (functional), and if other cell types also carry CAR, and cannot evaluate CAR-T phenotype (Table 16.1).

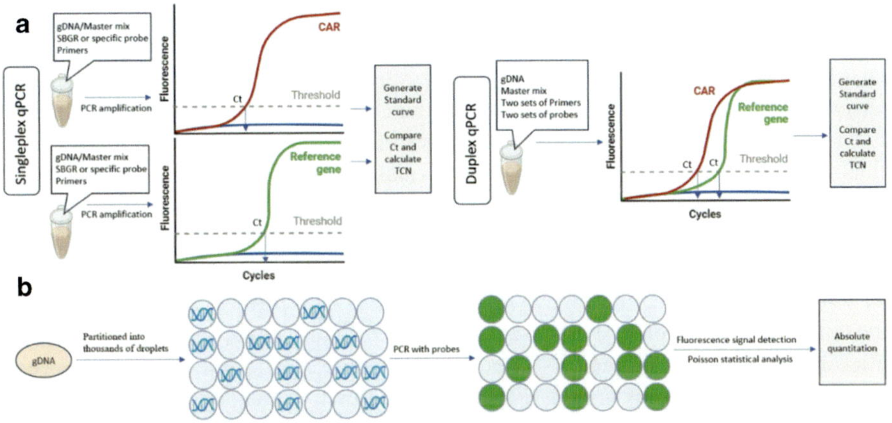

Fig. 16.3 CAR transgene copy number (TCN) detection by real-time quantitative PCR (qPCR) and digital PCR (dPCR). (**a**) qPCR amplifies the target gene sequence from genomic DNA (gDNA) and measures the fluorescent signal at the end of each cycle. The copy number of the target is calculated by its cycle threshold (Ct) compared with standards from a standard curve. In the singleplex assay, the CAR transgene and reference gene are amplified separately, allowing the use of either a sequence-specific probe or a general fluorescent double-stranded DNA-binding dye, such as SYBR Green (SBGR). In the duplex assay, CAR transgene and the reference gene are amplified in the same reaction system using two sets of specific primers/probes. (**b**) In a dPCR assay, the gDNA sample is partitioned into thousands of droplets where the PCR amplification occurs. Each droplet contains zero or one target template. After amplification, droplets containing the template are detected by fluorescence and read as positive, and droplets without a fluorescence signal are read as negative. Poisson statistical analysis of the binary data generates absolute quantitation of the target sequence

Method Development and Critical Reagents

There are two types of setups for a qPCR assay: singleplex and multiplex. In a singleplex assay, the target gene and reference gene (normalizer) are amplified separately, so that they do not interfere with each other. Multiplex qPCR assays allow simultaneous detection of both the transgene and the reference gene in one system, providing benefits of reduced consumption of samples and reagents, and decreased inter-assay variation. The reference gene used to normalize TCN values should be consistently and reproducibly detected at the level expected for a given amount of gDNA extracted from normal diploid cells. Both singleplex and duplex qPCR assays were developed for CAR-T detection. An anti-CD19 CAR assay with two qPCR reactions amplifying the FMC63 region of anti-CD19 CAR and GAPDH separately achieved a detection limit of 10 CAR TCNs/μL blood [32]. A duplex qPCR assay targeting anti-CD19 CAR and RPPH1 (normalizer) achieved similar efficiency to the corresponding singleplex setup [33].

The optimization of a qPCR assay includes evaluating PCR efficiency, temperatures of the reaction, and the LOD and LLOQ. PCR efficiency refers to how effectively the target DNA is amplified in each cycle, and it is typically measured by the slope of a standard curve generated from a series of dilutions from a positive sample. A slope of −3.32 on a log scale corresponds to an amplification efficiency of 100%, meaning that the amount of PCR product doubles with each cycle. Efficiency should be targeted to at least 90% [34], and an efficiency within a range of 90–110% (standard curve slope −3.6 to −3.1) is considered acceptable historically for a typical qPCR assay [35]. If a PCR efficiency significantly exceeds 100%, possible causes include contamination, aberrant product formation, and pipetting mistakes.

Critical reagents for CAR-T qPCR assays include primers, probes, master mix, gDNA extraction reagents, calibrators, and quality controls. A generic qPCR assay targeting the provirus sequence of the viral vector or a shared CAR junction sequence can be used for research studies. For clinical studies, the primers and probes should be designed to target the specific transgene sequences, especially the scFv region or the junction of two different genes. The primers and probes can be chosen based on the published assays. For an original design, the process starts in silico by checking available DNA sequence databases. The selected primer/probe sets are then evaluated by testing a set of created positive and negative samples. The PCR product should be confirmed by size and sequence to ensure specific amplification by selected primers. The selection of primers and assay optimization can follow the published standard procedures [36]. It is important to optimize the gDNA extraction procedure for the best yield and high quality. Column-based extraction kits should be avoided because of the clotting issue commonly seen with biological specimens. The selection of the master mix also affects the efficiency and robustness of a qPCR assay. Many different master mixes are commercially available, and the selection should be determined through experiments.

Specimens, Standards and Controls, Sample Stability

The specimens for CAR-T qPCR assays include CAR-T products, patients' post-infusion PB, and, less commonly, BM, CSF, or lymph nodes. Given the commonly present lymphopenia, the gDNA yield is usually low for the PB samples from CAR-T-treated patients. The minimal amount of gDNA needed for each qPCR reaction should be determined. It is recommended that the standard calibrators should include at least six levels in triplicate, spanning the quantitation range and including LLOQ and upper limit of quantitation (ULOQ). For a qPCR assay targeting the CAR transgene, the standard calibrators and quality controls are made from negative human gDNA samples spiked with plasmids encoding the CAR transgene. For a reference gene qPCR assay, the standard calibrators and quality controls are generated by spiking plasmids encoding the reference gene into surrogate mammalian gDNA samples. The linear plasmids should be as pure as possible because any contamination will likely lead to inaccurate concentration measurement. The stability of specimens, calibrators, and control samples should be assessed for freeze/thaw, short-term, and long-term storage, and proper storage and freeze/thaw conditions should be written in the protocol.

Reporting Units and Sensitivity

The commonly used reporting unit for qPCR assays is copies of the target gene per microgram of gDNA. This unit may not accurately represent the CAR-T cellular kinetics because of the dramatic changes in blood gDNA levels due to lymphocyte-depletion treatment before CAR-T infusion and rapid CAR-T expansion after infusion [37]. The unit of copies per milliliter of blood or microgram of tissue is likely more appropriate for characterizing CAR-T cellular kinetics [37, 38]. If possible, the results should be reported using both units for a clinical study.

LOB, LOD, and LLOQ are required for the sensitivity evaluation of qPCR assays intended for evaluating CAR-T cellular kinetics. They should be measured during method development and confirmed in method validation following the guidelines published [39, 40]. The US FDA recommends that, for preclinical or clinical assessment of a gene therapy product, the qPCR assay should have a LLOQ of ≤50 copies/μg gDNA [41]. This sensitivity should be the target for a qPCR assay developed for CAR-T cellular kinetics. The assay sensitivity is affected by the amount of gDNA used for the PCR reaction. Therefore, minimal and maximal amounts of gDNA for each reaction should be determined during method development.

Specificity, Accuracy, and Precision

Specificity, accuracy, and precision should be determined during method development and confirmed at method validation. Specificity is the key consideration for selecting ideal primers and probes at the method development stage. The selected primer/probe sets should be evaluated by testing a set of generated positive and negative samples. The PCR product should be confirmed by size and sequence. Each reaction should include a negative control to monitor assay specificity and possible contamination. Accuracy and precision should be evaluated by repeated tests using representative samples (human gDNA for CAR and rat gDNA for reference gene) spiked with positive material with resulting concentrations across the analytical ranges. The positive material used for this purpose can be the CAR-T products or plasmids as described for calibrators and quality controls. The assessment should include at least six independent runs in triplicate with sample concentrations including ULOQ, a high-level control, a mid-level control, a low-level control, and LLOQ [42, 43]. The acceptance criteria can be defined through statistical analysis of the results of multiple experimental runs. It is ideal to compare the results to those performed on the split samples using another method or by another laboratory.

Validation

The validation of qPCR assays can follow the general rules of published regulatory guidance for quantitative bioanalytical methods [44–46]. However, these guidelines address the validation process of bioanalytical methods with a focus on chromatographic assays and ligand binding assays, and may not apply to certain parameters of qPCR assays. More specific recommendations for qPCR and dPCR have been developed by American Association of Pharmaceutical Scientists (AAPS) workshops and published recently [35, 42], and they are a good resource to consult for the development and validation of CAR-T qPCR or dPCR assays.

CAR T-Cell Detection by dPCR

dPCR is a relatively new PCR technique characterized by extensive sample splitting and Poisson statistical analysis [47]. The sample is partitioned into thousands of tiny droplets, where the target DNA sequence is amplified with a setup similar to qPCR. The fluorescence signal (positive or negative) is collected for each droplet at the endpoint of the reaction, and the Poisson statistical analysis of the data generates absolute quantitation of the target (Fig. 16.3b). dPCR has become a preferred technique in some research and clinical studies because of its analytical advantages compared with qPCR (Table 16.1). It provides absolute quantitation without the need for a calibrating curve. It is less susceptible to the presence of PCR inhibitors and shows increased precision and sensitivity. The drawbacks of dPCR include its smaller analytic range, longer running time, and higher cost compared with qPCR.

Several published studies have demonstrated that dPCR is a better method than qPCR in anti-CD19 CAR detection and quantitation [17, 48, 49]. Using a series of dilutional standards and PB samples from CAR-T-treated patients, a Chinese team assessed the key performance parameters of both the dPCR and qPCR assays they developed. The same primer/probe sets targeting anti-CD19 CAR and POP4 (reference gene) were used in both assays. They found that the two methods demonstrated good correlation and linearity across the analytical range, and dPCR showed higher precision and lower LOD [48]. A recently published duplex dPCR assay targeting the FMC63 region of anti-CD19 CAR and JAK2 (reference gene) tested samples collected at various time points post-CAR-T infusion from patients with B-cell lymphoma. The results demonstrated that dPCR had a higher sensitivity (0.01%) than FCM (0.1%) and qPCR assay (1%) [17]. Another recently published study described dPCR assays for three anti-CD19 CAR-T products, targeting the junction region between the transmembrane and intracellular signaling domains. These assays demonstrated high sensitivity (LOD: 20 copies/μg DNA) and robust quantification of CAR-Ts from a variety of specimens [49]. Similar to qPCR, the results expressed as copy numbers per microgram gDNA should be interpreted in view of cell populations in the samples since they are highly impacted by the proportion of non-CAR-T cell types in the assessed tissue.

dPCR shares the same principles for assay development and method validation with qPCR [35, 42], with a few exceptions. dPCR offers absolute quantification and does not need calibrating curves to extrapolate the copy numbers of transgenes and reference genes. Given the absence of a standard curve, dPCR should have a quality control sample at the LLOQ level to verify the performance of each run at that limit.

CAR T-Cell Cellular Kinetics and Persistence In Vivo

CAR-Ts are different from other therapeutic antibodies or small molecules, which decrease in vivo over time. CAR-Ts are "living drugs" that can grow in vivo with rapid expansion after infusion and persist for months or even years. The characteristics of the CAR-T cellular kinetics are associated with clinical therapeutic efficacy and toxicity, and therefore, evaluation of CAR-T cellular kinetics is clinically important. The parameters of CAR-T cellular kinetics include the area under the curve from day 0 to day 28 post-infusion (AUC0–28d), peak/maximum concentration (*C*max), the time when *C*max is observed (*T*max), the last time when CAR-T is detected (Tlast), the concentration of CAR-Ts in the last detectable sample (Clast), and the half-life of CAR-T (T1/2).

After infusion, the anti-CD19 CAR-Ts usually undergo a fast expansion till days 7–14, followed by a rapid decrease till day 20 by FCM and/or PCR-based detection assays (Fig. 16.4) [50–53]. There may be a slight difference in expansion rate among the CAR-Ts with different co-stimulatory domains [53]. Many studies have demonstrated a positive correlation between CAR T-cell expansion and therapeutic responses, that is, higher *C*max and/or larger AUC0-28d by FCM or qPCR/dPCR assays in well-responding patients than those in non-responding patients [50–52, 54–57]. However, no convincing association between peak expansion and therapeutic responses has been found in a few studies [53, 58–60]. This discordance may be attributed to the differences in the number of patients included, features of the patients (disease type/location and treatment history), or study design and methodology. Higher tumor burden is usually associated with greater CAR-T expansion and more severe CRS and ICANS [13, 51, 54]. There is no association identified between the dose of CAR-Ts infused and in vivo peak CAR-T expansion [51, 59].

Anti-CD19 CAR-Ts target malignant CD19+ B cells as well as normal B cells, leading to B-cell aplasia. Therefore, B-cell aplasia can be used as a surrogate marker for functional persistence of CD19-targeted CAR-Ts. Loss of B-cell aplasia is associated with an increased risk of CD19+ relapse in B-ALL patients with anti-CD19 CAR-T treatment [61, 62]. The application of sensitive PCR-based CAR detection assays makes low-level CAR-T detection and CAR-T long-term persistence monitoring possible. Indeed, CAR-Ts can persist in vivo for a long time, and they can be

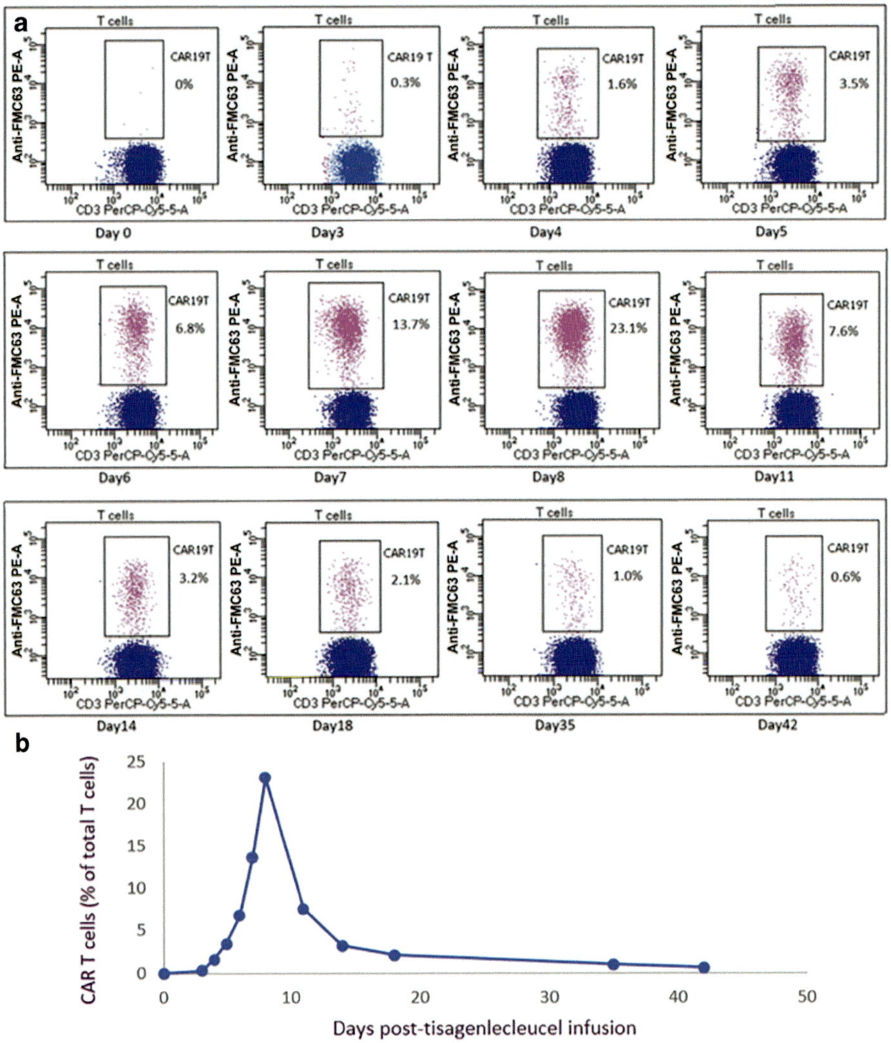

Fig. 16.4 CAR T-cell cellular kinetics by flow cytometry analysis. (**a**) Dot plots and CAR T-cell values from day 0 to day 42 post-tisagenlecleucel infusion. (**b**) The curve shows dynamic changes of CAR T-cell numbers after tisagenlecleucel infusion

detected years after infusion [13, 63]. The longer persistence is associated with better event-free survival [13, 63].

CAR T-Cell Phenotypic Characterization and Its Association with Therapeutic Response

The proliferation and survival abilities of the CAR-Ts are critically important to CAR-T therapeutic effectiveness, and they are affected by the differentiation status of the cells. A higher complete response rate is associated with increased frequency of CD27+CD45RO-CD8+ T cells in leukapheresis products [52, 64]. In the studies of CD19-targeted CAR-T treatments, the responder and non-responder patients exhibited different gene expression profiles in T cell differentiation and metabolism [52, 65]. Specifically, CAR-T products from responders of CLL patients displayed increased expression in memory-related genes, while those from non-responders showed increased gene expression involved in effector T-cell differentiation, glycolysis, exhaustion, and apoptosis [52]. The CAR-T products from large B-cell lymphoma patients with good responses demonstrated higher frequencies of memory CD8+ T cells than those from patients with partial or no response, and high-grade ICANS was associated with the presence of a rare monocyte-like cell population [65]. The expression of exhaustion markers PD1, TIM3, and LAG3 in the leukapheresis and/or CAR-T products has been associated with reduced efficacy of CAR-T treatments in several studies [52, 55, 65].

After infusion, CAR-Ts encounter the targeted antigen, become activated, and undergo rapid expansion (Fig. 16.4). At *T*max, CAR-Ts usually show a reduced CD4/CD8 ratio, an increase in effector memory T-cells, decreased proportion of central memory T-cells, and the acquisition of an activated and exhausted phenotype [53, 66, 67]. Elevation of CAR-T-regulatory cells is associated with therapy failure or early relapse [58, 68]. Interestingly, different from pre-infusion CAR-Ts, increased expression of PD1 and LAG3 in CD4+ CAR-Ts at *T*max has been found to be associated with increased event-free survival [53]. CD107a, also known as lysosomal-associated membrane protein-1, correlates with the cytolytic activity of T-cells when expressed on the cell surface. The reduction in CD107a in CD8+ CAR-Ts at *T*max correlated with increased event-free survival [53].

Immunogenicity of CAR T-Cells and Laboratory Detection

The expressed components of CAR constructs can induce humoral and cellular immune responses, which can cause a safety issue, and may negatively impact CAR-T expansion and persistence as well as clinical response [69, 70]. The non-human sequences in the CAR constructs, such as the scFv domain, are the major culprit for CAR immunogenicity [71, 72]. In most reported cases, especially in patients with relapse after CAR-T therapy, the immune response was against the scFv of murine origin. Cytotoxic T cells targeting CAR have also been detected, and their presence has been associated with immunological rejection of CAR-Ts, leading to disease progression [73]. Immune response against CAR-Ts impedes the success of repeat dosing and affects the therapeutic efficacy. However, some studies showed no significant impact of CAR immunogenicity on CAR-T expansion and CAR-T therapeutic response. The study in patients treated with tisagenlecleucel demonstrated a high frequency (>80%) of pre-existing anti-murine CAR (mCAR) antibodies and over 30% of the patients showing infusion-induced or boosted humoral immunogenicity [51]. The pre-existing or treatment-induced anti-mCAR19 antibodies did not affect efficacy, safety, cellular kinetics of tisagenlecleucel, or duration of remission [50, 51, 74]. The CAR-Ts in patients with identified anti-CAR cellular immune response showed sustained anti-leukemic effects, raising the question about the significant impact of immune rejection on treatment outcomes [54]. Therefore, the clinical significance of CAR immunogenicity should be further studied, and it may vary depending on the type of CAR-T used, disease type, patient conditions, and extent of the immune response.

The humoral immunogenicity can be detected by ligand-binding assays. The patient's serum is added to wells of a plate coated with the recombinant CAR protein. Following incubation and wash steps, the bound antibody is detected by an enzymatic, fluorescent, or chemiluminescent readout method. However, the recombinant CAR protein may not accurately represent the CAR physical structure expressed on the cell surface in vivo. FCM is likely a better method for this purpose [75]. The patients' serum or plasma samples are incubated with CAR-expressing cell lines, and the anti-CAR antibodies are then detected with fluorochrome-conjugated anti-human IgG monoclonal antibodies. The assay should include a non-transfected cell line sample to measure nonspecific binding. The pre-infusion specimen should be evaluated to detect pre-existing anti-CAR antibodies. Data can be reported qualitatively (positive or negative) or semi-quantitatively as the expression level. The results are compared to and often normalized by pre-infusion levels for measuring CAR-T therapy-induced immune response. The method development and validation of CAR immunogenicity assays should follow the FDA regulatory guidelines [76].

Conclusion

CAR-T analyses evaluate the quality of CAR-T products, monitor CAR-T expansion and persistence in vivo, and characterize the phenotypes of CAR-Ts. These analyses play a critical role in the success and prognostic prediction of CAR-T therapies. The commonly used methods for detecting CAR-Ts include FCM, qPCR, and dPCR. Substantial variation exists in these methods across different laboratories and clinical trials, highlighting the need for standardization and regulatory guidelines. Consensus and guidelines are also needed regarding the selection of testing methods, test frequencies, test parameters, and how to apply the results to clinical practice.

References

1. June CH, O'Connor RS, Kawalekar OU, Ghassemi S, Milone MC. CAR T cell immunotherapy for human cancer. Science. 2018;359(6382):1361–5. https://doi.org/10.1126/science.aar6711. PMID: 29567707.
2. Rafiq S, Hackett CS, Brentjens RJ. Engineering strategies to overcome the current roadblocks in CAR T cell therapy. Nat Rev Clin Oncol. 2020;17(3):147–67. https://doi.org/10.1038/s41571-019-0297-y. Epub 2019 Dec 17. PMID: 31848460; PMCID: PMC7223338.
3. Tokarew N, Ogonek J, Endres S, von Bergwelt-Baildon M, Kobold S. Teaching an old dog new tricks: next-generation CAR T cells. Br J Cancer. 2019;120(1):26–37. https://doi.org/10.1038/s41416-018-0325-1. Epub 2018 Nov 9. PMID: 30413825; PMCID: PMC6325111.
4. Maryamchik E, Gallagher KME, Preffer FI, Kadauke S, Maus MV. New directions in chimeric antigen receptor T cell [CAR-T] therapy and related flow cytometry. Cytometry B Clin Cytom. 2020;98(4):299–327. https://doi.org/10.1002/cyto.b.21880. Epub 2020 Apr 30. PMID: 32352629.
5. Maude SL, Frey N, Shaw PA, et al. Chimeric antigen receptor T cells for sustained remissions in leukemia. N Engl J Med. 2014;371(16):1507–17. https://doi.org/10.1056/NEJMoa1407222. Erratum in: N Engl J Med. 2016;374(10):998. https://doi.org/10.1056/NEJMx160005. PMID: 25317870; PMCID: PMC4267531.
6. Maude SL, Laetsch TW, Buechner J, et al. Tisagenlecleucel in children and young adults with B-cell lymphoblastic leukemia. N Engl J Med. 2018;378(5):439–48. https://doi.org/10.1056/NEJMoa1709866. PMID: 29385370; PMCID: PMC5996391.
7. Chen YJ, Abila B, Mostafa Kamel Y. CAR-T: what is next? Cancers (Basel). 2023;15(3):663. https://doi.org/10.3390/cancers15030663. PMID: 36765623; PMCID: PMC9913679.
8. Brudno JN, Kochenderfer JN. Recent advances in CAR T-cell toxicity: mechanisms, manifestations and management. Blood Rev. 2019;34:45–55. https://doi.org/10.1016/j.blre.2018.11.002. Epub 2018 Nov 14. PMID: 30528964; PMCID: PMC6628697.
9. Hu Y, Huang J. The chimeric antigen receptor detection toolkit. Front Immunol. 2020;11:1770. https://doi.org/10.3389/fimmu.2020.01770. PMID: 32849635; PMCID: PMC7431616.
10. Turicek DP, Giordani VM, Moraly J, Taylor N, Shah NN. CAR T-cell detection scoping review: an essential biomarker in critical need of standardization. J Immunother Cancer. 2023;11(5):e006596. https://doi.org/10.1136/jitc-2022-006596. PMID: 37217245; PMCID: PMC10230989.
11. Demaret J, Varlet P, Trauet J, et al. Monitoring CAR T-cells using flow cytometry. Cytometry B Clin Cytom. 2021;100(2):218–24. https://doi.org/10.1002/cyto.b.21941. Epub 2020 Aug 25. PMID: 32841511.
12. Schanda N, Sauer T, Kunz A, et al. Sensitivity and specificity of CD19.CAR-T cell detection by flow cytometry and PCR. Cells. 2021;10(11):3208. https://doi.org/10.3390/cells10113208. PMID: 34831430; PMCID: PMC8621201.
13. Mueller KT, Maude SL, Porter DL, Frey N, Wood P, Han X, Waldron E, Chakraborty A, Awasthi R, Levine BL, Melenhorst JJ, Grupp SA, June CH, Lacey SF. Cellular kinetics of CTL019 in relapsed/refractory B-cell acute lymphoblastic leukemia and chronic lymphocytic leukemia. Blood. 2017;130(21):2317–25. https://doi.org/10.1182/blood-2017-06-786129. Epub 2017 Sep 21. PMID: 28935694; PMCID: PMC5731220.
14. Peinelt A, Bremm M, Kreyenberg H, et al. Monitoring of circulating CAR T cells: validation of a flow cytometric assay, cellular kinetics, and phenotype analysis following tisagenlecleucel. Front Immunol. 2022;13:830773. https://doi.org/10.3389/fimmu.2022.830773. PMID: 35309367; PMCID: PMC8926389.
15. Zaninelli S, Meli C, Borleri G, et al. Optimization and validation of in vivo flow cytometry chimeric antigen receptor T cell detection method using CD19his indirect staining. Cytometry A. 2024;105(2):112–23. https://doi.org/10.1002/cyto.a.24796. Epub 2023 Sep 27. PMID: 37707318.

16. Valdivieso-Shephard JL, Matas-Pérez E, et al. The challenge of standardizing CAR-T cell monitoring: a comparison of two flow-cytometry methods and correlation with qPCR technique. Cytometry A. 2024;105(5):368–75. https://doi.org/10.1002/cyto.a.24825. Epub 2024 Feb 7. PMID: 38327134.
17. de la Iglesia-San Sebastián I, Carbonell D, Bastos-Oreiro M, et al. Digital PCR improves sensitivity and quantification in monitoring CAR-T cells in B cell lymphoma patients. Transplant Cell Ther. 2024;30(3):306.e1–306.e12. https://doi.org/10.1016/j.jtct.2023.12.672. Epub 2024 Jan 5. PMID: 38184148.
18. Sarikonda G, Pahuja A, Kalfoglou C, Burns K, Nguyen K, Ch'en IL, Pollner R, Tangri S, Dakappagari N. Monitoring CAR-T cell kinetics in clinical trials by multiparametric flow cytometry: benefits and challenges. Cytometry B Clin Cytom. 2021;100(1):72–8. https://doi.org/10.1002/cyto.b.21891. Epub 2020 Jun 23. PMID: 32573972.
19. Eurofins Viracor. ExPeCT™ expansion and persistence of CAR T assay. https://www.eurofins-viracor.com/test-menu/33285-car-t-expect-chimeric-antigen-receptor-persistence-and-expansion-test-cd19-fmc63. Accessed 15 Sept 2025.
20. Fehse B, Badbaran A, Berger C, Sonntag T, Riecken K, Geffken M, et al. Digital PCR assays for precise quantification of CD19-CAR-T cells after treatment with axicabtagene ciloleucel. Mol Ther Methods Clin Dev. 2020;16:172–8. https://doi.org/10.1016/j.omtm.2019.12.018. PMID: 32055645; PMCID: PMC7005515.
21. CLSI 2021; Clinical and Laboratory Standards Institute (CLSI). Validation of assays performed by flow cytometry, CLSI guideline H62. 1st ed. Wayne: Clinical and Laboratory Standards Institute; 2021.
22. Selliah N, Eck S, Green C, Oldaker T, Stewart J, Vitaliti A, Litwin V. Flow cytometry method validation protocols. Curr Protoc Cytom. 2019;87(1):e53. https://doi.org/10.1002/cpcy.53. Epub 2018 Nov 12. PMID: 30418706.
23. Sommer U, Eck S, Marszalek L, Stewart JJ, Bradford J, McCloskey TW, Green C, Vitaliti A, Oldaker T, Litwin V. High-sensitivity flow cytometric assays: considerations for design control and analytical validation for identification of rare events. Cytometry B Clin Cytom. 2021;100(1):42–51. https://doi.org/10.1002/cyto.b.21949. Epub 2020 Sep 17. PMID: 32940947.
24. Sarikonda G, Mathieu M, Natalia M, et al. Best practices for the development, analytical validation and clinical implementation of flow cytometric methods for chimeric antigen receptor T cell analyses. Cytometry B Clin Cytom. 2021;100(1):79–91. https://doi.org/10.1002/cyto.b.21985. Epub 2020 Dec 29. PMID: 33373096.
25. Zheng Z, Chinnasamy N, Morgan RA. Protein L: a novel reagent for the detection of chimeric antigen receptor (CAR) expression by flow cytometry. J Transl Med. 2012;10:29. https://doi.org/10.1186/1479-5876-10-29. PMID: 22330761; PMCID: PMC3299624.
26. Kochenderfer JN, Feldman SA, Zhao Y, Xu H, Black MA, Morgan RA, Wilson WH, Rosenberg SA. Construction and preclinical evaluation of an anti-CD19 chimeric antigen receptor. J Immunother. 2009;32(7):689–702. https://doi.org/10.1097/CJI.0b013e3181ac6138. PMID: 19561539; PMCID: PMC2747302.
27. Jena B, Maiti S, Huls H, Singh H, Lee DA, Champlin RE, Cooper LJ. Chimeric antigen receptor (CAR)-specific monoclonal antibody to detect CD19-specific T cells in clinical trials. PLoS One. 2013;8(3):e57838. https://doi.org/10.1371/journal.pone.0057838. Epub 2013 Mar 1. PMID: 23469246; PMCID: PMC3585808.
28. Ruella M, Barrett DM, Kenderian SS, et al. Dual CD19 and CD123 targeting prevents antigen-loss relapses after CD19-directed immunotherapies. J Clin Invest. 2016;126(10):3814–26. https://doi.org/10.1172/JCI87366. Epub 2016 Aug 29. PMID: 27571406; PMCID: PMC5096828.
29. Johansson U, Gallagher K, Burgoyne V, Maus MV, Casey KS, Brini GG, et al. Detection of CAR-T19 cells in peripheral blood and cerebrospinal fluid: an assay applicable to routine diagnostic laboratories. Cytometry B Clin Cytom. 2021;100(6):622–31. https://doi.org/10.1002/cyto.b.22005. Epub 2021 Apr 29. PMID: 33915021.

30. Ruella M, Xu J, Barrett DM, et al. Induction of resistance to chimeric antigen receptor T cell therapy by transduction of a single leukemic B cell. Nat Med. 2018;24(10):1499–503. https://doi.org/10.1038/s41591-018-0201-9. Epub 2018 Oct 1. PMID: 30275568; PMCID: PMC6511988.
31. Wood B, Jevremovic D, Béné MC, Yan M, Jacobs P, Litwin V, ICSH/ICCS Working Group. Validation of cell-based fluorescence assays: practice guidelines from the ICSH and ICCS—part V—assay performance criteria. Cytometry B Clin Cytom. 2013;84(5):315–23. https://doi.org/10.1002/cyto.b.21108. PMID: 24022854.
32. Wang H, Du X, Chen WH, Lou J, Xiao HL, Pan YM, Chen H, An N, Zhang QX. Establishment of a quantitative polymerase chain reaction assay for monitoring chimeric antigen receptor T cells in peripheral blood. Transplant Proc. 2018;50(1):104–9. https://doi.org/10.1016/j.transproceed.2017.11.028. PMID: 29407291.
33. Kunz A, Gern U, Schmitt A, et al. Optimized assessment of qPCR-based vector copy numbers as a safety parameter for GMP-grade CAR T cells and monitoring of frequency in patients. Mol Ther Methods Clin Dev. 2020;17:448–54. https://doi.org/10.1016/j.omtm.2020.02.003. PMID: 32201711; PMCID: PMC7078460.
34. Svec D, Tichopad A, Novosadova V, Pfaffl MW, Kubista M. How good is a PCR efficiency estimate: recommendations for precise and robust qPCR efficiency assessments. Biomol Detect Quantif. 2015;3:9–16. https://doi.org/10.1016/j.bdq.2015.01.005. PMID: 27077029; PMCID: PMC4822216.
35. Hays A, Islam R, Matys K, Williams D. Best practices in qPCR and dPCR validation in regulated bioanalytical laboratories. AAPS J. 2022;24(2):36. https://doi.org/10.1208/s12248-022-00686-1. Erratum in: AAPS J. 2022;24(3):55. https://doi.org/10.1208/s12248-022-00705-1. PMID: 35194700.
36. Bustin S, Huggett J. qPCR primer design revisited. Biomol Detect Quantif. 2017;14:19–28. https://doi.org/10.1016/j.bdq.2017.11.001. PMID: 29201647; PMCID: PMC5702850.
37. Yamamoto S, Matsumoto SI, Goto A, Ugajin M, Nakayama M, Moriya Y, Hirabayashi H. Quantitative PCR methodology with a volume-based unit for the sophisticated cellular kinetic evaluation of chimeric antigen receptor T cells. Sci Rep. 2020;10(1):17884. https://doi.org/10.1038/s41598-020-74927-8. PMID: 33087808; PMCID: PMC7578827.
38. Hays A, Durham J, Gullick B, Rudemiller N, Schneider T. Bioanalytical assay strategies and considerations for measuring cellular kinetics. Int J Mol Sci. 2022;24(1):695. https://doi.org/10.3390/ijms24010695. PMID: 36614138; PMCID: PMC9820866.
39. Forootan A, Sjöback R, Björkman J, Sjögreen B, Linz L, Kubista M. Methods to determine limit of detection and limit of quantification in quantitative real-time PCR (qPCR). Biomol Detect Quantif. 2017;12:1–6. https://doi.org/10.1016/j.bdq.2017.04.001. PMID: 28702366; PMCID: PMC5496743.
40. Bustin SA, Benes V, Garson JA, Hellemans J, Huggett J, Kubista M, Mueller R, Nolan T, Pfaffl MW, Shipley GL, Vandesompele J, Wittwer CT. The MIQE guidelines: minimum information for publication of quantitative real-time PCR experiments. Clin Chem. 2009;55(4):611–22. https://doi.org/10.1373/clinchem.2008.112797. Epub 2009 Feb 26. PMID: 19246619.
41. US FDA. Long term follow-up after administration of human gene therapy products. 2020. https://www.fda.gov/regulatory-information/search-fda-guidance-documents/long-term-follow-after-administration-human-gene-therapy-products. Accessed 28 Nov 2024.
42. Hays A, Wissel M, Colletti K, et al. Recommendations for method development and validation of qPCR and dPCR assays in support of cell and gene therapy drug development. AAPS J. 2024;26(1):24. https://doi.org/10.1208/s12248-023-00880-9. PMID: 38316745.
43. Yang TY, Doddareddy R. Considerations in the development and validation of real-time quantitative polymerase chain reaction and its application in regulated bioanalysis to characterize the cellular kinetics of CAR-T products in clinical studies. Bioanalysis. 2021;13(2):115–28. https://doi.org/10.4155/bio-2020-0221. Epub 2020 Dec 23. PMID: 33356555.
44. European Medicines Agency. Guideline on bioanalytical method validation. 2011. https://www.ema.europa.eu/en/bioanalytical-method-validation-scientific-guideline. Accessed 28 Nov 2024.

45. US FDA. Bioanalytical method validation guidance for industry. 2018. https://www.fda.gov/media/70858/download. Accessed 28 Nov 2024.
46. ICH harmonized guideline: bioanalytical method validation and study sample analysis M10. Guidance 2022. Available online: https://database.ich.org/sites/default/files/M10_Guideline_Step4_2022_0524.pdf
47. Huggett JF, Whale A. Digital PCR as a novel technology and its potential implications for molecular diagnostics. Clin Chem. 2013;59:1691–3.
48. Lou Y, Chen C, Long X, Gu J, Xiao M, Wang D, Zhou X, Li T, Hong Z, Li C, Zhou J, Chen L. Detection and quantification of chimeric antigen receptor transgene copy number by droplet digital PCR versus real-time PCR. J Mol Diagn. 2020;22(5):699–707. https://doi.org/10.1016/j.jmoldx.2020.02.007. PMID: 32409121.
49. Wiedemann G, Bacher U, Joncourt R, Solly F, Widmer CC, Zeerleder S, Novak U, Pabst T, Porret NA. A comprehensive ddPCR strategy for sensitive and reliable monitoring of CAR-T cell kinetics in clinical applications. Int J Mol Sci. 2024;25(16):8556. https://doi.org/10.3390/ijms25168556. PMID: 39201242; PMCID: PMC11354041.
50. Mueller KT, Waldron E, Sickert D, Grupp SA, Maude SL, Levine JE, et al. Impact of humoral immunogenicity (anti-mCAR19 anti-bodies) on CTL019 cellular kinetics, efficacy, and safety. Blood. 2017;130:1281.
51. Mueller KT, Waldron E, Grupp SA, et al. Clinical pharmacology of tisagenlecleucel in B-cell acute lymphoblastic leukemia. Clin Cancer Res. 2018;24(24):6175–84. https://doi.org/10.1158/1078-0432.CCR-18-0758. Epub 2018 Sep 6. PMID: 30190371; PMCID: PMC7433345.
52. Fraietta JA, Lacey SF, Orlando EJ, et al. Determinants of response and resistance to CD19 chimeric antigen receptor (CAR) T cell therapy of chronic lymphocytic leukemia. Nat Med. 2018;24(5):563–71. https://doi.org/10.1038/s41591-018-0010-1. Epub 2018 Apr 30. Erratum in: Nat Med. 2021;27(3):561. https://doi.org/10.1038/s41591-021-01248-2. PMID: 29713085; PMCID: PMC6117613.
53. García-Calderón CB, Sierro-Martínez B, García-Guerrero E, et al. Monitoring of kinetics and exhaustion markers of circulating CAR-T cells as early predictive factors in patients with B-cell malignancies. Front Immunol. 2023;14:1152498. https://doi.org/10.3389/fimmu.2023.1152498. PMID: 37122702; PMCID: PMC10140355.
54. Lee DW, Kochenderfer JN, Stetler-Stevenson M, et al. T cells expressing CD19 chimeric antigen receptors for acute lymphoblastic leukaemia in children and young adults: a phase 1 dose-escalation trial. Lancet. 2015;385(9967):517–28. https://doi.org/10.1016/S0140-6736(14)61403-3. Epub 2014 Oct 13. PMID: 25319501; PMCID: PMC7065359.
55. Finney OC, Brakke HM, Rawlings-Rhea S, Hicks R, Doolittle D, Lopez M, Futrell RB, Orentas RJ, Li D, Gardner RA, Jensen MC. CD19 CAR T cell product and disease attributes predict leukemia remission durability. J Clin Invest. 2019;129(5):2123–32. https://doi.org/10.1172/JCI125423. PMID: 30860496; PMCID: PMC6486329.
56. Monfrini C, Stella F, Aragona V, et al. Phenotypic composition of commercial anti-CD19 CAR T cells affects in vivo expansion and disease response in patients with large B-cell lymphoma. Clin Cancer Res. 2022;28(15):3378–86. https://doi.org/10.1158/1078-0432.CCR-22-0164. PMID: 35583610; PMCID: PMC9662896.
57. Cappell KM, Kochenderfer JN. Long-term outcomes following CAR T cell therapy: what we know so far. Nat Rev Clin Oncol. 2023;20(6):359–71. https://doi.org/10.1038/s41571-023-00754-1. Epub 2023 Apr 13. PMID: 37055515; PMCID: PMC10100620.
58. Good Z, Spiegel JY, Sahaf B, et al. Post-infusion CAR T_{Reg} cells identify patients resistant to CD19-CAR therapy. Nat Med. 2022;28(9):1860–71. https://doi.org/10.1038/s41591-022-01960-7. Epub 2022 Sep 12. PMID: 36097223; PMCID: PMC10917089.
59. Schuster SJ, Bishop MR, Tam CS, et al. Tisagenlecleucel in adult relapsed or refractory diffuse large B-cell lymphoma. N Engl J Med. 2019;380(1):45–56. https://doi.org/10.1056/NEJMoa1804980. Epub 2018 Dec 1. PMID: 30501490.
60. Sauter CS, Senechal B, Rivière I, et al. CD19 CAR T cells following autologous transplantation in poor-risk relapsed and refractory B-cell non-Hodgkin lymphoma. Blood.

2019;134(7):626–35. https://doi.org/10.1182/blood.2018883421. Epub 2019 Jul 1. PMID: 31262783; PMCID: PMC6695562.

61. Gabelli M, Oporto-Espuelas M, Burridge S, Chu J, Farish S, Hedges E, et al. Maintenance therapy for early loss of B-cell aplasia after anti-CD19 CAR T-cell therapy. Blood Adv. 2024;8(8):1959–63. https://doi.org/10.1182/bloodadvances.2023011168. PMID: 37820111; PMCID: PMC11021820.
62. Molinos-Quintana Á, Alonso-Saladrigues A, Herrero B, Caballero-Velázquez T, Galán-Gómez V, Panesso M, et al. Impact of disease burden and late loss of B cell aplasia on the risk of relapse after CD19 chimeric antigen receptor T cell (Tisagenlecleucel) infusion in pediatric and young adult patients with relapse/refractory acute lymphoblastic leukemia: role of B-cell monitoring. Front Immunol. 2024;14:1280580. https://doi.org/10.3389/fimmu.2023.1280580. Erratum in: Front Immunol. 2024;15:1373852. https://doi.org/10.3389/fimmu.2024.1373852. PMID: 38292483; PMCID: PMC10825008.
63. Porter DL, Hwang WT, Frey NV, et al. Chimeric antigen receptor T cells persist and induce sustained remissions in relapsed refractory chronic lymphocytic leukemia. Sci Transl Med. 2015;7(303):303ra139. https://doi.org/10.1126/scitranslmed.aac5415. PMID: 26333935; PMCID: PMC5909068.
64. Cohen AD, Garfall AL, Stadtmauer EA, et al. B cell maturation antigen-specific CAR T cells are clinically active in multiple myeloma. J Clin Invest. 2019;129(6):2210–21. https://doi.org/10.1172/JCI126397. PMID: 30896447; PMCID: PMC6546468.
65. Deng Q, Han G, Puebla-Osorio N, et al. Characteristics of anti-CD19 CAR T cell infusion products associated with efficacy and toxicity in patients with large B cell lymphomas. Nat Med. 2020;26(12):1878–87. https://doi.org/10.1038/s41591-020-1061-7. Epub 2020 Oct 5. PMID: 33020644; PMCID: PMC8446909.
66. Talleur AC, Qudeimat A, Métais JY, et al. Preferential expansion of CD8+ CD19-CAR T cells postinfusion and the role of disease burden on outcome in pediatric B-ALL. Blood Adv. 2022;6(21):5737–49. https://doi.org/10.1182/bloodadvances.2021006293. PMID: 35446934; PMCID: PMC9647829.
67. Paixão EA, Barros LRC, Fassoni AC, Almeida RC. Modeling patient-specific CAR-T cell dynamics: multiphasic kinetics via phenotypic differentiation. Cancers (Basel). 2022;14(22):5576. https://doi.org/10.3390/cancers14225576. PMID: 36428671; PMCID: PMC9688514.
68. Haradhvala NJ, Leick MB, Maurer K, et al. Distinct cellular dynamics associated with response to CAR-T therapy for refractory B cell lymphoma. Nat Med. 2022;28(9):1848–59. https://doi.org/10.1038/s41591-022-01959-0. Epub 2022 Sep 12. PMID: 36097221; PMCID: PMC9509487.
69. Gorovits B, Koren E. Immunogenicity of chimeric antigen receptor T-cell therapeutics. BioDrugs. 2019;33(3):275–84. https://doi.org/10.1007/s40259-019-00354-5. PMID: 31069709.
70. Khan AN, Chowdhury A, Karulkar A, Jaiswal AK, Banik A, Asija S, Purwar R. Immunogenicity of CAR-T cell therapeutics: evidence, mechanism and mitigation. Front Immunol. 2022;13:886546. https://doi.org/10.3389/fimmu.2022.886546. PMID: 35677038; PMCID: PMC9169153.
71. Hege KM, Bergsland EK, Fisher GA, Nemunaitis JJ, Warren RS, McArthur JG, Lin AA, Schlom J, June CH, Sherwin SA. Safety, tumor trafficking and immunogenicity of chimeric antigen receptor (CAR)-T cells specific for TAG-72 in colorectal cancer. J Immunother Cancer. 2017;5:22. https://doi.org/10.1186/s40425-017-0222-9. PMID: 28344808; PMCID: PMC5360066.
72. Lamers CH, Willemsen R, van Elzakker P, et al. Immune responses to transgene and retroviral vector in patients treated with ex vivo-engineered T cells. Blood. 2011;117(1):72–82. https://doi.org/10.1182/blood-2010-07-294520. Epub 2010 Oct 1. PMID: 20889925.
73. Turtle CJ, Hanafi LA, Berger C, et al. CD19 CAR-T cells of defined CD4+:CD8+ composition in adult B cell ALL patients. J Clin Invest. 2016;126(6):2123–38. https://doi.org/10.1172/JCI85309. Epub 2016 Apr 25. PMID: 27111235; PMCID: PMC4887159.

74. Awasthi R, Pacaud L, Waldron E, et al. Tisagenlecleucel cellular kinetics, dose, and immunogenicity in relation to clinical factors in relapsed/refractory DLBCL. Blood Adv. 2020;4(3):560–72. https://doi.org/10.1182/bloodadvances.2019000525. PMID: 32045475; PMCID: PMC7013261.
75. Potthoff B, McBlane F, Spindeldreher S, Sickert D. A cell-based immunogenicity assay to detect antibodies against chimeric antigen receptor expressed by tisagenlecleucel. J Immunol Methods. 2020;476:112692. https://doi.org/10.1016/j.jim.2019.112692. Epub 2019 Nov 1. PMID: 31678267.
76. US FDA. Guidance for industry: immunogenicity testing of therapeutic protein products—503 developing and validating assays for anti-drug antibody detection. 2019. https://www.fda.gov/regulatory-information/search-fda-guidance-documents/immunogenicity-testing-therapeutic-protein-products-developing-and-validating-assays-anti-drugs. Accessed 28 Nov 2024.

Post-transplant Bone Marrow Engraftment Monitoring

17

Ibrahim Ahmed and Elena A. Repnikova

Introduction

Allogeneic hematopoietic stem cell transplantation (aHSCT) is a vital therapeutic treatment option and long-term disease control for various hematological malignancies. The success of aHSCT relies on the successful engraftment of donor cells and the effective elimination of recipient cells, which is assessed through chimerism testing. Given that relapse is the primary cause of mortality following aHSCT, the detection of recipient cells is important in patients with hematological malignancies. Early detection of relapse can facilitate timely intervention. Chimerism analysis coupled with measurable residual disease (MRD) monitoring appears to be a key tool for evaluating treatment response and risk stratification for patients with acute lymphoblastic leukemia and acute myeloid leukemia [1–3].

In 1959, Dr. Edward Donnall Thomas and his team conducted the first successful bone marrow transplantation in two patients diagnosed with acute lymphoblastic leukemia. These patients received total body irradiation followed by a bone marrow infusion. Their health parameters were restored to normal 2 weeks following infusion. However, several months later, both patients died from a leukemia recurrence [4]. Presently, monitoring of chimerism is a necessary procedure for patients following aHSCT. The assessment of chimerism is based on the analysis of genetic differences between donor and recipient cells. Analysis of short tandem repeats (STR) is the primary method utilized for post-transplant monitoring of donor

I. Ahmed
Division of Hematology, Oncology, and Blood and Marrow Transplant, Children's Mercy Kansas City, University of Missouri-Kansas City School of Medicine, Kansas City, MO, USA

E. A. Repnikova (✉)
Department of Pathology and Laboratory Medicine, Children's Mercy Kansas City, University of Missouri-Kansas City School of Medicine, Kansas City, MO, USA
e-mail: erepnikova@cmh.edu

W. Li (ed.), *Laboratory Assessments of Pediatric Leukemia*,
https://doi.org/10.1007/978-3-032-26557-9_17

engraftment and chimerism assessment. This approach facilitates early detection of disease relapse, evaluates the level of engraftment, and offers valuable insights into graft-versus-host disease (GVHD) and graft-versus-tumor (GVT) effects, thereby aiding in timely therapeutic intervention [5].

Overview of Chimerism Analysis Techniques

One of the early methods for the routine monitoring of chimerism involved analysis of erythrocyte antigens using hemagglutination assay. While this method is robust and reproducible, it has a significant drawback. This limitation arises from the prolonged persistence of recipient erythrocytes and the frequent occurrence of matching blood types between donor and recipient. As such, this method is not currently employed in routine clinical practice for chimerism monitoring, as it does not adequately assess chimerism in a particular cell lineage [6]. Additionally, this testing method has insufficient informative markers and decreased sensitivity [7].

Another technique used to monitor chimerism is flow cytometry analysis. This approach utilizes monoclonal antibodies targeted against specific erythrocyte antigens. However, this method can only be applied to the recipients who have not undergone blood transfusions.

Fluorescence in situ hybridization (FISH), a widely used cytogenetic analysis, has been used to assess the degree of chimerism in either sorted or non-sorted peripheral blood or bone marrow cells. This method relies on the visualization of fluorescence signals from the X and Y chromosomes in nuclei of interphase cells using probes which recognize repetitive sequences on these chromosomes. FISH is a well-established technique, with sensitivity to detect chimerism of up to ~0.5% which enables rapid screening of a large number of cells. The main disadvantage of this method, however, is that it is only useful for monitoring engraftment in transplants with opposite sex donors [8].

Of the molecular-based methods for engraftment monitoring, quantitative polymerase chain reaction (PCR) analysis, digital-droplet PCR, and PCR analysis of short tandem repeats (STR-PCR) offer high sensitivity for chimerism detection, but each has its limitations. Quantitative real-time PCR (qPCR) for the detection of single nucleotide polymorphisms (SNPs) or short deletions/insertions (In/del) has a sensitivity of 0.1%; however, in a case of a related donor–recipient transplant, the amplification panel may not be sufficient to identify unique markers to distinguish between donor and recipient [9].

Digital droplet PCR (ddPCR) analysis is an attractive approach to lineage-specific monitoring of chimerism in aHSCT patients with a sensitivity of nearly 0.01%. However, this method has certain limitations in clinical practice, as it necessitates a minimum amount of DNA of approximately 50–75 ng. This requirement is often challenging to meet, particularly in patients who have undergone aHSCT and may present with cytopenia.

PCR analysis of short tandem repeats (STR-PCR) constitutes the gold standard method for chimerism quantification. This method is quantitative, requires little

Table 17.1 Comparison between methods for chimerism detection in patients with aHSCT

Method	Sensitivity	Advantages	Limitations
Hemagglutination assay	5%	Reproducibility	Limited to analysis of only erythrocyte antigens
Flow cytometry analysis	1%	Reproducibility	Technically challenging, expensive, only lineage-specific
Fluorescent in situ hybridization	0.5–2%	High sensitivity	Only can be used for opposite sex donor–recipient
STR-based fragment analysis	1–5%	Reproducibility, quick turn around time, low DNA input	Cannot be used for identical twins
Quantitative PCR analysis	0.1%	High sensitivity	Unable to use in a related donor–recipient pairs
Digital droplet PCR	0.01%	Single cell assay, high sensitivity	Costly, requires higher input of DNA
Next-generation sequencing	0.01–0.05%	High sensitivity, applicable for monozygotic twin pairs	Costly, requires batching for low price, long turnaround time

amount of input DNA (~2–10 ng), and relies on simultaneous amplification of multiple short-tandem repeats in the genome. It provides a quick and accurate assessment of the contribution of both donor and/or recipient hematopoietic cells in post-transplantation specimens and has a sensitivity of ~1–5% [10].

Recent advancements in next-generation sequencing (NGS) technology have introduced a more sensitive alternative to short tandem repeat (STR) analysis. Chimerism testing by NGS was reported with excellent assay performance, high sensitivity and accuracy, similar to a combined qPCR/STR strategy. However, reported sensitivity of NGS chimerism varies depending on the selection of marker types and sequencing platforms. Additionally, cost, turnaround time, and availability of sufficient informative markers are critical factors in implementing this assay in the clinical setting [11] (Table 17.1).

DNA Polymorphism Repeat Analysis as a Tool to Monitor Engraftment

With advancements in molecular techniques and genome sequencing, researchers have identified several types of genomic polymorphisms. These include single nucleotide polymorphisms (SNPs), insertion/deletions (InDels), and microsatellites (variable number tandem repeats (VNTR) and short tandem repeats (STR)), which are predominantly located in the noncoding regions of the genome. The initial DNA analysis method utilizing sequence polymorphisms was restriction fragment length polymorphism (RFLP), which involves the digestion of genomic DNA with restriction endonucleases. However, RFLP analysis was often time-consuming,

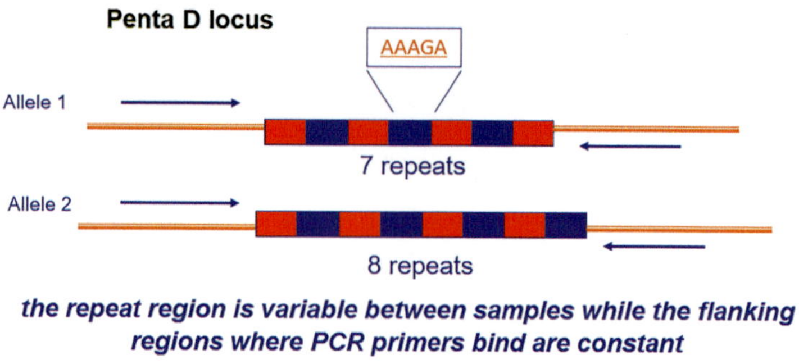

Fig. 17.1 An example of a Penta D locus, which is characterized by a pentanucleotide expansion located on chromosome 21. In this illustration, one allele contains 7 repeats while the other has 8 repeats. The PCR primers are designed to bind to the specific flanking regions of the STR locus and amplify the region containing the pentanucleotide repeats

labor-intensive, low in sensitivity, and required substantial amounts of high-quality DNA [7].

A significant advancement in chimerism monitoring occurred with the development of polymerase chain reaction (PCR) techniques. The molecular analysis of microsatellite markers amplified by PCR followed by fragment analysis has become the predominant method for chimerism testing. VNTRs were initially used for chimerism analysis. However, due to their limited number in the genome, it makes it difficult to distinguish certain donor/recipient pairs rendering this technique as non-informative for certain transplant pairs. STRs are short DNA sequences (2–6 base pairs) repeated multiple times in a head-to-tail manner within the genome (Fig. 17.1). In contrast to VNTR analysis, the STR-based method offers a significantly higher degree of polymorphism, making it more suitable for accurate chimerism detection and quantification. This method was quickly adopted in the diagnostics setting due to its rapidity, reliability, accuracy, and reproducibility. Additionally, this method required a low amount of DNA input (2–10 ng), which is essential for analyzing chimerism in low-frequency, limited-cell samples, such as in myeloid and lymphoid lineages.

Nonetheless, STR testing does have limitations, including a sensitivity range of 1–5%. Furthermore, analytical challenges may arise from issues such as allelic imbalance (preferential amplification of certain alleles), stutter peaks (PCR-generated artifacts resulting from strand slippage during DNA synthesis), allele dropouts, and non-template adenine addition, necessitating manual interpretation of results and analyst expertise.

Establishment of STR Informative Markers Prior to aHSCT

At the initial step prior to aHSCT, pre-transplant patient DNA and the corresponding donor DNA are first analyzed to identify the presence of genetic markers that are suitable for STR-based chimerism analysis after transplant. Initial analysis typically includes pre-transplant recipient DNA, donor DNA, and a known donor–recipient mixture, enabling a comprehensive review of all markers. This process facilitates the selection of informative markers for subsequent post-transplant analysis and the examination of artifacts and stutter peaks associated with all relevant loci. Extra attention needs to be paid to analysis of the markers in the recipient DNA as tumor cells may cause corresponding loss of an STR locus. This is a potential source of error in the interpretation of engraftment analysis, especially if only few informative loci are available to monitor engraftment.

To monitor engraftment, a panel of multiple STR loci from commercially available kits, like the "AmpFlSTR Identifiler" or Promega GenePrint®24 System which analyze multiple STRs across different chromosomes, is typically used. These loci allow for accurate distinction between donor and recipient DNA based on their unique allele variations at each locus. Commonly used polymorphic loci include Penta E, D18S51, D21S11, THO1, D3S1358, FGA, TPOX, D8S1179, vWA, Penta D, CSF1P0, D16S539, D7S820, D13S317, D5S818, D1S1656, D2S441, D2S1338, D10S1248, D12S391, D19S433, and D22S1045 and two nonpolymorphic loci Amelogenin and DYS391.

Main Steps of the Procedure

At first, PCR reactions are set up in a room separate from the thermal cycler and post-PCR analysis area. No amplified products are allowed in the PCR setup area. Aerosol barrier pipette tips are used for the setup of all PCR reactions to prevent cross contamination. A known, previously run sample is used to validate new reagents. Each reagent must display acceptable results before the reagent can be used for clinical casework.

Appropriate positive and negative controls must be run with each assay. Assay results should be reported only if all control samples yield expected results. A sensitivity control (generally, 95% donor and 5% recipient) should be used and evaluated with each run. Standard deviation and coefficient of variation should be tracked over time to evaluate variance. A minimum of three informative loci are routinely used in calculations. In the case of a closely related donor and recipient, an exception can be made to use fewer loci.

All reactions need to be optimized to avoid preferential amplification. The minimum amount of DNA is used as determined by the manufacturer to obtain optimal sensitivity. Preferential allele amplification is considered in the interpretation of results. Any heterozygous locus with an allele peak imbalance of less than 85% is typically not considered in analysis of the post sample. Locus amplification generally must exceed 1000 RFU (Relative Fluorescence Units) to be analyzed. Anything less will be considered on a case-by-case basis and may be rejected.

Following amplification, samples can be analyzed using an ABI DNA Sequencer (Applied Biosystems). Fragment size and peak area data are typically assessed using ABI software. Gene Mapper may serve as a secondary tool for calculating percentages in STR analysis. When utilizing Gene Mapper, peaks selected for chimerism calculations should be based on their position and stutter characteristics. Calculations can be performed either manually or with the assistance of automated software, such as ChimeRMarker™, offering an efficient alternative to manual methods (Fig. 17.2). The use of automated software significantly reduces analysis time and effectively accommodates increasing test volumes.

Data Analysis

The percentage of donor and recipient DNA can be quantified through STR analysis to assess the extent of bone marrow engraftment. The ratios of the peak areas of donor and recipient alleles at informative loci are utilized to determine the DNA percentages in post-transplant samples. The specific formulas for calculating the percentage of donor or recipient DNA depend on whether the informative loci are heterozygous or homozygous, as well as whether the donor and recipient share any alleles. In some samples, the recipient DNA can represent the minor component in post-transplant samples, and calculations most commonly focus on determining the percentage of recipient DNA. However, in some samples the recipient DNA will be the major component, and calculations would need to focus on determining the percentage of donor DNA. The percentage of recipient DNA can then be obtained by subtracting the percentage of donor DNA from 100%.

Percent donor is calculated by taking the area of the donor peak(s) and dividing by the total area of the donor and recipient peaks. The following guidelines should be used for calculations and determining if a marker is informative or not:

1. The peak is not the same as a stutter peak in either its own sample or the sample to which it is being compared.
2. The peak is not shared between the donor and the recipient.
3. The exception wherein a shared allele may be useable is if one of the samples has a second unshared allele that is not the same size as any stutter peaks.

Stutter Peaks: Stutter peaks are artifacts of PCR amplification that may arise from "slippage" during the PCR process. They are smaller by one or two repeat units or larger by one repeat unit than the actual peak for that locus. For example, a microsatellite marker comprised of a pentanucleotide repeat will generate stutter peaks that are five or ten base pairs smaller than the real peaks. As the alleles are sized in base pair units along the X-axis of the chromatograph, this type of stutter will be found 5 bp to the left of the real peak (Fig. 17.3). Any peak found to be the same size (in bp) or in the same position as another allele's stutter peak cannot be

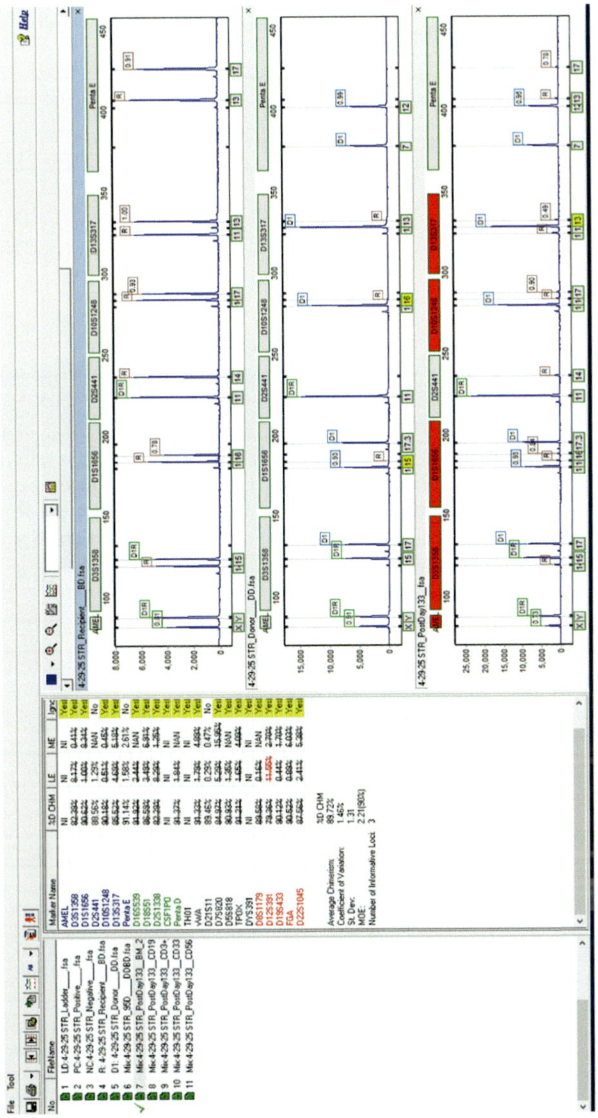

Fig. 17.2 Automated chimerism analysis allows to quickly and accurately analyze all STR loci, exclude stutter peaks from calculations as needed, and with the percentage of donor and recipient chimerism

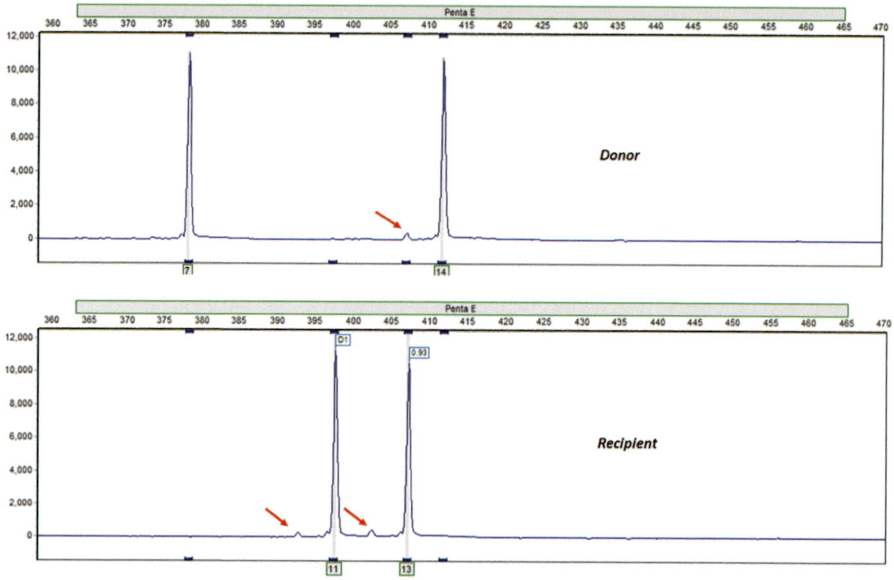

Fig. 17.3 Stutter peaks are artifacts of PCR amplification that may arise from "slippage" during the PCR process. Penta E, [AAAGA] pentanucleotide microsatellite shows heterozygous 7 and 14 repeat alleles for the Donor and heterozygous 11 and 13 repeat alleles for the Recipient. Red arrows indicate stutter peaks (13, 12 and 10 repeats) that are five base pairs smaller than the real peaks and are found to the left of the real peak

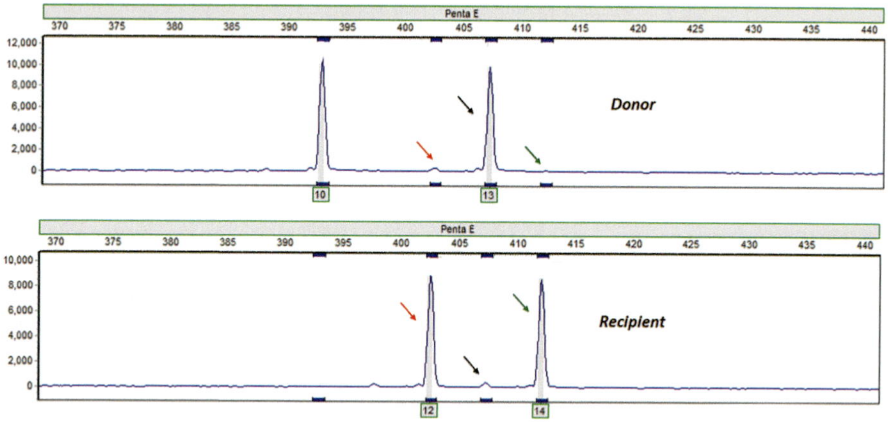

Fig. 17.4 The Recipient peak at size 12 is not suitable for chimerism analysis, as it is in stutter position of the largest donor peak. Similarly, the Donor peak at size 13 is unsuitable because it is a stutter peak of the largest Recipient peak at size 14. Additionally, it produces a forward stutter at size 14, which overlaps with the Recipient peak and may lead to inaccuracies in the Recipient chimerism calculation

used. As Fig. 17.4 illustrates, the recipient peak cannot be used because it is a stutter peak of the largest Donor peak. Also, the smallest Donor peak cannot be used because it is a stutter peak of the largest Recipient peak.

Assessment of Chimerism After Allogeneic Hematopoietic Stem Cell Transplantation

Following successful aHSCT, it is important to assess donor chimerism in the bone marrow and/or peripheral blood. The detection of greater than 95% donor chimerism in both myeloid and lymphoid lineages within the blood and bone marrow indicates complete donor chimerism [12]. Detection of 5–95% of donor chimerism for either one or both myeloid and lymphoid lineages in the bone marrow and blood is consistent with a mixed or partial chimerism; and <5% of donor chimerism for both myeloid and lymphoid lineages is considered with absent donor chimerism [13]. "Split chimerism" used to refer to when a complete donor engraftment is observed in some cell types (e.g. T-cells) and mixed chimerism consisting of Donor-derived and Recipient-derived cells is present in other cell types (e.g. myeloid cells) (Table 17.2) [14].

There are also some studies in which the mixed chimerism has been classified separately into transient, progressive, and stable mixed chimerism. In case of transient mixed chimerism, a mixed population of donor and recipient cells is observed within 1 year following aHSCT. This is further validated by the confirmation of complete chimerism. If the proportion of recipient cells increases by more than 15% within a 3-month period, this scenario is classified as progressive mixed chimerism. Conversely, stable mixed chimerism is characterized by the identification of less than 5% of recipient cells over a long period of time [15].

Assessing chimerism status is crucial to differentiate the graft status, and the likelihood of relapse. Loss of chimerism is associated with either primary graft failure due to lack of absolute neutrophil count (ANC) $\geq$ 500 with associated pancytopenia by D+30 for peripheral blood or bone marrow stem cell source or D+42 for umbilical cord blood stem cell source. A decline in hematopoietic function, characterized by the development of anemia, thrombocytopenia, and/or neutropenia requiring blood product support or growth factor administration, after achieving neutrophil and platelet engraftment, may be indicative of secondary graft failure

Table 17.2 Chimerism definition

	Donor chimerism	Recipient chimerism	Notes
Full chimerism	>95%	≤5%	For both myeloid and lymphoid lineages
Mixed chimerism	5–95%	95–5%	For either one or both myeloid and lymphoid lineages
Absent chimerism	<5%	≥95%	

associated with loss of chimerism or, in cases where full donor chimerism is maintained, suggestive of poor graft function [13].

Lineage-Specific Chimerism Testing

There are two primary methods for affinity cell enrichment: positive and negative. Positive enrichment involves isolating target cells through the interactions between surface antigens on the target cells and specific antibodies. Negative enrichment involves removing unwanted cell types, leaving the desired cells untouched in the supernatant.

Positive selection immunomagnetic cell separation techniques consist of directly labeling target cells with an antibody or ligand that recognizes a specific cell surface antigen. These antibodies or ligands are conjugated to magnetic particles, enabling the retention of labeled cells in the final isolated fraction when the sample is subjected to a magnetic field. A key characteristic of positive magnetic selection methods includes high purity of the isolated cells. However, these cells are usually bound by antibodies and magnetic particles and this method can sometimes pull additional cell populations from the negative fraction.

In the negative selection, immunomagnetic cell separation antibodies or ligands specifically label unwanted cell types for removal based on their surface proteins. These antibodies or ligands are conjugated to magnetic particles, enabling the depletion of labeled, unwanted cells from the final isolated fraction when the sample is exposed to a magnetic field. In this approach, the desired cells do not interact with antibodies or ligands and therefore remain free from particle binding. The main advantage of this method is an efficient and quick protocol requiring minimal sample manipulation. It leaves the desired cells unaffected and unbound by magnetic particles.

Most laboratories provide chimerism testing on specific cell subsets, while a few do not. Chimerism testing is most frequently offered on T cell populations, specifically selecting for CD3. Additionally, some laboratories perform tests on myeloid populations by selecting for markers such as CD33. Other populations tested by laboratories include B cells (selecting for CD19), NK cells (selecting for CD56), CD34+ cells, and CD14+ cells. Rarely, laboratories may perform sorting for CD71+, a marker of early erythroid precursors [11].

Protocol for Monitoring Chimerism

In the context of a stable clinical course, most transplant centers evaluate chimerism in conjunction with other diagnostic tests, typically using peripheral blood samples. This assessment generally begins around the time of engraftment and is performed routinely on days +30, +90, +180, and at 1 year post-aHSCT [16]. Despite the general consensus, the frequency and timing of chimerism testing may be influenced by the patient's relapse risk. Chimerism evaluation is primarily conducted to assess the success of aHSCT, confirm engraftment, evaluate relapse risk, and facilitate timely adjustments to therapeutic strategies before the emergence of clinical signs or symptoms [16–18].

Post-aHSCT chimerism follow-up involves the analysis of bone marrow aspirates and/or peripheral blood samples. The results should include assessments of total and sorted individual cell lineages, such as T-lymphocytes, B-lymphocytes, myeloid cells, and natural killer (NK) cells. Additionally, where applicable, analysis of sorted stem cells using specific markers should be performed and reported accordingly [16]. Immune cell lineage reconstitution following aHSCT exhibits variability. Neutrophil recovery typically occurs between days 14 and 30 post-transplant. Natural killer (NK) cell recovery generally occurs between days 30 and 100, followed by T cell recovery around day 100. B-cell recovery is observed approximately 1–2 years after the procedure [19].

The duration of chimerism monitoring following aHSCT varies considerably among transplant centers. Although a 5-year follow-up is generally recommended, each center develops its own protocols regarding the appropriate follow-up period. Acute graft-versus-host disease (aGVHD) has been linked to the presence of T cell (CD3+) donor full chimerism in patients undergoing reduced-intensity conditioning therapy [20] and is associated with a decreased overall incidence of disease relapse [21, 22]. Conversely, the presence of mixed T-cell chimerism correlates with an absence of grade 2 or higher aGVHD [20]. Mixed myeloid chimerism has been identified as a potential prognostic indicator for disease relapse in myeloid fibrosis, as documented by Srour et al. [23]. In the context of sickle cell disease, donor-derived myeloid chimerism levels directly correlate with post-transplant erythropoietic activity in recipients undergoing aHSCT. A minimum threshold of stable mixed myeloid lineage chimerism of 20–25% appears to be the minimal level required to sustain favorable transplant outcomes [24–26].

Despite the limited studies, the progressive loss of B-cell lineage of donor chimerism is highly associated with acute B-cell lineage leukemia relapse; and drop of donor *NK*-lineage chimerism may reflect eminent B-cell as well non-B-cell leukemia relapse [27].

Choice of Blood Versus Bone Marrow for Engraftment Monitoring

The selection of a sample type for chimerism evaluation in leukemic patients post-aHSCT is a crucial consideration. Most transplant centers typically favor peripheral blood as the sample source, as it offers a less invasive method of collection compared to bone marrow aspiration. However, it is important to acknowledge that there may be instances where chimerism levels in blood and bone marrow differ among certain patients.

For instance, in a study conducted by J. Stump et al. chimerism was compared between bone marrow and peripheral blood in patients with acute leukemia and other hematological disorders following aHSCT [28]. Notably, of the 49 patients evaluated, 8 exhibited discrepancies in chimerism levels between the two sample types. In these cases, no recipient cells were detected in the peripheral blood, while 1–18% of the cells in the bone marrow displayed the host genotype.

Furthermore, Rauwerdinck et al. published a retrospective study involving 42 patients to compare chimerism in bone marrow and peripheral blood [29]. Their findings revealed no significant differences in chimerism rates between the two sample types at 30, 60, and 90 days post-transplant. Similarly, a study by Bach et al. reported an average difference of ~2% between bone marrow and peripheral blood chimerism [30].

Conclusions

Quantitative assessment of chimerism status is vital for post-HSCT patient management. The optimal analytical method should be cost-effective, rapid, and straightforward to interpret. Additionally, the technique must demonstrate high reproducibility and minimal inter-sample variability. This is particularly critical during the early post-transplant period, where precise quantification of donor versus recipient DNA is essential for evaluating engraftment success and early detection of graft failure. Moreover, the method should allow for analysis across various leukocyte subsets, such as T lymphocytes, to yield comprehensive insights into disease monitoring. Finally, the assay must possess high analytical sensitivity to facilitate the early detection of relapse during subsequent post-transplant phases. Chimerism analysis utilizing PCR-based amplification of STR markers has become the most prevalent technique for assessing stem cell engraftment, surpassing many other methodologies. This widespread adoption is due in part to the affordability of genotyping chemistry kits, as well as the high degree of polymorphism inherent to STR markers, which enhances the likelihood of identifying informative loci for quantitative analysis. Employing these markers allows for rapid and reliable detection and quantification of chimerism levels during stem cell engraftment monitoring. Although this methodology has several limitations, such as selecting appropriate informative loci for chimerism assessment, distinguishing true peaks from stutter artifacts, achieving accurate allele genotyping, managing heterozygous imbalance, addressing PCR amplification bias, and standardizing the quantification process across multiple time points, patients, and cell types, it remains the most widely used for chimerism assessment. Implementation of automated chimerism analysis software increases speed and accuracy of analysis while providing an interface designed for ease of use by laboratory personnel. STR-based analysis continues to be considered the gold standard methodology for chimerism assessment.

Acknowledgment The authors would like to thank Yelisey Romanov for his critical review and valuable suggestions.

References

1. Berry DA, Zhou S, Higley H, et al. Association of minimal residual disease with clinical outcome in pediatric and adult acute lymphoblastic leukemia: a meta-analysis. JAMA Oncol. 2017;3:e170580.
2. Cryz A, Nagler A. The role of measurable residual disease (MRD) in hematopoietic stem cell transplantation for hematological malignancies focusing on acute leukemia. Int J Mol Sci. 2019;20(21):5362.
3. Zhang A, et al. Engraftment and measurable residual disease monitoring after hematopoietic stem cell transplantation: comparison of two chimerism test strategies, next-generation sequencing versus a combination of short-tandem repeats and quantitative PCR. J Mol Diagn. 2024;26(4):233–44.
4. Thomas ED, et al. Intravenous infusion of bone marrow in patients receiving radiation and chemotherapy. N Engl J Med. 1957;257(11):491–6.
5. Clark JR, et al. Monitoring of chimerism following allogeneic haematopoietic stem cell transplantation (HSCT): technical recommendations for the use of Short Tandem Repeat (STR) based techniques, on behalf of the United Kingdom National External Quality Assessment Service for Leucocyte Immunophenotyping Chimerism Working Group. Br J Haematol. 2015;168(1):26–37.
6. van Dijk BA, et al. Erythrocyte repopulation after allogeneic bone marrow transplantation: analysis using erythrocyte antigens. Transplantation. 1987;44(5):650–4.
7. Blouin AG, et al. A practical guide to chimerism analysis: review of the literature and testing practices worldwide. Hum Immunol. 2021;82(11):838–49.
8. Van Deerlin VM, Reshef R. Chimerism testing in allogeneic hematopoietic stem cell transplantation. In: Leonard DG, editor. Molecular pathology in clinical practice. Cham: Springer; 2016. p. 823–48.
9. Alizadeh M, et al. Quantitative assessment of hematopoietic chimerism after bone marrow transplantation by real time quantitative polymerase chain reaction. Blood. 2002;99(12):4618–25. PMID: 12036896.
10. Buño I, et al. A comparison of fluorescent in situ hybridization and multiplex short tandem repeat polymerase chain reaction for quantifying chimerism after stem cell transplantation. Haematologica. 2005;90:1373–9.
11. Blouin AG, et al. Performance characteristics of next-generation sequencing-based engraftment monitoring and microchimerism detection in allogeneic hematopoietic cell transplantation: a practical approach for clinical assay validation. J Mol Diagn. 2024;26(11):995–1006.
12. Bader P. Chapter 20: documentation of engraftment and chimerism after HSCT. In: Carreras E, Dufour C, Mohty M, Kröger N, editors. The EBMT handbook: hematopoietic stem cell transplantation and cellular therapies. 7th ed. Cham: Springer; 2019. p. 143–7. https://doi.org/10.1007/9783030022785_20.
13. Sureda A, Carpenter PA, Bacigalupo A, et al. Harmonizing definitions for hematopoietic recovery, graft rejection, graft failure, poor graft function, and donor chimerism in allogeneic hematopoietic cell transplantation: a report on behalf of the EBMT, ASTCT, CIBMTR, and APBMT. Bone Marrow Transplant. 2024;59(6):832–7. https://doi.org/10.1038/s41409-024-02251-0. Epub 2024 Mar 5. Erratum in: Bone Marrow Transplant. 2024;59(9):1335. https://doi.org/10.1038/s41409-024-02336-w. PMID: 38443706; PMCID: PMC11161398.
14. Sellmann L, Rabe K, Bünting I, Dammann E, Göhring G, Ganser A, et al. Diagnostic value of highly sensitive chimerism analysis after allogeneic stem cell transplantation. Bone Marrow Transplant. 2018;53(11):1457–65.
15. Gineikiene E, Stoskus M, Griskevicius L. Recent advances in quantitative chimerism analysis. Expert Rev Mol Diagn. 2009;9(8):817–32. https://doi.org/10.1586/erm.09.66. PMID: 19895227.

16. Bader P, Kreyenberg H, Hoelle W, Dueckers G, Handgretinger R, Lang P, Kremens B, Dilloo D, Sykora KW, Schrappe M, Niemeyer C, Von Stackelberg A, Gruhn B, Henze G, Greil J, Niethammer D, Dietz K, Beck JF, Klingebiel T. Increasing mixed chimerism is an important prognostic factor for unfavorable outcome in children with acute lymphoblastic leukemia after allogeneic stem-cell transplantation: possible role for pre-emptive immunotherapy? J Clin Oncol. 2004;22(9):1696–705. https://doi.org/10.1200/JCO.2004.05.198. PMID: 15117992.
17. Liou A, Wahlstrom JT, Dvorak CC, Horn BN. Safety of pre-emptive donor lymphocyte infusions (DLI) based on mixed chimerism (MC) in peripheral blood or bone marrow subsets in children undergoing hematopoietic stem cell transplant (HSCT) for hematologic malignancies. Bone Marrow Transplant. 2017;52(7):1057–9. https://doi.org/10.1038/bmt.2017.45. Epub 2017 Apr 10. PMID: 28394367.
18. Mollet I, Giannoli C, Rigal D, Dubois V. Étude de chimérisme post-greffe de cellules souches hématopoïétiques. Intérêt du tri cellulaire: revue générale [Chimerism analysis after allogeneic haematopoietic stem cell transplantation. Interest of cell sorting: general review]. Pathol Biol (Paris). 2012;60(2):143–8. French. https://doi.org/10.1016/j.patbio.2010.10.002. Epub 2010 Nov 30. PMID: 21123007.
19. Ogonek J, Kralj Juric M, Ghimire S, Varanasi PR, Holler E, Greinix H, Weissinger E. Immune reconstitution after allogeneic hematopoietic stem cell transplantation. Front Immunol. 2016;7:507. https://doi.org/10.3389/fimmu.2016.00507. PMID: 27909435; PMCID: PMC5112259.
20. El-Cheikh J, Vazquez A, Crocchiolo R, Furst S, Calmels B, Castagna L, Lemarie C, Granata A, Ladaique P, Oudin C, Faucher C, Chabannon C, Blaise D. Acute GVHD is a strong predictor of full donor CD3+ T cell chimerism after reduced intensity conditioning allogeneic stem cell transplantation. Am J Hematol. 2012;87(12):1074–8. https://doi.org/10.1002/ajh.23319. Epub 2012 Aug 22. PMID: 22911907.
21. Peterlin P, Delaunay J, Guillaume T, Gastinne T, Mahé B, Dubruille V, Blin N, Le Bourgeois A, Brissot E, Lodé L, Le Gouill S, Moreau P, Mohty M, Chevallier P. Complete donor T cell chimerism predicts lower relapse incidence after standard double umbilical cord blood reduced-intensity conditioning regimen allogeneic transplantation in adults. Biol Blood Marrow Transplant. 2015;21(1):180–4. https://doi.org/10.1016/j.bbmt.2014.08.018. Epub 2014 Aug 28. PMID: 25175796.
22. Yokohata E, Kuwatsuka Y, Ohashi H, Terakura S, Kawashima N, Seto A, Kurahashi S, Ozawa Y, Goto T, Imahashi N, Nishida T, Miyao K, Sakemura R, Kato T, Sawa M, Kohno A, Sao H, Iida H, Kiyoi H, Naoe T, Miyamura K, Murata M. Impact of T-cell chimerism on relapse after cord blood transplantation for hematological malignancies: Nagoya Blood and Marrow Transplantation Group study. Bone Marrow Transplant. 2017;52(4):612–4. https://doi.org/10.1038/bmt.2016.323. Epub 2017 Jan 9. PMID: 28067879.
23. Srour SA, Olson A, Ciurea SO, Desai P, Bashir Q, Oran B, Bose P, Mehta R, Patel KP, Pemmaraju N, Daver N, Verstovsek S, Champlin RE, Popat UR. Mixed myeloid chimerism and relapse of myelofibrosis after allogeneic stem cell transplantation. Haematologica. 2021;106(7):1988–90. https://doi.org/10.3324/haematol.2019.223503. PMID: 31296578; PMCID: PMC8252931.
24. Shah NC, Rangarajan HG, Ngwube A, Shenoy S. Mixed donor chimerism following stem cell transplantation for sickle cell disease. Curr Opin Hematol. 2023;30(6):187–93. https://doi.org/10.1097/MOH.0000000000000786. Epub 2023 Sep 1. PMID: 37694765.
25. Fitzhugh CD, Cordes S, Taylor T, Coles W, Roskom K, Link M, Hsieh MM, Tisdale JF. At least 20% donor myeloid chimerism is necessary to reverse the sickle phenotype after allogeneic HSCT. Blood. 2017;130(17):1946–8. https://doi.org/10.1182/blood-2017-03-772392. Epub 2017 Sep 8. PMID: 28887325; PMCID: PMC5659067.
26. Abraham A, Hsieh M, Eapen M, Fitzhugh C, Carreras J, Keesler D, Guilcher G, Kamani N, Walters MC, Boelens JJ, Tisdale J, Shenoy S, National Institutes of Health; Center for International Blood and Marrow Transplant Research. Relationship between mixed donor-recipient chimerism and disease recurrence after hematopoietic cell transplantation for sickle

cell disease. Biol Blood Marrow Transplant. 2017;23(12):2178–83. https://doi.org/10.1016/j.bbmt.2017.08.038. Epub 2017 Sep 4. PMID: 28882446; PMCID: PMC5782809.
27. Jiang Y, Wan L, Qin Y, Wang X, Yan S, Xie K, Wang C. Donor chimerism of B cells and nature killer cells provides useful information to predict hematologic relapse following allogeneic hematopoietic stem cell transplantation. PLoS One. 2015;10(7):e0133671. https://doi.org/10.1371/journal.pone.0133671. PMID: 26226104; PMCID: PMC4520605.
28. Stumph J, Vnencak-Jones CL, Koyama T, Frangoul H. Comparison of peripheral blood and bone marrow samples for detection of post-transplant mixed chimerism. Bone Marrow Transplant. 2008;41(6):589–90. https://doi.org/10.1038/sj.bmt.1705938. Epub 2007 Nov 26. PMID: 18037938.
29. Rauwerdink CA, Tsongalis GJ, Tosteson TD, Hill JM, Meehan KR. The practical application of chimerism analyses in allogeneic stem cell transplant recipients: blood chimerism is equivalent to marrow chimerism. Exp Mol Pathol. 2012;93(3):339–44. https://doi.org/10.1016/j.yexmp.2012.07.003. Epub 2012 Jul 28. PMID: 22850633.
30. Bach C, Steffen M, Roesler W, Winkler J, Mackensen A, Stachel KD, Metzler M, Spriewald BM. Systematic comparison of donor chimerism in peripheral blood and bone marrow after hematopoietic stem cell transplantation. Blood Cancer J. 2017;7(6):e566. https://doi.org/10.1038/bcj.2017.42. PMID: 28574489; PMCID: PMC5520393.

18 Human Leukocyte Antigen (HLA) Testing

Dharmendra Jain and Eszter Lázár-Molnár

Abbreviations

APC	antigen presenting cell
ARS	antigen recognition site
ART	assisted reproductive technology
CBU	cord blood unit
CDC	complement dependent cytotoxicity
CIBMTR	Center for International Blood and Marrow Transplant Research
DNA	deoxyribonucleic acid
dNTP	deoxynucleotide triphosphate
ddNTP	dideoxynucleotide triphosphate
DSA	donor-specific antibodies
FCXM	flow cytometric crossmatch
GvHD	graft-versus-host disease
GvL	graft-versus-leukemia
HD	haploidentical donor
HLA	human leukocyte antigen
IPD-IMGT/HLA	Immuno Polymorphism Database-ImMunoGeneTics/HLA
HvG	host versus graft
KIR	killer inhibitory receptor
LEL	low expression HLA loci
LoH	loss of heterozygosity
mHA	minor histocompatibility antigen

D. Jain (✉) · E. Lázár-Molnár
Department of Pathology, University of Utah, Salt Lake City, UT, USA

Histocompatibility & Immunogenetics Laboratory, Salt Lake City, UT, USA

Immunology Division, ARUP Laboratories, Salt Lake City, UT, USA
e-mail: Dharmendra.Jain@path.utah.edu

W. Li (ed.), *Laboratory Assessments of Pediatric Leukemia*,
https://doi.org/10.1007/978-3-032-26557-9_18

MHC	major histocompatibility complex
MFI	mean fluorescence intensity
NIMA	non-inherited maternal antigens
NK	natural killer
NMDP	national marrow donor program
OS	overall survival
PCR	polymerase chain reaction
PGT	preimplantation genetic testing
SAB	single antigen bead
SCT	stem cell transplantation
SNP	single nucleotide polymorphism
SSOP	sequence-specific oligonucleotide probe
SSP	sequence-specific primer
UTR	untranslated region
WHO	World Health Organization

Human Leukocyte Antigen: Characteristics and Functions

The role of human leukocyte antigen (HLA) was first identified in tissue compatibility for solid organ transplantation and was later extensively evaluated in hematopoietic stem cell transplantation (SCT) [1, 2]. HLA, also known as the major histocompatibility complex (MHC) in humans, is located on the short arm of chromosome 6 and comprises more than 200 genes grouped into HLA class I, II, and III regions. The classical HLA class I (HLA-A, -B, and -C), and class II (HLA-DR, -DQ, and -DP) genes are associated with histocompatibility, while the role of HLA class III and non-classical HLA genes in tissue compatibility has not been well established. The HLA class I molecule consists of 7 or 8 exons coding for a hypervariable alpha chain and a non-covalently linked beta-2 microglobulin subunit, and includes extracellular, transmembrane, and cytoplasmic domains. Exons 2 and 3 of HLA class I genes encode the α1 and α2 domains, which together form the peptide-binding domain, also known as the antigen recognition site (ARS), and referred to as such throughout this chapter. HLA class II molecules are heterodimers consisting of a hypervariable alpha, and a beta chain, both of which include external transmembrane and cytoplasmic domains. Exon 2 of both the alpha and beta chains encodes the ARS [3]. Despite their structural similarities, small variations in nucleotide and amino acid sequences make HLA genes highly polymorphic, with more than 41,000 HLA alleles identified as of 2025 [4]. The current HLA allele nomenclature consists of four fields, each separated by colons. The first field represents the type, or allele group, which often corresponds to the serological antigen, followed by the second field reflecting the subtype, displaying amino acid sequence variation that defines the specific allele. The third field reflects synonymous nucleotide variations in the coding region, while the last field indicates variations in intronic regions [5]. A unique characteristic of HLA is allele linkage disequilibrium, a phenomenon in which certain HLA alleles are tightly linked and inherited as haplotypes with minimal recombination, which increases HLA similarity among individuals within the same population. Additionally, HLA genes exhibit co-dominance, meaning that both the maternal and paternal HLA genes are expressed simultaneously on the cell surface [6].

The primary function of HLA molecules is to provide central tolerance during thymic education of T cells, allowing them to distinguish between self and non-self, and regulating immune responses through antigen presentation. Foreign antigens, such as viral, bacterial, or fungal proteins, as well as non-self HLA molecules, are captured in the ARS of HLA molecules and presented to T cells to initiate an adaptive immune response [7]. However, the presentation of non-self HLA molecules from donor allograft cells triggers an undesired immune response against the allograft. Sensitization to foreign HLA molecules can occur through pregnancy, blood transfusion, or allotransplantation. Foreign HLA can be presented via three pathways: the direct pathway, where the recipient's T cells recognize intact donor HLA molecules on the surface of donor antigen presenting cells (APC); the indirect pathway, where the recipient's APCs process and present donor-derived antigens to recipient T cells; and the semi-direct pathway, where recipient APCs acquire intact donor HLA molecules but, rather than presentation as processed allopeptide, is re-presented as conformationally intact protein to recipient T cells. Allorecognition leads to an adaptive immune response, involving the generation of alloreactive T cells that mount a cellular response, as well as alloreactive B cells differentiating into plasma cells that produce antibodies to foreign HLA antigens [8].

In the context of transplantation, HLA antibodies can bind to the allograft and mediate rejection via complement activation, or antibody-dependent cytotoxicity. A re-exposure to the same foreign antigen can lead to memory response that appears faster and is more intense than a primary immune response. Therefore, the presence of pre-formed donor-specific HLA antibodies (DSA) is a contraindication for both solid organ and stem cell transplantation (SCT). Particularly in SCT, donor-derived alloreactive T cells can mount an immune response against mismatched HLA antigens in the recipient, leading to graft versus host disease (GvHD), which highlights the importance of HLA matching between donor-recipient pairs. The two main attributes of HLA compatibility are either the absence of mismatched HLA alleles/antigens between the donor and recipient or absence of specific HLA antibodies in the recipient to the HLA antigens of the donor [9].

HLA Typing Methods

HLA testing methodologies have evolved over the last 50 years from serology-based methods such as complement-dependent cellular cytotoxicity (CDC), to recently introduced third-generation sequencing methods. The serological typing methods and some earlier iterations of molecular methods like sequence-specific primer (SSP) polymerase chain reaction (PCR), and PCR followed by melting curve analysis do not meet the current standards of HLA typing requirements for SCT and will not be discussed further in this chapter. The methods discussed here are commonly used in clinical histocompatibility laboratories and meet the current recommendations for HLA typing in SCT.

Solid Phase Assays

The sequence-specific oligonucleotide probe (SSOP) hybridization method is the most common bead-based solid phase assay used in clinical laboratories. Briefly, HLA genes are first amplified using PCR with biotinylated primers targeting each specific HLA locus. The amplified biotinylated product is then hybridized with a bead array, where each bead is coated with unique probes designed to detect the most common specific HLA alleles. After washing away unbound PCR products, the biotin-labeled amplified product is detected using a streptavidin-phycoerythrin conjugate. The bead mixture is then analyzed with a Luminex cytometer to identify the amplified HLA product. Allele assignment is performed using specialized software (HLA Fusion from OneLambda/ThermoFisher Scientific, and MATCH IT!® Antibody Analysis from Immucor/Werfen). The intensity of fluorescence on each bead is measured and the software will determine positive or negative reactions based on the strength of the fluorescence signals, compared to negative and positive controls. The probes used in this method do not cover all the exons of the HLA genes and therefore may not identify variations outside the regions analyzed. Additionally, any variation, for example, single nucleotide polymorphism (SNP), beyond the probe binding site may not be detected. Therefore, the presence of a rare or novel allele cannot definitively be determined by this method and the sample will need to be reflexed to sequence-based testing methods.

With the extended exon coverage and increased probe quantity, the SSOP method mostly provides intermediate resolution HLA typing, identifying the common and well-documented HLA alleles or at least narrow down the HLA allele assignments. The rapid turnaround time of 3–5 h makes this assay well-suited for expedited HLA typing, initial typing to identify potential related donors from family members, and meeting the requirements for confirmatory testing in SCT candidates [10].

Sequencing Assays

HLA typing using deoxyribonucleic acid (DNA) sequencing is considered more precise as it accounts for the variability at single nucleotide level and therefore can differentiate between closely related HLA alleles that differ by only one or a few nucleotides. As it can determine the exact nucleotide sequence of a gene or a region of a gene, it is considered the gold standard for HLA allele identification. With the recent introduction of the newer methods, the DNA sequencing-based HLA typing methods have revolutionized the field. Advanced DNA-based sequencing methods, such as massive parallel sequencing, can also be employed for the identification and characterization of novel alleles.

Sanger Sequencing

HLA typing by Sanger sequencing relies on chain termination, where DNA synthesis is randomly halted by the incorporation of modified nucleotides (dideoxynucleotide triphosphates, ddNTPs), preventing further nucleotide addition. The terminating nucleotide at the end of various DNA fragments is detected either by gel electrophoresis (conventional) or capillary electrophoresis. In capillary electrophoresis, fluorochrome-labeled terminating nucleotides (ddATP, ddTTP, ddGTP, ddCTP, each labeled with different fluorochrome) at the end of the fragments are detected as they pass through the capillary. During the sequencing process, single-stranded DNA is annealed with a primer, and DNA polymerase begins incorporating new nucleotides at the 3′ end of the elongating DNA chain. The chain continues to grow when normal nucleotides (deoxynucleotide triphosphates, dNTPs) are added, but terminates when a modified nucleotide (ddNTP) is incorporated. The resulting oligonucleotides of varying lengths are then separated by electrophoresis. As DNA fragments pass through the capillary, a laser excites the fluorescent dye attached to the fragments, causing them to fluoresce at specific wavelengths. This fluorescence is measured and translated by the detector into nucleotide assignments (A, T, G, or C), producing the DNA consensus sequence.

The consensus sequence is then aligned with the reference HLA database (IPD-HLA/IMGT) to identify the HLA allele. Because both alleles at each locus are sequenced simultaneously, there is often a high degree of ambiguity (i.e., alternative genotypes) due to the inability to determine the cis/trans linkage of polymorphic motifs at heterozygous positions. To resolve such ambiguities, either HLA typing of additional family members or reflex testing using SSP or SSO methods may be necessary. Similar to the SSO method, Sanger sequencing typically covers the exons encoding the ARS, so variations outside these regions may go undetected, limiting the identification of novel alleles. Since each sample is sequenced and analyzed individually, Sanger sequencing is not a high-throughput method and has a relatively longer turnaround time compared to some of the advanced sequencing methods discussed below [11].

Massive Parallel Sequencing

This method, also known as second-generation or next-generation sequencing (NGS), relies on sequencing during DNA synthesis, where new sequence information is captured each time, a nucleotide is added. The key steps include amplification of the entire HLA gene locus through long-range PCR, typically covering most exons, introns, and sometimes untranslated regions (UTRs), followed by library preparation, sequencing, and detection [12, 13].

Two different approaches are commonly used to prepare library for sequence-based HLA typing [14]. In the first approach, genomic DNA is amplified using primers specific to each HLA gene. The amplified DNA is subsequently fragmented using enzymes, and short nucleotide adapters are ligated to the resulting fragments. These adapters serve as binding sites to the sequencing flow cell, providing annealing sites for the sequencing primers. The adapters also include an index, a short sequence unique to each adapter, which allows for barcoding, enabling multiple samples to be processed on the same flow cell (multiplexing). To achieve uniform fragment lengths, a size selection method is subsequently applied. This method has challenges of allelic dropouts and although high resolution, it is limited in capturing all the genetic variations across the HLA gene [14, 15].

An alternative approach to library preparation involves the selective capture of targeted HLA genes using probe hybridization. In this method, genomic DNA is first fragmented, then ligated to sequencing adapters containing unique molecular identifiers or barcodes. Biotinylated probes specific to HLA gene regions are then hybridized to the adapter-ligated DNA and captured using streptavidin-coated magnetic beads. The enriched DNA fragments are subsequently PCR amplified to prepare them for sequencing. The hybrid capture methods enable better phasing when combined with third-generation long-read sequencing methods like Oxford Nanopore and PacBio sequencing platforms, described below [16].

The sequencing chemistry and detection methods vary depending on the instrument on which the sequencing takes place. For instance, on the Ion Torrent platform (Thermo Fisher Scientific), H^+ ions are released with the incorporation of each nucleotide, and these are measured as pH changes using semiconductors [13, 15]. In the Illumina platform (Illumina, Inc.), nucleotides are conjugated with fluorescent dyes, and each added nucleotide emits a specific fluorescent signal, which is captured by a camera [14].

One of the advantages of NGS is its ability to sequence millions of DNA fragments simultaneously in a single run. The sequencing reads are then demultiplexed (sorted) for each HLA locus for each sample in the batch, based on the specific adapter/index sequences. These short, overlapping sequences are combined to form a consensus sequence (de novo assembly), which is then aligned with a reference sequence to determine the HLA allele. Because each nucleotide is sequenced multiple times (read depth), NGS produces highly reliable results, compensating for errors from amplification, sequencing reactions, or random occurrences. Due to its ability to provide fully phased sequences, NGS can also resolve the phasing issues encountered with Sanger sequencing. Additionally, the comprehensive coverage of the HLA gene, combined with the ability to phase variants and distinguish true variants from sequencing noise due to high read depths, enables the identification of novel alleles. However, phasing challenges may still arise if polymorphic sites are more than 1000 base pairs apart, as seen in HLA-DRB1 and -DPB1 alleles. Similarly, closely related alleles with few polymorphic differences and alleles containing homopolymer regions can pose challenges for accurate sequencing and allele assignment. While NGS offers high throughput due to multiplexing, it may not be ideal for sequencing individual samples in a short time frame, such as patients with acute myeloid leukemia (AML) who fail primary induction therapy and are considered for SCT [17].

Third-Generation Sequencing

Third-generation sequencing provides long-read sequencing, which is particularly useful for HLA typing since it allows for direct phasing to resolve cis-trans ambiguities for heterozygous positions that are at a longer distance from each other on the gene. In the context of HLA typing, two technologies have been evaluated in clinical laboratories.

Single-Molecule, Long-Read Sequencing

Single molecule, real-time (SMRT) sequencing (Pacific Biosciences of California, Inc.) is an ideal technology for generating unambiguous, phase-resolved imputation-free HLA typing. In the first step, the target-specific primers are used to amplify the HLA gene/s; however, unlike the other technologies special hairpin adapters are used to prepare a circular DNA template called as SMRTbell™. The hairpin adapters provide a universal primer binding site and initiation sequence within the circular template allowing the generation of both sense and antisense sequence from a single molecule. These library templates are then sequenced in a SMRT flow cell, which consists of millions of tiny chambers called zero-mode wave guides. These chambers channels light to the bottom, where the polymerase adds new bases labeled with unique fluorochromes that are detected during imaging. Upon incorporation of a nucleotide, a millisecond-scale imaging event detects the fluorescent signal. The fluorescent tag is then released from nucleotide and diffuses away, making room for the next nucleotide. The imaging process is synchronized with the nucleotide incorporation rate, enabling real-time identification of each base [14].

Due to the coverage of complete HLA class I genes and long amplicons of HLA class II genes, and by generating de novo, reference-free consensus sequences, it can identify variants in regulatory regions within 5′ UTRs, introns, and 3′ UTRs. This enables up to four-field HLA genotyping and makes the identification of novel alleles straightforward.

Nanopore Sequencing

Nanopore sequencing, (Oxford Nanopore Technologies PLC) is an emerging technology for HLA typing that offers several advantages over traditional sequencing methods. Unlike other platforms, nanopore sequencing reads long stretches of DNA in real-time by passing single-stranded DNA molecules through biological nanopores, embedded in a membrane [18]. As the DNA moves through the nanopore, changes in ionic current specific for each of the four bases are detected and translated into nucleotide sequences. Commercial kits have been optimized to type all 11 classical HLA loci in 3–5 h [19].

The basic workflow is similar to massively parallel sequencing, requiring DNA extraction, single-tube amplification, library preparation, and sequencing. However, the sequencing instrument is much more affordable compared to other sequencing platforms, requiring no initial investment in instrumentation, and its compact, portable design requires minimal space. Additional cost saving includes reusable flow cells, which can be employed three to ten times, depending on the number of loci tested and the availability of functional pores after each run.

The advantages of this technology include remarkably short turnaround time, especially when used for single-sample testing (3–5 h), while providing high-resolution sequencing covering long stretches of DNA. While software tools for HLA allele assignment from nanopore data keep evolving, interpreting the long, complex reads generated by this technology may require more advanced bioinformatics workflows [19, 20].

Methods of HLA Antibody Testing

The presence of DSA is associated with poor transplant outcomes. Historically, HLA antibodies were detected using functional assays such as NIH-CDC, but this method is now considered outdated due to low sensitivity, challenges of maintaining cell viability, and limitations of HLA antigen representation in the assay.

Antibody Screening and Identification Assays

The introduction of solid-phase bead-based assays revolutionized HLA antibody testing, providing substantially more sensitive, accurate, and reliable results for identifying HLA antibody specificities. Today, two main types of HLA antibody assays are commonly used in histocompatibility laboratories: HLA phenotype bead assays, which utilize native HLA antigens purified from donor cells, and single antigen bead (SAB) assays, which use beads coated with single recombinant HLA antigens for specific antibody identification. The testing procedure for both assays is similar. Briefly, patient serum is incubated with a pool of beads, each bead possessing a unique dye signature and coated with either a single HLA haplotype (phenotype bead assay) or a single recombinant HLA antigen (SAB assay). HLA antibody binding to the antigens on the beads is detected by secondary antibodies specific to the Fc fragment of human immunoglobulin G (IgG), conjugated with fluorescent tags. Luminex instruments or flow cytometers are used to detect and record the mean fluorescence intensity (MFI) from each single bead and determine antibody specificity [21, 22].

Crossmatch Assays

Determination of DSAs can be achieved through virtual or physical crossmatch assays. Most commonly virtual crossmatch is employed in SCT, by comparing the recipient's HLA antibody profile with the donor's HLA typing to determine the presence of DSA. Physical crossmatch may sometimes be used to confirm DSA by testing the binding of recipient antibodies to donor cells in vitro.

Physical Crossmatch Assays

Physical crossmatch assays are performed by mixing the recipient's serum with live donor lymphocytes in a test tube to detect the presence of DSAs. Traditional methods such as NIH-CDC [23] and its more sensitive variants—AMOS [24] and anti-human globulin (AHG)-CDC [25]—measured the functional impact of DSA through donor cell cytotoxicity, but are now rarely used in most histocompatibility laboratories due to their low sensitivity.

Flow cytometric crossmatch (FCXM) is now the standard method used in most clinical laboratories. In FCXM, recipient serum is mixed with donor lymphocytes, and after washing away unbound antibodies, fluorescently conjugated antibodies binding to T cells (CD3) and B cells (CD19), and to human IgG are added. The cells are analyzed on a flow cytometer, and MFI of anti-IgG binding to T and B cells is recorded and compared to known negative sera to evaluate DSA positivity [26].

Virtual Crossmatch

A virtual crossmatch is a computational approach used to predict the outcome of a physical crossmatch. It helps assess immunological risk without the need for a physical laboratory test, eliminating the requirement for live donor cells. It compares the recipient's known anti-HLA antibody profile (typically determined by solid-phase assays) with the donor's HLA typing to assess compatibility. The availability of intermediate to high-resolution HLA typing of the donor, combined with HLA antibody identification in the recipient, can enable virtual determination of HLA DSA presence [27]. With the widespread use of solid phase technologies, the virtual crossmatch strategy has been the primary method to assess HLA-DSA in SCT, and is particularly valuable for assessing compatibility in unrelated SCT, where donor cells are rarely available for crossmatching [28, 29].

HLA Testing for Stem Cell Transplantation

The success of allogeneic SCT is measured by overall survival (OS), episodes and severity of GvHD, and transplant-related mortality; these parameters can be significantly impacted by the patient's disease status (remission and relapse), comorbidities, age, sensitization, and infectious disease history. The donor's age, gender, stem cell source, and HLA compatibility also have an impact on transplant outcomes [30]. Patients matched with fully compatible donors across all classical HLA loci achieve the best clinical outcomes. Therefore, HLA typing for both recipients and donors is essential prior to SCT [31]. Delayed availability of HLA typing has been identified as a potential cause of transplant delay [32]. It is recommended that allogeneic transplant candidates undergo HLA typing before the formal donor search begins [33]. In addition, confirmatory or verification typing should be completed before the formal donor search begins, or before patient conditioning, marrow harvesting, or administration of hematopoietic cell mobilization agents, whichever occurs first. The list of HLA alleles keeps growing due to addition of newly discovered alleles [4]. A repeat typing is required if the prior test was performed over 2 years ago using non-sequencing methods, and an extended typing is mandated if it did not include all required HLA genes and exons within the previous 5 years [33].

The most commonly used specimen source for HLA typing is peripheral blood; however, it may not be an ideal source for pediatric patients due to the invasive nature of collection and the risk of suboptimal collection. Additionally, SCT candidates with diseases like acute leukemia and aplastic anemia tend to have somatic mutations in neoplastic or aplastic cells, spanning the short arm of chromosome 6 carrying the HLA genes. Mutations in this region can significantly affect the HLA typing results by causing impaired binding of the primers used in HLA typing assays, or leading to allele dropouts due to loss of heterozygosity (LoH) [34, 35]. For such cases, non-peripheral blood sources like buccal swabs, saliva, or less commonly, hair follicles or nails are preferred. Chemotherapy, often used to induce remission in SCT candidates, may cause oral mucositis [36]. As a result, saliva samples may be unsuitable for patients with mutations in neoplastic blast cells due to possible contamination from peripheral blood cells. Using two different sample sources for initial and verification typing is recommended when clinical details are unavailable [33].

Patient-donor HLA matching is of primary importance in SCT with unrelated donors. The primary interaction in SCT is between the ARS of MHC molecules with the T-cell receptor (TCR). HLA alleles or antigens with identical amino acid sequences in the ARS are considered matched (commonly referred to as being in the same P group). The amino acids in this domain are encoded by exons 2 and 3 for HLA class I, and by exon 2 for class II. Matching at the antigen recognition sites (ARS) represents the minimum standard for compatibility. DNA sequencing-based HLA typing that meets this standard is referred to as high-resolution typing, which is defined as the identification of HLA alleles that encode the same protein sequence within the ARS, while excluding non-expressed alleles listed in the common, intermediate, and well-documented (CIWD) database [37]. Achieving high-resolution typing requires that both patient and donor are tested by sequencing-based methods. The reported HLA genotyping profile should have a minimum two-field assignment according to the World Health Organization (WHO) nomenclature and per the national marrow donor program (NMDP) policies, and must contain: a) only one unambiguously assigned genotype or; b) multiple alternative genotypes if the primary genotype includes two common or intermediate alleles, and the other genotypes do not include any alleles listed as common or intermediate or any CIWD null alleles. HLA P and G group assignments are acceptable which define alleles sharing amino acid (P group) and/or nucleotide (G group) sequences for the ARS and do not contain any known non-expressed alleles [33]. It is required that the SCT candidate and donor undergo HLA typing for at least HLA-A, -B, -C, -DRB1, and -DPB1 loci. Although not mandatory, optimal typing that includes low expressing loci HLA-DRB3/4/5, -DQA1, -DQB1, and -DPA1 is highly recommended for a better match and to assist with DSA risk assessment [33, 38]. While HLA typing is generally not required for patients undergoing autologous SCT, it is still recommended to perform typing for HLA class I genes (HLA-A and HLA-B), which are expressed on platelets. This enables the selection of an HLA-compatible platelet donor in cases where the patient develops platelet refractoriness [39].

The timeline, and specimen source requirements for adult and pediatric SCT patients are the same, but there is a slight difference for HLA loci testing and confirmatory typing requirement for cord blood transplants. A high-resolution typing for HLA-A, B, C, and -DRB1 loci for both patient and cord blood units (CBU) is required. Unlike adult SCT candidates, the DPB1 typing is not mandatory for CBU. Additionally, the HLA confirmatory typing for CBU should be done using a sample from a segment attached to the CBU or should be performed on a sample from the bag itself if the segment is unavailable. In SCT with cord blood as a stem cell source, non-HLA factors like CBU quality and stem cell dose equally impact the outcome and need to be evaluated [40].

The risk of alloresponse is higher following allogeneic SCT from matched unrelated donors compared to matched related donors, largely due to minor histocompatibility antigens (mHAs), which are peptides presented by MHC molecules to T cells. Unrelated donor–recipient pairs matched for HLA phenotypes only share specific MHC antigen regions, whereas genotypically identical siblings potentially have matching genetic sequences across the entire MHC region. Although over 100 mHAs have been identified, data linking them to SCT outcomes is limited, and matching for mHAs is not currently used in clinical practice [41].

Patients from underrepresented or mixed ethnicities or those with rare HLA haplotypes face challenges in finding fully HLA-matched donors. In these cases, partially matched or haploidentical donors (sharing one haplotype) may be considered. For mismatched transplant pairs, testing for HLA antibodies before the formal search is crucial to avoid resource waste and delays, as HLA-DSA presence is linked to primary graft failure through antibody-dependent cellular cytotoxicity or CDC. Conducting HLA antibody analysis early in the search process minimizes graft failure risks in HLA-sensitized patients and aids in strategizing for highly sensitized patients who may require desensitization, if no compatible donor is available [42].

HLA Matching for Donor Selection

The overall success of SCT relies significantly on securing an optimal donor match, with critical considerations including donor availability, age, and infectious disease status. Most importantly, the extent of HLA compatibility between the recipient and donor is paramount in optimizing SCT outcomes. As the benefit of HLA matching decreases with the progression of malignant disease, the medical urgency of the transplant must be considered when searching for SCT donor, including alternative sub-optimal HLA matched donors, partially matched or haploidentical donors (HD) if clinically necessary [32, 43].

While numerous factors influence the search for an optimal donor for pediatric patients compared to adult SCT candidates such as age, stem cell source, and donor availability, the HLA matching criteria remain largely consistent between the two groups. However, differences emerge when CBUs are used as the stem cell source compared to peripheral blood or bone marrow. Since CBUs contain T cells that are less mature and typically less immunologically potent than those in peripheral blood or bone marrow, the risk of GvHD is notably lower with CBUs. Consequently, the requirements for HLA matching are less stringent for CBUs, offering greater flexibility in donor selection while maintaining acceptable outcomes [44]. A matched sibling donor is generally preferred for pediatric patients, as it supports better long-term survival. However, in cases where a sibling match is unavailable, unrelated donors or cord blood are frequently used. Cord blood is especially valuable in pediatrics due to its higher tolerance of HLA mismatches and rapid availability, in contrast to adult patients for whom the cell dose from cords is often insufficient for full engraftment. The use of HD (half-matched) donors is also more common in pediatric patients, as children generally experience lower risks of GvHD compared to adults, making this option more viable [45]. In pediatric patients, candidates for SCT include those with both malignant and non-malignant conditions. These conditions encompass, but are not limited to, bone marrow failure syndromes, inborn errors of metabolism and immunity, and hemoglobinopathies. For candidates with malignant diseases, a slight degree of HLA mismatching can be acceptable, as the graft-versus-leukemia (GvL) effect associated with alloreactivity can be beneficial in controlling disease remission. However, for candidates with non-malignant diseases, a fully HLA-matched donor is preferred to minimize alloreactivity, as the GvL effect does not provide therapeutic benefit and could increase the risk of GvHD.

In summary, HLA matching criteria are more flexible for pediatric patients, allowing the use of alternative donor types like haploidentical family members or cord blood to expedite transplantation. Adult patients, however, typically need stricter HLA matching, prioritizing fully matched unrelated donors to minimize GvHD and ensure a cell dose suitable for successful engraftment.

Essential HLA Matching Criteria

For SCT, a fully HLA-matched donor (10/10 match at HLA-A, -B, -C, -DRB1, and -DQB1) is ideal [46], yet timely access to such donors is limited by factors like the underrepresentation of certain ethnic groups in donor registries, as well as donor health and availability. Additionally, SCT urgency impacts donor selection, as the advantage of high-resolution HLA matching decreases with disease progression—often taking longer than needed to find a matched donor, which may make the patient ineligible for transplant. In such cases, alternative options like partially matched or HD become viable options [43].

Numerous algorithms exist to guide optimal HLA-compatible donor selection. An evidence-based framework developed by the NMDP, the Center for International Blood and Marrow Transplant Research (CIBMTR), and the NMDP Histocompatibility Advisory Group is widely accepted in the field [38]. This guideline is based on data from adult and pediatric recipients of first unrelated donor SCT. These guidelines prioritize younger, allele-level matched unrelated donors for HLA-A, -B, -C, and -DRB1 loci. Any single mismatch, whether at the allele or antigen level, significantly lowers OS [47]. Some alleles such as HLA-C*03:03 and C*03:04 have only a subtle difference that do not impact the physical and chemical structure of the HLA molecule and its bound peptides thus, such mismatches are acceptable [48, 49].

There is only a 20% chance of finding an unrelated donor that is also matched at HLA-DPB1 locus along with HLA-A, -B, -C, and -DRB1. This is due to weak linkage disequilibrium of HLA-DPB1 with other HLA loci. Not all DPB1 mismatches carry the same immunogenic potential in inducing T-cell response, due to variation in the amino acid sequences within the ARS. Thus, it is recommended to search for DPB1 permissive mismatch [50]. Three T-cell epitope (TCE) groups that vary in strength to induce immunogenicity have been recommended to be considered in finding a DPB1 permissive mismatch. This strategy can prevent excessive alloreactivity associated with acute GvHD while maintaining limited alloreactivity needed for a GvL effect [51, 52]. A free online tool is available at IPD-IMGT/HLA website for the prediction of immunogenecity of an HLA-DPB1 allele (Table 18.1)

Table 18.1 HLA matching and donor selection tools

	HLA tool	Use in donor evaluation	Uniform resource locator (URL)	References
1	DPB1 T Cell Epitope Algorithm v2.0	To predict immunogenicity of the HLA-DPB1 alleles	https://www.ebi.ac.uk/ipd/imgt/hla/matching/	[53]
2	Expression of DP Antigens Tool (ExPAT)	To determine expression level and experimental confirmation status of HLA-DPB1 alleles	https://dpb1-tce-expression.nmdp.org/	[54]
3	HLA-B Leader Mismatch Calculator	To compare mismatches in the leader sequences of patient and donor HLA-B alleles	https://www.ebi.ac.uk/ipd/imgt/hla/matching/b_leader/	[55]
4	HLA-B leader assessment tool (BLEAT)	To automate the assignment of leader genotypes, define HLA-B leader match statuses, and rank order candidate stem cell sources according to clinical risk	https://bleader.nmdp.org/	[56]
5	KIR Ligand Calculator	To identify KIR ligand mismatches and directionality of mismatches	https://www.ebi.ac.uk/ipd/kir/matching/ligand/	[57]

(continued)

Table 18.1 (continued)

	HLA tool	Use in donor evaluation	Uniform resource locator (URL)	References
6	Donor KIR B-content group calculator	To assign the HLA genotype as "Neutral," "Better," "Best" based on KIR B content to determine relapse protection seen in T-cell replete URD SCT for AML	https://www.ebi.ac.uk/ipd/kir/matching/b_content/	[58]
7	HLA-DQA1 and HLA-DQB1 Heterodimers Assessment (QLASSy) Tool	To analyze HLA-DQ heterodimer data for DQα-DQβ trans-heterodimer evaluation, HLA-DQ imputation, and HLA-DQ-featured source selection	https://dq-dimers.nmdp.org/	[59]

[53]. More recently, another model based on HLA-DP expression has been proposed that can predict the immunogenicity of HLA-DP allotypes in patients and donors and help identify permissive DPB1 mismatch pair. A single mismatch between a patient and a donor with a high-expression of HLA-DPB1 allele in recipient is considered unfavorable and high-risk, while a mismatch with a low-expression HLA-DPB1 allele in recipient is considered favorable and low-risk. The expression of HLA-DP is associated with the SNP at rs9277534 in the 3′ UTR, where the A nucleotide is linked to low expression and the G nucleotide to high expression [60]. This model is not fully validated and currently not used in clinical practice. An online Expression of DP Antigens Tool (ExPAT) can be used to determine the expression level and experimental confirmation status of HLA-DPB1 alleles, indicating whether their expression is experimentally validated or predicted (Table 18.1) [54].

Although low-expression HLA loci (LEL), including HLA-DRB3/4/5, -DQB1, and -DPB1, are not primary matching targets, efforts should be made to limit mismatches at these loci, as ≥3 mismatches are linked to higher transplant-related mortality and lower OS [61]. While it remained unclear for a long time if allele-level matching is superior to antigen matching at LELs or how mismatches at specific loci impact outcomes, a recent study showed a 7% lower survival rate for 8/8 transplants with a single HLA-DQB1 mismatch, compared to HLA-A, -B, -C, -DRB1, -DQB1 ("10/10") transplants, highlighting the significance of HLA matching at LELs [62].

Mismatches can be further assessed for directionality. In bidirectional mismatches, the recipient and donor carry different alleles, while unidirectional mismatches occur when either the donor or recipient is homozygous and the other is heterozygous. When the recipient is homozygous and the donor is heterozygous, the mismatch occurs in the host-versus-graft (HvG) direction, while a heterozygous recipient with a homozygous donor results in a graft-versus-host (GvH) mismatch. Mismatches in the GvH direction are associated with increased acute GvHD risk, making HvG-preferred mismatches more favorable [63]. However, HLA mismatches in the GVH or HVG direction were not associated with non-relapse-related mortality and survival in patients with umbilical cord blood transplantation [64].

Pre-formed HLA antibodies can be found in up to 33% of SCT candidates due to prior transfusions, or pregnancies in women. Pre-existing DSA have been linked to primary graft failure and delayed engraftment after unrelated and related haploidentical donor SCT [42, 65]. Hence, identification and routine monitoring of the candidates with circulating HLA antibodies and avoidance of donors carrying corresponding allo-antigens should be considered. Patients with DSA to low-expression loci may benefit from extended HLA typing of potential donors to include these loci. Desensitization to reduce DSA levels may be useful for patients without matched donors or for those requiring urgent transplants [66].

In pediatric patients, CBUs are often preferred due to lower dose requirements, reduced GvHD risk, and decreased need for T-cell depletion compared to peripheral blood stem cells [44]. Traditionally, CBU matching has required antigen-level matches at HLA-A and -B and allele-level matches at HLA-DRB1, with a 4/6 match considered acceptable. More recent HLA matching approaches are evaluating the inclusion of HLA-C and the potential for lower acceptable mismatches. For double cord blood unit transplantation, the HLA matching criteria used for selecting a single unit should also apply to each unit in the double-unit graft. Currently, there is no evidence to support considering HLA matching between the two units in the selection process [38].

Enhanced HLA Matching Criteria

The practice of transplanting across a partially matched or HD donor has increased in recent years, highlighting the need for tools that can identify HLA mismatched, yet permissive donors [67]. Studies have targeted identification of biomarkers and development of tools to improve outcomes for HLA mismatched transplants. While these may be applied for donor selection to some extent, they are not part of the current recommendations by NMDP.

HLA-B Leader Mismatch

Among all classical HLA genes, HLA-B exhibits the highest polymorphism, with over 10,000 alleles reported to date [4]. This extensive variation significantly reduces the probability of finding a fully HLA-matched donor. A unique sequence dimorphism exists at codon −21 in the leader sequence of exon 1 of HLA-B, resulting in either methionine (M) or threonine (T) and consequently patients having a MM, MT, or TT genotype [68]. This variation can influence T cell and natural killer (NK) cell-mediated immune responses, impacting GvHD risk following HLA-B mismatched transplants. Previous studies have shown that GvHD risk is notably lower in patients with only HLA-B allele/antigen mismatch, when both mismatched patient and donor HLA-B alleles share the same leader sequence type (both M or both T) compared to when the leader sequences differ. Patients with a shared allele containing an M leader sequence showed a significantly higher incidence of GvHD compared to those with shared T leader sequences, independent of the mismatched HLA-B allele leader sequence. Additionally, MM patients benefit more from an MT donor than from an MM donor. While HLA-B mismatching increases GvHD risk, identifying the specific polymorphic residues in recipient-donor antigen mismatches enables a more precise risk assessment and facilitates targeted post-transplant treatment strategies [69]. Online tools are available to compare mismatches in the leader sequences of patient and donor HLA-B alleles and to automate the assignment of leader genotypes, to define HLA-B leader match status [55], and rank candidate stem cell sources according to clinical risk (Table 18.1) [56].

HLA Matching in Patients with Loss of Heterozygosity (LoH)

In a healthy immune system, immune cells monitor and control neoplastic cells, preventing unchecked proliferation. However, neoplastic cells can evade immune surveillance through both intrinsic and extrinsic mechanisms [70]. A key intrinsic mechanism is copy-neutral loss of heterozygosity (CN-LoH), in which malignant cells lose certain HLA genes on chromosome 6 to avoid recognition by the immune system. In SCT, donor alloreactive T cells exert immune pressure on leukemic cells, leading some to develop immune escape mechanisms. This can involve the complete or partial loss of chromosome 6, or partial deletions within the HLA region, resulting in the loss of one or more HLA alleles, or entire HLA haplotype [35].

CN-LoH, often due to acquired uniparental disomy, involves deletions across the short arm of chromosome 6p, followed by duplication of the remaining chromosome. HLA loss is more prevalent in leukemias at relapse, particularly in cases following HLA-mismatched or HD SCT [71]. A graft-versus-host (GvH) directional mismatch in SCT offers the advantage of enhancing the GvL effect. This effect enables the donor's alloreactive T cells to target mismatched haplotypes or HLA alleles on the recipient's tumor cells, helping to control residual tumor presence and potential relapse. The loss of recipient-specific, non-shared HLA haplotypes prevents the activation, cytokine release, and cytotoxic activity of donor T cells against relapsed leukemic cells [35, 71]. In the context of the pediatric SCT candidates receiving CBU, the HLA LoH has not been observed as a major mechanism of relapse. Detection of possible LoH in SCT patients with disease relapse is critical for guiding treatment decisions [72]. Donor lymphocyte infusions which are used to combat the leukemic cells lose efficacy in producing GvL effects, while still posing a risk for GvHD, in which case alternative treatment options should be used. These options may include selecting an alternative HD donor who shares the lost HLA haplotype with the recipient, achieving complete haplotype mismatch with the leukemic cells [35]. Additionally, NK cell-based therapies could be considered, utilizing inhibitory killer-cell immunoglobulin-like receptor (KIR)-based approaches discussed below [73]. Additionally, NK cells with Chimeric antigen receptor (CAR-NK) targeting tumor-specific antigens may be used [74].

HLA Matching for Non-inherited Maternal Antigen

Key factors in selecting a HD donor include evaluating donor-specific antibodies (DSA) against the mismatched haplotype, the relationship between the transplant pair, and the presence of non-inherited maternal antigens (NIMA) [72, 75]. NIMA refers to the HLA antigens carried by a person's mother but not inherited by the individual. During pregnancy, exposure to NIMA occurs as fetal and maternal cells interact, which can lead to natural sensitization of the fetus to these maternal antigens and development of tolerance to these antigens [75]. It has been published that NIMA exposure in transplantation, especially with HD or mismatched related donors, may reduce the risk of GvHD, improve graft acceptance, and enhance OS. This "NIMA effect" is thought to arise from the immune system's pre-existing tolerance to these maternal antigens during feto-maternal interaction, resulting in a potentially less immunogenic response compared to unrelated mismatched donors [76].

HLA Matching to Enhance NK Cell Alloreactivity

Natural killer cells are innate lymphoid cells that maintain self-tolerance to autologous healthy cells through inhibitory receptors, while they can recognize and kill abnormal cells that have downregulated, or do not express self HLA class I molecules, also known as "missing-self" theory. NK cells bear polymorphic activating and inhibitory killer-cell immunoglobulin-like receptors (KIR) on their surface which interact with the HLA molecules [77]. In SCT, specific HLA matching strategies can be employed to enhance NK cell alloreactivity, which is beneficial for GvL effects while minimizing GvHD. This matching strategy is based on the fact that NK cells can be alloreactive when they express inhibitory KIR that is not engaged by the HLA class I molecules present on the cells of the recipient. Additionally, the use of NK cell/ KIR receptor compatibility is considered helpful during early post-transplant period of severe T-cell lymphopenia especially in T-cell depleted graft for anti-viral infection and GvL effect [78].

NK cells are crucial in eliminating residual malignant cells and facilitating immune reconstitution, particularly in haploidentical or partially HLA-matched transplants. NK cell donor selection approaches emphasize mismatching for specific KIR ligands, such as HLA-Cw or HLA-Bw4, to enhance donor NK cell activity against leukemic cells [73]. Intentional HLA-Cw mismatching and managing HLA-E interactions can further boost NK cell-mediated cytotoxicity in the recipient. Four models have been proposed for NK cell-based donor selection: (1) Ligand–Ligand Model, (2) Receptor–Ligand Mismatch Model, (3) Receptor–Ligand Education Model, and (4) B Haplotype/Activating KIR Model. Clinical strategies incorporating KIR-ligand mismatches have demonstrated reduced relapse, lower GvHD incidence, and improved OS rates in patients with acute myeloid leukemia (AML) [73]. An online tool can assist in identifying KIR ligand mismatches and determining the directionality of mismatch (Table 18.1) [57]. Additionally, selecting donors with a KIR B haplotype has shown to improve NK cell function as the group B haplotypes have more genes encoding activating KIR than group A haplotypes and are characterized by the presence of one or more of the following genes: KIR2DL5, KIR2DS1, KIR2DS2, KIR2DS3, KIR2DS5, and KIR3DS1 [79]. NK cells with a KIR B haplotype thus have a lower threshold for initiating alloresponse compared to other haplotypes. Therefore, donors with two or more B motifs are preferred, which can be automatically assessed using the online tool available on the IPD/IMGT HLA website (Table 18.1) [58]. Clinical laboratories' ability to use NK cell compatibility models largely depends on the availability of KIR typing, which is not yet widely accessible, and NK cell compatibility testing remains outside of mainstream clinical practice.

HLA Matching for Single HLA-DQB1-Mismatched Donors

HLA-DQ molecules are α/β heterodimers formed by pairing the α-chain protein product of DQA1 with the β-chain protein product of the companion DQB1 gene. HLA-DQ can be classified into two groups based on their DQα-DQβ heterodimer combinations. The α chains from DQA1*02, *03, *04, *05, and *06 alleles form stable heterodimers with the β chains from DQB1*02, *03, and *04 alleles (group 1 molecules), as do DQA1*01α with DQB1*05β and 06β (group 2 molecules); however, structural constraints do not favor trans-dimerization of G1 DQα with G2 DQβ, or G2 DQα with G1 DQβ [80].

Recent studies focused on understanding the risk profile associated with HLA-DQB1 mismatches in SCT identified that in HLA-9/10 single HLA-DQB1 mismatched SCT, possession of G2 in the patient was associated with higher mortality and risks were further increased if the HLA-DQB1 mismatch was a G2 molecule. Similarly, in HLA-10/10-matched unrelated donor SCT, possession of G2 molecules was associated with significantly higher mortality than the absence of any G2. This indicates the presence of cis- and trans-forms of HLA-DQ proteins in HLA-DQ mismatched SCT reflecting low- and high-risk HLA-DQ mismatches [62]. These data suggest that G2-positive patients may benefit from matching for the G2 molecule. Additionally, patients who have inherited two G1 or G2 haplotypes may benefit from complete HLA-DQ matching to lower the number of mismatched molecules arising from trans-dimerization. An automated online tool (QLASSy) is available for analyzing HLA-DQ heterodimer data for DQα-DQβ trans-heterodimer evaluation, HLA-DQ imputation, and HLA-DQ-featured source selection (Table 18.1) [59].

Preimplantation and Prenatal HLA Testing: Technical and Ethical Considerations

Patients undergoing SCT achieve the best clinical outcomes when they have HLA-matched donors. Options include finding a matched sibling donor, a matched unrelated adult donor, or a cord blood donor. Among these, matched sibling donors yield superior transplant outcomes, likely due to additional genetic similarities beyond HLA, including minor histocompatibility antigens. However, there is only a 25% probability of finding an HLA-matched sibling, creating a significant barrier to obtaining a matched related donor. In some cases, understanding the importance of matched donors has led parents to attempt natural conception and use prenatal diagnosis to determine HLA compatibility of the unborn baby, or to plan an HLA-matched pregnancy via preimplantation HLA testing during assisted reproductive technology (ART) [81]. However, planning an HLA-matched pregnancy involves both technical and ethical challenges.

The preimplantation genetic testing (PGT) workup for each couple includes blood sample analysis to verify any disease trait and identify the HLA type of both parents [81, 82]. Prenatal testing for HLA is performed on amniotic fluid or chorionic villi, both of which are invasive procedures and can be affected by maternal cell contamination. A maternal sample is typically tested in parallel to rule out contamination. Additionally, prenatal HLA testing is not widely available in histocompatibility laboratories, and while clinical genetics laboratories are experienced in handling prenatal samples, they may lack the expertise required for HLA interpretation. Over the years, HLA typing techniques for preimplantation embryos have advanced. Traditionally, linkage analysis of short tandem repeats (STRs) across the HLA region was used to identify matching haplotypes between embryos and the affected sibling. More recently, next-generation sequencing (NGS) on single blastomeres has achieved high-resolution HLA typing in 88.9% of alleles tested [82].

Given the low likelihood of having an HLA-identical sibling, multiple ART cycles and embryo tests are often needed to find a suitable match, making this a costly option compared to SCT with a matched unrelated donor. Testing is also not limited to HLA compatibility; it must confirm that the disease trait present in the affected sibling is absent. The overall process can take one to a few years, which may not align with the urgency of SCT for the affected child. Additionally, the clinical success rate of PGT-HLA is relatively low. Couples should be counseled about these limitations, as they often place significant hope in this option. The success of

SCT with a sibling donor relies on several factors beyond finding an HLA-matched embryo, including embryo quality, implantation success, the achievement of a full-term pregnancy, the health of the newborn, and their clinical suitability as a donor [83].

PGT-HLA raises various ethical considerations. Parents' motives in conceiving a child to save another can raise complex questions about the new child's role in the family. Selecting embryos for HLA compatibility rather than health status introduces debates about the ethics of genetic selection. There are also health risks for both the mother and the child from ART, biopsy, and donation procedures. Balancing the donor sibling's interests with the family's needs is challenging, as is considering the psychological impact on all family members. Genetic and psychological counseling can help address some of these concerns by helping parents examine their motivations and the potential effects on family dynamics [83].

In summary, the HLA system is essential for successful SCT by ensuring immune compatibility between donor and recipient. However, the high diversity of HLA genes makes it difficult to find fully matched donors, especially among different ethnic groups where certain HLA types are less common. Advances in HLA typing have improved accuracy and speed, helping to identify the best possible matches, even if a perfect match isn't available. New algorithms have enabled SCTs with partially matched donors to achieve outcomes similar to those with fully matched sibling donors. Despite these advances, finding a compatible donor remains challenging for many, particularly from underrepresented backgrounds. Enhanced matching strategies show promise for improving SCT results in cases with suboptimal matches, while assisted reproductive technology (ART) and preimplantation genetic testing (PGT) have also sparked interest in planning HLA-matched sibling donors. These approaches could expand donor options and make life-saving transplants more accessible.

References

1. Dausset J, Nenna A. Presence of leuko-agglutinin in the serum of a case of chronic agranulocytosis. C R Seances Soc Biol Fil. 1952;146(19–20):1539–41.
2. Speiser DE, et al. High resolution HLA matching associated with decreased mortality after unrelated bone marrow transplantation. Blood. 1996;87(10):4455–62.
3. Cruz-Tapias P, Castiblanco J, Anaya JM. Chapter 10: major histocompatibility complex: antigen processing and presentation. In: Anaya JM, Shoenfeld Y, Rojas-Villarraga A, et al., editors. Autoimmunity: from bench to bedside [Internet]. Bogota: El Rosario University Press; 2013. Available from: https://www.ncbi.nlm.nih.gov/books/NBK459467/.
4. Barker DJ, et al. The IPD-IMGT/HLA database. Nucleic Acids Res. 2023;51(D1):D1053–d1060.
5. Marsh SG, et al. Nomenclature for factors of the HLA system. Tissue Antigens. 2010;75(4):291–455.
6. Rock KL, Reits E, Neefjes J. Present yourself! By MHC class I and MHC class II molecules. Trends Immunol. 2016;37(11):724–37.
7. Bjorkman PJ, et al. The foreign antigen binding site and T cell recognition regions of class I histocompatibility antigens. Nature. 1987;329(6139):512–8.

8. Lin CM, Gill RG. Direct and indirect allograft recognition: pathways dictating graft rejection mechanisms. Curr Opin Organ Transplant. 2016;21(1):40–4.
9. Ziemann M, et al. Preformed donor-specific HLA antibodies in living and deceased donor transplantation: a multicenter study. Clin J Am Soc Nephrol. 2019;14(7):1056–66.
10. Testi M, Andreani M. Luminex-based methods in high-resolution HLA typing. Methods Mol Biol. 2015;1310:231–45.
11. Lazaro A, et al. Human leukocyte antigen (HLA) typing by DNA sequencing. In: Zachary AA, Leffell MS, editors. Transplantation immunology: methods and protocols. Totowa: Humana Press; 2013. p. 161–95.
12. Bentley G, et al. High-resolution, high-throughput HLA genotyping by next-generation sequencing. Tissue Antigens. 2009;74(5):393–403.
13. Wittig M, et al. Development of a high-resolution NGS-based HLA-typing and analysis pipeline. Nucleic Acids Res. 2015;43(11):e70.
14. Slatko BE, Gardner AF, Ausubel FM. Overview of next-generation sequencing technologies. Curr Protoc Mol Biol. 2018;122(1):e59.
15. Guerra SG, et al. Evaluation of Ion Torrent sequencing technology for rapid clinical human leucocyte antigen typing. Int J Immunogenet. 2018;45(4):230–5.
16. Brown NK, et al. Reduced PCR-generated errors from a hybrid capture-based NGS assay for HLA typing. Hum Immunol. 2021;82(4):296–301.
17. Othus M, et al. Fate of patients with newly diagnosed acute myeloid leukemia who fail primary induction therapy. Biol Blood Marrow Transplant. 2015;21(3):559–64.
18. Mayer SF, Cao C, Dal Peraro M. Biological nanopores for single-molecule sensing. iScience. 2022;25(4):104145.
19. Mosbruger TL, et al. Utilizing nanopore sequencing technology for the rapid and comprehensive characterization of eleven HLA loci; addressing the need for deceased donor expedited HLA typing. Hum Immunol. 2020;81(8):413–22.
20. Liu C. A long road/read to rapid high-resolution HLA typing: the nanopore perspective. Hum Immunol. 2021;82(7):488–95.
21. Colombo MB, et al. Luminex technology for anti-HLA antibody screening: evaluation of performance and of impact on laboratory routine. Cytometry B Clin Cytom. 2007;72(6):465–71.
22. Gebel HM, Bray RA. HLA antibody detection with solid phase assays: great expectations or expectations too great? Am J Transplant. 2014;14(9):1964–75.
23. Saito PK, et al. Complement-dependent cytotoxicity (CDC) to detect anti-HLA antibodies: old but gold. J Clin Lab Anal. 2014;28(4):275–80.
24. Amos DB, et al. A simple micro cytotoxicity test. Transplantation. 1969;7(3):220–3.
25. Fuller TC, et al. HLA alloantibodies and the mechanism of the antiglobulin-augmented lymphocytotoxicity procedure. Hum Immunol. 1997;56(1–2):94–105.
26. Bray RA, Lebeck LK, Gebel HM. The flow cytometric crossmatch. Dual-color analysis of T cell and B cell reactivities. Transplantation. 1989;48(5):834–40.
27. Rocha Y, et al. Crossmatch assays in transplantation: physical or virtual?: a review. Medicine (Baltimore). 2023;102(50):e36527.
28. Gladstone DE, Bettinotti MP. HLA donor-specific antibodies in allogeneic hematopoietic stem cell transplantation: challenges and opportunities. Hematology Am Soc Hematol Educ Program. 2017;2017(1):645–50.
29. Gutman JA, et al. Prospective monitoring for alloimmunization in cord blood transplantation: "virtual crossmatch" can be used to demonstrate donor-directed antibodies. Transplantation. 2009;87(3):415–8.
30. Jeon YW, et al. Risk factors predicting graft-versus-host disease and relapse-free survival after allogeneic hematopoietic stem cell transplantation in relapsed or refractory non-Hodgkin's lymphoma. Ann Hematol. 2019;98(7):1743–53.
31. Anasetti C. What are the most important donor and recipient factors affecting the outcome of related and unrelated allogeneic transplantation? Best Pract Res Clin Haematol. 2008;21(4):691–7.

32. Davis E, et al. Validation of an algorithm to predict the likelihood of an 8/8 HLA-matched unrelated donor at search initiation. Biol Blood Marrow Transplant. 2018;24(5):1057–62.
33. NMDP policy for HLA confirmatory typing requirements for unrelated adult donors and HLA typing requirement for patients (Number: P00079). Available at https://network.nmdp.org/policies-protocols/transplant-centers/confirmatory-typing-policy/. Accessed on 11 June 2024. Revision: 2.
34. Masuda K, et al. Loss or down-regulation of HLA class I expression at the allelic level in freshly isolated leukemic blasts. Cancer Sci. 2007;98(1):102–8.
35. Arnold PY. Review: HLA loss and detection in the setting of relapse from HLA-mismatched hematopoietic cell transplant. Hum Immunol. 2022;83(10):712–20.
36. Nakagaki M, et al. The incidence of severe oral mucositis in patients undergoing different conditioning regimens in haematopoietic stem cell transplantation. Support Care Cancer. 2022;30(11):9141–9.
37. Nunes E, et al. Definitions of histocompatibility typing terms. Blood. 2011;118(23):e180–3.
38. Dehn J, et al. Selection of unrelated donors and cord blood units for hematopoietic cell transplantation: guidelines from the NMDP/CIBMTR. Blood. 2019;134(12):924–34.
39. Kreuger AL, et al. HLA-matched platelet transfusions are effective only in refractory patients with positive HLA antibody screening. Transfusion. 2019;59(11):3303–7.
40. Yu N, et al. Current HLA testing recommendations to support HCT. Hum Immunol. 2022;83(10):665–73.
41. Spierings E, et al. Multicenter analyses demonstrate significant clinical effects of minor histocompatibility antigens on GvHD and GvL after HLA-matched related and unrelated hematopoietic stem cell transplantation. Biol Blood Marrow Transplant. 2013;19(8):1244–53.
42. Lima ACM, et al. Donor-specific HLA antibodies are associated with graft failure and delayed hematologic recovery after unrelated donor hematopoietic cell transplantation. Transplant Cell Ther. 2023;29(8):493.e1–493.e10.
43. Eapen M, et al. Mismatched related and unrelated donors for allogeneic hematopoietic cell transplantation for adults with hematologic malignancies. Biol Blood Marrow Transplant. 2014;20(10):1485–92.
44. Eapen M, et al. Effect of graft source on unrelated donor haemopoietic stem-cell transplantation in adults with acute leukaemia: a retrospective analysis. Lancet Oncol. 2010;11(7):653–60.
45. Eyrich M, Schulze H. HLA matching in pediatric stem cell transplantation. Transfus Med Hemother. 2019;46(5):348–55.
46. Yakoub-Agha I. Transplantations from HLA-identical siblings versus 10/10 HLA-matched unrelated donors. Semin Hematol. 2016;53(2):74–6.
47. Lee SJ, et al. High-resolution donor-recipient HLA matching contributes to the success of unrelated donor marrow transplantation. Blood. 2007;110(13):4576–83.
48. Fernández-Viña MA. HLA allotype expressivity in transplantation. Blood. 2014;124(26):3839–40.
49. Fernandez-Viña MA, et al. Identification of a permissible HLA mismatch in hematopoietic stem cell transplantation. Blood. 2014;123(8):1270–8.
50. Shaw BE, et al. The importance of HLA-DPB1 in unrelated donor hematopoietic cell transplantation. Blood. 2007;110(13):4560–6.
51. Fleischhauer K, et al. Effect of T-cell-epitope matching at HLA-DPB1 in recipients of unrelated-donor haemopoietic-cell transplantation: a retrospective study. Lancet Oncol. 2012;13(4):366–74.
52. Crivello P, et al. The impact of amino acid variability on alloreactivity defines a functional distance predictive of permissive HLA-DPB1 mismatches in hematopoietic stem cell transplantation. Biol Blood Marrow Transplant. 2015;21(2):233–41.
53. DPB1 T-cell epitope algorithm v2.0. Available at https://www.ebi.ac.uk/ipd/imgt/hla/matching/dpb_v2/. Accessed on 11 June 2024.
54. Expression of DP antigens tool (ExPAT). Available at https://dpb1-tce-expression.nmdp.org/. Accessed on 11 June 2024.

55. HLA-B leader mismatch calculator. Available at https://www.ebi.ac.uk/ipd/imgt/hla/matching/dpb_v2/. Accessed on 11 June 2024.
56. HLA-B leader assessment tool (BLEAT). Available at https://bleader.nmdp.org/. Accessed on 11 June 2024.
57. KIR ligand calculator. Available at https://www.ebi.ac.uk/ipd/kir/matching/ligand/. Accessed on 11 July 2024.
58. Donor KIR B-content group calculator. Available at https://www.ebi.ac.uk/ipd/kir/matching/b_content/. Accessed on 11 July 2024.
59. HLA-DQA1 and HLA-DQB1 heterodimers assessment (QLASSy) tool. Available at https://dq-dimers.nmdp.org/. Accessed on 26 Apr 2025.
60. Petersdorf EW, et al. High HLA-DP expression and graft-versus-host disease. N Engl J Med. 2015;373(7):599–609.
61. Fernández-Viña MA, et al. Multiple mismatches at the low expression HLA loci DP, DQ, and DRB3/4/5 associate with adverse outcomes in hematopoietic stem cell transplantation. Blood. 2013;121(22):4603–10.
62. Petersdorf EW, et al. HLA-DQ heterodimers in hematopoietic cell transplantation. Blood. 2022;139(20):3009–17.
63. Hurley CK, et al. The impact of HLA unidirectional mismatches on the outcome of myeloablative hematopoietic stem cell transplantation with unrelated donors. Blood. 2013;121(23):4800–6.
64. Cunha R, et al. Impact of HLA mismatch direction on outcomes after umbilical cord blood transplantation for hematological malignant disorders: a retrospective Eurocord-EBMT analysis. Bone Marrow Transplant. 2014;49(1):24–9.
65. Lima ACM, et al. The impact of donor-specific anti-human leukocyte antigen antibodies in salvage haploidentical hematopoietic cell transplantation with posttransplant cyclophosphamide in patients with nonmalignant disorders. Hla. 2021;97(6):493–504.
66. Kongtim P, et al. ASTCT consensus recommendations on testing and treatment of patients with donor-specific anti-HLA antibodies. Transplant Cell Ther. 2024;30(12):1139–54.
67. Cusatis R, et al. Current trends and outcomes in cellular therapy activity in the United States, including prospective patient-reported outcomes data collection in the Center for International Blood and Marrow Transplant Research Registry. Transplant Cell Ther. 2024;30(9):917.e1–917.e12.
68. Petersdorf EW, et al. Role of HLA-B exon 1 in graft-versus-host disease after unrelated haemopoietic cell transplantation: a retrospective cohort study. Lancet Haematol. 2020;7(1):e50–60.
69. Petersdorf EW, et al. HLA-B leader and survivorship after HLA-mismatched unrelated donor transplantation. Blood. 2020;136(3):362–9.
70. Rovatti PE, et al. Mechanisms of leukemia immune evasion and their role in relapse after haploidentical hematopoietic cell transplantation. Front Immunol. 2020;11:147.
71. Vago L, et al. Loss of mismatched HLA in leukemia after stem-cell transplantation. N Engl J Med. 2009;361(5):478–88.
72. Wang A, et al. Clinical characteristics and outcome analysis for HLA loss patients following partially mismatched related donor transplantation using HLA chimerism for loss of heterozygosity analysis by next-generation sequencing. Cell Transplant. 2022;31:9636897221102902.
73. Jennifer Zhang Q. Donor selection based on NK alloreactivity for patients with hematological malignancies. Hum Immunol. 2022;83(10):695–703.
74. Myers JA, Miller JS. Exploring the NK cell platform for cancer immunotherapy. Nat Rev Clin Oncol. 2021;18(2):85–100.
75. Hirayama M, Azuma E, Komada Y. Tolerogenic effect of non-inherited maternal antigens in hematopoietic stem cell transplantation. Front Immunol. 2012;3:135.
76. Tang FF, et al. Comparison of the clinical outcomes between NIMA-mismatched and NIPA-mismatched haploidentical hematopoietic stem cell transplantation for patients with hematological malignancies. Bone Marrow Transplant. 2021;56(11):2723–31.
77. Sivori S, et al. Human NK cells: surface receptors, inhibitory checkpoints, and translational applications. Cell Mol Immunol. 2019;16(5):430–41.

78. Palmer JM, et al. Clinical relevance of natural killer cells following hematopoietic stem cell transplantation. J Cancer. 2013;4(1):25–35.
79. Hsu KC, et al. The killer cell immunoglobulin-like receptor (KIR) genomic region: gene-order, haplotypes and allelic polymorphism. Immunol Rev. 2002;190:40–52.
80. Tollefsen S, et al. Structural and functional studies of trans-encoded HLA-DQ2.3 (DQA1*03:01/DQB1*02:01) protein molecule. J Biol Chem. 2012;287(17):13611–9.
81. De Rycke M, et al. Preimplantation genetic testing with HLA matching: from counseling to birth and beyond. J Hum Genet. 2020;65(5):445–54.
82. Rafati M, et al. Preimplantation high-resolution HLA sequencing using next generation sequencing. Biol Blood Marrow Transplant. 2018;24(8):1575–80.
83. Kaye DK. Addressing ethical issues related to prenatal diagnostic procedures. Matern Health Neonatol Perinatol. 2023;9(1):1.

Coagulation Abnormalities in Leukemia 19

Sara McElroy and Gabor Oroszi

Introduction

In the 1950s, a distinct form of acute myeloid leukemia (AML) that demonstrated a severe, fatal hemorrhagic tendency was described in the literature for the first time. The blood smears of these patients were notable for the presence of promyelocytes and the disease was named acute promyelocytic leukemia (APL). During the work-up of these patients, they were found to have low fibrinogen and other clotting factors primarily from plasmin-mediated proteolysis [1]. Since that time, much has been elucidated regarding the detection of, mechanism for, and management of the unique coagulopathy in APL. Variable coagulopathy has also been demonstrated in many other acute leukemias in childhood secondary to processes including disseminated intravascular coagulation (DIC), sepsis, liver dysfunction, and platelet dysfunction. In contrast to the risk of hemorrhage, many patients will develop thrombosis due to various risk factors including the central venous line and medications they receive during therapy. Management of the coagulopathic patient with leukemia includes caution with or consideration of delaying procedures and blood product and/or medication administration to normalize the coagulation status and treat the underlying leukemia. Management of thrombosis presents significant challenges due to the combined bleeding risk from anticoagulation and

S. McElroy (✉)
Division of Hematology/Oncology/Bone Marrow Transplant, Children's Mercy Kansas City, University of Missouri-Kansas City School of Medicine, Kansas City, MO, USA
e-mail: smmcelroy@cmh.edu

G. Oroszi
Department of Pathology and Laboratory Medicine, Children's Mercy Kansas City, University of Missouri-Kansas City School of Medicine, Kansas City, MO, USA

W. Li (ed.), *Laboratory Assessments of Pediatric Leukemia*,
https://doi.org/10.1007/978-3-032-26557-9_19

thrombocytopenia with or without coagulopathy. Though there have been some advances in coagulation testing, the routine coagulation parameters, prothrombin time (PT), international normalized ratio (INR), activated partial thromboplastin time (aPTT), fibrinogen, and D-dimer, make up the primary laboratory studies that are obtained and help define the bleeding risk in patients with leukemia. There is great value in being able to interpret these studies individually and collectively to synthesize the overall coagulation status of each individual patient.

Testing the Coagulation System

No discussion related to thrombosis and hemostasis is complete without an overview of testing the coagulation system, as there are many nuances to the laboratory testing that should be considered before ordering tests and subsequently in the interpretation of the tests. Screening for abnormalities in the coagulation pathway can be done by using specific laboratory tests. The starting place for evaluating the coagulation system is with basic coagulation laboratory assays.

Standard Coagulation Assays

Many coagulation laboratory tests are functional, measuring how long a clot takes to form. This is true of the PT, aPTT, thrombin time (TT), and fibrinogen activity (Clauss). The PT measures the extrinsic and common pathways of the coagulation cascade that includes Factors II, V, VII, X, and fibrinogen. It is expressed in the number of seconds it takes for a clot to form after thromboplastin (a complex of tissue factor [TF] and phospholipid) and calcium chloride ($CaCl_2$) are added to the patient's platelet-poor plasma. Due to variations in the PT results with different thromboplastin reagents and instruments, it is recommended that PT results be converted to an INR. INR is a patient's PT result expressed as a ratio to a normal population, which is adjusted for the sensitivity of the thromboplastin used. The aPTT measures the intrinsic and common pathways of the coagulation cascade that includes Factors II, V, VIII, IX, X, XI, XII, and fibrinogen. It is expressed in the number of seconds it takes for a clot to form after partial thromboplastin (surface activator and phospholipid) and $CaCl_2$ are added to the patient's platelet-poor plasma. The TT measures the time it takes for a clot to form when thrombin is added to patient's plasma and therefore measures fibrinogen's conversion to fibrin. Fibrinogen can be determined with a variety of testing techniques including quantifying the level of the antigen itself or functional assays to measure the activity. D-dimer assay is commonly used to assess fibrinolysis that is part of screening for DIC. D-dimer is a specific fibrin degradation product (FDP) formed exclusively from the breakdown of the fibrin polymer covalently cross-linked (by FXIII) between adjacent D-domains. Of note, elevated D-dimer can be detected in many clinical settings, and it is not specific for DIC. In addition to testing procoagulant levels, anticoagulant proteins can also be measured, such as antithrombin (AT), Protein C, or Protein S [2, 3].

If a patient's PT or aPTT is prolonged, subsequent testing can determine the underlying cause of the prolongation. An initial test is commonly a mixing study where the patient's plasma is mixed with normal plasma. After pooling the two plasmas, the PT or aPTT is run again on the combination. If the PT/aPTT has corrected and remained corrected after the incubated mix, that suggests that a factor deficiency is the likely cause of the patient's abnormal test. If the PT/aPTT does not correct (remains prolonged), that suggests that an inhibitor in the sample is the likely cause of the abnormality. Examples of inhibitors include anticoagulant medications or autoantibodies present in the plasma [2].

Sometimes, a routine coagulation assay is used alone to monitor the anticoagulant effect of a medication a patient is taking. This is true of the INR for patients on Vitamin K antagonists [3]. But, especially in the case of leukemia, multiple tests are run and interpreted together to obtain a full picture of the overall coagulation status of the patient. This is certainly true in disseminated intravascular coagulation (DIC) where a combination of PT/INR, aPTT, fibrinogen, platelet count, and D-dimer are evaluated.

In leukemia, coagulation abnormalities may be complex and can encompass bleeding risk, clotting risk, both, or a balance between the two. The conventional coagulation tests do not measure the interactions between all components (such as platelets, FXIII) of the hemostatic system and often fall short of displaying a clear picture of what is happening physiologically with regard to bleeding and clotting [4, 5]. The standard coagulation tests PT/INR, aPTT, fibrinogen, platelet count, D-dimer, and AT have shown to be poorly predictive of the bleeding and/or clotting risk in individual patients. INR alone has an association with bleeding in patients with leukemia but is not necessarily predictive. None of these tests demonstrate a clear association with thrombosis. D-dimer approaches are predictive in one study, though ultimately fall short [6]. A similar study found it is not reliable for predicting venous thromboembolism (VTE) in patients with leukemia likely because they have an elevated D-dimer at baseline, making it difficult to interpret the test in this setting. This study also investigated if inflammatory markers or indicators of infection or organ dysfunction could be used to predict bleeding risk but found they also could not [7].

Viscoelastic Testing

Global hemostasis assays are relatively newer tests compared to conventional coagulation assays and may start to be used with greater frequency in patients with leukemia. There are complex interactions between the various components of the coagulation system and the limitations of isolating a single part of that system to determine risk in a patient is evident. Global hemostasis assays have the potential to better evaluate the overall balance in a patient, whether that is more toward bleeding or clotting.

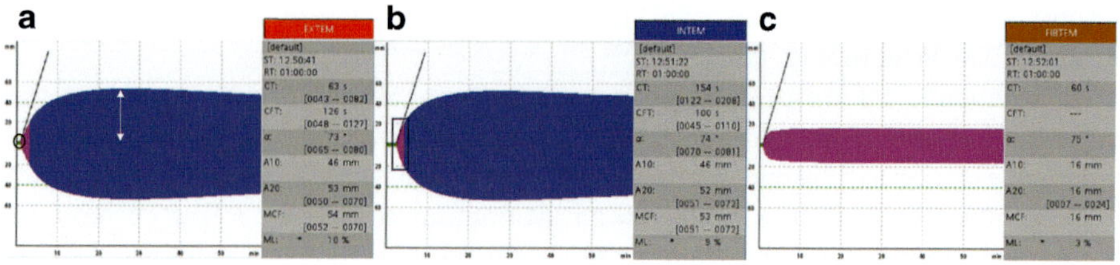

Fig. 19.1 *CT* clotting time (circled in EXTEM): The time it takes for a clot to start forming; measures secondary hemostasis. *CFT* clot formation time (boxed in INTEM): The time from initiation of clot formation to achieving a certain amplitude; combination of secondary hemostasis, platelet, and fibrin contribution. A10, A20: Measure the amplitude of the clot at various timepoints during the test (10 min, 20 min). *MCF* maximum clot firmness (double arrow): The maximum amplitude of the clot; measures the quality of the clot (i.e., platelets, fibrin, FXIII). *ML* maximum lysis: The percentage of clot that lyses by the end of the test, measures fibrinolysis. (**a**) EXTEM: Corresponds to the extrinsic and common pathway of the coagulation cascade. (**b**) INTEM: Corresponds to the intrinsic and common pathway of the coagulation cascade. (**c**) FIBTEM: Corresponds to the fibrinogen contribution to the clot independent of platelets. Not pictured, HEPTEM: Corrects for the presence of heparin in the sample; APTEM: Corrects for the presence of fibrinolysis in the sample

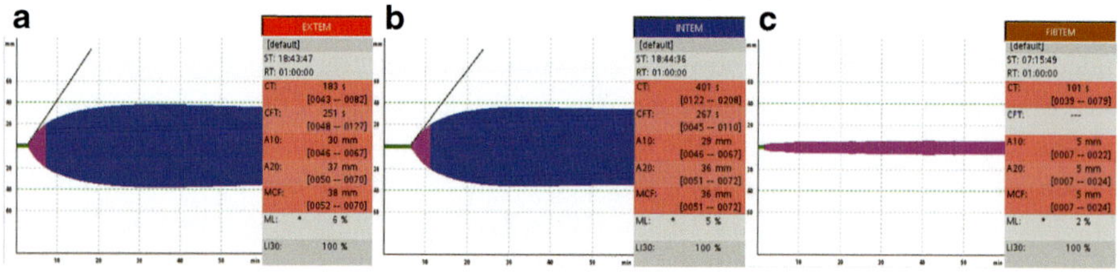

Fig. 19.2 This ROTEM® shows prolonged CT in both EXTEM and INTEM suggesting both the extrinsic and intrinsic pathways of the coagulation cascade are likely impacted. The CFT is prolonged and the MCF is low in EXTEM and INTEM indicating that platelets and/or fibrinogen are low/dysfunctional. The MCF is low in FIBTEM indicating that the fibrinogen contribution is insufficient. ML is normal in each test indicating that there is no hyperfibrinolysis in the sample. *CFT* clot formation time, *CT* clot time, *MCF* maximum clot firmness, *ML* maximum lysis

Thromboelastography (TEG) and rotational thromboelastometry (ROTEM®) are whole blood tests that measure clot formation, clot lysis, and the viscoelastic strength of a clot (see Figs. 19.1 and 19.2). They can simultaneously test the interactions of many aspects of coagulation including coagulation factors, fibrinogen, platelets, and anticoagulant medications. They are rapid, can be employed as point-of-care tests, and result much faster than standard coagulation tests. They provide a visual representation of a clot, in addition to numerical values [8]. Classically, these tests have been used in cardiac surgery, liver transplantation, the intensive care unit (ICU) and trauma patients, and are particularly amenable to those clinical situations because they are faster than standard coagulation assays and are often readily available in operating rooms and the ICU [5]. In particular, there is value in their ability to quickly determine what blood product is needed for a bleeding patient in those circumstances. However, there is great potential for various other uses as TEG/ROTEM® is being incorporated more widely into the coagulation testing arsenal [8].

Several studies have been done using TEG/ROTEM® in patients with leukemia to attempt to characterize the complexity of their coagulation and compare them to standard coagulation assays. TEG demonstrated that coagulation status in patients with AML at diagnosis is variable, ranging from hypercoagulable to hypocoagulable. During chemotherapy, TEG more commonly displayed hypocoagulability, which is likely due to a combination of thrombocytopenia as well as platelet dysfunction, whereas, after chemotherapy, TEG found hypercoagulability [9]. In ROTEM® testing, in theory, the clotting time (CT) on extrinsic thromboelastometry (EXTEM) is analogous to the PT, and the CT on intrinsic thromboelastometry (INTEM) is analogous to the aPTT; however, in acute lymphoblastic leukemia (ALL) these may not actually correlate well. In fact, oftentimes the PT and the aPTT are prolonged but the CT for EXTEM and INTEM are normal. Between the two, ROTEM® may be a better indicator of the true coagulation status of the patient when compared to the PT, aPTT, and fibrinogen. ROTEM® may also show changes in the days leading up to a VTE event, such as shortening of the CT [4]. TEG demonstrated similar findings in AML, with a poor correlation between standard coagulation tests and global hemostasis assays, and may be better able to determine bleeding risk in patients with thrombocytopenia, as some methodologies are able to demonstrate platelet dysfunction that may be more reflective of the bleeding risk than a simply low platelet count [5]. There is potential for using a combination of platelet count and TEG to determine the risk of hemorrhage and the need for platelet transfusion in patients with thrombocytopenia [9].

Platelet Function Testing

Platelet count alone may not be sufficient to determine the bleeding risk of a patient and obtaining platelet aggregation and secretion studies may be more reflective of this risk. Standard ways to measure platelet aggregation such as whole blood aggregometry (WBA) and light transmission aggregometry (LTA) often cannot be used in patients with malignancy and receiving therapy due to chemotherapy-induced thrombocytopenia. Other methods of measuring platelet aggregation and activation are needed that are independent of platelet count, such as flow cytometry [10].

General Coagulation Abnormalities in Leukemia

The following section will discuss the general coagulation abnormalities that can occur during a patient's journey through leukemia from diagnosis throughout treatment. Later in the chapter, there will be a dedicated discussion to specific leukemia subtypes and treatments or medications used in leukemia with coagulation ramifications. However, it is important to remember that coagulopathy can occur in leukemia of any form and at any timepoint before, during, or after therapy.

Disseminated Intravascular Coagulation (DIC)

DIC is present in a third of patients with acute leukemia [11]. While there is a well-known association of DIC with particular subtypes, it can present in any patient with leukemia. In children, 3.1% of patients with acute lymphoblastic leukemia (ALL) and 13.8% of patients with AML have abnormal coagulation studies at diagnosis [12]. DIC is a pathologic process characterized by exaggerated intravascular activation of coagulation with subsequent excessive thrombin generation, leading to fibrin deposition and fibrinolysis on a level that the body's natural mechanisms for confining coagulation locally are overwhelmed (see Fig. 19.3) [13, 14]. This leads to thrombosis, which is often microvascular, but can also be overt. Thrombosis subsequently might cause organ dysfunction in essentially any body system and consumption of platelets and factors in the coagulation cascade. Patients with DIC tend to have bleeding due to consumption causing acquired factor deficiencies. A contributor to widespread activation of coagulation is tissue factor (TF) release from damaged cells, which, physiologically, is known to initiate coagulation through the extrinsic pathway of the coagulation cascade [15]. At diagnosis, children with ALL may have elevated D-dimer and thrombin–antithrombin (TAT) complexes in their circulation, indicating increased generation of thrombin and the downstream effect

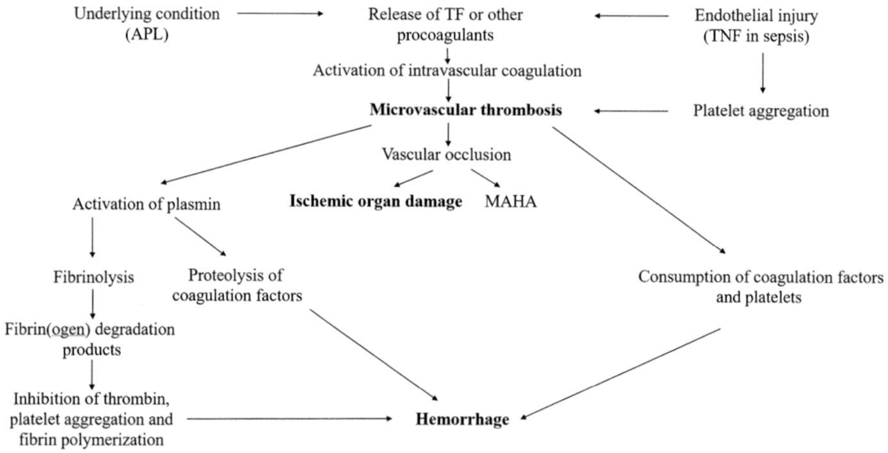

Fig. 19.3 Disseminated intravascular coagulation mechanism. *APL* acute promyelocytic leukemia, *MAHA* microangiopathic hemolytic anemia, *TF* tissue factor, *TNF* tumor necrosis factor. (Adapted from: Bleeding and Thrombosing Diseases Conference and Workshop, October 6–8, 2021; Mayo Medical Laboratories, Intravascular Coagulation and Hyperfibrinolysis Presentation by Dr. Ashrani; Chapter 14: Red Blood Cell and Bleeding Disorders in Robbins and Cotran Pathologic Basis of Disease, Professional Edition, 10th Edition, 2021)

of fibrin clot formation. During the first phase of chemotherapy, these levels normalize. At diagnosis, there are also increased levels of inflammatory cytokines, such as tumor necrosis factor (TNF) alpha and interleukin 6 (IL6), consistent with an inflammatory state in acute leukemia. Though this could be due to the leukemia itself, infection/sepsis is often present at onset of leukemia and would certainly contribute to the presence of these cytokines, as well [16]. These cytokine levels, subsequently decrease during the first phase of therapy. Inflammation contributes to coagulopathy in several ways including inhibiting fibrinolysis by increasing PAI-1, inducing expression of TF, and decreasing expression of thrombomodulin (TM), thus promoting activation of the coagulation cascade. In addition, by increasing expression of adhesion molecules on endothelial cells, leukocyte adhesion is enhanced that might cause endothelial cell damage via reactive oxygen species and proteases. PAI-1 and P-selectin increase during chemotherapy. P-selectin is related to cell adhesion and has been shown previously to predict risk of VTE when there are elevated levels, specifically in patients with malignancy [17].

DIC is a clinical and laboratory diagnosis, based on findings of coagulopathy and/or fibrinolysis. No single laboratory test can accurately confirm or eliminate the diagnosis. In the laboratory, the diagnosis of DIC can be supported based on a combination of tests. Since DIC is a consumptive coagulopathy, patients acquire factor deficiencies leading to the prolongation of the PT and aPTT, low fibrinogen, in addition to low platelets [13]. The formation of thrombi leads to fibrinolysis and explains why increases in fibrin degradation products, such as D-dimer, are seen. Intravascular thrombi can cause fragmentation of red blood cells, leading to the presence of increased schistocytes on peripheral blood smears. When comparing patients with acute leukemia with and without DIC, the patients with DIC have lower platelet counts, longer PT, lower fibrinogen, and higher D-dimer. D-dimer is significantly elevated in patients with DIC but may also be elevated in patients with leukemia without DIC due to other factors, such as inflammation or stress [11]. Multiorgan dysfunction as a result of thrombosis of the microvasculature can cause laboratory abnormalities associated with damage or dysfunction of the particular organs or organ systems that have been affected.

There are various scoring systems that have been validated for use in adults to determine whether DIC is present. These scoring systems are necessary because no one lab test is sufficient to make a diagnosis of DIC. They typically combine PT, aPTT, platelet count, fibrinogen, and D-dimer or other fibrin degradation products. Scoring systems may be extrapolated to children but should be interpreted with caution as they are not validated in the pediatric population. A commonly used one is the International Society on Thrombosis and Hemostasis (ISTH) Scoring System (see Table 19.1) [18].

Clinically, patients often present with bleeding, essentially anywhere. Bleeding frequently occurs in mucocutaneous areas, presenting as bruising, petechiae, epistaxis, or heavy menstrual bleeding. Bleeding in internal organs is not uncommon in hematologic malignancies. Patients with myelodysplastic syndrome (MDS) have more gastrointestinal, genitourinary, and pulmonary bleeding, in contrast to patients with nonmalignant thrombocytopenia such as immune-mediated thrombocytopenia

Table 19.1 ISTH DIC scoring system

Laboratory parameter	Result	Score
Platelet count	>100 × 10^3/μL <100 × 10^3/μL <50 × 10^3/μL	0 1 2
Prothrombin time	<3 s prolonged 3–6 s prolonged >6 s prolonged	0 1 2
Fibrinogen	>100 mg/dL <100 mg/dL	0 1
D-dimer/fibrin degradation products	No increase Moderate increase Strong increase	0 2 3

Scoring: ≥5 is consistent with overt DIC
DIC disseminated intravascular coagulation, *ISTH* International Society of Thrombosis and Hemostasis

Table 19.2 Differentiating acute and chronic DIC based on clinical associations and laboratory tests

	Acute DIC	Chronic DIC
Causative condition	Trauma, sepsis, malignancy, ABO-incompatible pRBC transfusion	Malignancy
Presenting symptoms	Hemorrhage	Venous thromboembolism
Platelets	Decreased	Variable
PT	Prolonged	Normal
aPTT	Prolonged	Normal
Thrombin time	Prolonged	Normal or slightly prolonged
Fibrinogen	Decreased	Normal or elevated
D-dimer/fibrin degradation products	Elevated	Elevated

aPTT activated partial thromboplastin time, *DIC* disseminated intravascular coagulation, *pRBC* packed red blood cell, *PT* prothrombin time

(ITP), where the bleeding is often localized to the mucosa and skin [16]. Aside from bleeding, because of thrombosis in the microvasculature, end organ dysfunction can occur in almost any body system with subsequent associated symptoms. Common organs affected include the kidneys, liver, and brain. Patients will also frequently have hypotension [13].

Chronic DIC is an entity where coagulation is activated for a longer period of time. It does lead to excess thrombin formation, as in acute DIC; however, the body is better able to compensate for the consumption of coagulation factors and platelets, so thrombosis predominates over bleeding manifestations. This does occur in malignancies. Laboratory abnormalities such as prolonged PT, aPTT, and low platelet count can be present, but are usually not as pronounced as in acute DIC (see Table 19.2) [13, 14].

Initially, it was thought that DIC at diagnosis was rare in ALL, except in the cases of infection or shock. A study from 1978 described a series of atypical patients with ALL who had coagulopathy. One occurred shortly after starting chemotherapy and was presumed to be secondary to lysis of leukemia blasts. The chemotherapy itself was implicated in two of the patients with DIC, which will be discussed in further detail later in the chapter. This study found several factors that were more likely to lead to DIC in children with ALL including treatment with asparaginase, higher disease burden, rapid lysis of blast cells, or the possibility of having tumor cells that were not actually lymphocytic in origin. The example provided for the last factor was leukemia identified as ALL based on phenotype but then found to have the Philadelphia chromosome leading to the BCR-ABL fusion gene. At the time, this was presumed to not be a true case of ALL, but rather a blast crisis of chronic myelogenous leukemia (CML) [19]. In ALL, though, general coagulation abnormalities, which tend to be milder than that of APL, are present in 15.4–16% of patients at diagnosis and rise to 24.4–36% when considering the full timeframe at diagnosis and treatment. Patients with DIC tend to have splenomegaly and a higher white blood cell (WBC) count at diagnosis than patients without DIC [20, 21]. Other factors associated with higher rates of DIC in ALL include being on antibiotics before admission and high-risk leukemia [20]. Within ALL, patients with the T-cell phenotype may be more likely to have DIC, found in up to 4.1% at diagnosis, though the coagulopathy in these patients is typically mild [21, 22]. Distinctive from APL, which has low fibrinogen, the fibrinogen level is often normal or elevated in T-cell ALL [22]. There is potential for DIC to become more pronounced after initial chemotherapy administration, which may be secondary to lysis of blast cells [23]. For patients who develop DIC after starting chemotherapy, they seem to have already had a more hypercoagulable state, as evidenced by higher FDP prior to initiating chemotherapy. Their labs demonstrate thrombin generation and hypofibrinogenemia, though less than in APL. They do not show the characteristic decrease in AT [20]. There is a risk of severe bleeding in patients with ALL and coagulopathy, but it is less common to see hemorrhagic deaths, but patients with DIC have a higher percentage of death during induction chemotherapy [20, 21]. Essentially, it is vital to evaluate for the presence of DIC, or any level of coagulopathy, in a patient newly diagnosed with leukemia [11].

Sepsis-Induced Coagulopathy

Patients with leukemia are considered functionally immunocompromised at diagnosis because of malignant cell production taking over the normal trilineage hematopoiesis in the bone marrow, causing a major decrease in functioning white blood cells. Most chemotherapy causes immunocompromise, as well, through its nondiscriminatory action on rapidly growing and dividing cells, impacting the bone marrow's ability to produce white blood cells. It is well known that patients with leukemia are at risk for severe infection that can cause sepsis. Coagulopathy is common in sepsis but does not always reach the designation of DIC [24]. Sepsis-induced coagulopathy can appear very similarly to the coagulopathy seen in patients as a direct result of leukemia. And, in fact the pathophysiologic mechanisms for sepsis-induced DIC are similar to leukemia-induced DIC (see above and Fig. 19.1). However, one particular difference is fibrinogen, which was less helpful early on in identifying sepsis-induced coagulopathy because of its acute phase-reactant properties. Fibrinogen is characteristically low in DIC, but early in sepsis, fibrinogen will be elevated. Late in sepsis-induced coagulopathy, though, fibrinogen will trend down.

Liver Dysfunction

Liver disease is another cause of coagulopathy that can look similar to DIC. The vast majority of coagulation factors, procoagulant and anticoagulant, are made in the liver by the hepatocytes. A notable exception is Factor VIII, which is produced by the endothelial cells of the hepatic sinusoids. When the liver is malfunctioning, there is a subsequent decrease in production of all of those coagulation factors. There may be a decrease in procoagulant factors and anticoagulant factors, so patients may be at increased risk for bleeding or sometimes for clotting. Additionally, there may be a proportional decrease in both, leading to an overall balanced state of coagulation in terms of thrombin generation. Patients with higher leukemia blast cell counts in the blood tended to have more liver dysfunction and lower levels of Protein C and AT. The decrease in these anticoagulants is felt to be attributable to liver dysfunction, rather than to DIC. This is supported by the finding that Protein C and AT levels are not significantly different between patients with leukemia both with and without DIC [25]. Differentiating between DIC and liver disease coagulopathy can be done through looking at Factor VIII, which is not made in the liver parenchyma. It is expected to be normal or elevated in liver disease, whereas it is low in DIC since it is being consumed [13].

Platelet Dysfunction

Platelet count alone is not sufficient to determine the bleeding risk of a patient with leukemia. It is possible that platelet dysfunction is a major part of the bleeding risk in thrombocytopenic patients with leukemia, so measuring platelet function through platelet aggregation and secretion studies may be more likely to determine that risk [10]. The functional abnormalities seen in patients with leukemia receiving chemotherapy encompass platelet aggregation, adhesion, and secretion, as evidenced by decreased activation markers on the platelets and receptors on the platelet surface [26].

Thrombosis

Thromboembolism is a complication of acute leukemia during therapy with an overall incidence of 2–12% and equal incidence between ALL and AML [26–28]. In children, the venous thromboembolism (VTE) rate in leukemia is reported as 3–36.7%. Frequently, thrombosis occurs within the first month after diagnosis, or even right before diagnosis [29]. Patients with thromboembolism often have many hypercoagulable risk factors including the important risk factor of having a central venous catheter (CVC) in place. The most common VTE is CVC-associated, which makes up half of VTE events. The other half is made up of deep vein thrombosis (DVT) and pulmonary embolism (PE). Endothelial dysfunction contributes to hypercoagulability in these patients. Markers of endothelial dysfunction increase during chemotherapy, whereas markers of inflammation and thrombin generation decrease. Leukemia cells themselves and some therapeutic agents lead to hypercoagulability [16]. Patients with AML who had evidence of DIC when they were initially diagnosed are more likely to develop thrombosis [30]. D-dimer is particularly predictive. New research has come out looking at gene expression and epigenetic modification in patients who develop VTE. In an ALL study, patients who had a VTE within 6 weeks of diagnosis were found to have upregulation of genes associated with neutrophil extracellular traps (NET), like *CXCL8*; platelet activation, like *PF4*; and coagulation, like *VWF* [31]. This finding will likely prompt additional study into other genetic drivers of coagulation in the setting of leukemia and may be able to assist clinicians in predicting the patients who are at higher risk of developing VTE and might benefit from prophylactic measures.

Leukemia Subtypes Commonly Associated with Coagulation Ramifications

Acute Promyelocytic Leukemia

Acute promyelocytic leukemia (APL) is the classic leukemia diagnosis that is associated with coagulopathy. APL is characterized by a t(15;17) translocation leading to the *PML-RARA* fusion gene that stands for ProMyelocytic Leukemia protein and Retinoic acid receptor alpha [32, 33]. APL is determined to be high or low risk for treatment failure based on the white blood cell count at presentation with $10 \times 10^3/\mu L$ being the cutoff. A WBC of at least $10 \times 10^3/\mu L$ also appears to be related to an elevated bleeding risk [34]. In the bone marrow, promyelocytes are hypergranular. The less common microgranular variant can present with a much higher WBC and is harder to differentiate from other subtypes of AML. APL may require treatment with conventional chemotherapy but is also treated differently than other subtypes of leukemia with the initiation of all trans-retinoic acid (ATRA) and arsenic trioxide (ATO) immediately upon diagnosis [33].

Studies have demonstrated a wide range of coagulopathy incidence in patients with APL, predominantly from primary fibrinolysis, though it can encompass secondary fibrinolysis and DIC. The actual incidence of DIC in APL is difficult to determine due to the variation in each study's definition of DIC. One study reports an incidence of DIC in 28.9% of patients, but also found that 69.9% of patients had coagulation lab abnormalities that did not qualify as DIC, while 60.2% of patients had hypofibrinogenemia [35]. Another study, which used the ISTH DIC scoring system, reported coagulopathy consistent with DIC was found in 77.6% of patients with APL [32]. Patients with a higher WBC count and/or a higher percentage of tumor cells in the bone marrow may have more significant coagulopathy [31–34]. Other factors showing potentially higher risk of bleeding include elevated lactate dehydrogenase (LDH), low fibrinogen, low performance status, and high creatinine [32, 34]. A higher WBC count has also shown an association with early death [36].

Laboratory abnormalities demonstrating coagulopathy include low platelets, prolonged PT and aPTT, high D-dimer, and low fibrinogen. Typically, the anticoagulants Protein C, Protein S, and AT are normal, which is distinct from DIC secondary to other causes [33]. A prolonged PT is the lab value most correlated with clinical bleeding, and is highly predictive of clinical bleeding; however, some patients do not have significant prolongation of the PT or aPTT [32]. Patients with non-APL AML have a more similar laboratory profile to patients with DIC from infection, whereas patients with APL have a distinctive coagulation profile, consistent with primary fibrinolysis rather than DIC, characterized by more significantly elevated D-dimer levels and lower levels of fibrinogen [37]. Patients with APL have higher levels than patients with other subtypes of AML of the acute phase reactants, total iron binding capacity (TIBC), transferrin, triglycerides, and cholesterol, but have lower erythrocyte sedimentation rates (ESR) and WBC count [37]. The standard score of 5 to identify overt DIC on the ISTH DIC scoring system has not been shown to be as helpful in predicting the patients with APL who are at highest risk of hemorrhage, likely because the vast majority (close to 90%) of patients with APL meet criteria for overt DIC [34]. The ISTH DIC score originated from patients with DIC from sepsis or trauma and is most accurate and predictive when used for those clinical scenarios. APL is distinct from these conditions due to a different mechanism of coagulopathy: primary fibrinolysis versus DIC. Leukemia, itself, is also different from these conditions relevant to the DIC score in that thrombocytopenia may already be present independent of coagulopathy due to bone marrow infiltration and/or from chemotherapy. This gives an automatic 1 or 2 points for patients with leukemia on this scoring system but may not actually be attributable to DIC. Because of this difference, there is likely a different cutoff required to identify DIC using the ISTH scoring system in APL as compared to other causes of DIC. One study proposes using a cutoff of 6 rather than 5, as they found that scores of at least 6 were more predictive of significant or life-threatening hemorrhage [36].

The pathophysiology for primary fibrinolysis in APL is due to Annexin 2 expressed on the surface of malignant APL cells forming a complex with tissue plasminogen activator (tPA) and plasminogen provoking cleavage of plasminogen to plasmin, and subsequent fibrinolysis. The malignant cells in APL also express tissue factor (TF) and cancer procoagulant (CP) on their cell surface that contribute to coagulopathy. TF and CP, which are pro-thrombotic, initiate coagulation leading to thrombin generation. These two processes happening concurrently lead to consumption of coagulation factors and increased risk of bleeding [34]. As previously discussed, the platelet count is potentially low for other reasons besides consumption, including leukemic infiltration of the bone marrow and chemotherapy. APL coagulopathy demonstrates less microthrombosis than traditional DIC, which seems to be due to primary fibrinolysis being the major driver in the APL phenotype, in contrast to DIC. Contributors include the APL blast cells creating more activators of fibrinolysis including tissue plasminogen activator (tPA), urokinase plasminogen activator (uPA), and urokinase-type plasminogen activator receptor (uPAR). APL cells also produce inflammatory cytokines, making the body hypercoagulable [33].

Clinically, there is a high bleeding incidence in patients with APL of 22.4% with over half of those patients having severe bleeding. When bleeding occurs in the lungs or brain, the mortality rate is extremely high, approaching 100% in one study [32, 33]. Central nervous system (CNS) bleeding makes up about 2/3 of the patients with severe or fatal hemorrhage and pulmonary bleeding makes up the other 1/3 [33]. Bleeding into the CNS also introduces a potential area with increased risk for relapse after a patient has achieved remission [33, 36]. Other common sites of bleeding include the gastrointestinal tract, retina, and uterus. Despite therapy advances over the years, hemorrhage remains a leading cause of early death in APL. When patients diagnosed with APL have an induction failure, the most common cause is hemorrhagic death during induction [34]. Mortality in induction secondary to hemorrhage occurs in 3.7–13% of patients, and in children, specifically, the early death rate is 4% [33, 34]. Because of the severe coagulopathy and the association with mortality, APL is considered a medical emergency at diagnosis.

Patients with APL can have thrombosis as well, in 10–20% [33, 38]. As previously mentioned, TF and CP are expressed on the malignant cells, and likely contribute to this increased risk. The patients who develop thrombosis have lower ISTH DIC scores than patients who do not. Thrombosis occurs in patients after they start therapy for APL. Factors that are shown to be associated with increased risk for thrombosis include male sex, lower DIC score (<5), the bcr3 isoform, and having *FLT3*-ITD. *FLT3*-ITD seems to be the most significant risk factor [38].

Treatment is aimed first at addressing the underlying cause by administering ATRA to combat the leukemia [33]. Making a quick and accurate diagnosis is extremely important for these patients, because ATRA treatment leads to rapid resolution of bleeding symptoms and should be administered as soon as APL is suspected or confirmed [32, 34]. ATRA leads to differentiation of the promyelocytes. ATRA improves coagulopathy specifically through decreasing expression of the coagulopathy-inducing surface markers including TF, Annexin 2, and CP [33, 35]. ATRA does not lead to decrease in inflammatory cytokines. Within about 2 weeks of instituting treatment, the coagulopathy in APL has at least improved if not resolved completely. Thrombocytopenia is slower to improve than the other coagulopathy markers, though likely due to the other mechanisms leading to low platelets including chemotherapy and bone marrow infiltration [33, 35]. Arsenic trioxide treatment leads to apoptosis of leukemia cells and is another medication utilized in the treatment of patients with APL, but it does not seem to have as much of an effect on coagulopathy as ATRA does [33].

Beyond treating the underlying cause, supportive care measures with transfusions may be needed for patients with APL before therapy can be started or until the resolution of coagulopathy. Coagulation labs should be monitored closely at diagnosis and throughout induction to determine the bleeding risk and when a patient may need a transfusion [33]. A mainstay of supportive care includes replacing fibrinogen by administering cryoprecipitate and replacing platelets with a platelet transfusion. The other factor deficiencies can be replaced with fresh frozen plasma (FFP), although there is some controversy in this setting. On one hand, PT and aPTT prolongation are highly predictive of bleeding and FFP has the potential to improve that [32]. But, the prolonged PT and aPTT in patients with APL may be mostly due to hypofibrinogenemia, so cryoprecipitate is likely a better first option. Additionally, because there can be prothrombotic tendency concurrent with the bleeding risk, FFP could lead to increased risk of thrombosis [33]. It is difficult to set transfusion thresholds as they are variable depending on the clinical situation but generally, platelets are kept greater than $30 \times 10^3/\mu L$ and fibrinogen greater than 100–150 mg/dL. Delaying invasive procedures until the bleeding risk has been mitigated, if possible, is recommended [33, 34]. Some patients may require consideration of other means of decreasing the WBC besides ATRA including conventional chemotherapy or the use of hydroxyurea [34]. Other medication options that have been considered include antifibrinolytics, especially since fibrinolysis is a major contributor to the bleeding tendency, although the data is not strong for their use in this setting. Recombinant Factor VII product has shown some efficacy in bleeding but not in mortality [33, 34]. Anticoagulation has not been studied extensively, but it has not seemed to be particularly beneficial, so is not routinely recommended [33].

AML with t(8;16)

There is a distinct form of non-APL AML that has a t(8;16) translocation and presents with coagulopathy including DIC or fibrinolysis in over half of patients at diagnosis [39, 40]. When early death occurs, over half of the time it is due to severe hemorrhage. Coagulopathy at diagnosis is a factor leading to a poorer prognosis in these patients. The t(8;16) translocation is rare, occurring in <1% of patients diagnosed with AML. This genetic mutation can occur both de novo and as a treatment-related AML [40]. The malignant cells typically show monocytic differentiation or myelomonocytic differentiation [40]. The distinctive finding in the bone marrow in this form of AML is erythrophagocytosis [39, 41]. Other characteristics of this type of leukemia include a *KAT6A (MYST)-CREBBP* fusion gene [40, 41]. On flow cytometry, the blast cells do not express CD34, which is the same as APL, and CD117 and CD33 are often negative. A differentiating marker on flow cytometry is human leukocyte antigen DR isotope (HLA-DR), which is usually positive in AML with t(8;16) whereas it is not in APL. It is important to differentiate these types of leukemia, because ATRA does not treat AML with t(8;16). Patients may mistakenly be started on ATRA prior to an official diagnosis because of the signs of coagulopathy that overlap with those of APL, but coagulopathy does not improve in patients with t(8;16) who receive ATRA. When this scenario has been reported in one paper, once ATRA was discontinued and conventional AML chemotherapy began, the coagulopathy resolved [41]. It is important to pursue urgent treatment in patients with AML with t(8;16) because of the risk of early death from hemorrhage, but the rarity of the diagnosis and the clinical similarity to APL make early identification and proper treatment of this entity challenging [40].

AML with Mutated NPM1

One additional AML subtype that is known to present with DIC with similar findings to APL is AML with mutated *NPM1*. Besides the *NPM1* mutation, they can have co-occurrence of other genetic mutations, such as *TET2* or *IDH1/2* mutations, but they do not have t(15;17) translocation or the PML-RARA fusion gene. Clinically, AML with mutated *NPM1* presents with elevated D-dimer and low platelets. Patients with DIC in AML with mutated *NPM1* tend to have much higher white blood cell counts. A markedly elevated WBC count with coagulopathy should raise the concern for this subtype of AML. However, some patients with APL will have a higher WBC count, especially patients with the microgranular variant [33, 42]. AML with *NPM1* mutation is considered an APL-like diagnosis but is not treated the same as APL. ATRA is not effective for these patients [43].

Treatment of Leukemia with Coagulation Ramifications

L-asparaginase is a chemotherapy medication used in the treatment of ALL that has many possible adverse effects [44]. It is included in various cycles of therapy for ALL including induction. The L-asparaginase product initially used was a bacterial form from *Escherichia coli* (*E. coli*). A product from a different bacterium, *Erwinia*, has also been used. Improvements to the development of L-asparaginase came later primarily through pegylation, which has increased the half-life of the medication [44]. Lymphoblasts are dependent on extracellular sources of L-asparagine for protein synthesis. L-asparaginase catalyzes depletion of the circulating pool of L-asparagine, which leads to arrest of protein synthesis. This is highly effective in harming leukemia cells, but also impacts protein synthesis in some healthy cells leading to decreased levels of several essential proteins in the coagulation pathway such as protein C, protein S, plasminogen, fibrinogen, and AT [43–46]. Hypofibrinogenemia to a level of less than 100 mg/dL is common in patients after taking asparaginase, occurring in over half of patients receiving the medication, though bleeding symptoms are often minimal. AT levels decrease in all patients and can get down to less than 50% in up to 67% of patients. AT levels decrease by the fifth day after L-asparaginase administration and take at least 3 weeks to normalize [47].

Some practitioners monitor fibrinogen and AT levels after L-asparaginase administration and replace fibrinogen if it is less than a threshold, some recommending 100 mg/dL, others 50–60 mg/dL. Some monitor AT levels and replace if it is less than 60% [45, 47, 48]. The effects of L-asparaginase are distinct from DIC and care should be taken to confirm L-asparaginase coagulopathy versus DIC primarily for potential therapeutic considerations [45]. Though fibrinogen can reasonably be replaced in either scenario, AT, which would not be administered in DIC, is a consideration in L-asparaginase-associated coagulopathy [45, 47]. AT replacement may be effective in reducing thrombosis risk [49]. Most practitioners do not routinely utilize prophylactic anticoagulation after L-asparaginase administration and including it in management of these patients is controversial [48]. Anticoagulation is challenging in these patients for various reasons. Heparin and low molecular weight heparin (LMWH) are AT dependent, and AT is deficient in patients after L-asparaginase, so these anticoagulants may not be efficacious in this setting. Warfarin is extremely difficult to use in children with cancer because of dietary factors and medication interactions. However, LMWH can be considered if the platelet count is not severely low. It has been shown to be effective in reducing thrombosis frequency, superior to unfractionated heparin, and with low bleeding risk [45, 49].

Chimeric antigen receptor T-cells (CAR-T) are used in the treatment of patients with relapsed and/or refractory acute leukemia and have been associated with coagulation abnormalities after administration. Coagulopathy occurs in over half of patients after CAR-T, with the lab abnormalities most commonly being elevated D-dimer and fibrin degradation products and decreased fibrinogen [50, 51]. Coagulopathy is more common in patients with severe cytokine release syndrome (CRS) and is sometimes even classified as overt DIC [51]. Coagulopathy is most notable about 2–3 weeks after infusion of the product. Risk factors for the development of coagulopathy post infusion include multiple prior treatment courses for leukemia that has relapsed several times, higher disease burden in ALL at the time of infusion, and more marked thrombocytopenia [50]. Toxicity secondary to CAR-T classically is either cytokine release syndrome (CRS) or immune effector cell-associated neurotoxicity syndrome (ICANS). CRS is an inflammatory state with noted elevations in pro-inflammatory cytokines and subsequent development of coagulopathy [51, 52]. CRS often co-occurs in patients with coagulopathy, and the higher the grade of CRS, the worse the coagulopathy is [50]. In a study analyzing coagulopathy after CAR-T, all patients who were found to have overt DIC on laboratory evaluation also had clinical and laboratory evidence of severe CRS [51]. The inflammation and cytokines that are secreted in CRS cause endothelial activation that plays a major role in the activation of coagulation due to increased expression of TF [50, 51].

Most patients who develop coagulopathy after CAR-T therapy will have resolution without requiring intervention. But, a quarter of patients, especially patients with overt DIC, will require supportive care measures with cryoprecipitate transfusion or prothrombin complex concentrates [50]. Patients who develop more severe DIC will have microthrombosis that can lead to multiorgan dysfunction and may be a major cause of mortality. Death after CAR-T that is not related to relapse of the primary disease is often related to DIC. Severe CRS and DIC should be monitored very closely, and appropriate treatment initiated to prevent severe complications and death. Management of the CRS, apart from the coagulopathy, is vital, as the mainstay of DIC management is to treat the underlying causative problem [51].

In a patient being treated for relapsed/refractory hematologic malignancy with clinical deterioration, there are many possible factors at play that could be causing worsening of their symptoms, and it is important to be able to accurately identify the cause, so that appropriate treatment can be implemented. In patients after CAR-T, there may be clinical worsening due to CRS, but they can also have an elevated inflammatory state due to sepsis with many overlapping clinical features, yet the treatments for these two entities are quite different. There was a study done looking at ways to differentiate between CRS and sepsis through various combinations of biomarkers found in the circulation of patients with one of these clinical scenarios. They compared biomarkers related to endothelial dysfunction and coagulopathy in patients after CAR-T infusion versus patients with sepsis. They found that, although vWF (von Willebrand factor) antigen and PAI-1 are elevated in patients with CAR-T toxicity, they are significantly higher in patients with sepsis, and this finding could potentially be used in the future to differentiate between the two processes [52].

Besides these two notable therapies with coagulation effects, there are several other medications to highlight. *Idarubicin* is a chemotherapeutic agent used in the treatment of AML. An in vitro study showed that after idarubicin administration, there is an increase in procoagulant activity at the cellular level with higher levels of TF and phosphatidylserine (PS) found on endothelial and tumor cell surfaces after treatment. They also found elevated levels of thrombomodulin (TM) on endothelial and tumor cell surfaces, though, which is anticoagulant. PS is noted to be procoagulant because it is part of the lipid bilayer of cells and when it gets exposed from damage or apoptosis of the cells, it results in TF exposure into the circulation. Overall, it seems that TF and PS effects may be more potent than the TM effect so that the overall balance is procoagulant for patients treated with Idarubicin [53]. *Dasatinib*, a medication used in the treatment of Philadelphia-chromosome positive leukemia, has been associated with an increased bleeding risk and is likely due to its effects on platelet function [54]. Patients receiving *blinatumomab* have elevations of fibrinogen and D-dimer levels after the infusion has started, but these abnormalities are transient and self-resolve without intervention [55]. Leukocytapheresis is a treatment modality occasionally used to decrease the malignant blast count in a patient presenting with new onset acute leukemia and a markedly elevated WBC count. The leukocytapheresis procedure might lead to a decrease in the platelet count by up to 50%, which should be monitored closely and intervened with platelet transfusions due to the bleeding risk. There are no notable changes in coagulation lab tests after leukapheresis [56]. Many other chemotherapy medications cause thrombocytopenia due to their effect on rapidly growing and dividing cells in the bone marrow (myelotoxicity).

Management of Coagulopathy

The management of specific coagulopathies has been touched on in previous sections, but the general management of coagulation abnormalities in the setting of leukemia is important to consider. Most of the data regarding management is taken from studies and clinical experience in APL, but some of the findings and recommendations can be extrapolated to other subtypes of leukemia, as well.

As previously noted, and classically known by practitioners, the management of DIC should begin with treating the underlying cause. In APL, this is accomplished by starting ATRA immediately when a diagnosis of APL is suspected [57]. ATRA is effective in decreasing the blast count, but it has also shown to improve coagulopathy even before the WBC count has decreased. An in vitro study demonstrated it has the ability to decrease tumor cell surface expression of TF and increase expression of TM [45, 58]. In patients with other subtypes of acute leukemia, ATRA will not be an effective treatment, but instituting the appropriate therapy for the patient's diagnosis is paramount. Supportive care measures include giving cryoprecipitate, platelets, and FFP to keep fibrinogen >100–150 mg/dL, platelets >30–50 × $10^3/\mu L$ or 20–30 × $10^3/\mu L$, and INR <1.5 [45, 57]. Some recommend a lower platelet threshold of 10–20 × $10^3/\mu L$ in patients who are not actively bleeding and increasing the threshold to 50 × $10^3/\mu L$ in patients with bleeding [45, 59]. It is recommended to monitor coagulation labs at least daily until all abnormalities resolve. Invasive procedures should be avoided if at all possible while coagulopathy is present. For other medications such as anticoagulants or antifibrinolytics, there are small studies that suggest their use in this setting but no proven clinical trials to support a recommendation for either. Use of antifibrinolytics, in particular tranexamic acid (TXA), has been described in acute leukemia with varying efficacy, but with some patients having thrombotic complications. TXA has successfully controlled bleeding symptoms in some cases, but care should be used in this setting [60]. Anticoagulation is not typically used because of the risk of hemorrhage [45]. There are no recommendations for recombinant activated Factor VII products or prothrombin complex concentrates. While they may be helpful for patients with hemorrhage, the possible increase in thrombosis risk is generally considered too high [45, 57].

In Japan, recombinant TM has been used to treat patients with DIC from sepsis with some success. Thrombomodulin is present on several cell types in the body, especially endothelial cells, and is a thrombin receptor. When thrombin binds to TM, its function is reversed and becomes an anticoagulant. Its effect is activation of protein C, the natural anticoagulant that inactivates Factors Va and VIIIa in the prothrombinase and intrinsic tenase complexes, respectively, of the coagulation cascade. TM also has anti-inflammatory properties. No clinical trials have been done for recombinant TM in the management of leukemia-associated DIC, so there are no current recommendations for its use in this setting [45]. For adult patients with leukemia treated with TM who had bleeding symptoms, 55% had resolution or improvement in the bleeding symptoms secondary to DIC. DIC resolved in 55.9% with the DIC score and coagulation tests, in general, improving significantly [61]. There are case reports of children who have been treated with TM with success. In one instance, the patient had a very high WBC and was considered high risk for DIC. They were given thrombomodulin and did not have any hemostasis/thrombosis complications [62].

Thrombosis is associated with increased mortality in patients with cancer and management of this complication is important to consider to decrease mortality [63]. Managing a patient who develops thrombosis during treatment for leukemia is challenging because of the coexisting significant bleeding risk primarily due to thrombocytopenia. Unfractionated heparin is a recommendation to consider for sicker patients requiring continuous infusion of an anticoagulant [57]. Recommendations regarding the use of LMWH in this setting suggest using a tiered approach depending on the platelet count. When the platelet count is >50 × 10^3/μL, target an LMWH level of 0.5–1.0 IU/mL and when the platelet count drops below 50 × 10^3/μL, reduce the LMWH dose by half. If the platelet count falls below 20 × 10^3/μL, discontinue LMWH [57, 59, 63]. Direct oral anticoagulants (DOAC) have not been extensively studied in this setting, but have potential use in these patients [59]. Because of the bleeding risk, there may be situations, such as some line-associated thromboses, where treatment may be deferred. Some older patients, though not generally children, will have placement of an inferior vena cava (IVC) filter to prevent pulmonary embolism (PE) while the bleeding risk is considered too high for anticoagulation [59, 63].

While it is rare, there are patients who have hereditary bleeding disorders and develop leukemia, and they are a particularly challenging patient population to manage due to the bleeding risk. Evidence in the literature regarding these patients is limited to case reports. Patients with Hemophilia have been managed with prophylactic factor replacement throughout therapy. During the first part of therapy, factor replacement was given daily and after remission, was spaced out to a prophylactic regimen [64]. A patient with von Willebrand disease was managed with platelet transfusions to keep platelets >20 × 10^3/μL and infusions of vWF-containing product every other day to keep vWF activity trough levels >12%. They also administered the antifibrinolytic agent TXA for mucosal bleeding complications. That patient unfortunately developed a basilic vein thrombosis but was not treated with anticoagulation because of the high risk of hemorrhage [65]. It is important to note that prior to a diagnosis of leukemia, these patients will likely have increased bleeding symptoms that could be mistakenly attributed to a complication of their bleeding disorder such as an inhibitor development. Remembering to keep a broad differential diagnosis is important, particularly where there is unexpected bleeding and if there are other symptoms present such as fevers or lymphadenopathy [64].

References

1. Hillestad LK. Acute promyelocytic leukemia. Acta Med Scand. 1957;159(3):189–94.
2. Winter WE, Flax SD, Harris NS. Coagulation testing in the core laboratory. Lab Med. 2017;48(4):295–313. https://doi.org/10.1093/labmed/lmx050.

3. Favaloro EJ, Pasalic L. Routine coagulation. Clin Lab Med. 2024;44(3):527–39. https://doi.org/10.1016/j.cll.2024.04.012. Epub 2024 Jun 4.
4. Burley K, Salem J, Phillips T, Reilly-Stitt C, Marks DI, Tunstall O, Moppett J, Mumford A, Bradbury CA. Evaluation of coagulopathy before and during induction chemotherapy for acute lymphoblastic leukaemia, including assessment of global clotting tests. Blood Cancer J. 2017;7(6):e574. https://doi.org/10.1038/bcj.2017.54. PMID: 28622302; PMCID: PMC5520401.
5. Raso S, Lucchesi A, Sardo M, et al. Global hemostasis assays in acute myeloid leukemia: results of an observational prospective study. Blood Transfus. 2024;22(1):65–74. https://doi.org/10.2450/BloodTransfus.575.
6. Russell L, Madsen MB, Dahl M, Kampmann P, Perner A. Prediction of bleeding and thrombosis by standard biochemical coagulation variables in haematological intensive care patients. Acta Anaesthesiol Scand. 2018;62(2):196–206. https://doi.org/10.1111/aas.13036.
7. Qdaisat A, Soud RA, Wu CC, et al. Poor performance of D-dimer in excluding venous thromboembolism among patients with lymphoma and leukemia. Haematologica. 2019;104(6):e265–8. https://doi.org/10.3324/haematol.2018.211466.
8. Whiting D, DiNardo JA. TEG and ROTEM: technology and clinical applications. Am J Hematol. 2014;89(2):228–32. https://doi.org/10.1002/ajh.23599.
9. Raso S, Lucchesi A, Sardo M, Annibali O, Sucato V, Ciaccio M, Vitale S, Dolce A, Giordano G, Siragusa S, Napolitano M. Global hemostasis assays in acute myeloid leukemia: results of an observational prospective study. Blood Transfus. 2024;22(1):65–74. https://doi.org/10.2450/BloodTransfus.575. Epub 2023 Jun 12. PMID: 37458717; PMCID: PMC10812886.
10. Just Vinholt P, Højrup Knudsen G, Sperling S, Frederiksen H, Nielsen C. Platelet function tests predict bleeding in patients with acute myeloid leukemia and thrombocytopenia. Am J Hematol. 2019;94(8):891–901. https://doi.org/10.1002/ajh.25512.
11. Aggarwal A, Mahajan D, Sharma P. Application of the International Society on Thrombosis and Haemostasis scoring system in evaluation of disseminated intravascular coagulation in patients with acute leukemias. South Asian J Cancer. 2021;10(4):241–5. Published 2021 Nov 24. https://doi.org/10.1055/s-0041-1733347.
12. Ribeiro RC, Pui CH. The clinical and biological correlates of coagulopathy in children with acute leukemia. J Clin Oncol. 1986;4(8):1212–8. https://doi.org/10.1200/JCO.1986.4.8.1212.
13. Bleeding and thrombosing diseases conference and workshop, October 6–8, 2021. Mayo Medical Laboratories, Intravascular Coagulation and Hyperfibrinolysis Presentation by Dr Ashrani.
14. Kumar V, Abbas AK, Fausto N, Aster JC. Red blood cell and bleeding disorders. In: Kumar V, Abbas AK, Fausto N, Aster JC, Des. Robbins and Cotran Pathologic Basis of Disease.10th ed. Philadelphia, PA: Elsevier. 2020:635–72.
15. Boral BM, Williams DJ, Boral LI. Disseminated intravascular coagulation. Am J Clin Pathol. 2016;146(6):670–80. https://doi.org/10.1093/ajcp/aqw195.
16. Giordano P, Molinari AC, Del Vecchio GC, et al. Prospective study of hemostatic alterations in children with acute lymphoblastic leukemia. Am J Hematol. 2010;85(5):325–30. https://doi.org/10.1002/ajh.21665.
17. Ay C, Simanek R, Vormittag R, et al. High plasma levels of soluble P-selectin are predictive of venous thromboembolism in cancer patients: results from the Vienna Cancer and Thrombosis Study (CATS). Blood. 2008;112(7):2703–8. https://doi.org/10.1182/blood-2008-02-142422.
18. Taylor FB Jr, Toh CH, Hoots WK, Wada H, Levi M. Scientific Subcommittee on Disseminated Intravascular Coagulation (DIC) of the International Society on Thrombosis and Haemostasis (ISTH). Towards definition, clinical and laboratory criteria, and a scoring system for disseminated intravascular coagulation. Thromb Haemost. 2001;86(5):1327–30.
19. Champion LA, Luddy RE, Schwartz AD. Disseminated intravascular coagulation in childhood acute lymphocytic leukemia with poor prognostic features. Cancer. 1978;41(4):1642–6. https://doi.org/10.1002/1097-0142(197804)41:4<1642::aid-cncr2820410456>3.0.co;2-r.

20. Higuchi T, Mori H, Niikura H, Omine M, Okada S, Terada H. Disseminated intravascular coagulation in acute lymphoblastic leukemia at presentation and in early phase of remission induction therapy. Ann Hematol. 1998;76(6):263–9. https://doi.org/10.1007/s002770050399.
21. Songthawee N, Chavananon S, Sripornsawan P, McNeil E, Chotsampancharoen T. Prevalence and risk factors of disseminated intravascular coagulation in childhood acute lymphoblastic leukemia. Pediatr Res. 2023;94(2):588–93. https://doi.org/10.1038/s41390-023-02475-8.
22. Li XY, Zhou YL, Zhang Y, et al. Coagulation profile in newly diagnosed T-cell acute lymphoblastic leukemia. Thromb Res. 2021;203:69–71. https://doi.org/10.1016/j.thromres.2021.04.013.
23. Mangal AK, Grossman L, Vickars L. Disseminated intravascular coagulation in acute monoblastic leukemia: response to heparin therapy. Can Med Assoc J. 1984;130(6):731–3.
24. Ding R, Wang Z, Lin Y, Liu B, Zhang Z, Ma X. Comparison of a new criteria for sepsis-induced coagulopathy and International Society on Thrombosis and Haemostasis disseminated intravascular coagulation score in critically ill patients with sepsis 3.0: a retrospective study. Blood Coagul Fibrinolysis. 2018;29(6):551–58. https://doi.org/10.1097/MBC.0000000000000075521.
25. Rodeghiero F, Mannucci PM, Viganò S, et al. Liver dysfunction rather than intravascular coagulation as the main cause of low protein C and antithrombin III in acute leukemia. Blood. 1984;63(4):965–9.
26. Bumbea H, Vladareanu AM, Dumitru I, et al. Platelet defects in acute myeloid leukemia-potential for hemorrhagic events. J Clin Med. 2021;11(1):118. Published 2021 Dec 26. https://doi.org/10.3390/jcm11010118.
27. Annibali O, Napolitano M, Avvisati G, Siragusa S. Incidence of venous thromboembolism and use of anticoagulation in hematological malignancies: critical review of the literature. Crit Rev Oncol Hematol. 2018;124:41–50. https://doi.org/10.1016/j.critrevonc.2018.02.003.
28. Mohren M, Markmann I, Jentsch-Ullrich K, Koenigsmann M, Lutze G, Franke A. Increased risk of venous thromboembolism in patients with acute leukaemia. Br J Cancer. 2006;94(2):200–2. https://doi.org/10.1038/sj.bjc.6602945.
29. De Stefano V, Sorà F, Rossi E, et al. The risk of thrombosis in patients with acute leukemia: occurrence of thrombosis at diagnosis and during treatment. J Thromb Haemost. 2005;3(9):1985–92. https://doi.org/10.1111/j.1538-7836.2005.01467.x.
30. Libourel EJ, Klerk CPW, van Norden Y, et al. Disseminated intravascular coagulation at diagnosis is a strong predictor for thrombosis in acute myeloid leukemia. Blood. 2016;128(14):1854–61. https://doi.org/10.1182/blood-2016-02-701094.
31. Pelland-Marcotte MC, Belaktib A, Droit A, et al. Molecular signatures associated with venous thromboembolism in children with acute lymphoblastic leukemia. J Thromb Haemost. 2025;23(3):1009–22. https://doi.org/10.1016/j.jtha.2024.12.007.
32. Chang H, Kuo MC, Shih LY, et al. Clinical bleeding events and laboratory coagulation profiles in acute promyelocytic leukemia. Eur J Haematol. 2012;88(4):321–8. https://doi.org/10.1111/j.1600-0609.2011.01747.x.
33. Breen KA, Grimwade D, Hunt BJ. The pathogenesis and management of the coagulopathy of acute promyelocytic leukaemia. Br J Haematol. 2012;156(1):24–36. https://doi.org/10.1111/j.1365-2141.2011.08922.x.
34. Naymagon L, Mascarenhas J. Hemorrhage in acute promyelocytic leukemia: can it be predicted and prevented? Leuk Res. 2020;94:106356. https://doi.org/10.1016/j.leukres.2020.106356.
35. Zhu HH, Guo ZP, Jia JS, Jiang Q, Jiang H, Huang XJ. The impact of oral arsenic and all-trans-retinoic acid on coagulopathy in acute promyelocytic leukemia. Leuk Res. 2018;65:14–9. https://doi.org/10.1016/j.leukres.2017.11.009.
36. Rajpurkar M, Alonzo TA, Wang YC, et al. Risk markers for significant bleeding and thrombosis in pediatric acute promyelocytic leukemia; report from the Children's Oncology Group study AAML0631. J Pediatr Hematol Oncol. 2019;41(1):51–5. https://doi.org/10.1097/MPH.0000000000001280.
37. Lee HJ, Park HJ, Kim HW, Park SG. Comparison of laboratory characteristics between acute promyelocytic leukemia and other subtypes of acute myeloid leukemia with disseminated intra-

vascular coagulation. Blood Res. 2013;48(4):250–3. https://doi.org/10.5045/br.2013.48.4.250. Epub 2013 Dec 24. PMID: 24466548; PMCID: PMC3894382.
38. Mitrovic M, Suvajdzic N, Elezovic I, et al. Thrombotic events in acute promyelocytic leukemia. Thromb Res. 2015;135(4):588–93. https://doi.org/10.1016/j.thromres.2014.11.026.
39. Sun T, Wu E. Acute monoblastic leukemia with t(8;16): a distinct clinicopathologic entity; report of a case and review of the literature. Am J Hematol. 2001;66(3):207–12. https://doi.org/10.1002/1096-8652(200103)66:3<207::aid-ajh1046>3.0.co;2-q.
40. Kayser S, Hills RK, Langova R, et al. Characteristics and outcome of patients with acute myeloid leukaemia and t(8;16)(p11;p13): results from an International Collaborative Study. Br J Haematol. 2021;192(5):832–42. https://doi.org/10.1111/bjh.17336.
41. Hastings A, Apperley JF, Nadal-Melsio E, Brown L, Bain BJ. Acute myeloid leukemia with a severe coagulopathy and t(8;16)(p11;p13). Am J Hematol. 2021;96(1):163–4. https://doi.org/10.1002/ajh.25903.
42. Nagendra S, Meyerson H, Skallerud G, Rosenthal N. Leukemias resembling acute promyelocytic leukemia, microgranular variant. Am J Clin Pathol. 2002;117(4):651–7. https://doi.org/10.1309/KD1G-NUR1-J75P-HQ28.
43. Arana Rosainz MJ, Nguyen N, Wahed A, et al. Acute myeloid leukemia with mutated NPM1 mimics acute promyelocytic leukemia presentation. Int J Lab Hematol. 2021;43(2):218–26. https://doi.org/10.1111/ijlh.13357.
44. Stock W, Douer D, DeAngelo DJ, et al. Prevention and management of asparaginase/pegasparaginase-associated toxicities in adults and older adolescents: recommendations of an expert panel. Leuk Lymphoma. 2011;52(12):2237–53. https://doi.org/10.3109/10428194.2011.596963.
45. Ten Cate H, Leader A. Management of disseminated intravascular coagulation in acute leukemias. Hamostaseologie. 2021;41(2):120–6. https://doi.org/10.1055/a-1393-8302.
46. Caruso V, Iacoviello L, Di Castelnuovo A, et al. Thrombotic complications in childhood acute lymphoblastic leukemia: a meta-analysis of 17 prospective studies comprising 1752 pediatric patients. Blood. 2006;108(7):2216–22. https://doi.org/10.1182/blood-2006-04-015511.
47. Douer D, Yampolsky H, Cohen LJ, et al. Pharmacodynamics and safety of intravenous pegaspargase during remission induction in adults aged 55 years or younger with newly diagnosed acute lymphoblastic leukemia. Blood. 2007;109(7):2744–50. https://doi.org/10.1182/blood-2006-07-035006.
48. Greenmyer JR, Wyatt KD, Rodriguez V, Ashrani AA, Warad D. Management practices for asparaginase-associated coagulopathy: a survey of pediatric oncologists. J Pediatr Hematol Oncol. 2022;44(8):e1023–8. https://doi.org/10.1097/MPH.0000000000002396.
49. Greiner J, Schrappe M, Claviez A, et al. THROMBOTECT—a randomized study comparing low molecular weight heparin, antithrombin and unfractionated heparin for thromboprophylaxis during induction therapy of acute lymphoblastic leukemia in children and adolescents. Haematologica. 2019;104(4):756–65. https://doi.org/10.3324/haematol.2018.194175.
50. Wang Y, Qi K, Cheng H, et al. Coagulation disorders after chimeric antigen receptor T cell therapy: analysis of 100 patients with relapsed and refractory hematologic malignancies. Biol Blood Marrow Transplant. 2020;26(5):865–75. https://doi.org/10.1016/j.bbmt.2019.11.027.
51. Jiang H, Liu L, Guo T, et al. Improving the safety of CAR-T cell therapy by controlling CRS-related coagulopathy. Ann Hematol. 2019;98(7):1721–32. https://doi.org/10.1007/s00277-019-03685-z.
52. Moreno-Castaño AB, Fernández S, Ventosa H, et al. Characterization of the endotheliopathy, innate-immune activation and hemostatic imbalance underlying CAR-T cell toxicities: laboratory tools for an early and differential diagnosis. J Immunother Cancer. 2023;11(4):e006365. https://doi.org/10.1136/jitc-2022-006365.
53. Tsunaka M, Shinki H, Koyama T. Cell-based evaluation of changes in coagulation activity induced by antineoplastic drugs for the treatment of acute myeloid leukemia. PLoS One. 2017;12(4):e0175765. Published 2017 Apr 13. https://doi.org/10.1371/journal.pone.0175765.

54. Beke Debreceni I, Mezei G, Batár P, Illés Á, Kappelmayer J. Dasatinib inhibits procoagulant and clot retracting activities of human platelets. Int J Mol Sci. 2019;20(21):5430. Published 2019 Oct 31. https://doi.org/10.3390/ijms20215430.
55. Locatelli F, Markovic A, Klinger M, Zeng T, Zugmaier G. Transient and fully reversible changes in laboratory parameters and modifications of the cytokine profile during blinatumomab treatment in children with relapsed or refractory B-cell acute lymphoblastic leukemia. Pediatr Blood Cancer. 2023. Published online May 28, 2023; https://doi.org/10.1002/pbc.30435.
56. Villgran V, Agha M, Raptis A, et al. Leukapheresis in patients newly diagnosed with acute myeloid leukemia. Transfus Apher Sci. 2016;55(2):216–20. https://doi.org/10.1016/j.transci.2016.07.001.
57. Sanz MA, Montesinos P. Advances in the management of coagulopathy in acute promyelocytic leukemia. Thromb Res. 2020;191(Suppl 1):S63–7. https://doi.org/10.1016/S0049-3848(20)30399-6.
58. Koyama T, Hirosawa S, Kawamata N, Tohda S, Aoki N. All-trans retinoic acid upregulates thrombomodulin and downregulates tissue-factor expression in acute promyelocytic leukemia cells: distinct expression of thrombomodulin and tissue factor in human leukemic cells. Blood. 1994;84(9):3001–9.
59. Falanga A, Rickles FR. Management of Thrombohemorrhagic Syndromes (THS) in hematologic malignancies. Hematology Am Soc Hematol Educ Program. 2007:165–71. https://doi.org/10.1182/asheducation-2007.1.165.
60. Koseki M, Asada N, Uryu H, Takeuchi M, Asakura H, Matsue K. Successful combined use of tranexamic acid and unfractionated heparin for life-threatening bleeding associated with intravascular coagulation in a patient with chronic myelogenous leukemia in blast crisis. Int J Hematol. 2007;86(5):403–6. https://doi.org/10.1007/BF02983996.
61. Asakura H, Takahashi H, Tsuji H, et al. Post-marketing surveillance of thrombomodulin alfa, a novel treatment of disseminated intravascular coagulation—safety and efficacy in 1,032 patients with hematologic malignancy. Thromb Res. 2014;133(3):364–70. https://doi.org/10.1016/j.thromres.2013.12.033.
62. Saito A, Okamoto Y, Seki Y, et al. DIC complicating APL successfully treated with recombinant thrombomodulin alfa. J Pediatr Hematol Oncol. 2016;38(6):e189–90. https://doi.org/10.1097/MPH.0000000000000585.
63. Rickles FR, Falanga A, Montesinos P, Sanz MA, Brenner B, Barbui T. Bleeding and thrombosis in acute leukemia: what does the future of therapy look like? [published correction appears in Thromb Res. 2008;123(1):187–90]. Thromb Res. 2007;120(Suppl 2):S99–S106. https://doi.org/10.1016/S0049-3848(07)70137-8.
64. Zülfikar B. Two patients with haemophilia and acute leukaemia. Haemophilia. 2002;8(5):698–702. https://doi.org/10.1046/j.1365-2516.2002.00660.x.
65. Dillon J, Mykytiv V, Keenan C, et al. Management of a patient with acute myeloid leukaemia with a diagnosis of type 2 von Willebrand disease and a novel variant within the von Willebrand factor (VWF) gene. Br J Haematol. 2022;199(2):e5–7. https://doi.org/10.1111/bjh.18390.

Acute Leukemias of Ambiguous Lineage 20

Olga Kagan Weinberg and Weina Chen

Definitions

Acute leukemias of ambiguous lineage (ALAL) are a group of leukemias in which neoplastic blasts constitute ≥20% of the total cells (based on morphology) and do not show differentiation along a single lineage, either lack clear evidence of commitment to the myeloid, B-cell lymphoid, or T-lymphoid lineages (acute undifferentiated leukemia, AUL), or demonstrate evidence of commitment to more than one lineage (mixed phenotype acute leukemia, MPAL) [1–6]. Leukemias that can be classified into other clinically or genetically defined categories should not be considered MPAL despite meeting the lineage criteria [1].

MPAL includes both biphenotypic leukemia, where a single blast population expresses markers from more than one lineage, and bilineal leukemia, where separate distinct populations of blasts each show a single, but different lineage. In most cases, the blast populations show various subsets, some with biphenotypic pattern and some with a single immunophenotype. Based on the lineage markers expressed on the blast cells, MPAL can also be further divided into B/Myeloid, T/Myeloid, B/T, B/T/Myeloid, and other rare subtypes.

O. K. Weinberg · W. Chen (✉)
Department of Pathology, University of Texas Southwestern Medical Center, Dallas, TX, USA
e-mail: Olga.weinberg@UTSouthwestern.edu

W. Li (ed.), *Laboratory Assessments of Pediatric Leukemia*,
https://doi.org/10.1007/978-3-032-26557-9_20

Evolving Diagnostic Criteria

Initial classification systems of MPAL utilized a scoring system whereby certain lineage markers were assigned points, and the first scoring system was described by Catovsky et al. [6] The European Group for the Immunologic Characterization of Leukemias (EGIL) further modified the Catovsky system, primarily by changing weight assigned to certain markers [7, 8] (Table 20.1). The 3rd edition of the World Health Organization (WHO) Classification (2001 WHO) endorsed this system, and the 4th edition of the WHO classification (2008 WHO) eliminated a scoring system and sought to simplify the diagnosis by reducing the specific lineage markers necessary to ascribe a lineage and combined biphenotypic leukemias and bilineal leukemias within the MPAL category [9, 10]. The 4th revised edition of WHO classification (2017 WHO) further refined the criteria by requirement of strong expression of lineage-defining markers [10]. The 5th edition of WHO (WHO-HEM5, 2022) and the International Consensus Classification (ICC) of acute leukemias continued utilizing lineage-defining markers outlined in the 2017 WHO classification and included more genetically defined subtypes [1, 2, 11] (Tables 20.2 and 20.3). Both updated classifications further strengthened MPAL diagnostic criteria by providing guidelines on the definition of strong expression of lineage-defining markers.

Table 20.1 European Group for the Immunological Characterization of Leukemias (EGIL) scoring system for biphenotypic acute leukemia

Points	B-lineage	T-lineage	Myeloid lineage
2	CD79a, cIgM, cCD22	CD3, TCR-α/β, TCR-γ/δ	MPO, lysozyme
1	CD19, CD10, CD20	CD2, CD5, CD8, CD10	CD13, CD33, CDw65, CD117
0.5	TdT, CD24	TdT, CD7, CD1a	CD14, CD15, CD64

Table 20.2 WHO-HEM5 classification of acute leukemia of ambiguous lineage entities

Acute leukemia of ambiguous lineage with defining genetic abnormalities
Mixed-phenotype acute leukemia with *BCR::ABL1* fusion
Mixed-phenotype acute leukemia with *KMT2A* rearrangement
Mixed-phenotype acute leukemia with *ZNF384* rearrangement
Acute leukemia of ambiguous lineage with *BCL11B* rearrangement
Acute leukemia of ambiguous lineage with other defined genetic alterations
Acute leukemia of ambiguous lineage, immunophenotypically defined
Mixed-phenotype acute leukemia, B/myeloid
Mixed-phenotype acute leukemia, T/myeloid
Mixed-phenotype acute leukemia, rare types
Acute leukemia of ambiguous lineage, not otherwise specified
Acute undifferentiated leukemia

Table 20.3 International Consensus Classification (ICC) classification of acute leukemia of ambiguous lineage entities

MPAL with defining genetic alterations
MPAL with *BCR::ABL1*
MPAL, with t(v;11q23.3); *KMT2A* rearrangement
MPAL with *ZNF384* rearrangement
MPAL with *BCL11B* activation
MPAL with defining immunophenotypic changes
B/Myeloid MPAL
T/Myeloid MPAL
B/T/Myeloid MPAL
B/T MPAL
Acute undifferentiated leukemia (AUL)
ALAL, not otherwise specified (NOS)

Epidemiology

The reported frequency of MPAL depends on the classification used. Earlier studies utilizing EGIL criteria reported that biphenotypic acute leukemia comprised up to 5% of acute leukemias [12]. The updated WHO classifications led to a decreased number of MPAL cases, and in the two largest case series using the WHO 2008 criteria, MPAL cases accounted for between 0.5% and 2.4% of all leukemias [13]. In a large study of pediatric and adult patients with acute leukemia, 1.6% of patients were diagnosed with MPAL with a bimodal age distribution [14, 15]. Because of its rarity, little is known about the frequency of AUL. Using the SEER database, age-adjusted AUL incidence rate of 1.34 per million person-years has been reported [16] but appears to have decreased over time, likely due to refined diagnostic criteria.

Clinical Features

The clinical manifestations of MPAL generally overlap with those seen in other forms of acute leukemia. Most patients present with signs and symptoms of bone marrow failure, including fatigue, weakness, recurrent infections, or bleeding, which reflect varying degrees of pancytopenia. Other findings may relate to the accumulation of leukemic cells in peripheral blood, bone marrow, or extramedullary sites (e.g., abdominal fullness from splenomegaly and bone pain).

Diagnostic Criteria and Lineage Assignment

The diagnosis of ALAL requires the presence of ≥20% blasts (based on the morphologic assessment) in peripheral blood or marrow, blasts with the immunophenotype that fulfils the lineage assignment criteria (Table 20.4), and the leukemia being excluded from other clinically or genetically defined categories (detailed in section "Differential diagnosis").

Blasts in MPAL are morphologically diverse and range in size with variable cytoplasm, and in some cases, two or three separate blast populations with distinctive size, morphology, and phenotype can be identified (Fig. 20.1). In cases with completely separate blast populations (in bilineal or trilineal MPAL cases), each abnormal progenitor population only needs to meet the immunophenotypic criteria for single lineage acute leukemia, expression of myeloperoxidase (MPO) is not required for myeloid lineage blast population, and the numerical blast criterion only applies to aggregate. Notably, there is a discrepancy between the WHO-HEM5 and the ICC regarding whether there is a minimum percentage of each neoplastic blast component. ICC classification proposes that in cases with small aberrant clones of divergent lineage composing ≥5% of all cells, a diagnosis of MPAL could be rendered if clear immunophenotypic aberrancies are identified. For cases with aberrant clones that represent <5% of all cells, a diagnosis should be based on the major leukemic population with a descriptive modifier [2]. In contrast, WHO-HEM5 permits the diagnosis of MPAL regardless of the percentage of the individual aberrant blast population (i.e., no minimum percentage for either blast component) as long as the percentage of the total blast populations is ≥20% of all cells (by morphology) [1]. Whether applying the ICC or the WHO-HEM5 guidelines, it is essential to document a minor population of leukemic blasts of divergent lineage, as this population may become predominant after therapy (as illustrated in an example case in

Table 20.4 Markers used in lineage assignment in both WHO-HEM5 and ICC classifications

B-lineage[a]	Strong CD19 *and*	1 or more marker expression: CD10, CD22, or CD79a
	Weak CD19 *and*	2 more strongly expressed: CD10, CD22, CD79a[b]
	Considering immunohistochemical stains for B-lineage	PAX5, OCT2, BOB1
T-lineage[a]	CD3 (surface or cytoplasmic)[c]	
Myeloid lineage[a]	MPO	
	Monocytic differentiation	NSE, CD64, CD11c, CD14, or lysozyme

[a]Per the WHO-HEM5, normal counterparts are B-cell progenitors, mature T-cells, and neutrophils for B-, T-, and myeloid (non-monocytic)-lineage assignment, respectively. Per the ICC, normal counterparts are stage 1 B-cell progenitors (or mature B-cells) and mature T-cells for B- and T-lineage assignment, respectively. The threshold for MPO has not yet been established in the ICC
[b]CD79a cannot be used as a criterion for B-lineage assignment in the diagnosis of B/T MPAL
[c]Using CD3 epsilon-chain antibody

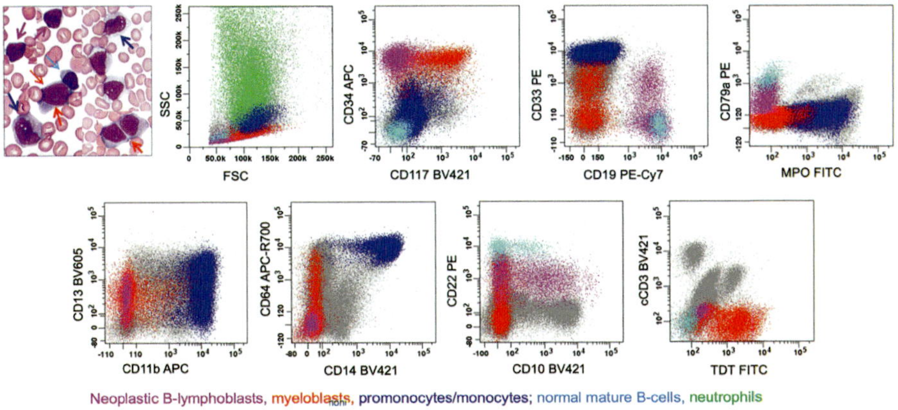

Fig. 20.1 *BCR::ABL1* rearranged B/myeloid (bilineal) MPAL with myeloid predominance. This is a case of bilineal MPAL with three distinctly discrete neoplastic blast populations showing differentiation along B-lymphoid and myeloid (neutrophilic and monocytic) lineages. Morphologically, lymphoblasts have medium-sized nuclei (violet arrows), myeloblasts have large-sized blasts with fine chromatin and moderate amount of cytoplasm (red arrows), and neoplastic monocytes have large, folded nuclei and moderate amount of cytoplasm (blue arrows, some with the feature of promonocytes). By immunophenotype, the neoplastic B-lymphoid blasts (in violet) express CD34, CD10 (partial), TdT, B-cell markers (CD19, CD22, and CD79a), and myeloid associated markers (partial CD13 and CD33), but lack expression of CD3, CD11b, CD14, CD117, CD64, or MPO. The neoplastic myeloblasts (in red) express CD34, MPO (partial), CD13, CD33 (partial), and CD64 (partial), but lack expression of CD14, B-cell markers, or CD3. The neoplastic promonocytes/monocytes (in blue) express CD11b, CD13 (partial), CD14, CD33, and CD64, and MPO, but lack expression of CD3 (surface and cytoplasmic, sCD3 and cCD3), CD34, CD117, or B-cell markers. Color code: violet, neoplastic B-lymphoblasts; red, neoplastic myeloblasts; blue, neoplastic monocytes; green, neutrophils; and cyan, normal mature B-cells

Fig. 20.2), and this minor leukemic population can have significant therapeutic and prognostic implications. Future studies are warranted to address the differences between the two classifications and to establish a consensus on diagnostic criteria.

Extensive immunophenotyping is essential for an accurate diagnosis of ALAL. Lineage assignment is best performed by flow cytometric immunophenotyping to evaluate the intensity and pattern of expression of lineage-defining markers and to correlate the patterns of antigen expression on one or more cell populations; for details in flow cytometric immunophenotyping on ALAL, please refer to review articles on this topic [17, 18]. Immunohistochemical stains may be used to show expression of lineage-associated antigens such as MPO, CD3, and PAX5 (Table 20.4), although discriminating leukemic populations from normal cells may be difficult in a case with only a low percentage of neoplastic blasts.

Both the WHO-HEM5 and the ICC stress that the assignment of lineage is dependent on the intensity of expression of lineage-defining markers on the lineage being assessed. Specifically, the strong antigen expression requires the intensity of these markers on "a proportion of the blasts" exceeding the 50% of the intensity level seen on normal counterparts per the WHO-HEM5 or similar to the level

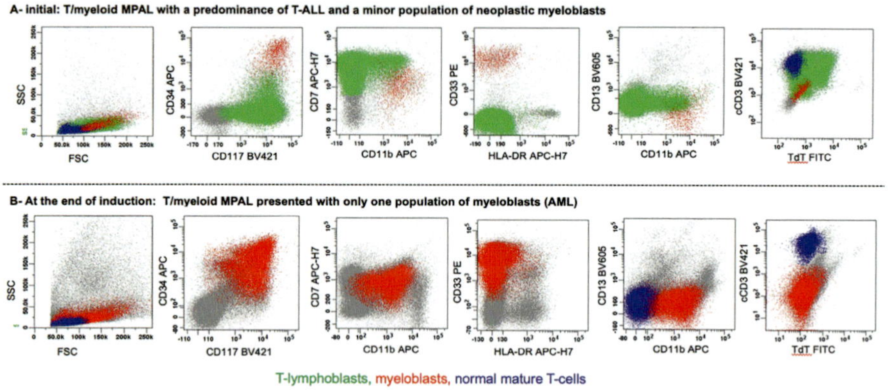

Fig. 20.2 T/myeloid MPAL with T-lymphoid predominance (bilineal with a minor population of neoplastic myeloblasts, <5%) progressing into acute myeloid leukemia (AML). (**a**) At diagnosis, there are two separate discrete neoplastic blast populations, a large population (78%) of T-lymphoblasts and a minor population (0.8%) of neoplastic myeloblasts. T-lymphoblasts (in green) are positive for CD7, CD117, CD11b (in a small subset), cCD3, and TdT, but negative for CD34, CD13, CD33, or human leukocyte antigen–DR isotype (HLA-DR). Neoplastic CD34+/CD117+/CD33+ myeloblasts (in red) have an aberrant expression of CD7/CD11b and loss of CD13/HLA-DR. (**b**) At the end of induction, T-lymphoblasts are undetectable, but neoplastic myeloblasts are significantly expanded (becoming AML) and retain the same immunophenotype as observed at initial T/myeloid MPAL, displaying aberrant expression of CD7/CD11b along with loss of CD13/HLA-DR. Color code: green, T lymphoblasts; red, neoplastic myeloblasts; blue, normal T cells

observed on normal counterparts per the ICC (Table 20.4 and Fig. 20.3). However, both classifications do not clearly provide *a threshold for* "a proportion of the blasts" exceeding those intensity cutoff levels. To enhance the specificity of lineage assignment, both classifications state that MPAL cases typically show immunophenotypic heterogeneity, including complex displays with bright to weak expression of lineage-defining markers on subpopulations of blasts (Fig. 20.3). The WHO-HEM5 further emphasizes a coordinated expression pattern of multiple antigens along the same lineage. For example, the combined and coordinated expression of multiple myeloid markers (such as CD117 and CD33) on MPO-expressed blasts is more strongly associated with myeloid lineage commitment than the expression of each antigen individually.

Assignment of B-lineage requires strong CD19 expression on blasts in addition to strong expression of at least one other B-lineage marker, or if only weak CD19 is present, two additional markers are required. The most specific marker for B-lineage leukemias is CD19; however, it can be detected in other entities including t(8;21)(q22;q22)/*RUNX1::RUNX1T1* rearranged acute myeloid leukemia (AML), which preclude its use as the sole lineage assignment marker [19, 20]. Another B-cell marker CD79a is seen early in B-cells and is retained through plasmacytic differentiation; however, its expression is not unique to acute leukemias of B-lineage, as CD79a is also expressed in T-lymphoblastic leukemia (T-ALL) [21, 22]. WHO-HEM5 specifies that CD79a cannot be used as a criterion for B-lineage assignment

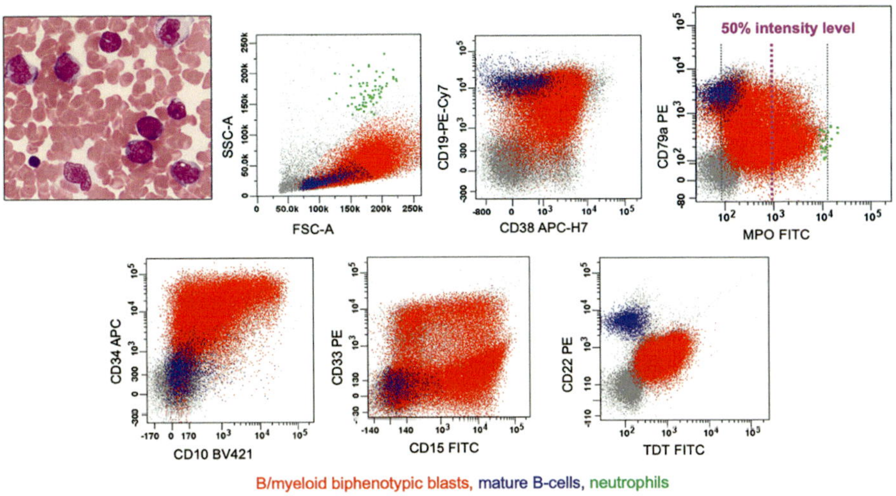

Fig. 20.3 B/myeloid MPAL (biphenotypic, demonstrating immunophenotypic features of lineage assignment on the intensity and heterogenous pattern of antigen expression per the WHO-HEM5 and the ICC). This is a case of biphenotypic MPAL with a single blast population showing differentiation along B-lymphoid and myeloid lineages and illustrating the strong expression of lineage-defining markers. Morphologically, these blasts are medium-sized with a high N/C ratio, irregular nuclei, occasional distinct nucleoli, and scant to moderate amount of cytoplasm. By immunophenotype, B/myeloid CD34(+) blasts (in red) have *strong* expression of B-lineage-defining markers (CD19, CD22, and CD79a) and myeloid lineage-defining marker (MPO) with the intensity in a subset of blasts exceeding the 50% of the normal counterparts (by WHO-HEM5) or similar to the level of normal counterparts (by ICC). Heterogenous pattern of antigen expression is manifested as strong to weak expression of lineage-defining markers (MPO, CD10, and CD19) on subpopulations of blasts and MPO is expressed along with coordinate expression of other myeloid lineage-associated markers (partial CD15 and CD33). The enlarged plot shows the midpoint (i.e., 50% expression intensity level in a log-axis) of the dynamic range for MPO expression established using the midpoint of the neutrophils (in green) as the positive control and the midpoint of the mature lymphocytes (in blue) as the negative control. Color code: red, neoplastic B/myeloid biphenotypic blasts; blue, mature B-cells; green, neutrophils

in the diagnosis of B/T MPAL. Similarly, CD10 is expressed early in B-cell and T-cell development and is also detected in a subset of T-lymphoblastic leukemia (T-ALL), making it less specific for assigning B-lineage. Cytoplasmic expression of CD22 is detected in most cases of B-lymphoblastic leukemia/lymphoma (B-ALL), but its expression in basophils and dendritic cells makes it less specific for assigning B-lineage [23, 24] if a thorough evaluation to exclude CD22 expression originating from basophils and dendritic cells is not carried out.

For T-lineage, blasts must express strong CD3 (using the CD3 epsilon-chain antibody) on the surface or within the cytoplasm. If antibody reactive with the CD3-zeta chain is used, the presence of natural killer (NK)-cells should be excluded. Other T-cell markers, including CD2, CD4, CD5, CD7, CD8, and T-cell receptor (TCR) α/β, have been used in prior scoring systems; however, CD2 and CD7 are commonly found expressed on blasts for leukemias that otherwise are consistent with AML, while CD4 is expressed on early granulocytic precursors and on monocytic and dendritic precursors [23, 24].

Myeloid lineage is assigned when blasts express strong myeloperoxidase (MPO), or at least two of the following monocytic markers: non-specific esterase, CD11c, CD14, CD64, or lysozyme. MPO has long been considered the most specific marker for myeloid lineage leukemias [25]. MPO expression by immunohistochemistry, cytochemistry, or flow cytometry, or monocytic differentiation, is considered a requirement for assigning the myeloid lineage when considering a diagnosis of MPAL. Although older studies suggest a cutoff of 3% MPO expression for cytochemistry based on expert opinion, no formally established cutoff guidelines (for flow cytometry) exist by the ICC [26–30]. The issue is further compounded by the availability of many MPO clones, known non-specific staining patterns, and lack of criteria for evaluating the stains and lack of consistent data (Table 20.5). According to the WHO-HEM5, the hallmark of myeloid/non-monocytic lineage is the strong expression of MPO on aberrant blasts that exceeds 50% of intensity level what is observed on mature neutrophils (its expression relative to positive control). Notably, dim expression of MPO (not reaching the 50% intensity threshold of neutrophils) can be seen in otherwise typical B-lymphoblastic leukemia/lymphoma (B-ALL) that has relatively homogenous expression of strong CD19 and CD10 (Fig. 20.6); these cases are not currently considered B/myeloid MPAL [1, 2, 31].

AUL is defined by lack of clear differentiation along any hematolymphoid lineage. The blasts must not express any lineage-defining markers, such as CD3, CD19, and MPO, and they cannot express more than one lineage-associated marker for any specific lineage. A comprehensive immunophenotypic analysis is required

Table 20.5 Myeloperoxidase antibodies used and the cutoff recommended in various studies[a]

Study	Antibody	Threshold recommendations
	Flow cytometry (clone used not reported)	>10%
Arber et al. [27]	Immunohistochemistry (IHC) 1:1000 dilution (Dako, Carpinteria, CA), polyclonal and monoclonal MPO antibody (clone MPO-7; 1:100 dilution; Dako)	≥5%
Ahuja et al. [28]	IHC: anti-human MPO (Thermo Scientific, United Kingdom)	3% for cytochemistry and 10% for IHC
Oberley et al. [29]	Flow cytometry: MPO (clone 8E6; Life Tech, Waltham, MA) IHC (clone 59A5; Leica Biosystems, Newcastle, United Kingdom) plus cytochemistry	>20% for flow 3% cytochemistry
Guy et al. [26]	Flow cytometry: monoclonal antibody (Dako or Immunotech), fluorescein isothiocyanate (FITC)	>13% (if using isotype control) >28% (if using internal control: lymphocytes)
Matutes et al. [15]	Flow cytometry: monoclonal MPO (clone used not reported)	>10%

[a]These cutoffs for the percentage of MPO-positive cells by flow cytometry were established relative to the negative/isotype control, in contrast to the determination of “strong” versus “weak” MPO expression relative to the positive controls on neutrophils in the WHO-HEM5

to exclude rare/unusual neoplasms of plasmacytoid dendritic, erythrocytic, megakaryocytic, and basophilic cell lineages.

Genetic and Molecular Findings

The majority (60–90%) of MPAL cases have an abnormal karyotype [13, 15, 32–39]. The most common abnormalities are rearrangements of t(9;22)/*BCR::ABL1* and t(v;11q23)/*KMT2A* that form discrete subgroups of MPAL. MPALs with *KMT2A* rearrangement are more common in the pediatric group (infants), while MPALs with *BCR::ABL1* are more common in adults [40]. In addition, other cytogenetic abnormalities, particularly observed in the B/myeloid subtype, include del(1)(p32), trisomy 4, 12p11.2 abnormalities, and del(6q). Recent studies have performed genomic analyses of MPAL cases and have found that gene mutations are a mixture of those commonly seen in both AML and acute lymphoblastic leukemia (ALL). In 2012, Yan et al. reported deletions of the ALL-associated gene, *IKZF1,* as well as mutations of AML-associated epigenetic modifiers, *TET2, EZH2,* and *ASXL1*, in B/myeloid leukemias [13]. In 2016, Eckstein and colleagues performed whole exome sequencing on 23 cases of MPAL and found similar mutations and identified AML-associated *DNMT3A*, *WT1* mutations as well as frequent *NOTCH1* mutations in cases with a T-lineage component, suggesting genetic overlap with T-ALL [41]. In a series of 31 cases, Takahashi et al. reported genomic anomalies and methylation patterns in a comparison of T/Myeloid and B/Myeloid MPALs with AML, T-ALL, and B-ALL, and demonstrated that MPAL could be further subclassified into ALL-like MPAL and AML-like MPAL [38]. Similarly, in a recent series of 25 cases, Zheng et al. reported that B/myeloid and T/myeloid MPALs share the AML, B-ALL, and T-ALL genotype in association with the myeloid-, B-lymphoid-, and T-lymphoid-lineage predominance, respectively (i.e., genomic landscape of MPAL associated with immunophenotypic/lineage predominance) [39]. In a study of pediatric and adult patients, Xiao and colleagues identified recurrent and largely mutually exclusive alterations in *PHF6, DNMT3A,* and *WT1* in MPAL cases with T-cell antigen expression [32]. A series of B/T MPALs have identified recurrent acquired aberrations, including mutations in *PHF6* and the Janus Kinase–signal transducer and activator of transcription (JAK-STAT) and rat sarcoma (refers to the RAS family of proto-oncogenes) (RAS) signaling pathways [34, 42].

Whole exome and genome sequencing in a cohort of 115 pediatric MPAL/ALAL cases identified *WT1, FLT3, RUNX1*, and *PHF6* mutations are among the most recurrent alteration in pediatric T/myeloid MPAL [36]. Fusion genes involving the *ZNF384* transcription factor gene were identified in nearly 50% of cases and especially predominant in B/myeloid MPAL (Fig. 20.4). ZNF384 fusions are also common in B-ALL [43, 44], supporting the notion that genomic alteration plays a critical role in classifying certain subtypes of leukemia. ALAL with rearrangements leading to deregulation of *BCL11B* (*BCL11B*-activated) comprises 10–15% of MPAL and is further enriched in patients with MPAL, T/myeloid cases,

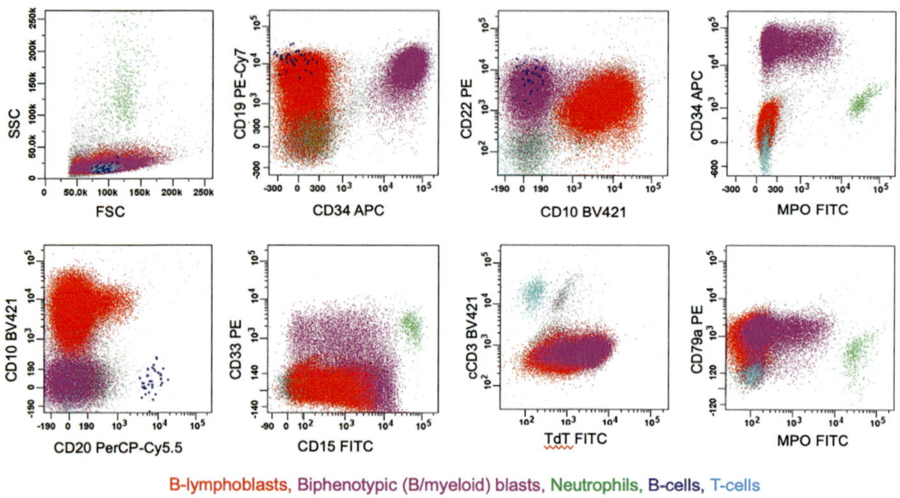

Fig. 20.4 *EP300::ZNF384* rearranged B/myeloid MPAL (bilineal/biphenotypic). This is a case of bilineal leukemia with two distinctly discrete blast populations with differentiation of one of them into a biphenotypic subpopulation. The neoplastic B-lymphoblasts (in red) express CD10, CD19, CD22, CD79a, CD15, and TdT but lack CD20, CD34, CD33, CD117, or MPO. The neoplastic B/myeloid blasts (in violet) express CD34, CD10 (in a small subset), CD15, CD33 (partial+), CD19 (strong in a subset), CD22, CD79a, and MPO (strong in a subset) but lack CD20. Color code: red, B-cells; violet, B/myeloid biphenotypic blasts; green, neutrophils; blue, mature B-cells; and cyan, T-cells

representing up to one-third of this population [35, 45, 46]. Unlike the *BCL11B* alterations described for T-ALL, the 14q32 structural variants identified in ALAL usually leave the *BCL11B* coding region intact. These alterations involve juxtaposition of super enhancers active in hematopoietic stem cells to *BCL11B*, or in 20% of cases, amplification of a 2 kb region distal to *BCL11B* resulting in the generation of a neoenhancer that deregulates and increases *BCL11B* expression. Based on these recent findings, the WHO-HEM5 and ICC recognize two new entities with defined genetic alterations, which include MPAL with *ZNF384* rearrangements and *BCL11B* activation [1, 2, 11].

Additionally, the WHO-HEM5 adds a new rare subtype of T/megakaryocytic (T/Mk) MPAL that occurs in infants and young children. The clinicopathological features overlap with those of pediatric non-Down syndrome, *CBFA2T3::GLIS2* fusion positive acute megakaryoblastic leukemia (AMKL) [47–51]. Most patients with T/Mk MPAL harbor *CBFA2T3::GLIS2* or rarely *CBFA2T3::GLIS3*, and have an extremely poor prognosis. A defining immunophenotypic feature distinguishing T/Mk MPAL from AMKL is the expression of strong CD3 in a proportion of blasts in T/Mk MPAL; typically, cCD3 is the only T-lineage marker expressed within the T-lineage and presence of two or more megakaryocytic markers (CD41, CD61, or CD42b) although the WHO-HEM5 criteria has not yet specified immunophenotypic criterion for assigning the megakaryocytic lineage.

B/T MPAL is another rare subtype of MPAL that is more commonly occurring in children than in adults [34, 42, 52, 53]. The clinicopathologic and genetic profiles

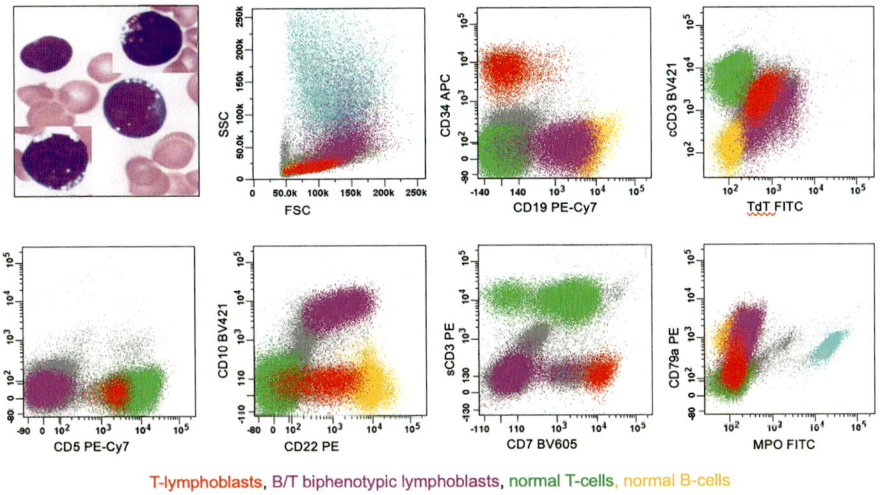

Fig. 20.5 B/T MPAL with codominance of B- and T-lineage cells (bilineal/biphenotypic). This is a case of bilineal leukemia with two distinctly discrete neoplastic populations, T-lymphoblasts and B/T biphenotypic lymphoblasts. Morphologically, medium-sized to large blasts have moderately condensed chromatin, irregular nuclei, small or inconspicuous nucleoli, and scant cytoplasm, some with cytoplasmic vacuoles. Immunophenotypically, T-lymphoblasts (in red) express cCD3, CD5 (dim), CD7, CD22 (partial), CD34, and TdT, but lack expression of CD1a, sCD3, CD19, or MPO, an immunophenotype characteristic of early T-cell progenitor-ALL (ETP-ALL). B/T biphenotypic lymphoblasts (in violet) express cCD3, CD10, CD19 (strong but slightly dimmer than normal B-cells), CD22, and TdT, but lack expression of sCD3, CD5, CD34, or MPO. By immunocytochemistry, lymphoblasts co-express CD3, PAX5, and TdT (not shown). Color codes: red, T-lymphoblasts; violet, B/T biphenotypic lymphoblasts; green, T-cells; yellow, mature B-cells; and cyan, neutrophils

are characterized by young patients with a male predominance, frequent extramedullary involvement, and most cases harboring T-ALL-like genotype. Immunophenotypically, blasts co-express both B- and T-cell lineage-defining markers (Fig. 20.5). Blasts express strong CD19 with strong expression of ≥1 other B-cell marker including CD22 [34, 42]. Notably, CD79a is not considered a B-lineage-defining marker in diagnosing B/T MPAL since CD79a can be also expressed in T-ALL [1, 21].

Clinical Course

It has been widely recognized that the clinical outcome of ALAL is markedly adverse and variable. Patients with MPAL with *BCR::ABL1* may ultimately benefit from addition of a tyrosine kinase inhibitor [54, 55]. Clinical outcomes of children with MPAL tend to be better when compared to adults with MPAL, with a higher overall survival (OS) and fewer relapses [15, 54]. The currently recommended treatment approach for MPAL in both pediatric and adult patients is induction therapy with an ALL regimen based on the retrospective studies using the EGIL or WHO criterion (4th Edition) that show patients beginning therapy with an ALL-type induction regimen were significantly more likely to achieve a complete remission [54–57]. This approach seems appropriate for the majority of patients, as most MPAL patients (60–70%) could be classified as ALL-like MPAL based on gene alterations and methylation profiles with associated lymphoid lineage predominance [38, 39, 52]. However, an ALL-based regimen might not be optimal for all MPAL patients because 30–40% of MPAL could be classified as AML-like MPAL. The debate on the most appropriate induction regimen remains unresolved regarding whether initial therapy should be based on immunophenotype, cytogenetics, or molecular biology. Future MPAL research is essential to establish biologically and lineage-informed therapy selection guidelines and to integrate molecular-targeted therapies (Fig. 20.6).

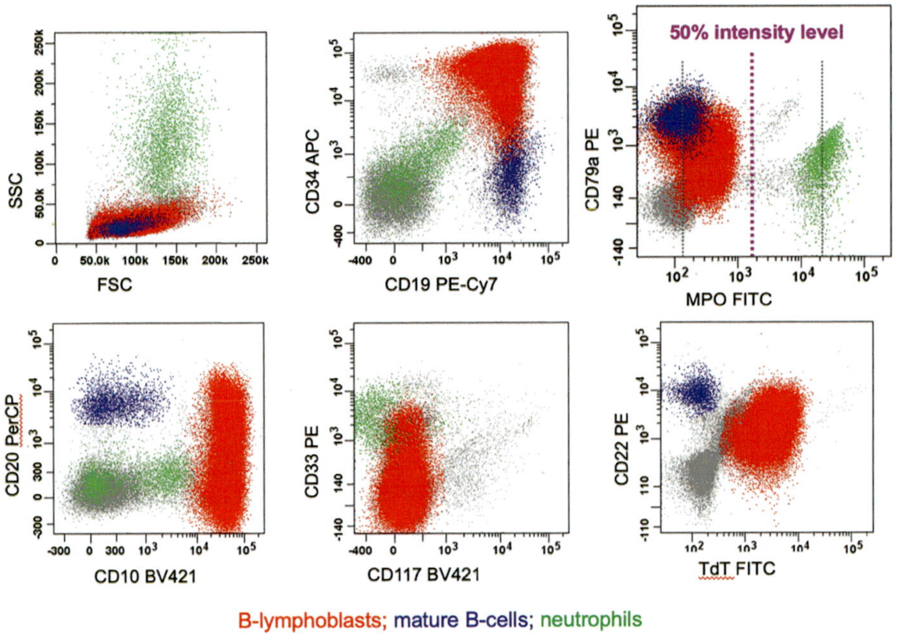

Fig. 20.6 B-lymphoblastic leukemia with dim myeloperoxidase (MPO) (B-ALL with MPO^{dim}): B-lymphoblasts (in red) express B-cell markers (CD19, CD20 [partial], CD22, and CD79a), CD10, CD34, and TdT, but lack expression of myeloid markers (CD33 [most], CD117, or MPO [as defined by MPAL-lineage-defining marker expression criteria per the WHO-HEM5]). While a large proportion of the B-lymphoblasts show dim MPO expression, no proportion of the B-lymphoblasts reach the 50% intensity level of neutrophils. Color codes: red, neoplastic B lymphoblasts; blue, mature B-cells; and green, granulocytes

Differential Diagnosis

The primary challenge in diagnosing cases of MPAL is ruling out other clinically and genetically defined neoplasms that demonstrate an acute leukemia with mixed lineage phenotype (MPAL-like immunophenotype) (Fig. 20.7). A careful review of patient history is thus essential, and for example, patients with a history of chronic myeloid leukemia (CML) who develop blast crisis with mixed phenotype should not be diagnosed as MPAL with t(9;22)/*BCR::ABL1* fusion. Similarly, patients with CML in blast crisis with lineage switch are also excluded from this category. AML cases with t(8;21)(q22;q22.1)/*RUNX1::RUNX1T1* fusion often express B-lineage markers, including CD19, PAX5, and CD79a, and care should be taken to not diagnose MPAL in this setting. Myeloid/lymphoid neoplasms with *FGFR1* rearrangement are a group of hematopoietic neoplasms that can present as acute leukemias expressing mixed lineage markers but should not be diagnosed as MPAL. Cytogenetic abnormalities and molecular findings diagnostic of AML with myelodysplasia-related cytogenetic abnormalities or myelodysplasia-related mutation (introduced in the WHO-HEM5/ICC criteria) also preclude diagnosis of MPAL [1, 2]. Such a diagnosis could be potentially modified in such a way as to highlight the immunophenotype (i.e., AML with myelodysplasia-related gene mutations and a mixed B/myeloid immunophenotype). However, it remains highly controversial as to whether to include or exclude these cases from MPAL category, particularly those MPAL cases with lymphoid predominant immunophenotype and harboring ALL-like genotype. More studies are necessary to investigate the impact of these new criteria on the boundary between AML and MPAL categories and refine the MPAL diagnostic criteria.

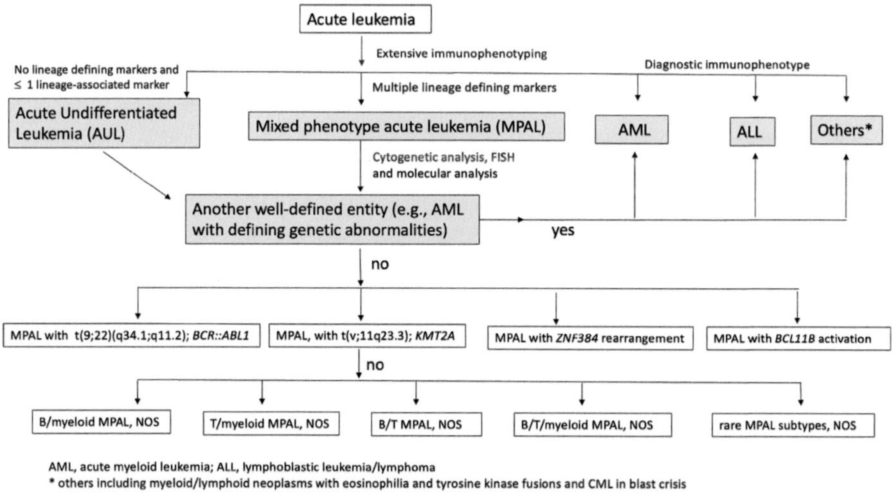

Fig. 20.7 Diagnostic algorithms for acute leukemias. Diagnosis of MPAL is required to rule out other clinically or genetically defined categories, such as AML with defining genetic abnormalities, myeloid/lymphoid neoplasms with eosinophilia and tyrosine kinase fusions, and CML in blast crisis

References

1. Khoury JD, Solary E, Abla O, et al. The 5th edition of the World Health Organization classification of haematolymphoid tumours: myeloid and histiocytic/dendritic neoplasms. Leukemia. 2022;36(7):1703–19.
2. Weinberg OK, Arber DA, Dohner H, et al. The International Consensus Classification of acute leukemias of ambiguous lineage. Blood. 2023;141(18):2275–7.
3. Weinberg OK, Arber DA. Mixed-phenotype acute leukemia: historical overview and a new definition. Leukemia. 2010;24(11):1844–51.
4. Bene MC, Porwit A. Acute leukemias of ambiguous lineage. Semin Diagn Pathol. 2012;29(1):12–8.
5. Charles NJ, Boyer DF. Mixed-phenotype acute leukemia: diagnostic criteria and pitfalls. Arch Pathol Lab Med. 2017;141(11):1462–8.
6. Catovsky D, Matutes E, Buccheri V, et al. A classification of acute leukaemia for the 1990s. Ann Hematol. 1991;62(1):16–21.
7. Bene MC, Castoldi G, Knapp W, et al. Proposals for the immunological classification of acute leukemias. European Group for the Immunological Characterization of Leukemias (EGIL). Leukemia. 1995;9(10):1783–6.
8. Bene MC, Bernier M, Casasnovas RO, et al. The reliability and specificity of c-kit for the diagnosis of acute myeloid leukemias and undifferentiated leukemias. The European Group for the Immunological Classification of Leukemias (EGIL). Blood. 1998;92(2):596–9.
9. Jaffe ES, Harris NL, Stein H, et al. WHO classification of tumours of haematopoietic and lymphoid tissues. Lyon: International Agency for Research on Cancer Press; 2001.
10. Borowitz MJ, Bene M-C, Harris NL, Porwit A, Matutes E, Arber DA. Acute leukaemias of ambiguous lineage. In: Swerdlow SH, Campo E, Harris NL, Jaffe ES, Pileri SA, Stein H, Thiele J, Arber DA, Hasserjian RP, Le Beau MM, Orazi A, Siebert R, editors. WHO classification of tumours of haematopoietic and lymphoid tissues. Revised 4th ed. Lyon: IARC Press; 2017. p. 180–7.
11. Arber DA, Orazi A, Hasserjian RP, et al. International consensus classification of myeloid neoplasms and acute leukemias: integrating morphologic, clinical, and genomic data. Blood. 2022;140(11):1200–28.
12. Owaidah TM, Al Beihany A, Iqbal MA, Elkum N, Roberts GT. Cytogenetics, molecular and ultrastructural characteristics of biphenotypic acute leukemia identified by the EGIL scoring system. Leukemia. 2006;20(4):620–6.
13. Yan L, Ping N, Zhu M, et al. Clinical, immunophenotypic, cytogenetic, and molecular genetic features in 117 adult patients with mixed-phenotype acute leukemia defined by WHO-2008 classification. Haematologica. 2012;97(11):1708–12.
14. Weinberg OK, Seetharam M, Ren L, Alizadeh A, Arber DA. Mixed phenotype acute leukemia: a study of 61 cases using World Health Organization and European Group for the Immunological Classification of Leukaemias criteria. Am J Clin Pathol. 2014;142(6):803–8.
15. Matutes E, Pickl WF, Van't Veer M, et al. Mixed-phenotype acute leukemia: clinical and laboratory features and outcome in 100 patients defined according to the WHO 2008 classification. Blood. 2011;117(11):3163–71.
16. Arber DA, Borowitz MJ, Cessna M, et al. Initial diagnostic workup of acute leukemia: guideline from the College of American Pathologists and the American Society of Hematology. Arch Pathol Lab Med. 2017;141(10):1342–93.
17. Fuda F, Chen W. Acute leukemia of ambiguous lineage: diagnosis and evaluation by flow cytometry. Cancers (Basel). 2025;17(5):871.
18. Porwit A, Bene MC. Multiparameter flow cytometry applications in the diagnosis of mixed phenotype acute leukemia. Cytometry B Clin Cytom. 2019;96(3):183–94.
19. Anderson KC, Bates MP, Slaughenhoupt BL, Pinkus GS, Schlossman SF, Nadler LM. Expression of human B cell-associated antigens on leukemias and lymphomas: a model of human B cell differentiation. Blood. 1984;63(6):1424–33.

20. Ball ED, Davis RB, Griffin JD, et al. Prognostic value of lymphocyte surface markers in acute myeloid leukemia. Blood. 1991;77(10):2242–50.
21. Shuyu E, Jelloul FZ, Nahmod KA, et al. Acute lymphoblastic leukaemia with T- and B-lineage defining markers. Pathology. 2025;57(6):739–45.
22. Arber DA, Jenkins KA, Slovak ML. CD79 alpha expression in acute myeloid leukemia. High frequency of expression in acute promyelocytic leukemia. Am J Pathol. 1996;149(4):1105–10.
23. Janossy G, Coustan-Smith E, Campana D. The reliability of cytoplasmic CD3 and CD22 antigen expression in the immunodiagnosis of acute leukemia: a study of 500 cases. Leukemia. 1989;3(3):170–81.
24. Sato N, Kishi K, Toba K, et al. Simultaneous expression of CD13, CD22 and CD25 is related to the expression of fc epsilon R1 in non-lymphoid leukemia. Leuk Res. 2004;28(7):691–8.
25. Buccheri V, Shetty V, Yoshida N, Morilla R, Matutes E, Catovsky D. The role of an anti-myeloperoxidase antibody in the diagnosis and classification of acute leukaemia: a comparison with light and electron microscopy cytochemistry. Br J Haematol. 1992;80(1):62–8.
26. Guy J, Antony-Debre I, Benayoun E, et al. Flow cytometry thresholds of myeloperoxidase detection to discriminate between acute lymphoblastic or myeloblastic leukaemia. Br J Haematol. 2013;161(4):551–5.
27. Arber DA, Snyder DS, Fine M, Dagis A, Niland J, Slovak ML. Myeloperoxidase immunoreactivity in adult acute lymphoblastic leukemia. Am J Clin Pathol. 2001;116(1):25–33.
28. Ahuja A, Tyagi S, Seth T, et al. Comparison of immunohistochemistry, cytochemistry, and flow cytometry in AML for myeloperoxidase detection. Indian J Hematol Blood Transfus. 2018;34(2):233–9.
29. Oberley MJ, Li S, Orgel E, Phei Wee C, Hagiya A, O'Gorman MRG. Clinical significance of isolated myeloperoxidase expression in pediatric B-lymphoblastic leukemia. Am J Clin Pathol. 2017;147(4):374–81.
30. Patel SS, Weinberg OK. Diagnostic workup of acute leukemias of ambiguous lineage. Am J Hematol. 2020;95(6):718–22.
31. Weinberg OK, Dennis J, Zia H, et al. Adult mixed phenotype acute leukemia (MPAL): B/myeloid MPAL(isoMPO) is distinct from other MPAL subtypes. Int J Lab Hematol. 2023;45(2):170–8.
32. Xiao W, Bharadwaj M, Levine M, et al. PHF6 and DNMT3A mutations are enriched in distinct subgroups of mixed phenotype acute leukemia with T-lineage differentiation. Blood Adv. 2018;2(23):3526–39.
33. Wang Q, Cai WZ, Wang QR, et al. Integrative genomic and transcriptomic profiling reveals distinct molecular subsets in adult mixed phenotype acute leukemia. Am J Hematol. 2022;98(1):66–78.
34. Mi X, Griffin G, Lee W, et al. Genomic and clinical characterization of B/T mixed phenotype acute leukemia reveals recurrent features and T-ALL like mutations. Am J Hematol. 2018;93(11):1358–67.
35. Montefiori LE, Bendig S, Gu Z, et al. Enhancer hijacking drives oncogenic BCL11B expression in lineage-ambiguous stem cell leukemia. Cancer Discov. 2021;11(11):2846–67.
36. Alexander TB, Gu Z, Iacobucci I, et al. The genetic basis and cell of origin of mixed phenotype acute leukaemia. Nature. 2018;562(7727):373–9.
37. Manola KN. Cytogenetic abnormalities in acute leukaemia of ambiguous lineage: an overview. Br J Haematol. 2013;163(1):24–39.
38. Takahashi K, Wang F, Morita K, et al. Integrative genomic analysis of adult mixed phenotype acute leukemia delineates lineage associated molecular subtypes. Nat Commun. 2018;9(1):2670.
39. Zheng R, Gagan JR, Botten GA, et al. Genomic landscape of mixed phenotype acute leukemia associated with immunophenotypic lineage predominance: impact on diagnosis and treatment. Eur J Haematol. 2025;114(6):1041–51.
40. Mejstrikova E, Volejnikova J, Fronkova E, et al. Prognosis of children with mixed phenotype acute leukemia treated on the basis of consistent immunophenotypic criteria. Haematologica. 2010;95(6):928–35.

41. Eckstein OS, Wang L, Punia JN, et al. Mixed-phenotype acute leukemia (MPAL) exhibits frequent mutations in DNMT3A and activated signaling genes. Exp Hematol. 2016;44(8):740–4.
42. Zheng R, Fuda F, Gagan JR, et al. Genomic heterogeneity within B/T mixed phenotype acute leukemia in a context of an immunophenotype. Leuk Res Rep. 2024;21:100410.
43. Hirabayashi S, Ohki K, Nakabayashi K, et al. ZNF384-related fusion genes define a subgroup of childhood B-cell precursor acute lymphoblastic leukemia with a characteristic immunotype. Haematologica. 2017;102(1):118–29.
44. Zhu L, Bai W, Cheng Q, Fang J. ZNF384-related fusion genes in acute lymphoblastic leukemia. Cancer Control. 2023;30:10732748231182787.
45. Di Giacomo D, La Starza R, Gorello P, et al. 14q32 rearrangements deregulating BCL11B mark a distinct subgroup of T-lymphoid and myeloid immature acute leukemia. Blood. 2021;138(9):773–84.
46. Wang W, Beird H, Kroll CJ, et al. T(6;14)(q25;q32) involves BCL11B and is highly associated with mixed-phenotype acute leukemia, T/myeloid. Leukemia. 2020;34(9):2509–12.
47. Rossi JG, Rubio P, Alonso CN, et al. Cytoplasmic CD3 expression in infant acute megakaryoblastic leukemia: a new ambiguous lineage subtype? Leuk Res. 2018;71:6–12.
48. Klairmont MM, Choi JK. Mixed-phenotype acute leukemia, T/megakaryoblastic. Blood. 2018;132(22):2418.
49. Panda D, Chatterjee G, Sardana R, et al. Utility of CD36 as a novel addition to the immunophenotypic signature of RAM-phenotype acute myeloid leukemia and study of its clinicopathological characteristics. Cytometry B Clin Cytom. 2021;100(2):206–17.
50. Chen Wongworawat Y, Eskandari G, Gaikwad A, et al. Frequent detection of CBFA2T3::GLIS2 fusion and RAM-phenotype in pediatric non-Down syndrome acute megakaryoblastic leukemia: a possible novel relationship with aberrant cytoplasmic CD3 expression. Leuk Lymphoma. 2023;64(2):462–7.
51. Khanlari M, Wang L, Bolen CY, et al. CBFA2T3::GLIS2-positive acute leukemia with RAM and mixed T/megakaryocytic phenotype. EJHaem. 2023;4(3):765–9.
52. Wang Q, Cai WZ, Wang QR, et al. Integrative genomic and transcriptomic profiling reveals distinct molecular subsets in adult mixed phenotype acute leukemia. Am J Hematol. 2023;98(1):66–78.
53. Han L, Nguyen VT, Zheng R, et al. B/T mixed phenotype acute leukemia revealing immunophenotypic lineage-genotype associations and frequent myelodysplasia-related cytogenetic/gene abnormalities: implication for diagnosis and treatment. Ann Diagn Pathol. 2025;80:152540.
54. Maruffi M, Sposto R, Oberley MJ, Kysh L, Orgel E. Therapy for children and adults with mixed phenotype acute leukemia: a systematic review and meta-analysis. Leukemia. 2018;32(7):1515–28.
55. Orgel E, Alexander TB, Wood BL, et al. Mixed-phenotype acute leukemia: a cohort and consensus research strategy from the Children's Oncology Group Acute Leukemia of Ambiguous Lineage Task Force. Cancer. 2020;126(3):593–601.
56. Hrusak O, de Haas V, Stancikova J, et al. International cooperative study identifies treatment strategy in childhood ambiguous lineage leukemia. Blood. 2018;132(3):264–76.
57. Shi R, Munker R. Survival of patients with mixed phenotype acute leukemias: a large population-based study. Leuk Res. 2015;39(6):606–16.

Juvenile Myelomonocytic Leukemia 21

Kimberly H. Hein, Mrinal M. Patnaik, and M. Tarek Elghetany

Introduction

Juvenile myelomonocytic leukemia (JMML) is a rare myeloproliferative neoplasm in young children with an annual incidence of 1.2 cases per million children [1–4]. The neoplasm is characterized by leukocytosis with granulocytosis with left shift, monocytosis, and organ infiltration. Children are typically diagnosed around 2 years of age [4, 5]. Only 5% are diagnosed after the age of 4 years, while 9% are diagnosed when they are less than 4 months old [5]. The neoplasm had been classified as a myeloproliferative/myelodysplastic overlap neoplasm in previous World Health Organization (WHO) Classifications [6]. However, the most recent fifth edition of WHO Classification in 2022 (print edition published 2024) has classified JMML as a myeloproliferative neoplasm [1]. In parallel, the recent International Consensus Classification (ICC) has classified JMML under a special category called "Pediatric Disorders and/or Germline Mutation-Associated Disorders." [7, 8] The vast majority of cases are

K. H. Hein · M. T. Elghetany (✉)
Department of Pathology, Baylor College of Medicine, Texas Children's Hospital, Houston, TX, USA
e-mail: txelghet@texaschildrens.org

M. M. Patnaik
Division of Hematology, Department of Internal Medicine, Mayo Clinic, Rochester, MN, USA

W. Li (ed.), *Laboratory Assessments of Pediatric Leukemia*,
https://doi.org/10.1007/978-3-032-26557-9_21

associated with hyperactivation of the Rat Sarcoma Virus (RAS) signaling pathway (see below). Although most cases are secondary to somatic mutations involving the RAS pathway, germline mutations such as neurofibromatosis type 1 (*NF1* gene) and CBL syndrome caused by alterations in the *CBL* gene (Casitas B-lineage Lymphoma gene) have been associated with the development of JMML. These germline-associated JMMLs account for approximately 25% of cases [9].

Clinical Presentations

JMML has no specific clinical symptoms besides possible abdominal distension due to splenomegaly. The symptoms are mostly related to abnormal leukocyte function, anemia, thrombocytopenia, neoplastic cell infiltration causing organomegaly, and inflammation, sometimes autoimmune manifestation. As such patients can present with fever and pallor, with some presenting symptoms similar to an upper respiratory tract infection, including dry cough. Uncommon presentations include skin lesions, easy bleeding, and gastrointestinal symptoms [5, 10]. Physical exam shows splenomegaly in 90% of cases, with hepatomegaly also being common in 80% of cases. In 50% of patients, lymphadenopathy can be seen, with approximately 30% demonstrating a skin rash [4, 5, 10]. This neoplasm can also present with tonsillar enlargement, myeloid sarcoma of the central nervous system (CNS]), diabetes insipidus, and facial palsy [5]. In the context of germline genetic syndromes, additional physical findings may be related to the germline syndrome, such as café-au-lait spots in patients with neurofibromatosis type 1 [11].

Peripheral Blood Findings and Bone Marrow Findings

Complete blood counts usually demonstrate leukocytosis (median total white blood cell [WBC] count is 25–30 × 10^9/L), monocytosis, anemia, and thrombocytopenia (Fig. 21.1) [4, 5]. On rare occasions, the WBC count may be normal, with an abnormal differential count reflecting monocytosis. Granulocytes usually show a left shift with occasional circulating blasts. The monocytosis can be marked and typically ≥1 × 10^9/L. [4, 5] On hemoglobin fractionation studies, increased hemoglobin F for age can be seen [5]. Some patients, particularly in association with CBL syndrome, may have immunologic features, such as increased immunoglobulins or autoantibodies [12]. On peripheral blood smears, the neutrophils may have abnormal morphologic changes, such as hypo-segmentation and pseudo-Pelger-Hüet forms. Myeloid precursors such as promyelocytes, myelocytes, and metamyelocytes are usually seen along with occasional eosinophilia and basophilia. Red blood cells are typically normocytic, with macrocytosis being more common with monosomy 7. Microcytosis is uncommon and only seen if there is concomitant thalassemia (trait)

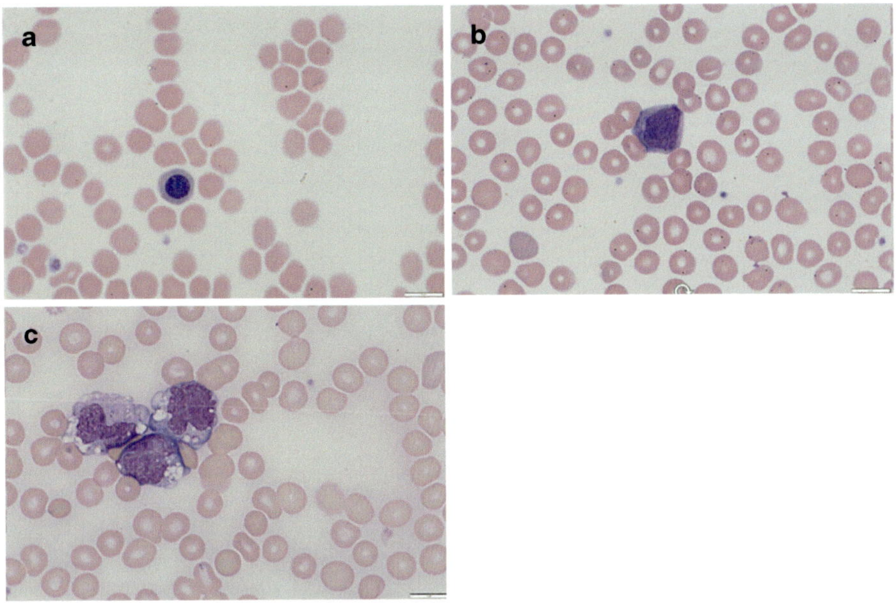

Fig. 21.1 (**a–c**) Giemsa stain of peripheral blood smear in JMML showing erythroid precursors (**a**: 1000× magnification), neutrophilic left shifts (**b**: 500× magnification), and monocytosis (**c**: 1000× magnification)

or iron deficiency [13]. Red blood cell precursors are common (nucleated red cells), sometimes with abnormal red blood cell morphologies such as dacrocytes.

On bone marrow aspirates and biopsies, there is usually increased bone marrow cellularity with a myeloid (granulocytic) predominance (Fig. 21.2). Monocytes typically comprise only 5–10% of the bone marrow cells. Monocytes can be identified on the biopsy using CD14, CD163, or CD68 immunohistochemical stains [1, 5]. Erythroid hyperplasia can be seen particularly in association with monosomy 7; these patients are usually anemic but without significant difference in hemoglobin levels from non-monosomy 7 patients [5]. The megakaryocytes are usually decreased in numbers, with normal morphology and without significant dysplastic features. Bone marrow dysplastic features may be seen in some cases. However, morphologic dysplastic features are not one of the diagnostic criteria in previous and recent classifications and also in several previous studies [1, 6–8, 10, 14]. Myeloblasts may be prominent but always less than 20%. In the presence of more than 20% myeloblasts, the diagnosis should be acute myeloid leukemia (AML).

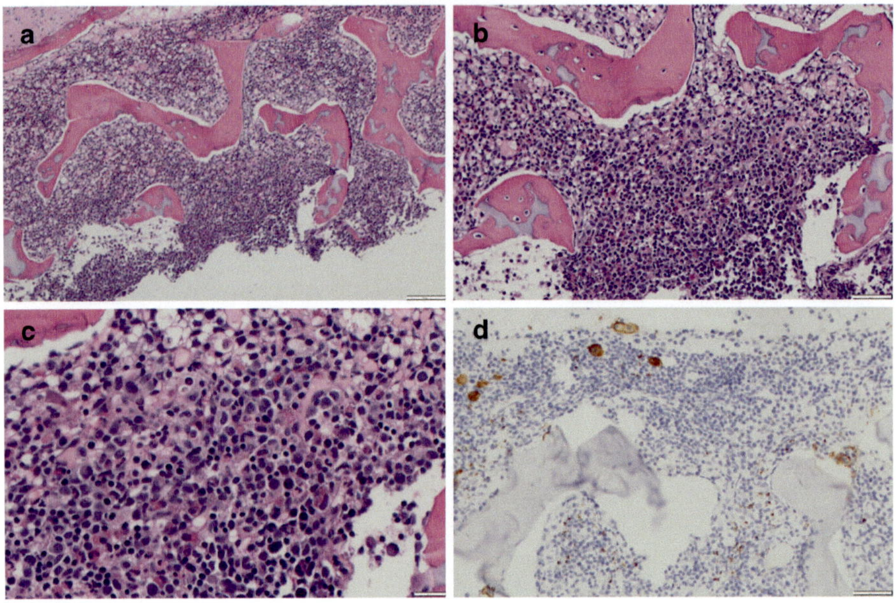

Fig. 21.2 (**a**–**c**) H&E-stained bone marrow sections showing increased bone marrow cellularity, with increased monocytes at (**a**) 100× magnification, (**b**) 200× magnification, and (**c**) 400× magnification. The bone marrow also showed (**d**) decreased megakaryocytes with normal morphology highlighted with CD61 immunohistochemical stain at 200× magnification

Flow cytometry of peripheral blood in JMML cases will show similar monocytosis and neutrophilia with a small myeloid blast percentage usually <2% in peripheral blood and < 20% in the bone marrow. Flow cytometry of the bone marrow can show an aberrant blast population expressing CD7 with decreased CD13 and CD33. Granulocytes can show abnormal maturation patterns on CD16/CD13 and absence of CD10 (Fig. 21.3). Also seen in occasional cases is increased B-cell hematogone populations similar to cases with Noonan syndrome JMML-like disorder [15].

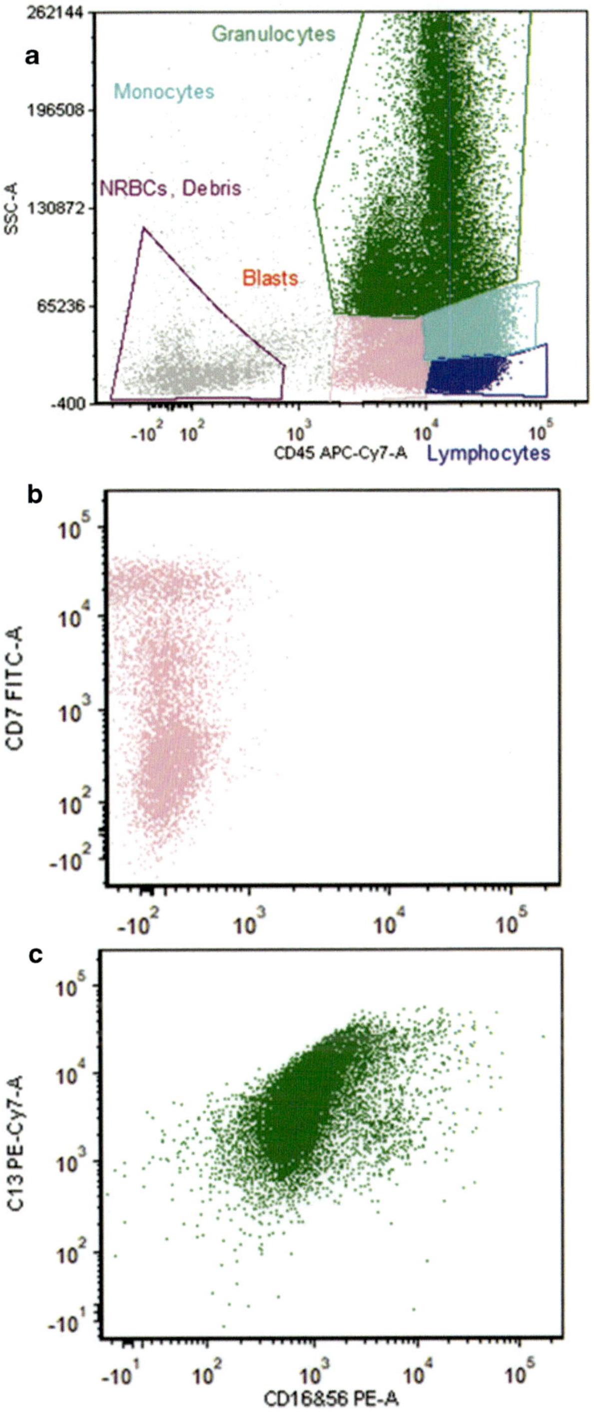

Fig. 21.3 (**a**–**c**) Flow cytometry of bone marrow in a JMML patient. Granulocytes are in green, blasts in pink, monocytes in aqua, and lymphocytes in blue. (**a**) CD45 vs SSC showing increased monocytes (6%), and a prominent myeloblast (10%) population in this case. (**b**) The blasts show partial CD7 expression. (**c**) The granulocytes show abnormal maturation and does not show the classic check mark sign on CD13 vs CD16&56, suggesting CD13 abnormal expression

Extramedullary Histopathology/Tissue Findings

JMML usually affects solid organs/tissues such as spleen, liver, lymph nodes, and skin. The leukemic cells include monocytes/histiocytes, myeloid precursors, and mature granulocytes and may form large aggregates resembling myeloid sarcoma. The leukemic cells tend to localize around vascular areas. This causes distinctive patterns of involvement. In the liver, the monocyte populations infiltrate the portal tracts and sinusoids. In the spleen, the cells usually localize to the red pulp. In the lymph node, the cells are usually in the interfollicular and sinusoidal areas. In the skin, the cells are in perivascular and peri-adnexal areas. In the lungs, the cells originate from the vascular bed and extend into the alveolar septa and the alveoli. As mentioned above, immunohistochemistry usually identifies monocyte populations demonstrating classic monocyte markers (CD163+, CD14+, CD68, with occasional expression of CD56), along with myeloid precursors (CD117+, CD34+).

Pathogenesis/Molecular Findings

Canonical RAS Pathway Alterations

JMML is driven by RAS oncogenesis, with >90% of patients having canonical RAS pathway/RAS pathway regulator mutations (*KRAS, NRAS, PTPN11, NF1, CBL*) [9]. Most commonly, patients present with somatic mutations in the RAS pathway regulator *PTPN11* (35–40%) [9]. Also, 10–15% of cases have mutation in *NRAS* and *KRAS*, each, respectively [9]. Other RAS pathway mutations are rare and include *RRAS2* or *RIT1* [9]. *NF1* alterations occur in 5–10% and *CBL* alterations in 12–15% [9]. These mutations and alterations lead to constitutional overactivation of the RAS signaling pathway (Fig. 21.4). While these mutations are somatic in nature, they occur very early in life, with 40% being identifiable at birth, implying an in-utero event leading to the mutagenesis [16]. This is partially responsible for the early life incidence of this disease. JMML in patients with germline alterations, such as *NF1* and *CBL*, is usually associated with loss of heterozygosity of the chromosomal regions harboring the genes (somatic copy number alteration [SCNA]) [17, 18]. As such, genetic testing is encouraged on non-hematopoietic tissues (skin fibroblasts or hair/nail-derived DNA) to identify germline mutations. Patients typically have only one RAS pathway mutation as they tend to be mutually exclusive but secondary mutations have occurred and are associated with tumor progression and poor outcomes. Also, 10–15% of patients have two mutations in the RAS pathway [9]. CBL-associated JMML does not typically have secondary mutation events but does demonstrate SCNA [18]. Non-RAS pathway mutations can also occur as secondary somatic mutations and are associated with poor outcomes. Secondary mutations are seen in approximately 30% of patients and include *SETBP1*, *ASXL1*, *EZH2*, *JAK3*, and *SH2B3*, although *SH2B3* has recently been

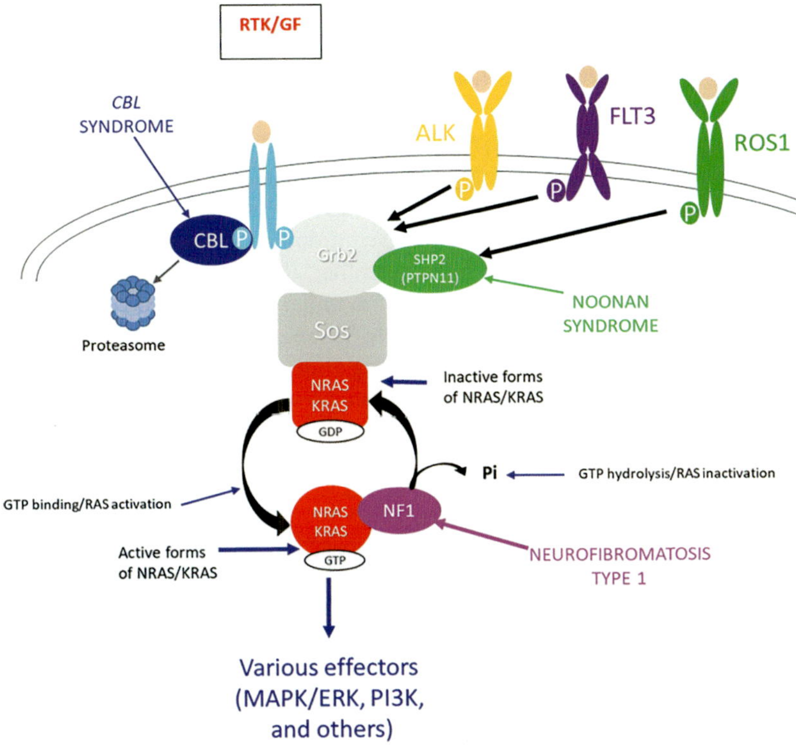

Fig. 21.4 Ras pathway. The pathway is activated by cellular membrane receptors: receptor tyrosine kinase/growth factor (RTK/GF), ALK, FLT3, or ROS1 that trigger adaptor proteins (GRB2 and SOS) to activate RAS by GTP binding, which leads to the effects of the RAS pathway activating/turning on downstream genes required for cell growth. NF1 protein normally inactivates *NRAS/KRAS* through GTP hydrolysis producing GDP inactive forms. Mutations can lead to the pathway being constantly activated and constantly activating other processes required for cell growth

reported as a driver mutation in itself [9, 19, 20]. DNA hypermethylation can be seen and is associated with a more aggressive clinical course and additional somatic mutations [21–24]. RAS engages with two major downstream effector signaling pathways, including RAF/MEK/ERK (mitogen activated protein kinase [MAPK]) and phosphatidylinositol-3-kinase (PI3K) cascades. These pathways are associated with specific cancer-related phenotypes, including transcriptional reprogramming, promoted cell survival and proliferation, suppressed apoptosis, and enhanced invasiveness of the cells.

Cytogenetic testing shows monosomy 7 in approximately 25% of cases, which is more common in KRAS-mutated diseases, while the majority (65–75%) of patients have a normal karyotype [5, 23].

Non-canonical RAS Pathway Alterations

Non-canonical *RAS* alterations have been reported in some patients with JMML features. This can be seen in patients with fusions in genes upstream of the RAS pathway (*ALK*, *PDGFRB*, *FLT3*, *PDGFRA*, *ROS1*, and *FIP1L1::RARA*) [9]. In one study, these fusions occurred in older children (median 59 months, range 56–153 months) and involved receptor tyrosine kinases allowing for targeted therapies with improved treatment responses (e.g., Crizotinib-*ALK/ROS1* inhibitor) [23]. Studies on the use of *ALK/ROS1* inhibitors in other JMML subtypes, including those with traditional RAS pathway mutations, are under investigation.

In the WHO 5th edition these patients with upstream genetic alterations are included in classic JMML due to their overlapping clinical and laboratory features, while the ICC consensus guidelines include them under JMML-like neoplasms [1, 7, 8, 25].

Diagnosis

JMML diagnosis requires the following criteria:

Clinical, hematological, and laboratory (all are required).

- Peripheral blood absolute monocyte count $\geq 1 \times 10^9$/L
- <20% blasts in peripheral blood and bone marrow
- Organ infiltration, typically splenomegaly*
- No *BCR::ABL1* fusion or Philadelphia chromosome
- No *KMT2A* (*MLL1*) gene rearrangement*

*ICC requires splenomegaly and does not require the exclusion of *KMT2A* rearrangements

Genetic criteria (1 required):

- Canonical RAS pathway mutation
  - Clonal somatic *PTPN11, KRAS, NRAS*
  - Clonal somatic/germline *NF1* mutation with loss of heterozygosity or compound heterozygosity
  - Clonal somatic/germline *CBL* mutation with loss of heterozygosity
- Non-canonical clonal RAS pathway pathogenic variant or fusions causing activation of genes upstream of the RAS pathway, such as *ALK*, *PDGFRB*, and *ROS1*

Other criteria (can be used if genetic testing is not available, at least 2 are required):

- Increased hemoglobin F for age
- Peripheral blood smear with erythroid and myeloid precursors
- Thrombocytopenia in the context of a hypercellular bone marrow
  - Decreased megakaryocytes
- Hypersensitivity of myeloid progenitors to GM-CSF

  Can test using methylcellulose as a clonogenic assay or measure STAT5 phosphorylation with and without low-dose GM-CSF administration**

**This can be tested by culturing the myeloid progenitors from suspected patients and seeing colony forming unit count curves before, with or without administration of granulocyte-macrophage colony stimulating factor, or by flow cytometry with anti-phosphorylated STAT5 antibody and comparing the expression profile of the myeloid progenitors before and after GM-CSF administration [26, 27].

The key diagnostic features include the peripheral blood monocytosis, low level of blasts, organ involvement, and RAS pathway mutations. In comparison to the revised 4th edition of the WHO (Table 21.1), the 5th edition allows for any organ involvement, not just splenomegaly to be diagnostic highlighting the capacity of JMML to infiltrate organs other than the spleen and bone marrow [1, 6]. The 5th edition also highlights the necessity to rule out *KMT2A* rearrangements as in the

Table 21.1 WHO fourth edition criteria

JMML diagnosis requires the following criteria:
Clinical, hematological, and laboratory (all are required)
Peripheral blood absolute monocyte count ≥1 × 10^9/L
<20% blasts in peripheral blood and bone marrow
Splenomegaly
No *BCR::ABL1* fusion or Philadelphia chromosome
Genetic criteria (1 required)
Canonical RAS pathway mutation
Clonal somatic *PTPN11*, *KRAS*, *NRAS*
Clonal somatic/germline *NF1* mutation with loss of heterozygosity or compound heterozygosity
Clonal somatic/germline *CBL* mutation with loss of heterozygosity
Other criteria (can be used if genetic testing is not available, at least 2 are required)
Monosomy 7 or any other chromosomal abnormality
≥2
Increased hemoglobin F for age
Peripheral blood smear with erythroid and myeloid precursors
Hypersensitivity of myeloid progenitors to GM-CSF
Can test using methylcellulose as a clonogenic assay or measure STAT5 phosphorylation with and without low-dose GM-CSF administration[a]

[a]This can be tested using culturing the myeloid progenitors from suspected patients and seeing colony forming unit count curves before with or without administration of granulocyte-macrophage colony stimulating factor, or by flow cytometry with anti-phosphorylated STAT5 antibody and comparing the expression profile of the myeloid progenitors before and after GM-CSF administration [26, 27]

current edition KMT2A arrangement AML can be diagnosed even with <20% blasts and has different prognostic impact in comparison to JMML [1]. Since JMML pathogenesis is characterized by hyperactive GM-CSF signal pathway, mostly through activation of the RAS pathway, it produces myelomonocytic proliferative features with leukocytosis and monocytosis and no obvious features of ineffective hematopoiesis. These features were the basis for moving JMML from myelodysplastic/myeloproliferative neoplasms to myeloproliferative neoplasms in the 2022 WHO Classification. This parallels the proliferative type of adult chronic myelomonocytic leukemia, which has significant proliferative features and is associated with secondary activation of RAS pathway and also increased sensitivity to GM-CSF [1, 28]. Monosomy 7 and other karyotype abnormalities were removed from the diagnostic criteria in the current WHO as 65% of cases will have normal karyotypes [1]. Additionally, monosomy 7 is now identified as being commonly associated with numerous other disorders such as GATA2-associated, SAMD9-associated, or SAMD9L-associated disorders [1].

When considering this diagnosis in practice, key diagnostic tests/specimens must be obtained. These include CBC with differential to assess for monocytosis and other CBC features, spleen exam/imaging to assess spleen size, and possibly bone marrow aspirate and biopsy to assess blast percentage and involvement. Bone marrow exam may not be necessary for the diagnosis if molecular and cytogenetics studies are available. Otherwise, bone marrow examination may be needed in order to apply the WHO criteria for bone marrow and to exclude the possibility of acute myeloid leukemia. Involved specimens should be sent for molecular testing to test for RAS pathway mutations, *BCR::ABL1* able fusions (via PCR or FISH), and *KMT2A* rearrangements (typically via FISH). Next generation sequencing (NGS) or multiplex PCR testing is typically required to identify the RAS pathway mutation. Genetic testing typically requires the collection of bone marrow aspirate in EDTA tubes as the most standard anticoagulant (most laboratories discourage the use of sodium heparin as an anticoagulant for molecular testing). Multiplex panels for RAS/RAF pathway mutations are available at many reference labs. In patients with other syndromic features, germline testing for NF1 or CBL with concomitant genotyping to assess for loss of heterozygosity (SNP genotyping or whole-genome copy number microarray-based testing) should be performed. This can be performed on peripheral blood collected in EDTA tubes at many places or may even require collection and culturing of skin fibroblasts depending on which testing institution or method is used, and may require referral to larger reference institutions. Additional testing such as cytogenetics/karyotype are also recommended to be performed on the bone marrow to allow for the assessment of chromosomal copy number variants. The current WHO classification recommends the following workflow for diagnosing JMML.

1. Patient manifesting with JMML-compatible clinical and hematological picture
2. Testing for BCR::ABL1 fusion gene and KMT2A gene rearrangement is negative

3. Test for RAS pathway driver gene mutation
   (a) Biallelic pathogenic alterations of *NF1*
   (b) Pathogenic *PTPN11* variant
   (c) Pathogenic *NRAS* variant
   (d) Pathogenic *KRAS* variant
   (e) Biallelic pathogenic (in some cases heterozygous only) variants involving the *CBL* gene
4. OR detection of a non-canonical genetic abnormality
   (a) Fusions leading to upstream RAS pathway activation (ALK, PDGFRB, and others)
   (b) Pathogenic variant in a non-canonical RAS pathway (RRAS or RRAS2) variant
5. Perform other laboratory testing if molecular testing is negative or unavailable
   (a) Hemoglobin fractionation studies with increased hemoglobin F for age
   (b) Peripheral blood smear with erythroid and myeloid precursors
   (c) Thrombocytopenia in the context of a hypercellular bone marrow
      (i) Decreased megakaryocytes
   (d) Hypersensitivity of myeloid progenitors to GM-CSF

Other Differential Diagnostic Considerations

Some disorders may have morphologic features similar to JMML. These disorders may be inherited or acquired, such as infections (EBV, CMV, HHV-6), leukocyte adhesion deficiency, infantile malignant osteopetrosis, and infective endocarditis and Wiskott-Aldrich Syndrome [29, 30]. Other differentials are acute myeloid leukemia with monocytic differentiation, which would have greater than 20% blasts and chronic myeloid leukemia (CML), which would have *BCR::ABL1* fusion.

JMML-Like Disorders in Children with Noonan Syndrome

In children with Noonan syndrome, a myeloproliferative disorder can sometimes occur starting shortly after birth and up to 4 years of life [31]. This is typically polyclonal, but more severe presentations mimicking JMML have been described [31, 32]. These patients usually have germline (not somatic) mutations in *PTPN11*, *KRAS*, *NRAS*, or *RIT1*. They usually have sustained monocytosis along with organ involvement, but unlike in classic JMML, this is usually transient in nature and resolves spontaneously usually in 2–3 years and the patients do not have somatic RAS pathway mutations [31]. This disorder differs from Down syndrome transient myeloproliferative disorder/transient abnormal myelopoiesis, which usually regresses within 3 months after birth and has morphologic features of acute leukemia, including increased blasts with a megakaryoblastic morphology/

immunophenotype, and is associated with *GATA1* mutations [33, 34]. There have been reports of patients with Noonan syndrome with prolonged monocytosis requiring long-term follow-up [32, 35].

RAS-Associated Autoimmune Leukoproliferative Disorder

RAS-associated autoimmune leukoproliferative disorder (RALD) is a non-malignant disorder that presents with features similar to JMML. It was first reported as an autoimmune lymphoproliferative syndrome (ALPS)-like disorder in 2007, in patients with similar features to ALPS without *FAS* mutations, harboring somatic *NRAS* mutations instead, and as such if ALPS is being worked up, patients should be screened for RAS mutations also [36]. They later reported that these patients did not always have the increased CD4–/CD8– double negative T-cells that is characteristic of ALPS, leading to the proposal of a new diagnostic category of RAS-associated autoimmune leukoproliferative disorder. Key features of RALD are monocytosis (relative or absolute) with splenomegaly. Patients have also reported cytopenias, lymphadenopathy, increased circulating B-cells, hypergammaglobulinemia, decreased complement, and autoimmunity with ANA positivity [37]. This condition should be considered in patients presenting with signs of autoimmunity and elevated WBC counts including increased monocytes. Similar to JMML, the male to female ratio is 1:1 and onset is typically at 2 years of age (reported cases range from 3 months to 36 years) [36, 37]. The autoimmunity can be severe enough to present as an early onset systemic lupus erythematosus (SLE)-like syndrome, and the diagnosis of RALD in these patients may be missed or delayed [38]. Bone marrow biopsies in these cases can show hypercellularity with increased myeloid to erythroid ratios without dysplasia or increase in blasts. Lymph node biopsies can show reactive follicular hyperplasia with focal progressive transformation of germinal centers [39]. Patients usually have gain-of-function somatic mutations in *KRAS* or *NRAS* involving canonical G12 and G13 codon sites, similar to what is seen in JMML [36]. Those with *NRAS* mutations typically present in infancy, while those with *KRAS* mutations present later on, usually as toddlers [36, 37]. Unlike JMML, RALD is non-malignant, is not associated with an increase in blasts, and does not have mutations/alterations in *CBL*, *NF1*, *PTPN11*, or monosomy 7. Some recent studies show that reduced IL-2 withdrawal-induced apoptosis can be seen in RALD, but there is limited research on whether this is present in JMML [37]. Approximately 10% of cases will progress to JMML but transformation can take years, therefore continued surveillance is critical. Rare progression to acute myeloid leukemia has been reported [36]. Treatment for RALD may include corticosteroid administration or immune modulators such as sirolimus for the management of cytopenias [37].

Table 21.2 Management of JMML

Ras pathway mutation	Frequency in JMML	Features	Recommendations for treatment
Somatic *NRAS*	10–15%	Varies	HSCT, watch-and-wait for some
Somatic *KRAS*	10–15%	Monosomy 7, autoimmune disorders	Azacitidine and/or HSCT
Somatic *PTPN11*	35%	Highest risk for unfavorable outcomes	Swift HSCT with pre-transplant azacitidine and low-intensity GVHD prophylaxis (may withdraw in absence), post-transplant azacitidine with donor lymphocyte infusions
Germline *NF1*	10–15%	Café-au-lait spots, older age at diagnosis, milder thrombocytopenia	Swift HSCT with pre-transplant azacitidine and low-intensity GVHD prophylaxis (may withdraw in absence)
Germline *CBL*	15%	Syndromic RAS-opathy features, autoimmunity, vasculitis	Watch-and-wait with HSCT if progress
Non-canonical	5–10%	RNA sequencing with rare activating kinase fusions	HSCT, patients need extended work-up for RAS-opathies; possible targeted therapy

Prognosis

Prognosis is better in younger-aged children. Adverse outcomes are associated with increasing age, >2 years of age, thrombocytopenia ($<33 \times 10^9$/L), elevation of hemoglobin F, and overexpression of LIN28B (detected via PCR RNA/microarray profiling) [23, 40]. A recent study of 119 JMML patients who underwent transplantation suggests the following adverse factors: age >2 years, monocyte count of >7.2 K/uL, the presence of at least one additional genetic alteration, and transplantation >6 months after the diagnosis [41]. JMML-like syndrome in Noonan syndrome may be transient or can develop into fulminant disease. The management of JMML differs depending on which mutation is identified (Table 21.2). It appears that the type of mutation generally predicts the course of disease and therefore the therapeutic approach. Earlier hematopoietic stem cell transplant (HSCT) may be required for patients with *PTPN11* or *NF1* mutations/alterations, while transplantation can be delayed with a watch-and-wait approach in those with *NRAS* mutations [42]. Without eventual HSCT, survival outcomes are <10% in some cases, with a post-HSCT relapse risk of approximately 25–35% [5, 41, 42].

Transformation

Patients with indolent JMML can suddenly undergo blast crisis and transformation into acute myeloid leukemia (AML), with up to 10% developing AML within 5 years of JMML diagnosis [4, 43]. Currently, there is limited data on what predisposes JMML patients to transform to AML, but increased hemoglobin F at presentation may be a predictor. This observation is strengthened by the fact that patients with Hgb F > 15% at presentation also have a higher PB and BM blast count [5]. In some patients, cytogenetic clonal evolution, especially monosomy 7, can be seen at blast transformation [44]. Cumulatively, 30% of JMML patients will eventually transform into AML [45]. This transformation can be seen in patients with duplication of mutated *KRAS* or *NRAS* that is acquired through uniparental disomy [9, 43]. Patients with known RAS-opathies have been identified as having more rapid progression to AML [46]. In these patients, both standard AML treatment regimens and HSCT have been used in the treatment with mixed success [44].

References

1. Elghetany MT, Patnaik M, Cavé H, De Vito R. Juvenile myelomonocytic leukaemia. In: Eric Solary E, Khoury JD, editors. WHO classification of haematolymphoid tumours. Lyon: International Agency for Research on Cancer; 2024.
2. Hasle H. Myelodysplastic syndromes in childhood—classification, epidemiology, and treatment. Leuk Lymphoma. 1994;13(1–2):11–26. https://doi.org/10.3109/10428199409051647.
3. Passmore SJ, Hann IM, Stiller CA, et al. Pediatric myelodysplasia: a study of 68 children and a new prognostic scoring system. Blood. 1995;85(7):1742–50.
4. Luna-Fineman S, Shannon KM, Atwater SK, et al. Myelodysplastic and myeloproliferative disorders of childhood: a study of 167 patients. Blood. 1999;93(2):459–66.
5. Niemeyer CM, Aricó M, Basso G, et al. Chronic myelomonocytic leukemia in childhood: a retrospective analysis of 110 cases. Blood. 1997;89(10):3534–43.
6. Swerldow SH, Campo E, Harris NL, Jaffe ES, Pileri SA, Stein H, Thiele J, editors. WHO classification of tumours of haematopoietic and lymphoid tissue. Revised 4th ed. Lyon: IARC; 2017.
7. Arber DA, Orazi A, Hasserjian RP, et al. International consensus classification of myeloid neoplasms and acute leukemias: integrating morphologic, clinical, and genomic data. Blood. 2022;140(11):1200–28. https://doi.org/10.1182/blood.2022015850.
8. Rudelius M, Weinberg OK, Niemeyer CM, Shimamura A, Calvo KR. The international consensus classification (ICC) of hematologic neoplasms with germline predisposition, pediatric myelodysplastic syndrome, and juvenile myelomonocytic leukemia. Virchows Arch. 2023;482(1):113–30. https://doi.org/10.1007/s00428-022-03447-9.
9. Niemeyer CM. JMML genomics and decisions. Hematology Am Soc Hematol Educ Program. 2018;2018(1):307–12. https://doi.org/10.1182/asheducation-2018.1.307.
10. Tufekci O, Kocak U, Kaya Z, et al. Juvenile myelomonocytic leukemia in Turkey: a retrospective analysis of sixty-five patients. Turk J Haematol. 2018;35(1):27–34. https://doi.org/10.4274/tjh.2017.0021.
11. Rauen KA. The RASopathies. Annu Rev Genomics Hum Genet. 2013;14:355–69. https://doi.org/10.1146/annurev-genom-091212-153523.
12. Hecht A, Meyer JA, Behnert A, et al. Molecular and phenotypic diversity of CBL-mutated juvenile myelomonocytic leukemia. Haematologica. 2022;107(1):178–86. https://doi.org/10.3324/haematol.2020.270595.

13. Fluhr S, Krombholz CF, Meier A, et al. Epigenetic dysregulation of the erythropoietic transcription factor KLF1 and the beta-like globin locus in juvenile myelomonocytic leukemia. Epigenetics. 2017;12(8):715–23. https://doi.org/10.1080/15592294.2017.1356959.
14. Aricó M, Biondi A, Ching-Hon P. Juvenile Myelomonocytic leukemia. Blood. 1997;90:479–88.
15. Nathany S, Chatterjee G, Ghai S, et al. Mutational landscape of juvenile myelomonocytic leukemia (JMML)—a real-world context. Int J Lab Hematol. 2021;43(6):1531–8. https://doi.org/10.1111/ijlh.13680.
16. Behnert A, Meyer J, Parsa J, et al. Exploring the genetic and epigenetic origins of juvenile myelomonocytic leukemia using newborn screening samples. Leukemia. 2022;36(1):279–82. https://doi.org/10.1038/s41375-021-01331-0.
17. Shannon KM, O'Connell P, Martin GA, et al. Loss of the normal *NF1* allele from the bone marrow of children with type 1 neurofibromatosis and malignant myeloid disorders. N Engl J Med. 1994;330(9):597–601. https://doi.org/10.1056/NEJM199403033300903.
18. Niemeyer CM, Kang MW, Shin DH, et al. Germline *CBL* mutations cause developmental abnormalities and predispose to juvenile myelomonocytic leukemia. Nat Genet. 2010;42(9):794–800. https://doi.org/10.1038/ng.641.
19. Arfeuille C, Vial Y, Cadenet M, et al. Germline bi-allelic *SH2B3/LNK* alteration predisposes to a neonatal juvenile myelomonocytic leukemia-like disorder. Haematologica. 2023; https://doi.org/10.3324/haematol.2023.283917.
20. Wintering A, Hecht A, Meyer J, Wong EB, Hübner J, Abelson S, et al. LNK/SH2B3 as a novel driver in juvenile myelomonocytic leukemia. Haematologica. 2024;109:2533–41.
21. Lipka DB, Witte T, Toth R, et al. RAS-pathway mutation patterns define epigenetic subclasses in juvenile myelomonocytic leukemia. Nat Commun. 2017;8(1):2126–w. https://doi.org/10.1038/s41467-017-02177-w.
22. Stieglitz E, Mazor T, Olshen AB, et al. Genome-wide DNA methylation is predictive of outcome in juvenile myelomonocytic leukemia. Nat Commun. 2017;8(1):2127–9. https://doi.org/10.1038/s41467-017-02178-9.
23. Murakami N, Okuno Y, Yoshida K, et al. Integrated molecular profiling of juvenile myelomonocytic leukemia. Blood. 2018;131(14):1576–86. https://doi.org/10.1182/blood-2017-07-798157.
24. Schonung M, Meyer J, Nollke P, et al. International consensus definition of DNA methylation subgroups in juvenile myelomonocytic leukemia. Clin Cancer Res. 2021;27(1):158–68. https://doi.org/10.1158/1078-0432.CCR-20-3184.
25. Elghetany MT, Cavé H, De Vito R, Patnaik MM, Solary E, Khoury JD. Juvenile myelomonocytic leukemia; moving forward. Leukemia. 2023;37:720–2.
26. Nishio N, Takahashi Y, Tanaka M, et al. Aberrant phosphorylation of STAT5 by granulocyte-macrophage colony-stimulating factor in infant cytomegalovirus infection mimicking juvenile myelomonocytic leukemia. Leuk Res. 2011;35(9):1261–4. https://doi.org/10.1016/j.leukres.2011.04.014.
27. Emanuel PD, Bates LJ, Castleberry RP, Gualtieri RJ, Zuckerman KS. Selective hypersensitivity to granulocyte-macrophage colony-stimulating factor by juvenile chronic myeloid leukemia hematopoietic progenitors. Blood. 1991;77(5):925–9.
28. Lasho T, Patnaik MM. Juvenile Myelomonocytic leukemia—a bona fide RASopathy syndrome. Best Pract Res Clin Haematol. 2020;33:101171.
29. Niemeyer CM, Fenu S, Hastle H, Mann G, Stary J, van Wering E. Differentiating juvenile Myelomonocytic leukemia from infectious disease. Blood. 1998;91:365–7.
30. Karow A, Baumann I, Niemeyer CM. Morphologic differential diagnosis of juvenile Myelomonocytic leukemia-Pitfalls apart from viral infection. J Pediatr Hematol Oncol. 2009;31:380.
31. Strullu M, Caye A, Lachenaud J, et al. Juvenile myelomonocytic leukaemia and Noonan syndrome. J Med Genet. 2014;51(10):689–97. https://doi.org/10.1136/jmedgenet-2014-102611.
32. Fukuda M, Horibe K, Miyajima Y, Matsumoto K, Nagashima M. Spontaneous remission of juvenile chronic myelomonocytic leukemia in an infant with Noonan syndrome. J Pediatr Hematol Oncol. 1997;19(2):177–9. https://doi.org/10.1097/00043426-199703000-00019.

33. Bhatnagar N, Nizery L, Tunstall O, Vyas P, Roberts I. Transient abnormal myelopoiesis and AML in Down syndrome: an update. Curr Hematol Malig Rep. 2016;11(5):333–41. https://doi.org/10.1007/s11899-016-0338-x.
34. Crispino JD. *GATA1* mutations in Down syndrome: implications for biology and diagnosis of children with transient myeloproliferative disorder and acute megakaryoblastic leukemia. Pediatr Blood Cancer. 2005;44(1):40–4. https://doi.org/10.1002/pbc.20066.
35. Bastida P, Garcia-Minaur S, Ezquieta B, Dapena JL, Sanchez de Toledo J. Myeloproliferative disorder in Noonan syndrome. J Pediatr Hematol Oncol. 2011;33(1):43. https://doi.org/10.1097/MPH.0b013e3181e7571e.
36. Neven Q, Boulanger C, Bruwier A, et al. Clinical spectrum of RAS-associated autoimmune leukoproliferative disorder (RALD). J Clin Immunol. 2021;41(1):51–8. https://doi.org/10.1007/s10875-020-00883-7.
37. Sullivan KE, Lambert M. RAS-associated autoimmune lymphoproliferative disorder. Br J Haematol. 2024;205(3):819–22. https://doi.org/10.1111/bjh.19564.
38. Wang W, Zhou Y, Zhong L, et al. RAS-associated autoimmune leukoproliferative disease (RALD) manifested with early-onset SLE-like syndrome: a case series of RALD in Chinese children. Pediatr Rheumatol Online J. 2019;17(1):55–1. https://doi.org/10.1186/s12969-019-0346-1.
39. Xie W, Fan G, Wiszniewska J, Press RD, Yang F. Histopathological and molecular findings in a patient with RAS-associated autoimmune leukoproliferative disorder. Human Pathol Rep. 2022;29:300670.
40. Helsmoortel HH, Bresolin S, Lammens T, et al. LIN28B overexpression defines a novel fetal-like subgroup of juvenile myelomonocytic leukemia. Blood. 2016;127(9):1163–72. https://doi.org/10.1182/blood-2015-09-667808.
41. Meyran D, Arfeuille C, Chevret S, Neven Q, Caye-Eude A, Lainey E, et al. A predictive classifier of poor prognosis in transplanted patients with juvenile myelomonocytic leukemia: a study on behalf of the Société Francophone de Greffe de Moelle et de Thérapie Cellulaire. Haematologica. 2024;109:2908–19.
42. Mayerhofer C, Niemeyer CM, Flotho C. Current treatment of juvenile myelomonocytic leukemia. J Clin Med. 2021;10(14):3084. https://doi.org/10.3390/jcm10143084.
43. Osumi T, Kato M, Ouchi-Uchiyama M, et al. Blastic transformation of juvenile myelomonocytic leukemia caused by the copy number gain of oncogenic *KRAS*. Pediatr Blood Cancer. 2017;64(9):e26496. Epub 2017 Feb 28. https://doi.org/10.1002/pbc.26496.
44. Honda Y, Tsuchida M, Zaike Y, et al. Clinical characteristics of 15 children with juvenile myelomonocytic leukaemia who developed blast crisis: MDS committee of Japanese Society of Paediatric Haematology/Oncology. Br J Haematol. 2014;165(5):682–7. https://doi.org/10.1111/bjh.12796.
45. Lachenaud J, Strullu M, Baruchel A, Cave H. Juvenile myelomonocytic leukemias. Bull Cancer. 2014;101(3):302–13. https://doi.org/10.1684/bdc.2014.1908.
46. Flex E, Jaiswal M, Pantaleoni F, et al. Activating mutations in *RRAS* underlie a phenotype within the RASopathy spectrum and contribute to leukaemogenesis. Hum Mol Genet. 2014;23(16):4315–27. https://doi.org/10.1093/hmg/ddu148.

Index

W. Li (ed.), *Laboratory Assessments of Pediatric Leukemia*,
https://doi.org/10.1007/978-3-032-26557-9

B

C

G

H

M

N

Q

R

GPSR Compliance

The European Union's (EU) General Product Safety Regulation (GPSR) is a set of rules that requires consumer products to be safe and our obligations to ensure this.

If you have any concerns about our products, you can contact us on ProductSafety@springernature.com

In case Publisher is established outside the EU, the EU authorized representative is:

Springer Nature Customer Service Center GmbH
Europaplatz 3
69115 Heidelberg, Germany

Batch number: 10756373

Printed by Printforce, the Netherlands